ANNUAL PROGRESS IN
CHILD PSYCHIATRY AND
CHILD DEVELOPMENT
1993

ANNUAL PROGRESS IN CHILD PSYCHIATRY AND CHILD DEVELOPMENT 1993

Edited by

MARGARET E. HERTZIG, M.D.

Associate Professor of Psychiatry
Cornell University Medical College

and

ELLEN A. FARBER, Ph.D.

Assistant Professor of Psychology in Psychiatry
Cornell University Medical College

BRUNNER/MAZEL *Publishers* ● **New York**

Library of Congress Card No. 68-23452
ISBN 0-87630-729-2
ISSN 0066-4030

Published by
BRUNNER/MAZEL, Inc.
19 Union Square West
New York, New York 10003

Manufactured in the United States of America
10 9 8 7 6 5 4 3 2 1

CONTENTS

ANNUAL PROGRESS IN
CHILD PSYCHIATRY AND
CHILD DEVELOPMENT
1993

Part I

DEVELOPMENTAL STUDIES

This section represents a diverse group of papers. The first by Meltzoff and Moore adds to our growing body of knowledge on the capacities of very young infants. Several new studies are presented on the imitative capacities of infants from 6 weeks to 3 months of age. Meltzoff and Moore contend that early facial imitation is not reflexive motor movement but is diagnostic of early social cognition. They studied the functional significance of early imitation by manipulating three factors: person, movement, and age. The questions studied were: (1) Do infants differentially imitate mothers versus strangers? (2) Can 6-week-old infants imitate both static postures and dynamic gestures? and (3) What are the developmental changes in imitation? Does imitation decline at 2 to 3 months of age when reflexes drop out? Their findings are used to suggest that early imitation serves an identity function, that is, that imitation is a way by which young infants know and communicate with persons as opposed to things.

In the second paper, Charlotte Patterson reviews the literature on children reared by lesbian and gay parents. Studying children reared by gay or lesbian parents raises questions relevant for developmental theory and social policy. There are two general questions addressed with respect to developmental theory. First, what is the impact of nontraditional family arrangements on development? Second, does nontraditional parenting challenge existing theories of psychosocial/psychosexual development? With respect to social policy, research on the effects of gay parenting can inform child custody, adoption, and foster care policies. The number of gay families openly raising children has increased substantially in the last few years. In several well-publicized cases, when gays have attempted to adopt children after foster-parenting them, an uproar ensued about the fitness of such individuals as parents. The arguments were rooted in emotion rather than empiricism. Patterson's review indicates that being raised by gay parents has little impact on children's social adjustment, in general, and gender identity or sexual orientation, specifically.

One methodological limitation of many pervious studies is that comparisons were of children reared by divorced lesbian mothers versus children of divorced heterosexual mothers. Both groups of children would have been exposed to male and female parents early on in their development. In recent years, there have been more children raised by lesbian mothers who chose to conceive or adopt children in the context of a lesbian relationship. Children raised exclusively in the context of gay relationships may show different patterns of adaptation from children born

1

into male-female marriages. Another question to be raised about the existing studies is whether the samples are biased. If many families are "in the closet," are only the most militant or those most comfortable with their sexuality being studied?

Although research in this area is relatively sparse and the studies have methodological limitations, this review raises a variety of interesting questions which should be addressed in future research. One area worth pursuing is a within-group analysis of gay families to determine what factors/processes account for successful and unsuccessful adaptation. Are the developmental pathways similar for children in "traditional" and nontraditional families?

The third article in this section is a normative study of children's short-term reactions to the death of a parent. Little is known about children's reactions in the months following a parent's death. The small literature on the impact of parental death is biased by the use of psychiatric samples. Silverman and Worden followed a group of 125 6- to 17-year-old children in the four months following a parent's death. Families were identified through funeral parlors; thus, they comprised a nonclinical sample. The surviving parents completed the Child Behavior Checklist for an assessment of emotional and behavioral problems, and the children provided self-reports of perceived competence and locus of control. Interviews provided additional information on affective and behavioral responses at the time of the death, the funeral, and in the months subsequent.

This descriptive study fills a void by discussing normal bereavement patterns. The information presented by Silverman and Worden can enhance the clinician's ability to determine if a child's reaction is within normal limits. Although the families were followed until two years after the death, this paper reports on reactions in the first four months following a parent's death. The paper describes the daily changes that occur in children's lives, as well as specific reactions to the funeral and the ways that children maintain a connection to the deceased parent. The behavior problem data is intriguing. Obviously pre-death data is unavailable; it is likely that some children with behavior problems had difficulty prior to the death. Of significance though is the fact that very few children had clinically elevated CBCLs. The scale with the highest number of children showing clinical elevations was Somatization.

The final paper in this section is an innovative study assessing psychophysiological responses during the Adult Attachment Interview (AAI). It also presents the use of Q-sorting for scoring the AAI along dimensions of security/anxiety and deactivation/hyperactivation. Individuals who are insecure develop strategies to regulate access to attachment information. Similar to the avoidant infant whose behavior signifies a shifting of attention away from attachment-eliciting conditions, adults have been observed to use "deactivating" strategies. Using a measure of skin conductance, Dozier and Kobak present the first documentation that individuals who employ deactivating attachment strategies are experiencing conflict during the Attachment Interview.

The AAI scoring system developed by Mary Main and her colleagues results in classifications in one of four overall categories: autonomous, dismissing, preoccupied, and unresolved. Kobak and his colleagues proposed that two continuous dimensions, secure/anxious and deactivating/hyperactivating, can be used to describe the first three states of mind—autonomous, dismissing, and preoccupied. These dimensions are coded using a Q-sort procedure rather than the rating scales and overall categories. Of particular interest in this study were persons in the dismissing category who devalue the importance of relationships, report extremely positive relationships with their parents, and downplay the influence of childhood experience on their development. The elevation in skin conductance levels associated with devaluing suggests that the subject is effortfully engaged in diverting attention from attachment issues and that they have not fully deactivated the attachment system. Correlations between deactivation and rises in skin conductance were particularly evident during questions about how the current personality has been influenced by early relationships, a task that requires the individual both to access early attachment memories and to make those experiences relevant to the self. Persons who find it difficult to direct attention to attachment experiences may be more likely to avoid situations such as insight-oriented psychotherapy, which focus on these issues.

1

Early Imitation Within a Functional Framework: The Importance of Person Identity, Movement, and Development

Andrew N. Meltzoff and M. Keith Moore

University of Washington, Seattle

Facial imitation was investigated in infants 6 weeks and 2 to 3 months of age. Three findings emerged: (a) early imitation did not vary as a function of familiarity with the model—infants imitated a stranger as well as their own mothers; (b) infants imitated both static facial postures and dynamic facial gestures; and (c) there was no disappearance of facial imitation in the 2- to 3-month age range, contrary to previous reports. Two broad theoretical points are developed. First, a proposal is made about the social and psychological functions that early imitation serves in infants' encounters with people. It is argued that infants deploy imitation to enrich their understanding of persons and actions and that early imitation is used for communicative purposes. Second, a theoretical bridge is formed between early imitation and the "object concept." The bridge is formed by considering the fundamental role that identity plays in infants' understanding of people and things. One of the psychological functions that early imitation subserves is to identify people. Infants use the nonverbal behavior of people as an identifier of who they are and use imitation as a means of verifying this identity. Data and theory are adduced in favor of viewing early imitation as an act of social cognition.

Reprinted with permission from *Infant Behavior and Development*, 1992, Vol. 15, 479–505. Copyright © 1992 by Ablex Publishing Corporation.

This research was supported by a grant from the National Institute of Child Health and Human Development (HD-22514). We gratefully acknowledge the assistance of Calle Fisher, Craig Harris, Becky Alder, Margaret Hampson, and Christy Loberg in the conduct of this research and thank the mothers and infants who participated. Thanks also to Patricia Kuhl and Alison Gopnik for providing valuable comments on an earlier draft and to Paul Sampson for statistical advice. The order of authorship of this article is alphabetical; the work was thoroughly collaborative.

Classic developmental theories consider the imitation of facial actions to be a landmark achievement that first emerges at about 8 to 12 months of age (e.g., Piaget, 1962). It is not that younger infants are considered nonimitative, but rather that there is a specific delay or deficit in facial imitation in particular. Other types of imitation, notably hand movements, are said to occur with facility before 6 months. The special psychological problem posed by facial imitation is that infants must connect the self and other in a unique way: They must match an act they see another perform with one of their own that they cannot see. The mechanism underlying other types of imitation such as manual imitation is not difficult to imagine: Infants can see both the model's hand and their own hands, and thus direct visual guidance is possible. Such visual guidance is impossible for facial imitation: How do infants bridge the gap between a visible and non-visible face?

Perhaps because this question poses such a challenge, most theorists found it convenient to accept the view that facial imitation first becomes possible at about 1 year. There have been few principled accounts, however, of why facial imitation should first emerge at that particular age and not earlier. Piaget (1962) addressed this issue by saying that facial imitation was not an isolated reaction but was embedded within other aspects of infant cognition. In particular Piaget saw a deep connection between imitation using nonvisible body parts (faces) and the capacity to find nonvisible objects (Stage 4 object permanence). Although there are numerous differences between the tasks, Piaget's insight was that their synchronous emergence at 8 to 12 months was causally related, not merely correlative. Both tap an underlying advance in the capacity to go beyond strictly sense-based impressions. One can imagine more socially rooted hypotheses, but this is the classical cognitive explanation for the emergence of facial imitation at 8 to 12 months of age.

Meltzoff and Moore (1977) challenged the consensus about the late emergence of facial imitation by reporting that 12- to 21-day-old infants imitated tongue protrusion, mouth opening, and lip protrusion. A further study (Meltzoff & Moore, 1983a) replicated these findings of early imitation and showed that this was an innate capacity: The mean age of the subjects in the latter study was 32 hours old, and the youngest was 42 minutes old at the time of test. Other work from our laboratory showed that neonates were not restricted to oral imitation (Meltzoff & Moore, 1989; see also Meltzoff & Moore, 1977, Study 1). The early matching effect has now been replicated and extended in new directions by independent investigators using a variety of test techniques. Numerous studies have replicated the tongue-protrusion and mouth-opening effects in infants less than 2 months old (Abravanel & Sigafoos, 1984; Fontaine, 1984; Heimann, Nelson, & Schaller, 1989; Heimann & Schaller, 1985; Jacobson, 1979; Kaitz, Meschulach-Sarfaty, Auerbach, & Eidelman, 1988; Legerstee, 1991; Reissland,

1988; Vinter, 1986). Early matching has also been reported for emotional expressions (Field et al., 1983; Field, Goldstein, Vaga-Lahr, & Porter, 1986; Field, Woodson, Greenberg, & Cohen, 1982) and a variety of other gestures, including eye blinking, cheek movements, and hand gestures (Fontaine, 1984; Vinter, 1986). It has been reported that there may be individual differences in the tendency to imitate (Abravanel & Sigafoos, 1984; Field et al., 1986; Heimann, 1989, 1991; Heimann et al., 1989) and that imitation is specific to people, with inanimate objects failing to yield matching responses (Abravanel & DeYong, 1991; Legerstee, 1991), although the data are mixed on the latter point (Jacobson, 1979). Thus, the phenomenon of early matching reported by Meltzoff and Moore has been upheld and broadened: A range of adult facial displays does elicit similar behavior in infants. The issue now becomes how best to character-ize the infant's reaction. What is the mechanism underlying early matching? What function does it serve? What meaning does it have for the infant? What motivates them to copy in the first place?

There are two principal schools of thought on how to interpret the findings. For the purposes of sharpening the debate, we will dub these the "reflexive" and "social-cognition" views. They suggest different mechanisms for linking the adult's act and the infant's, as well as a different functional significance and mean-ing of the behavior. Regarding mechanism, the first view holds that the adult's dis-play automatically triggers or "releases" a present motor packet analogous to the way that a sudden postural change causes a Moro reaction (Abravanel & Sigafoos, 1984; Bjorklund, 1987; Jacobson, 1979). According to the second view, the inter-modal equivalence between the adult's act and the infant's is taken into account by the infant (Meltzoff & Moore, 1977, 1983a, 1989; Meltzoff, Kuhl, & Moore, 1991). Regarding functional significance and meaning, the reflexive view pro-poses that early imitation does not serve any intrapsychic function for the infant. In contrast, Meltzoff and Moore (1985) held that young infants deploy imitation as a means of enriching their apprehension of people through reenacting their actions, and that even in early infancy imitation is used for social-communicative purposes. We suggest that early facial imitation is interwoven within a larger fab-ric of intentionality, representation, cross-modal coordination, and communica-tion. It is diagnostic of early social cognition, not reflexive motor movement.

We report here experiments on the nature and functional significance of early imitation that manipulated three important factors: person, movement, and age. We were interested in exploring how imitation is used by the child and the func-tion it serves in encounters with people. Thus, the question immediately arose as to whether young infants would differentially imitate mothers versus strangers. To date, there has been no systematic work directly comparing the efficacy of stran-gers versus the mother in eliciting early imitation. Are young infants more advanced in their imitation of mothers? One might predict that infants would imitate the familiar, affectively laden mother with greater facility than a stranger. The opposite view has its attractions. A stranger might elicit superior imitation as part of infants' exploring the interactive "properties" of this unknown entity. From a methodological perspective, it is useful to investigate the generalizability of the matching effect across people. Our experiments not only used a stranger, but also the infants' own mothers as demonstrators in a laboratory setting.

Second, these experiments explored the importance of stimulus motion to early imitation by presenting both dynamic gestures and static postures as models. Is there any evidence that 6-week-old infants can mimic static *facial forms* in addition to the *dynamic gestures* that are usually presented? Previous work with static postures revealed null results using newborns (Vinter, 1986); older infants might respond differently. We investigated two questions: (a) Is a static display a sufficient stimulus for eliciting imitation? and (b) If so, is the matching response so finely differentiated that, for example, static mouth-opening displays will yield *longer* mouth-opening acts than would a dynamic mouth-opening demonstration? The latter would suggest that temporal aspects of the display can be mimicked in addition to the spatial aspects (gestural types), which is relevant to the issue of underlying mechanism. Such a fine-grained correspondence to the model would not be compatible with the idea that imitation is a global reflex.

The third focus is on developmental changes in imitation. A cardinal finding used to support the reflexive model is the report that imitation occurring in the neonatal period disappears or declines at approximately 2 to 3 months of age (e.g., Abravanel & Sigafoos, 1984; Bjorklund, 1987; Field et al., 1986; Fontaine, 1984; Maratos, 1982). These data are often assimilated to the reflexive view by proposing that the initial imitation drops out in concert with the inhibition of other reflexive responses. However, the actual data are more complex. For example, using emotional expressions as stimuli, Field et al. found no absolute disappearance of imitation at any age tested in the first 6 months (age range tested = 2–6 months). It is possible that emotional expressions follow a different time course or are mediated by different processes than the elementary facial gestures of mouth opening and tongue protrusion: Some sort of affect contagion or empathic mood matching may be responsible for the duplication of these emotional expressions during the "drop-out" period. The simple but powerful fact is that, to date, no one has been successful in eliciting tongue-protrusion and mouth-opening imitation in the 2- to 3-month-old age group, and this has fueled the reflexive account for these gestures. We examined the reported absence of such imitation at this age by using a new test paradigm, one specifically designed to motivate imitation in infants in ways that will be described later. On the basis of a new study with 2- to 3-month-olds, we suggest that older infants' social-communicative efforts often displace imitative responding to simple facial gestures. We argue that the apparent drop out of these gestures is not due to a change in competence as postulated by the reflexive account, but rather to performance changes that can be reversed using novel designs that pose cognitive challenges to these older infants. Field et al. (1986) were cognizant of this possibility: "Future studies are needed to determine whether these apparent decreases in imitative behavior are real or simply an artifact of a limited paradigm" (p. 421).

Pilot Experiment: Proposal for a Relation Between Imitation and Rules for Object Identity

The manipulation of person, movement, and age were all straightforward extensions of work in the literature. However, using these manipulations in the pilot experiment led to some new hypotheses about the meaning and use of imitation for the child. We now believe that infants use imitation as a tool to help resolve issues concerning person identity. When an adult plays an imitation game with an infant, the infant remembers the person-act link and uses it when reencountering the person at a different time. In particular, the infant will often "probe" the person by producing the appropriate gesture.

These ideas about infants using imitation to probe the identity of a person emerged because in the pilot experiments ($N = 48$), we presented infants with two models: the mother and a stranger. Infants saw one person perform the mouth-opening demonstration and then the second person perform the tongue-protrusion demonstration. Infants acted in an interesting and surprising way when the first person disappeared and the other person appeared and began presenting the new gesture. Infants often stared at the second person and then intently produced what the *first* model had demonstrated. For example, the mother would demonstrate a mouth-opening gesture and the infant might provide some small reaction, but when the mother departed and the tongue-protruding stranger appeared, then suddenly, the infant would respond with a cluster of intensive mouth openings. We took this to mean that the sight of the adult gesture was not a simple trigger, because it was the "wrong" gesture that seemed to be triggered: Infants were not matching what was present before them, but what they remembered being shown.

We began to think it was the infant's interpretation of the stimulus and not the literal stimulus in front of them that was critical in governing these early reactions. Intensive study of the data records and videotapes revealed an interesting dichotomy among the subjects. The data revealed that the subset of infants who were imitating the current person in front of them were the ones who had visually tracked the entrances and exits of the people. The infants who had not visually tracked the approaches and departures tended to be the ones who responded with a burst of the previous person's gesture when confronted with the new person. The idea that emerged was that the infants who had not visually tracked the switch in people were thereby put in a state of conflict or ambiguity as to the identity of the new person (a face was presented in the same place as the first, but looked different; was it a new or the old person?), and they were using the previous person's gesture as a nonverbal probe of identity. As will be discussed later, this idea introduces a fundamentally new way of conceiving of the functional aspects of early imitation. It also suggests ways of modifying the two-person procedure to sharpen infants' responding. The next experiment was designed to ensure that infants had multiple, nonconflicting cues for identifying the experimenter and mother as separate people.

EXPERIMENT 1

The pilot experiment suggested that 6-week-old infants performed poorly on a two-person imitation situation when they did not track the movements of the different people who were to be imitated. The essential change between the pilot experiment and Experiment 1 was to ensure that all infants visually tracked the movements of the people so that they had full evidence that the person who was serving as the model had changed. With reduced conflict about the identity of the person, we predicted that infants would more systematically match what they presently saw. At a theoretical level, the logic for this change is tied to previous work concerning the criteria for object identity over time, how one distinguishes a fundamentally new object from an old object with its features (and thus appearance) changed. Michotte (1962; Thinès, Costall, & Butterworth, 1991) and Gibson (1966, 1979) might describe the object transitions and substitutions that occurred in the pilot work (and many naturalistic situations) as follows: There is an object in front of the infant, then after a period with broken sensory contact (for infants who did not track the adults), infants encounter an object of similar overall configuration in the same place as the first one. Michotte discovered that even adults are confused about the identity of objects under such conditions: Is it the same object with transformed features or a different object in the same place? We reasoned that if infants in the pilot experiment had identity questions of this sort, then the new procedures, in which infants are led to visually track the exchanges, would help clarify the situation. Philosophical analysis has established that such spatiotemporal tracking of objects is critical for determining their true identity (Strawson, 1959; Wiggins, 1967, 1980); visual tracking of objects has been found to be a powerful factor in young infants' determination of object identity (Bower, 1982, 1989; Moore, Borton, & Darby, 1978; Moore & Meltzoff, 1978; Piaget, 1954).

In Experiment 1, the pilot procedures were modified to require that infants visually track the movement of each adult to and from the test chamber. Using this procedure, we tested whether 6-week-old infants could differentially imitate in such a two-person situation, whether they could switch actions to follow what

each person demonstrated. The more specific aims of the experiment were to evaluate whether one person (mother or stranger) was the superior elicitor of imitation, and similarly, whether the movement factor had a significant effect on
infants' responding.

Method

Subjects. Subjects were 32 infants with a mean age of 6.12 weeks old (range =
5.71–6.43, *SD* = .23). They were recruited from the University's computerized
subject pool containing primarily white middle-class families. Pre-established
subject characteristics for admission into the study were: normal birthweight
(2.5–4.5 kg), normal length of gestation (40 ± 3 weeks), and no known visual
or motor disorders. The mean birthweight was 3.59 kg (range = 2.67–4.45, *SD*
= .39). The mean length of gestation was 40.30 weeks (range = 37.71–42.14,
SD = 1.00). All but one of the subjects were white. Twenty-five additional infants
were tested but dropped from the study due to fussing (11), hiccoughing, spitting,
choking uncontrollably (10), sleeping (1), or having a bowel movement during the
test (3).

Test environment and apparatus. Testing took place within a two-room suite. One
room was a waiting area where parents could feed and change their infants; the
other contained a three-sided test chamber. The walls of the chamber were lined
with gray paper, and the ceiling was papered with the same material. The infant
sat in the open end of the chamber and faced the rear wall, which was 2.6 m away.
The rear wall had a small hole cut in it to allow for videotaping by an assistant
who stood behind it. A small light located above (25 cm) and behind (15 cm) the
infant was used to spotlight the experimenter's face during the test. The experimenter's face was directly in front of the infant's at a distance of about 30 to 35
cm. The luminance of the experimenter's face was approximately 1.04 log cd/m^2,
and the luminance of the background 2.5 cm to the right of the experimenter's
face was approximately 1.01 log cd/m^2. The subject's reactions were videotaped
by a camera focused on the infant's oral region, with an image from the top of the
infant's head to about 5 cm below the chin. The experiment was electronically
timed by a character generator, the output of which was digitally displayed in a
small box located directly above the infant's head and also fed into the video
recorder, such that the elapsed time (in 0.10-s increments) was electronically
mixed in as a permanent time code for scoring purposes.

Stimuli and experimental design. The study used a repeated-measures design in
which each infant acted as his or her own control. Each infant was exposed to two
gestures, mouth opening and tongue protrusion. Each infant was exposed to two
actors, mother and stranger. For each infant, one of the actors (mother or stranger)
demonstrated one type of gesture (mouth opening or tongue protrusion), and the

other actor demonstrated the other gesture. Each actor presented the specified gesture in both movement formats: once as a dynamic gesture (e.g., the mouth was opened and closed at a prescribed rate) and once as a static gesture (e.g., the mouth was simply held open). Counterbalancing was achieved by systemically alternating the displays such that a mouth-opening trial was always alternated with a tongue-protrusion trial. This yielded the following eight test sequences (in which, *MO* = adult mouth-opening trial; *TP* = adult tongue-protrusion trial; mom = mother as the model; stranger = stranger as model; dyn = dynamic display; stat = static display):

$$
\begin{array}{llllllll}
\text{MO6}_{(mom/dyn)} & \to & \text{TP}_{(stranger/stat)} & \to & \text{MO}_{(mom/stat)} & \to & \text{TP}_{(stranger/dyn)} \\
\text{MO}_{(mom/stat)} & \to & \text{TP}_{(stranger/dyn)} & \to & \text{MO}_{(mom/dyn)} & \to & \text{TP}_{(stranger/stat)} \\
\text{MO}_{(stranger/dyn)} & \to & \text{TP}_{(mom/stat)} & \to & \text{MO}_{(stranger/stat)} & \to & \text{TP}_{(mom/dyn)} \\
\text{MO}_{(stranger/stat)} & \to & \text{TP}_{(mom/dyn)} & \to & \text{MO}_{(stranger/dyn)} & \to & \text{TP}_{(mom/stat)} \\
\text{TP}_{(mom/dyn)} & \to & \text{MO}_{(stranger/stat)} & \to & \text{TP}_{(mom/stat)} & \to & \text{MO}_{(stranger/dyn)} \\
\text{TP}_{(mom/stat)} & \to & \text{MO}_{(stranger/dyn)} & \to & \text{TP}_{(mom/dyn)} & \to & \text{MO}_{(stranger/stat)} \\
\text{TP}_{(stranger/dyn)} & \to & \text{MO}_{(mom/stat)} & \to & \text{TP}_{(stranger/stat)} & \to & \text{MO}_{(mom/dyn)} \\
\text{TP}_{(stranger/stat)} & \to & \text{MO}_{(mom/dyn)} & \to & \text{TP}_{(stranger/dyn)} & \to & \text{MO}_{(mom/stat)} \\
\end{array}
$$

Four infants (two of each sex) were randomly assigned to each of these eight sequences. Each trial (e.g., $\text{MO}_{(mom/dyn)}$) was of 90-s duration. Previous research indicated that infant attention and responsivity were maximized if a short period of adult gesturing was alternated with a short pause (Legerstee, 1991; Meltzoff & Moore, 1983a, 1983b; Meltzoff et al., 1991). Thus, within a 90-s trial, the adult displayed the target act for 15 s and then presented a neutral face pose for 15 s, and so on for the 90-s period. For the dynamic gestures, the prescribed rate of gesturing was four times in the 15-s interval; for the static displays, the actor simply held a pose (full mouth opening or full tongue protrusion) for the 15-s interval.

In order to maximize the perceptual distinction between the mother and the stranger, the stranger was the opposite gender of the mother (an adult male), wore a pair of glasses if the mother did not typically wear them, and adopted a different hairline than the mother (accomplished by wearing a fitted, knit cap if she had bushy hair that stood out from the skull line). All three of these factors—gender, glasses, and external hairline—have been designated as salient cues for facial discrimination and recognition in experiments ranging from neonates to adults (Bushnell, 1982; Carey & Diamond, 1977; Fagan & Singer, 1979; Haith, Bergman, & Moore, 1977; Young & Ellis, 1989).

Procedure. The infants did not see the stranger's face (the "experimental stimulus") before the test, so that it would remain novel. Rather, a research assistant greeted the parents and provided instructions about the mechanics of the upcom-

ing test. While seated in the waiting area, the assistant asked the mother to practice mouth opening and tongue protruding at the prescribed rate, which was done
while the infant was turned away and thus could not see her acts. The mothers
were instructed that these facial gestures were to be presented silently and that
they were not to laugh, talk, smile, nod, make mock-surprise faces (uncontrolled
mouth openings) or lick their lips (uncontrolled tongue protrusions) during the
test. Mothers were also asked not to engage in facial games with their infants in
the waiting room before the test so as not to "bore" their infants with such games,
and the research assistant ensured that these directions were followed. Finally,
mothers were instructed that to enter and exit the three-sided test chamber they
and the stranger would both need to proceed in a similar way. The adults were
seated on a stool with wheels (much like a dentist's or pediatrician's stool) before
they entered the test chamber. Once the subject fixated the adult, he or she rolled
in on the stool to the spot in front of the child from which the gesture was presented. After presenting the gesture of 90 s, the adults rolled out of the test chamber continuing the same path that they had used to come in. The mother entered
and exited on a path in the opposite direction of the stranger (direction of entrance
and departure randomized across infants), so there was no shared path of motion
for the mother and stranger. It was required that infants visually track the adults'
movement to and from the test chamber. The adult only moved as quickly as
allowed by the infant: If the adult began to roll to or from the test chamber and
the infant looked away from the adult, the adult temporarily stopped and attracted
the infant's attention. Attention was attracted by shaking a rattle or calling the
infant's name. Once the infant refixated, the adult continued.

  After the mother was satisfied that she understood the full procedure (maternal
instructions typically took about 15 min), the infant was carried to the test chamber. A standard 90-s acclimation period was used for all infants. Infants were
seated comfortably in the infant chair (a padded seat inclined 30° off the horizon-
tal) and then left on their own to explore visually the homogeneous gray test
chamber. Some infants would catch sight of the screen edges and a very few would
notice the camera lens, but most seemed to habituate rapidly to the new surround.
At the end of the 90-s acclimation period, the fixed-time stimulus-presentation
sequence commenced.

Scoring and behavioral definitions. The videotapes of the subjects consisted of
close-up images of the infants' faces with no picture or record of the adult's display. The subjects were coded in a random order by a scorer who remained blind
to which actor or gesture had been shown to the infant in any given segment. A
microanalytic scoring procedure was used in which the scorer viewed the videotapes in real time, slow motion, and frame by frame at her choosing. The scorer's
task was to record all instances of infant mouth openings and tongue protrusions,
identifying them by the time code that was part of the videotape record.

Operational definitions of the target behaviors were provided. They were adapted from Meltzoff and Moore's (1983a, 1989) scoring criteria, but modified slightly to accommodate the older age of the subject.

The onset of a "tongue protrusion" was operationally defined as a clear forward thrust of the tongue such that the tongue tip crossed the back edge of the lower lip. For those cases in which the tongue was being retracted but was not yet behind the lip when a second tongue thrust occurred, the first tongue protrusion was terminated with the initiation of the second. A "mouth opening" was defined as a separation of the lips that had four characteristics: (a) initiated by an abrupt drop of the jaw; (b) lips opened along the entire width including the corners of the mouth so that space (in the form of a black region on the video monitor) could clearly be seen; (c) executed in a unitary motion so that the lip separation was greater than or equal to the width of the lower lip; and (d) fulfilled the foregoing criteria in silence and more than 1.5 s before a vocalization was produced (such acts look like a separate behavioral unit and not simply a concomitant of vocalizing, cooing, or calling out). The termination of a mouth opening was defined by the end of the closing movement of the lips or the initiation of another criterial mouth opening. Any infant behavior that occurred during occasional yawning, sneezing, choking, spitting, or swallowing was not counted by the scorer.

Dependent measures and analysis plan. Four measures served as dependent variables: (a) frequency of infant tongue protrusion; (b) frequency of infant mouth opening; (c) overall duration of infant mouth opening (total time that the infant exhibited mouth opening, measured in seconds to one decimal place); and (d) longest mouth-opening act (the infant's longest single mouth-opening act, measured in seconds to one decimal place). These measures were calculated for each of the infant's four 90-s trials, and in the case that the analysis called for combining the data across two trials, the data were summed (e.g., the frequency of tongue protrusion across two trials was the sum of the frequencies in each of the two separate trials). No attempt was made to obtain the two duration measurements for the infant tongue protrusions.

Intra- and interscorer agreement was assessed by rescoring 12 randomly selected 90-s trials (approximately 10% of the study). Agreement was high for each of the four infant measures as assessed by both correlations and the kappa statistic. The correlation between the original and reliability scorings for the 12 trials averaged .94 across the measures, ranging from .84 to .99. The kappa statistic is an index of agreement that incorporates a correction for chance and assesses point-to-point agreement in the scoring records (Applebaum & McCall, 1983; Bakeman & Gottman, 1986; Cohen, 1960). Values greater than .75 are considered to be excellent agreement (Fleiss, 1981). The obtained values averaged .86, ranging from .80 to .93.

In line with most other studies of early imitation, the bulk of the analyses relied on nonparametric statistical approaches, because the assumptions underlying parametric statistics could not clearly be met using these behavioral measures on young infants (e.g., Abravanel & Sigafoos, 1984; Fontaine, 1984; Heimann et al., 1989; Heimann & Schaller, 1985; Meltzoff & Moore, 1977, 1983a, 1989; Vinter, 1986). One-tailed tests were used to assess whether infants' reactions to the adult gesture were in accord with the hypothesis of infant imitation.

Results

Overall results: Repeated-measures analyses. The overall results provided evidence for imitation (Table 1). The number of infant tongue protrusions was significantly greater to the TP demonstration than to the MO demonstration, $z = 2.58$, $p < .01$, using a Wilcoxon matched-pairs signed-ranks test. Infants produced a greater number of mouth openings to the MO demonstration than to the TP demonstration, but this did not reach significance, $p < .13$, Wilcoxon test. The duration of the infant mouth-opening measure was greater to the MO demonstration than to the TP demonstration, $z = 1.80$, $p < .05$, Wilcoxon test. Finally, the longest mouth-opening act was greater to the MO demonstration than to the TP demonstration, $z = 1.77$, $p < .05$, Wilcoxon test.

A more detailed analysis of imitation at the level of individual subject is provided by simultaneously taking into account two different categories of infant behaviors (tongue protrusions and mouth openings). With regard to tongue protrusions, each infant can produce a greater frequency of tongue protrusions to the adult TP display (indicated as a "+"), or to the MO display (indicated as a "−"), or can produce an equal frequency of tongue protrusions to both displays (indicated as a "0"). Similarly, for mouth openings, each infant can produce a greater frequency of mouth openings to the MO display (+) or to the TP display (−), or can produce an equal frequency to both (0). Infants who produced more tongue

TABLE 1
Infant Behaviors as a Function of the Adult Displays (6-Week-Old Infants)

Infant Behavior	MO Display			TP Display		
	M	(SD)	Median	M	(SD)	Median
Tongue Protrusions	6.69	(5.91)	4.50	10.84	(9.15)	7.50**
Mouth Openings						
Frequency	5.88	(6.97)	3.00	4.88	(6.12)	2.00
Duration	13.40	(15.87)	7.30	10.35	(14.82)	4.25*
Longest Act	6.04	(6.49)	4.35	4.34	(4.34)	3.45*

Note N = 32. Significance assessed by Wilcoxin matched-pairs signed-ranks tests.
*p < .05. **p < .o1.

protrusions to the TP display and more mouth openings to the MO display were classified as " + +" responders, and so on. An exhaustive categorization of the 32 subjects in terms of their individual response frequency patterns is presented in the first row of data in Table 2. A one-sample chi-square test shows that the distribution of the 32 subjects across the response patterns cannot be accounted for by chance, $X^2(5, N = 32) = 23.88, p < .001$. The hypothesis of imitation is most stringently tested by comparing the number of infants falling into the most extreme cells of this distribution (+ + vs.– –). The subjects who were categorized as + + had, by definition, systematically switched their behavior and matched both adult displays. Conversely, infants who were categorized as —had systematically mismatched both displays. Under the null hypothesis, there is an equal probability of infants falling in either the + + or the – – category. The data reveal 15 infants with the + + profile as compared to 6 with the – – profile, $p < .05$ using a binomial test, thus providing support for the hypothesis of imitation. The same analyses can be conducted using the duration of infant mouth opening and the longest mouth-opening act (instead of frequency) to measure the infant mouth-opening response. Both yield significant effects, with the extreme cells (+ + vs. – –) being 16 versus 4, $p < .01$, and 15 versus 4, $p < .01$, respectively (Table 2).

First trial data: Independent groups comparisons and interactions between factors. The type of adult display shown in the first 90-s trial was counterbalanced across subjects. These "first trial" data can be analyzed to assess whether separate groups of infants significantly varied as a function of treatment during the first 90-s exposure. It also makes sense to decompose the first trials into finer subdivisions, for example, examining whether the imitation effect was stronger to the

TABLE 2
Number of Infants as a Function of Response Pattern (6-Week-Old Infants)

Infant Behaviors	Response Patterns[a]							
	+ +	+ 0	0 +	+ –	– +	0 –	– 0	– –
Tongue protrusion and mouth opening (frequency)	15	4	0	4	1	2	0	6
Tongue protrusion and mouth opening (duration)	16	0	1	7	3	1	0	4
Tongue protrusion and mouth opening (longest act)	15	1	1	7	3	1	0	4

[a] Response patterns based on ordered pairs depicting the two infant behaviors in the order: tongue protrusions, mouth openings. + = a matching response, – = a mismatching response, 0 = an equal response to both displays. Each row in the table adds to 32, because there were 32 subjects in the experiment.

mother than to the stranger, or to the dynamic versus static displays. The value of the first trial data for answering such questions is that infants have not yet seen the other types of demonstrations, and thus the eliciting properties of a single type of display taken in isolation can be directly determined.

To assess the main effects of imitation in the first trial data, the subjects who saw the tongue protrusion ($n = 16$) were contrasted with the subjects who saw the mouth opening ($n = 16$). As can be seen in Table 3, infants produced more tongue protrusions to the TP demonstration than to the MO demonstration, $z = 1.70$, $p < .05$, Mann-Whitney U test. There was no significant difference in mouth-opening frequency as a function of demonstration, although the effect was in the predicted direction ($p < .13$, Mann-Whitney test). The other measures of infant mouth opening were more discriminating. Infants produced a longer duration of mouth opening to the MO demonstration than to the TP demonstration, $z = 1.71$, $p < .05$, Mann-Whitney test. Also, the longest mouth-opening act was greater to the MO demonstration than to TP demonstration, $z = 1.88$, $p < .05$, Mann-Whitney test.

These first trial data can also be used to examine the interactions between the stimulus manipulations in this experiment. It is not possible to investigate interactions between factors using a nonparametric analysis of the data (Siegel, 1956), but an analysis of variance (ANOVA) serves this purpose and will yield interpretable results even if the assumptions underlying this approach are not fully satisfied, especially if there are independent groups with the same number of cases in each sample as is the case in this experiment (Hays, 1981; Winer, 1971). Such an approach was adopted here to examine the influence of person and movement on imitative responding. A three-way ANOVA was conducted using person (mother/stranger) x movement (dynamic/static) x gesture (mouth opening/tongue protrusion) demonstrated to the subject.

The results reveal no three-way interactions (person x movement x gesture) for

TABLE 3
First Trial Data as a Function of the Adult Displays (6-Week-Old Infants)

Infant Behavior	MO Display			TP Display		
	M	(SD)	Median	M	(SD)	Median
Tongue Protrusions	3.88	(5.16)	2.00	6.75	(5.88)	5.00*
Mouth Openings						
Frequency	4.06	(4.20)	3.00	2.19	(2.32)	2.00
Duration	9.95	(9.47)	9.20	3.81	(4.70)	2.60*
Longest Act	4.13	(4.34)	3.20	1.73	(1.44)	1.70*

*$p < .05$, Mann-Whitney U tests; $n = 16$ versuds $n = 16$.

any of the infant measures (tongue protrusions or the three mouth-opening measures), with all $Fs(1, 24) < 1.0$, and ps ranging from .38–.90. The data displayed in Table 4 address the person x gesture interaction; they assess whether infants imitate mothers more than strangers. The ANOVA revealed no person x gesture interaction for the tongue-protrusion measure, $F(1, 24) < 1.0, p > .95$. As can be seen, the frequency of tongue protrusion was greater to the TP demonstration than to the MO demonstration in the case in which the mother served as model ($M = 6.50$ vs. 3.75); this was also true in the case that the stranger served as the model ($M = 7.00$ vs. 4.00). In both cases, the scores of infants presented with the TP demonstration exceed those presented with the MO demonstration, as predicted by the hypothesis of imitation. The same analyses were run using the measure of mouth-opening frequency, duration, and longest act, and again no person x gesture interaction emerged, with all $Fs(1, 24) < 1.0$, and ps ranging from .60 to .92. Reference to Table 4 shows the reason quite clearly: Whether one isolates just the mother as model or just the stranger as model, the effects are all in the same direction. There is more infant mouth opening to the mouth opening gesture than to the tongue protrusion gesture, as predicted by the hypothesis of imitation, and this is true regardless of who serves as model. In summary, Table 4 presents eight opportunities for examining the gesture effect (two persons x four measures), and all of those eight contrasts are in the direction predicted by the hypothesis of imitation. Thus, imitation is not modified by which person serves as the model.

The ANOVA approach also yielded information concerning a movement x gesture interaction. This interaction was not significant for the tongue-protrusion measure, $F(1, 24) < 1.0, p > .52$, or for the mouth-opening frequency, $F(1, 24) = 2.03, p > .16$, or mouth-opening longest act, $F(1, 24) = 2.63, p > .11$. However, there was a trend toward a movement x gesture interaction for the mouth-opening duration measure, $F(1, 24) = 3.38, p < .08$. Inspection of the

TABLE 4
First Trial Means (Standard Deviations) Showing Effects of Person x Gesture
(6-Week-Old Infants)

Infant Behavior	Mother				Stranger			
	MO		TP		MO		TP	
Tongue Protrusions	3.75	(3.99)	6.50	(5.63)	4.00	(6.41)	7.00	(6.50)
Mouth Openings								
Frequency	4.25	(5.26)	2.50	(2.93)	3.88	(3.18)	1.88	(1.64)
Duration	10.19	(11.05)	4.82	(6.28)	9.71	(8.35)	2.79	(2.36)
Longest Act	3.80	(2.58)	2.00	(1.82)	4.46	(5.79)	1.46	(0.98)

data (Table 5) indicates that this was because the MO$_{(stat)}$ manipulation elicited extremely long mouth-opening durations. Pairwise comparisons showed that the MO$_{(stat)}$ group produced significantly longer mouth-opening durations than did each of the other groups taken individually (all $ps < .05$ by Mann-Whitney tests), and identical results were obtained using a parametric Newman-Keuls test. On average, the duration of infant mouth opening to MO$_{(stat)}$ group was 14.66 s, which was more than twice that to the MO$_{(dyn)}$ ($M = 5.24$ s) and almost four times that to either TP$_{(stat)}$ ($M = 3.75$ s) or TP$_{(dyn)}$ ($M = 3.86$ s). This pattern of results indicates that infants were responsive to both the durational and form characteristics of the displays: They responded to the adult's static MO demonstration with significantly longer mouth-opening durations of their own; they did not respond to the adult's static TP demonstration (or other displays) in this manner. The most extreme mouth-opening durations were in response to the mouth-opening-in-static-form demonstration.

EXPERIMENT 2: EXPLORING DEVELOPMENT—EXTENSION TO 2- TO 3-MONTH-OLDS

Previous work suggested that there is a "drop-out" of facial imitation after the early period, beginning at approximately the second or third postnatal month (e.g., Abravanel & Sigafoos, 1984; Bjorklund, 1987; Maratos, 1982). A variety of theoretical interpretations have been offered, but the time course and explanation for this phenomenon is not settled. The specific purpose of the second experiment was to see how infants in the 2-to 3-month age range would fare in a study of facial imitation using the current design. Would the new procedures developed in Experiment 1 be useful in motivating imitation in this older age group? Or would the results fall to chance, as suggested in the previous reports, and if so, could we discern why?

TABLE 5
First Trial Means (Standard Deviations) Showing Effects of Movement x Gesture (6-Week-Old Infants)

Infant Behavior	Dynamic				Static			
	MO		TP		MO		TP	
Tongue Protrusions	4.62	(6.63)	6.13	(6.20)	3.13	(3.44)	7.37	(5.90)
Mouth Openings								
Frequency	2.50	(2.73)	2.38	(2.50)	5.63	(4.98)	2.00	(2.27)
Duration	5.24	(5.71)	3.86	(4.95)	14.66	(10.43)	3.75	(4.77)
Longest Act	2.29	(2.36)	1.72	(1.64)	5.97	(5.21)	1.74	(1.33)

Method

Subjects. The subjects were 16 infants ranging in age from 9.29 to 12.29 weeks old $M = 10.59$, $SD = 1.00$). They were recruited in the same manner and met the same selection criteria for birthweight and length of gestation as described in Experiment 1. One additional selection criterion became obvious before the experiment began, in piloting this extension to older infants. It became clear that at this age some parents had developed habitual facial routines, sometimes including tonguing and mouthing games with their infants. Such parent-child games have been amply described in the social-developmental literature (Bruner, 1975; Papoušek & Papoušek, 1986; Stern, 1985; Trevarthen, 1979). Obviously, an experiment on facial imitation using the mother as the stimulus would be confounded if the mother already had a well-rehearsed routine of this type. Piaget (1962) avoided developing oral routines with his subjects and called trained mimicry "pseudoimitation." Following Piaget's logic, the parents of prospective subjects were interviewed to see if they had developed games in which they commonly mimicked their infants' mouth openings or tongue protrusions, and those who did were not admitted into the experiment in order to avoid Piaget's pseudoimitation. The mean birthweight of the final sample was 3.59 kg (range $= 3.12–4.42$, $SD = .33$). The mean length of gestation was 40.62 weeks (range $= 37.71–42.86$, $SD = 1.39$). All the subjects were white. An additional three infants were tested but were dropped from the study due to excessive fussing.

Stimuli, design, procedure, and scoring. The stimuli, design, and procedure were identical to Experiment 1. The subjects were scored from videotape as previously described. Intra- and interobserver agreement were assessed by rescoring a randomly selected 15% of the trials. Scoring agreement for the four infant measures as assessed by correlations averaged .97, ranging from .93 to .99, and by kappas averaged .88, ranging from .79 to .97.

Results

The repeated-measures design yields strong evidence for imitation at this age, as shown in Table 6. There was a significantly greater number of tongue protrusions to the TP demonstration than to the MO demonstration, $z = 2.76$, $p < .01$, Wilcoxon test. Similarly, there was a greater number of mouth openings to the MO demonstration than to the TP demonstration, $z = 2.31$, $p < .05$, Wilcoxon test. There was significantly longer duration of mouth opening to the MO than to the TP demonstration, $z = 2.17$, $p < .05$, Wilcoxon test. An infant's longest mouth-opening act tended to be produced in response to the MO as opposed to the TP demonstration, $z = 2.10$, $p < .05$, Wilcoxon test.

TABLE 6
Infant Behaviors as a Function of the Adult Displays (2- to 3-Month-Old Infants)

Infant Behavior	MO Display			TP Display		
	M	(SD)	Median	M	(SD)	Median
Tongue Protrusions	9.44	(6.84)	8.00	13.81	(10.02)	11.00**
Mouth Openings						
Frequency	6.81	(5.29)	6.50	4.63	(4.76)	3.00*
Duration	15.44	(15.10)	11.40	7.57	(8.41)	5.05*
Longest Act	7.48	(8.57)	4.25	3.59	(2.65)	3.00*

Note N = 32. Significance assessed by Wilcoxin matched-pairs signed-ranks tests.
*$p < .05$. **$p < .o1$.

The imitation effect can also be examined in more detail at the level of individual subjects, as described in Experiment 1. Each individual infant can produce a greater frequency of tongue protrusions to the adult TP display (+), or to the adult mouth-opening display (–), or can produce an equal frequency to both displays (0). A similar casting can be done for the mouth-opening responses. Infants who produced more tongue protrusions to the TP display and more mouth openings to the MO display were classified as " + + " responders, and so on. Table 7 (p. 22) exhaustively categorizes the 16 subjects as a function of their individual response patterns. The hypothesis of imitation is most stringently tested by comparing the number of infants falling into the most extreme cells of this distribution (+ + versus – –). Subjects categorized as + + had switched their behavior and matched both adult displays; conversely, infants categorized as – – had systematically mismatched both displays. Under the null hypothesis, it is equiprobable for infants to fall into either the + + or the – – cell. The data reveal 7 infants with the + + profile as compared to only 1 with the – – profile, $p < .05$ using a binomial test. The identical analysis can be conducted using the duration of infant mouth opening or the longest mouth-opening act (instead of frequency) to quantify the infant mouth-opening response. The resulting profiles are also shown in Table 7; both yield significant effects, with the extreme cells (+ + vs. – –) being 9 versus 2 and 8 versus 1, respectively, both $ps < .05$.

The first trial analyses in this experiment were not discriminative, possibly because the first trials did not benefit from using each infant as his or her own control, which was utilized in the foregoing repeated-measures tests, and because the overall number of subjects for the independent groups comparisons was small ($n = 8$ seeing TP vs. 8 seeing MO). The main effects assessing imitation were in the predicted direction for each of the four behavioral measures, but none showed significant differences, all $ps > .23$, Mann-Whitney tests. There were no main effects either for person (mother vs. stranger) or for move-

TABLE 7
Number of Infants as a Function of Response Pattern (2- to 3-Month-Old Infants)

Infant Behaviors	Response Patterns[a]							
	+ +	+0	0+	+ −	− +	0−	−0	− −
Tongue protrusion and mouth opening (frequency)	7	4	1	2	1	0	0	1
Tongue protrusion and mouth opening (duration)	9	1	1	3	0	0	0	2
Tongue protrusion and mouth opening (longest act)	8	2	1	3	1	0	0	1

[a] Response patterns based on ordered pairs depicting the two infant behaviors in the order: tongue protrusions, mouth openings. + = a matching response, − = a mismatching response, 0 = an equal response to both displays. Each row in the table adds to 16, because there were 16 subjects in the experiment.

ment (dynamic vs. static) for any of the four infant measures, all $ps > .45$, Mann-Whitney tests; interactions could not be assessed because the cell sizes were too small.

GENERAL DISCUSSION

This research contributes three empirical findings to the early imitation literature: (a) early imitation does not significantly vary as a function of familiarity with the model—infants imitate a stranger as well as their own mothers; (b) infants can imitate static facial postures as well as dynamic gestures; and (c) there is no necessary loss of facial imitation at 2 to 3 months of age due to a drop out of neonatal reflexes—using this design, infants in this age group imitated as well or better than did younger subjects. Beyond these empirical findings, we will develop arguments concerning the function that early imitation serves in infants' encounters with people. In particular, the connection between imitation and person identity is elaborated, and evidence is adduced for viewing imitation as an act of social cognition rather than a fixed reflex. We will sketch a model in which imitation serves an *identity function*. In our view, imitative reenactments and the sharing of behavioral states are a fundamental means by which young infants know and communicate with "persons" as opposed to "things."

The Role of Person and Movement

One question examined in this research was whether the person who served as the model, mother or stranger, had a significant impact on imitation. This was directly tested using the first trial data in Experiment 1. For this comparison, the infants only saw one person: for half, it was the mother; for the other half, it was the stranger. The results showed significant imitation in the first trials, and moreover, that the imitative effect was not modified by whether the model was mother or stranger. This finding is of interest for both theoretical and methodological reasons. Methodologically, it is valuable to know that a group of "experimenters" who were essentially uninformed about the purpose of the experiment, and who each visited the laboratory for an hour or less, are as effective in eliciting the response as the trained experimenter. It demonstrates a generalizability of the effect across the people who serve as models. Theoretically, it is noteworthy that for infants in this young age group, imitating requires no special relationship or attachment to the person or even perceptual familiarity with the person's face. The person who served as model made no significant difference to imitative responding, although infants this age can discriminate their own mother from a stranger (Bushnell, Sai, & Mullin, 1989; Field, Cohen, Garcia, & Greenberg, 1984; Walton, Bower, & Bower, 1992; S. de Schonen, personal communication, 1992). Thus, the basis of imitation lies in stimulus attributes that are shared by both familiar maternal faces and a novel male face. It seems likely, however, that at some point in infancy, familiarity with a person and especially the shared interactive experience with that person would influence how imitation is used in that dyad; such a developmental change in imitative reactions would be interesting to examine in longitudinal work (Bandura, 1969; Bower, 1979; Uzgiris, 1981; Watson, 1972).

The research also investigated infants' reactions to static facial displays. The first-trial results of Experiment 1 showed that the average duration of infant mouth opening to the MO demonstration was 14.66 s, more than twice that to the $MO_{(dyn)}$ demonstration (5.24 s) and nearly four times that to either the $TP_{(stat)}$ or $TP_{(dyn)}$ demonstrations (3.75 s and 3.86 s, respectively). Two inferences can be drawn. First, the finding that $MO_{(stat)}$ elicited longer infant mouth opening than $TP_{(stat)}$ indicates that the form of the gesture (mouth opening vs. tongue protrusion) is critical even in the context of a nonmoving display. The increase in mouth-opening duration is not attributable to the "static-ness" per se, as if all static facial postures are indistinguishable to infants and result in lengthy infant mouth openings: Both $MO_{(stat)}$ and $TP_{(stat)}$ were equally static, and yet the former elicited 14.66 s of the target response and the latter only 3.75 s, which differed significantly. Second, temporal parameters are not wholly ignored by the infant. When the type of gesture is controlled, infants produced significantly longer mouth opening to one kind of adult mouth opening (static) than the other kind of mouth opening (dynamic). In brief, the infants matched both the form and the temporal aspects of the adult's demonstration. This is relevant for theory because so fine a differentiation between such closely related displays—two different types of mouth openings—is neither predicted by, nor compatible with, the notion of early imitation as a simple global reflex.

The results also weigh against a strong version of the hypothesis that imitation in the first few months of life is based *solely* on a visual analysis of movement per se and that form information plays a negligible role (e.g., Vinter, 1986). Vinter's data showed no imitation of static gestures in newborns averaging 4 days old (although the same study found significant imitation of moving gestures). Our data show that 6-week-old infants are capable of imitating static postures. Three developmental changes could account for this. First, between 4 days and 6 weeks of age there could be growth in peripheral systems; visual constraints could prevent newborns from extracting the relevant form information from nonmoving faces, in which case they would not be expected to imitate them (cf. Banks & Salapatek, 1981; Braddick & Atkinson, 1988). Second, there may also be growth in perceptual-motor "translation" capacities and the understanding of human acts. Six-week-olds may be able to match target postures without seeing the transitions: For 6-week-olds, a final configurational state may adequately specify the temporally organized body transformations needed to achieve the end state, although it does not do so innately. Third, nonmoving faces may lack social meaning for newborns; they may be objects to stare at but not to interact with. By 6 weeks, infants may interpret even static postures as socially relevant human acts that support social responding.

The finding that imitation can be tapped using duration measures (overall duration of mouth opening and longest act) casts new light on previous research. Most previous work has been limited to measuring movement frequency. Our results show that the duration measures are a more discriminating measure of mouth-opening imitation. We can now see that the exclusive reliance on frequency, the weakest of the measures used in these experiments, might account for null effects in some past studies (see also Meltzoff & Moore, 1983b). The duration code potentially provides a way of improving the sensitivity of future studies of early imitation. At a more theoretical level, there is no a priori reason to assume that infants will encode adult MO demonstrations in terms of frequency versus duration of the act. Indeed, the fact that infants were so attentive to mouth-opening duration invites an interesting speculation: Because people talk to infants (repeated mouth openings), the most novel aspects of the experimental stimulus may be the slow, long-duration aspects of the mouth-openings, and this may be true even of the dynamic demonstrations (which are performed far more slowly than speech articulations). Infants may be picking out and imitating aspects of the display based partly upon what they have experienced as "normal" and "expected" acts for human faces, underscoring the way in which imitation may be influenced by early interpersonal experience and development.

On Imitative Drop-Out: The Role of Social-Communicative Factors

In Experiment 2, using 2- to 3-month-olds, the data from the overall tests using subjects as their own controls provided strong evidence for imitation. We did not find imitation everywhere, however; the first-trial data were not discriminative, and observations of the infants suggest why. These older infants had expectations about face-to-face encounters and were especially likely to "greet" people when they first saw them, trying out motor routines as if to engage in a nonverbal interchange (cf. Bruner, 1975, 1983; Brazelton & Tronick, 1980; Fogel, 1991; Stern, 1985; Trevarten, 1979; Trevarthen & Marwick, 1986). The motor routines varied across children, probably depending on family games, but the variability worked to undermine the first-trial, between-subjects comparisons.

The literature contains two principal accounts of the "drop-out" of facial imitation in the 2- to 3-month age range; this research suggests a third interpretation of the same data. According to the first view, neonatal imitation is based on simple reflexes; development brings reflexive inhibition, hence the drop-out (Abravanel & Sigafoos, 1984; Bjorklund, 1987). A second view is that the neonatal period can be described as one of the perceptual unity (Bower, 1982, 1989); development brings a differentiation into the separate modalities, hence early imitation (along with neonatal reaching, auditory-visual spatial location, and other skills) drops out and is later reconstituted through a coordination of the now-differentiated modalities. Both the reflexive and the modality differentiation views highlight the inevitable, maturationally based drop-out of facial imitation.

The third view suggested here is that *social factors* play a more central role in the previously reported disappearance of imitation (cf. Field et al., 1986; Kugiumutzakis, 1985). From an observational viewpoint, the most striking developmental change in infant responding was that the older infants initially tried out all sorts of games on the adult (Piaget, 1952, 1954, would call them "magical procedures") and pursued them more vigorously than the younger infants. Such social games and solicitations serve to obscure imitation in this older age group initially, although after the initial social solicitations, infants generally settled down and engaged in imitation. Our repeated-measures design is thus more effective than a one-time test, because it measured the infant over an extended period and used each infant as his or her own control. This solved two problems presented by this older population, high intersubject variability and the initiation of social games with the experimenter. Relatedly, the gestures were shown in time-locked manner rather than being contingent on infants' behavior. This format may help shift older infants away from their routinized social-interactive games (e.g., smiling and cooing; see Watson, 1972) and focus them on watching and reacting to the particular experimental gestures under test.

Another possible reason for the efficacy of the experimental design is that it specified for the infant the category of adult behavior that was being demonstrated. Why should an older, socially adept infant focus on a single elementary act, for example, a mouth opening? Cohen and Caputo (1978) argued that multiexemplar variation will serve to "instruct the infant to respond to some feature or attribute common to all members of the category" (p. 1). The use of multiexemplar variation has proven to be a powerful stimulus manipulation (Cohen & Strauss, 1979; Fagan, 1976, 1979; Hayne, Rovee-Collier, & Perris, 1987; Kuhl, 1983; Reznick & Kagan, 1983; Ruff, 1978; Walker, Owsley, Megaw-Nyce, Gibson, & Bahrick, 1980). Yet, in all studies reporting imitative drop-out, infants were presented repetitions of an act with no variation. Such designs would not be expected to emphasize the "mouth openness" of the display for the infant. The current design provided each infant with within-category variation (both static and dynamic exemplars of the same underlying behavioral category). Simultaneously, and at least as importantly, the design highlighted intercategory differences. Person 1 performed one type of gesture (the mouth opening or tongue protrusion, but not both), and person 2 performed the other gesture. Thus, a specific gesture was paired with a specific person. In all the previous repeated-measures studies used with this age group, one experimenter performed both gestures, which can confuse infants and dampen imitation.

We are thus suggesting that older infants initially respond to people by engaging in social games. These games supersede infant imitation, hence the apparent drop-out. The current procedures served to focus the older infants on the narrower imitation task by using a noncontingent demonstration, highlighting intercategory differences, and providing variation in the exemplars of the target action. We conclude that the previously reported drop-out is not due to a fundamental loss of imitative competence but to the fact that social and motivational factors mask that competence.

Linking Imitation, Identity, and Representation: Towards a New Theory of the Function of Early Imitation

By putting together what we know from both the pilot and final experiments, we can now offer some new ideas about the meaning, motive, and functional significance of early imitation. These ideas situate early imitation within a broader psychological framework than simple reflexes. We intend to show how infant imitation contributes to theories of early social cognition and informs discussions about infants' earliest and most basic notions of persons.

A comprehensive view of early imitation needs to explain the conditions under which infants imitate, as well as those in which they do not. The reflexive account falls short in this regard. Imitation is not always elicited either in our work or that of others; it does not behave like an automatic and ubiquitous reflex. A model that considers imitation an act of primitive social cognition fares better by stressing the functional uses of imitation to infants. The pilot experiment revealed that infants who did not visually track adults as they appeared and disappeared, inspected the new person, and then intently performed the actions shown by the *previous* person. This suggests to us that the adult gestures are not simple sign stimuli that automatically trigger the infant's behavior, because the wrong act is often "triggered" by the sight of the new gesture. In contemplating this pattern of counterimitation (we now see it as deferred imitation), we have found it useful to consider two interrelated ideas: (a) young infants do not have a fully developed system for determining person identity; and (b) infants use actions, including facial gestures, as part of assimilating, "knowing," and communicating with a person.

Part 1 concerns infants' *rules for identity*. It holds that young infants may have questions about the identity of the person in a two-person situation. We attempted to clarify this by having the two people look different; however, there was no requirement that infants in the pilot experiment fully track the adults as they walked to and from the test chamber, and this may have led to ambiguity about the identity of the person. Indeed, philosophical analysis has shown that featural differences in objects, or for that matter featural similarity, is no guarantee as to the true identity of the objects (Hirsch, 1982; Strawson, 1959).[1] Two encounters with an object may appear different and yet be of the same object; conversely, two encounters may look the same and be of different objects. For example, two featurally identical coffee cups may be different objects; conversely, a person wearing a kerchief does not become a different entity, but merely the self-same person, featurally transformed. Logically, object and person identity are not reducible to featural similitude. Thus, it is plausible that infants can be confused about the identity of persons in a multiperson situation involving their appearance and disappearance. In fact, this would not be an uncommon event for young infants (Moore & Meltzoff, 1978). What action might they take to clarify such conflicts?

Part 2 concerns infants' *use of nonverbal gestures to clarify ambiguities about the identity of persons*. This point draws on the Piagetian-Wernerian notion of knowing-through-action (Piaget, 1952; Werner & Kaplan, 1963). According to that thesis, the young infant does not apprehend an object, for example, a rattle, as a fully differentiated and categorized object, but rather as a somewhat un-differentiated form-function unit, as "something-that-shakes or is-shakable." Perceptual objects are not fully differentiated or known independent of the actions

---

[1]The type of identity we are highlighting is not at the level of feature discrimination and visual appearance per se. Rather, it concerns what philosophers call numerical or particular identity (Strawson, 1959) and we have called unique identity in the context of object-concept development (Moore & Meltzoff, 1978). The examples used in the text should help to further clarify this issue.

they afford. When infants see a rattle again they will try to shake it as a way of understanding or recognizing it. By analogy we propose that when infants reencounter a person, they try to reinstitute the action that was connected with this person as a way of apprehending the person. If infants are confused or ambiguous about the identity of a new person who is perceptually present, they will be particularly motivated to test whether this person has the same behavioral properties as the old one, whether he or she acts the same, because the body actions and expressive behavior of people are identifiers of who they are. We are thus hypothesizing that one function of early imitation is to probe the identity of the person in front of the infant. We think infants use nonverbal gestures as the functional equivalent of the query: "Are you the one who does tongue protrusion?"

This functional use of imitation explains why the infants who did not track the change in demonstrator in the pilot experiment were so intent on duplicating the absent person's gesture. It was their way of comparing the past person with the present person, to probe whether identity was maintained despite a change in appearance or whether this was a new person. Experiment 1 was designed to reduce identity ambiguity by supplementing the featural information with spatiotemporal information about person identity. The new procedures ensured that the adults moved on two distinctly different paths and that infants fully tracked the movements of the adults to and from the test chamber. The adults were different both by featural and by spatiotemporal criteria. Thus, there was no question as to their different identity, and in this case, a significant number of infants switched responses so as to mimic the new person.

The foregoing theoretical analysis of the multiperson situation may also explain some aspects of imitation when only a single person is used. It has been reported that infants respond poorly if the adult repeatedly and unceasingly presents the target gesture (Meltzoff & Moore, 1983a, 1983b, 1985), a point also noted by Legerstee (1991). For this reason, we use a "burst-pause" procedure in which the experimenter alternates between a set of target gestures and a passive-face pose. We believe that the burst-pause procedure is especially effective because when the adult stops gesturing, the infants are confronted with a mismatch between their current perception of the model and their memory representation. We think the infant generates a matching response in order to reinstate the absent event (the gesturing), to make it perceptually present again. Thus, the pause in the adult's behavior gives the infant a problem to work through: the conflict between the world-as-represented and the here-and-now as presented to the visual system. This mismatch between perception and representation motivates the infant to action, and consequently, observable imitation. It is just because young infants can act from stored memories of absent realities—just because their behavior is not based solely on the stimulus before them—that their imitative acts may sometimes go unnoticed.

REFERENCES

Abravanel, E., & DeYong, N. G. (1991). Does object modeling elicit imitative-like gestures from young infants? *Journal of Experimental Child Psychology, 52*, 22–40.

Abravanel, E., & Sigafoos, A. D. (1984). Exploring the presence of imitation during early infancy. *Child Development, 55*, 381–392.

Applebaum, M. I., & McCall, R. B. (1983). Design and analysis in developmental psychology. In W. Kessen (Ed.), *Handbook of child psychology* (Vol. 1). New York: Wiley.

Bakeman, R., & Gottman, J. M. (1986). *Observing interaction: An introduction to sequential analysis.* Cambridge: Cambridge University Press.

Bandura, A. (1969). Social-learning theory of identifactory processes. In D. A. Goslin (Ed.), *Handbook of socialization theory and research.* Chicago: Rand McNally.

Banks, M. S., & Salapatek, P. (1981). Infant pattern vision: A new approach based on the contrast sensitivity function. *Journal of Experimental Child Psychology, 31*, 1–45.

Bjorklund, D. F. (1987). A note on neonatal imitation. *Developmental Review, 7*, 86–92.

Bower, T. G. R. (1979). *Human development.* San Francisco: W. H. Freeman.

Bower, T. G. R. (1982). *Development in infancy* (2nd ed.). San Francisco: W. H. Freeman.

Bower, T. G. R. (1989). *The rational infant: Learning in infancy.* San Francisco: W. H. Freeman.

Braddick, O., & Atkinson, J. (1988). Sensory selectivity, attentional control, and cross-channel integration in early visual development. In A. Yonas (Ed.), *The Minnesota symposia on child psychology: Vol. 20. Perceptual development in infancy.* Hillsdale, NJ: Erlbaum.

Brazelton, T. B., & Tronick, E. (1980). Preverbal communication between mothers and infants. In D. R. Olson (Ed.), *The social foundations of language and thought.* New York: Norton.

Bruner, J. S. (1975). From communication to language—A psychological perspective. *Cognition, 3*, 255–287.

Bruner, J. S. (1983). *Child's talk: Learning to use language.* New York: Norton.

Bushnell, I. W. R. (1982). Discrimination of faces by young infants. *Journal of Experimental Child Psychology, 33*, 298–308.

Bushnell, I. W. R., Sai, F., & Mullin, J. T. (1989). Neonatal recognition of the mother's face. *British Journal of Developmental Psychology, 7*, 3–15.

Carey, S., & Diamond, R. (1977). From piecemeal to configurational representation of faces. *Science, 195*, 312–314.

Cohen, J. (1960). A coefficient of agreement for nominal scales. *Educational and Psychological Measurement, 20*, 37–46.

Cohen, L. B., & Caputo, N. F. (1978, March). *Instructing infants to respond to perceptual categories.* Paper presented at the meeting of the Midwestern Psychological Association, Chicago.

Cohen, L. B., & Strauss, M. S. (1979). Concept acquisition in the human infant. *Child Development, 50*, 419–424.

Fagan, J. F., III. (1976). Infants' recognition of invariant features of faces. *Child Development, 47*, 627–638.

Fagan, J. F., III. (1979). The origins of facial pattern recognition. In M. H. Bornstein & W. Kessen (Eds.), *Psychological development from infancy: Image to intention.* Hillsdale, NJ: Erlbaum.

Fagan, J. F., III., & Singer, L. T. (1979). The role of simple feature differences in infants' recognition of faces. *Infant Behavior and Development, 2*, 39–45.

Field, T. M., Cohen, D., Garcia, R., & Greenberg, R. (1984). Mother-stranger face discrimination by the newborn. *Infant Behavior and Development, 7*, 19–25.

Field, T. M., Goldstein, S., Vaga-Lahr, N., & Porter, K. (1986). Changes in simitative behavior during early infancy. *Infant Behavior and Development, 9*, 415–421.

Field, T. M., Woodson, R., Cohen, D., Greenberg, R., Garcia, R., & Collins, E. (1983). Discrimination and imitation of facial expressions by term and preterm neonates. *Infant Behavior and Development, 6*, 485–489.

Field, T. M., Woodson, R., Greenberg, R., & Cohen, D. (1982). Discrimination and imitation of facial expressions by neonates. *Science, 218*, 179–181.

Fleiss, J. L. (1981). *Statistical methods for rates and proportions* (2nd ed.). New York: Wiley.

Fogel, A. (1991). *Infancy* (2nd ed.). New York: West Publishing.

Fontaine, R. (1984). Imitative skills between birth and six months. *Infant Behavior and Development, 7*, 323–333.

Gibson, J. J. (1966). *The senses considered as perceptual systems.* Boston: Houghton Mifflin.

Gibson, J. J. (1979). *The ecological approach to visual perception.* Boston: Houghton Mifflin.

Haith, M. M., Bergman, T., & Moore, M. J. (1977). Eye contact and face scanning in early infancy. *Science, 198*, 853–855.

Hayne, H., Rovee-Collier, C., & Perris, E. E. (1987). Categorization and memory retrieval by three-month-olds. *Child Development, 58*, 750–767.

Hays, W. L. (1981). *Statistics* (3rd ed.). New York: Holt, Rinehart & Winston.

Heimann, M. (1989). Neonatal imitation, gaze aversion, and mother-infant interaction. *Infant Behavior and Development, 12*, 495–505.

Heimann, M. (1991). Neonatal imitation: A social and biological phenomenon. In T. Archer & S. Hansen (Eds.), *Behavioral biology: The neuroendocrine axis.* Hillsdale, NJ: Erlbaum.

Heimann, M., Nelson, K. E., & Schaller, J. (1989). Neonatal imitation of tongue protrusion and mouth opening: Methodological aspects and evidence of early individual differences. *Scandinavian Journal of Psychology, 30*, 90–101.

Heimann, M., & Schaller, J. (1985). Imitative reactions among 14–21 day old infants. *Infant Mental Health Journal, 6*, 31–39.

Hirsch, E. (1982). *The concept of identity.* New York: Oxford University Press.

Jacobson, S. W. (1979). Matching behavior in the young infant. *Child Development, 50*, 425–430.

Kaitz, M., Meschulach-Sarfaty, O., Auerbach, J., & Eidelman, A. (1988). A reexamination of newborn's ability to imitate facial expressions. *Developmental Psychology, 24*, 3–7.

Kugiumutzakis, J. (1985). *Development of imitation during the first six months of life* (Uppsala Psychological Reports No. 377). Uppsala, Sweden: Uppsala University.

Kuhl, P. K. (1983). Perception of auditory equivalence classes for speech in early infancy. *Infant Behavior and Development, 6*, 263–285.

Legerstee, M. (1991). The role of person and object in eliciting early imitation. *Journal of Experimental Child Psychology, 51*, 423–433.

Maratos, O. (1982). Trends in the development of imitation in early infancy. In T. G. Bever (Ed.), *Regressions in mental development: Basic phenomena and theories*. Hillsdale, NJ: Erlbaum.

Meltzoff, A. N., Kuhl, P. K., & Moore, M. K. (1991). Perception, representation, and the control of action in newborns and young infants: Toward a new synthesis. In M. J. S. Weiss & P. R. Zelazo (Eds.), *Newborn attention: Biological constraints and the influence of experience*. Norwood, NJ: Ablex.

Meltzoff, A. N., & Moore, M. K. (1977). Imitation of facial and manual gestures by human neonates. *Science, 198*, 75–78.

Meltzoff, A. N., & Moore, M. K. (1983a). Newborn infants imitate adult facial gestures. *Child Development, 54*, 702–709.

Meltzoff, A. N., & Moore, M. K. (1983b). The origins of imitation in infancy: Paradigm, phenomena, and theories. In L. P. Lipsitt (Ed.), *Advances in infancy research* (Vol. 2). Norwood, NJ: Ablex.

Meltzoff, A. N., & Moore, M. K. (1985). Cognitive foundations and social functions of imitation and intermodal representation in infancy. In J. Mehler & R. Fox (Eds.), *Neonate cognition: Beyond the blooming, buzzing confusion*. Hillsdale, NJ: Erlbaum.

Meltzoff, A. N., & Moore, M. K. (1989). Imitation in newborn infants: Exploring the range of gestures imitated and the underlying mechanisms. *Developmental Psychology, 25*, 954–962.

Michotte, A. (1962). *Causalité, permanence, et réalité phénoménales* [Phenomenal causality, permanence, and reality]. Louvain: Publications Universitaires.

Moore, M. K., Borton, R., & Darby, B. L. (1978). Visual tracking in young infants: Evidence for object identity or object permanence? *Journal of Experimental Child Psychology, 25*, 183–198.

Moore, M. K., & Meltzoff, A. N. (1978). Object permanence, imitation, and language development in infancy: Toward a neo-Piagetian perspective on communicative and cognitive development. In F. D. Minifie & L. L. Lloyd (Eds.), *Communicative and cognitive abilities—Early behavioral assessment*. Baltimore, MD: University Park Press.

Papoušek, H., & Papoušek, M. (1986). Structure and dynamics of human communication at the beginning of life. *European Archives of Psychiatry and Neurological Sciences, 236*, 21–25.

Piaget, J. (1952). *The origins of intelligence in children.* New York: International Universities Press.

Piaget, J. (1954). *The construction of reality in the child.* New York: Basic Books.

Piaget, J. (1962). *Play, dreams and imitation in childhood.* New York: Norton.

Reissland, N. (1988). Neonatal imitation in the first hour of life: Observations in rural Nepal. *Developmental Psychology, 24,* 464–469.

Reznick, J. S., & Kagan, J. (1983). Category detection in infancy. In L. P. Lipsitt (Ed.), *Advances in infancy research* (Vol. 2). Norwood, NJ: Ablex.

Ruff, H. A. (1978). Infant recognition of the invariant form of objects. *Child Development, 49,* 293–306.

Siegel, S. (1956). *Nonparametric statistics for the behavioral sciences.* New York: McGraw-Hill.

Stern, D. N. (1985). *The interpersonal world of the infant.* New York: Basic Books.

Strawson, P. F. (1959). *Individuals: An essay in descriptive metaphysics.* London: Methuen.

Thinès, G., Costall, A., & Butterworth, G. (Eds.). (1991). *Michotte's experimental phenomenology of perception.* Hillsdale, NJ: Erlbaum.

Trevarthen, C. (1979). Communication and cooperation in early infancy: A description of primary intersubjectivity. In M. Bullowa (Ed.), *Before speech.* Cambridge: Cambridge University Press.

Trevarthen, C., & Marwick, H. (1986). Signs of motivation for speech in infants, and the nature of a mother's support for development of language. In B. Lindblom & R. Zetterström (Eds.), *Precursors of early speech.* New York: Stockton Press.

Uzgiris, I. C. (1981). Two functions of imitation during infancy. *International Journal of Behavioral Development, 4,* 1–12.

Vinter, A. (1986). The role of movement in eliciting early imitations. *Child Development, 57,* 66–71.

Walker, A. S., Owsley, C. J., Megaw-Nyce, J., Gibson, E. J., & Bahrick, L. E. (1980). Detection of elasticity as an invariant property of objects by young infants. *Perception, 9,* 713–718.

Walton, G. E., Bower, N. J. A., & Bower, T. G. R. (1992). Recognition of familiar faces by newborns. *Infant Behavior and Development, 15,* 265–269.

Watson, J. S. (1972). Smiling, cooing and the "game." *Merrill-Palmer Quarterly, 18,* 323–339.

Werner, H., & Kaplan, B. (1963). *Symbol formation: An organismic developmental approach to language and the expression of thought.* New York: Wiley.

Wiggins, D. (1967). *Identity and spatio-temporal continuity.* Oxford: Basil Blackwell.

Wiggins, D. (1980). *Sameness and substance.* Cambridge, MA: Harvard University Press.

Winer, B. J. (1971). *Statistical principles in experimental design* (2nd ed). New York: McGraw-Hill.

Young, A. W., & Ellis, H. D. (1989). *Handbook of research on face processing.* Amsterdam: North-Holland.

2

Children of Lesbian and Gay Parents

Charlotte J. Patterson

University of Virginia, Charlottesville

This paper reviews research evidence regarding the personal and social development of children with gay and lesbian parents. Beginning with estimates of the numbers of such children, sociocultural, theoretical, and legal reasons for attention to their development are then outlined. In this context, research studies on sexual identity, personal development, and social relationships among these children are then reviewed. These studies include assessment of possible differences between children with gay and lesbian parents. Research on these topics is relatively new, and many important questions have yet to be addressed. To date, however, there is no evidence that the development of children with lesbian or gay parents is compromised in any significant respect relative to that among children of heterosexual parents in otherwise comparable circumstances. Having begun to respond to heterosexist and homophobic questions posed by psychological theory, judicial opinion, and popular prejudice, child development researchers are now in a position also to explore a broader range of issues raised by the emergence of different kinds of gay and lesbian families.

What kinds of home environments best foster children's psychological adjustment and growth? No question is more central to the field of child development

Reprinted with permission from *Child Development*, 1992, Vol. 63, 1025–1042. Copyright © 1992 by The Society for Research in Child Development, Inc.

The first draft of this paper was written while the author was a scholar at the University of California at Berkeley; I wish to thank the Department of Psychology, the Institute of Human Development, and the Beatrice Bain Research Group for their hospitality during this period. I also wish to thank Cathy Cade, Deborah Cohn, Carolyn Cowan, Lin Gentemann, Larry Kurdek, Dan McPherson, Ritch Savin-Williams, and Melvin Wilson for their encouragement and for their comments on earlier versions of the paper.

research. Historically, researchers in the United States have often supposed that the most favorable home environments are provided by white, middle-class, two-parent families, in which the father is paid to work outside the home but the mother is not. Although rarely stated explicitly, it has most often been assumed that both parents in such families are heterosexual.

Given that decreasing numbers of American families fit the traditionally normative pattern (Hernandez, 1988; Laosa, 1988), it is not surprising that researchers have increasingly challenged implicit or explicit denigration of home environments that differ from it by virtue of race, ethnicity, income, household composition, and/or maternal employment (Harrison, Wilson, Pine, Chan, & Buriel, 1990; Hetherington & Arasteh, 1988; Hoffman, 1984; McLoyd, 1990, Spencer, Brookins, & Allen, 1985). Together with the authors of cross-cultural and historical studies (Cole, 1988; Elder, 1986; Rogoff, 1990), these researchers have highlighted the multiplicity of pathways through which healthy psychological development can take place and the diversity of home environments that can support such development.

In this article, I examine evidence from the social sciences regarding the personal and social development of children with gay and lesbian parents. Beginning with estimates of the numbers of such children, I then outline sociocultural, theoretical, and legal reasons that justify attention to their development. In this context, I then review research evidence on sexual identity, personal development, and social relationships among children of gay and/or lesbian parents. I first describe research on possible differences between children of gay or lesbian versus heterosexual parents; I then examine the beginnings of research on sources of diversity among children of gay and lesbian parents. In a final section, I draw a number of conclusions from the results of research to date and offer suggestions for future work.

HOW MANY CHILDREN OF LESBIAN OR GAY PARENTS ARE THERE?

How many children of gay and/or lesbian parents live in the United States today? No accurate answer to this question is available. Because of fear of discrimination in one or more domains of their lives, many gay men and lesbians take pains to conceal their sexual orientation (Blumenfeld & Raymond, 1988). It is especially difficult to locate gay and lesbian parents. Fearing that they would lose child custody and/or visitation rights if their sexual orientation were to be known, many lesbian and gay parents make special efforts to conceal their gay or lesbian identities (Lyons, 1983; Pagelow, 1980)—in some cases, even from their own children (Dunne, 1987; MacPike, 1989; Robinson & Barret, 1986).

Despite these difficulties, estimates of the numbers of gay and lesbian parents and children in the United States have been offered. Estimates of the number of lesbian mothers generally run from about 1 to 5 million (Falk, 1989; Gottman, 1990; Hoeffer, 1981; Pennington, 1987), and those for gay fathers from 1 to 3 million (Bozett, 1987; Gottman, 1990; Miller, 1979). Estimates of the numbers of children of gay or lesbian parents range from 6 million to 14 million (Bozett, 1987; Editors of the Harvard Law Review, 1990; Peterson, 1984; Schulenberg, 1985).[1]

In addition to those who became parents in the context of heterosexual marriages before coming out, growing numbers of lesbians and gay men are becoming parents after coming out. One recent estimate holds that 5,000 to 10,000 lesbians have borne children after coming out (Seligmann, 1990). The number of lesbians who are bearing children is also believed to be increasing (McCandlish, 1987; Pennington, 1987; Pies, 1985, 1990; Steckel, 1985). Additional avenues to parenthood, such as foster care, adoption, and coparenting, are also being explored increasingly both by lesbians and by gay men (Alpert, 1988; Pollack & Vaughn, 1987; Ricketts & Achtenberg, 1990; Rohrbaugh, 1988; Van Gelder, 1988). Estimates like those given above are therefore likely to underrepresent the actual numbers involved. Whatever the precise figures, it is clear that the numbers of children of gay or lesbian parents are substantial.

PERSPECTIVES ON CHILDREN OF GAY AND LESBIAN PARENTS

There are several perspectives from which interest in children of gay or lesbian parents has emerged. First, the phenomenon of openly gay or lesbian parents bearing and/or raising children represents a sociocultural innovation that is specific to the present historical era; as such, it raises questions about the impact of nontraditional family forms on child development. Second, from the standpoint of psychological theory, children of lesbian or gay parents—especially those born into gay or lesbian homes—pose a number of challenging questions for existing theories of psychosocial development. Finally, both in resolution of custody disputes and in administration of adoption and foster care policies, the legal system in the United States has frequently operated under strong but unverified assumptions about difficulties faced by children of lesbians and gay men, and there are impor-

---

[1]Such estimates can be based on extrapolations from what is known or believed about base rates in the population. According to Kinsey, Pomeroy, and Martin (1948) and others (see Blumenfeld & Raymond, 1988), approximately 10% of the 250 million people in the United States today can be considered gay or lesbian. According to large-scale survey studies (e.g., Bell & Weinberg, 1978; Saghir & Robins, 1973), about 10% of gay men and about 20% of lesbians are parents. Most have children from a heterosexual marriage that ended in divorce; many have more than one child. Calculations using these figures suggest that there are about 3–4 million gay or lesbian parents in the United States today. If, on average, each parent has two children, that would place the number of children of formerly married lesbians and gay men at about 6–8 million.

tant questions about the veridicality of such assumptions. I introduce key issues from each of these three perspectives below.

Social and Cultural Issues

The emergence of large numbers of openly self-identified gay men and lesbians is a recent historical phenomenon (Boswell, 1980; D'Emilio, 1983; Faderman, 1981, 1991). Although the beginnings of homophile organizations date to the 1950s and even earlier (D'Emilio, 1983; Faderman, 1991; Lauritsen & Thorstad, 1974), the origins of contemporary gay liberation movements are generally traced to police raids on the Stonewall bar in the Greenwich Village neighborhood of New York City in 1969, and to resistance shown by members of the gay community to these raids (Adam, 1987; D'Emilio, 1983). In the years since that time, increasing numbers of lesbians and gay men have abandoned secrecy, come out of the closet, and joined the movement for gay and lesbian rights (Blumenfeld & Raymond, 1988).

In the wake of increasing openness among lesbian and gay adults, a number of family forms are emerging in which one or more of a child's parents identify themselves as gay or lesbian (Baptiste, 1987; Bozett & Sussman, 1990; Pies, 1985). The largest numbers of these are families in which children were born in the context of a heterosexual relationship between the biological parents (Falk, 1989). These include families in which the parents divorce when the husband comes out as gay or when the wife comes out as lesbian, families in which the parents divorce when both the husband and the wife come out as gay or lesbian, and families in which one or both of the parents come out and they decide not to divorce. Parental acknowledgment of gay or lesbian identity may precede or follow decisions about divorce. The gay or lesbian parent may be either the residential or the nonresidential parent, or children may live part of the time in both homes. Gay or lesbian parents may be single, or they may have same-sex partners. A gay or lesbian parent's same-sex partner may or may not take up stepparenting relationships with the children. If the partner has also had children, the youngsters may also be cast into stepsibling relationships with one another.

In addition to children born in the context of heterosexual relationships, both single and coupled lesbians are believed increasingly to be giving birth to children (Pies, 1985, 1990; Steckel, 1985; Rohrbaugh, 1988; Van Gelder, 1988). The majority of such children are believed to be conceived through donor insemination (DI). Although techniques for successful DI have been known for many years, it is only relatively recently that DI with known or unknown sperm donors has become widely available to unmarried heterosexual women and to lesbians (Noble, 1987; Wolf, 1990). Lesbians who seek to become mothers using DI may choose a friend, relative, or acquaintance to be the sperm donor, or may choose instead to use sperm from an unknown donor. When sperm donors are known, they may take parental, avuncular, or other roles relative to children who are born using DI, or they may not (Pies, 1985; Van Gelder, 1988).

A number of gay men have also sought to become parents after coming out (Bigner & Bozett, 1990; Bozett, 1989; Ricketts & Achtenberg, 1990). Options pursued by these gay men include adoption and foster care of children to whom they are not biologically related. Through DI or through sexual intercourse, gay men may also become biological fathers of children whom they intend to coparent with a single woman (whether lesbian or heterosexual), with a lesbian couple, or with a gay male partner.

Although it is widely believed that family environments exert significant influences on children who grow up in them, authoritative scholarly treatments of such influences rarely consider children growing up in families with lesbian and/or gay parents (e.g., Jacob, 1987; Lamb, 1982; Parke, 1984). Given the multiplicity of new kinds of families among gay men and lesbians, and in view of their apparent vitality, child development researchers today are faced with remarkable opportunities to study the formation, growth, and impact of new family forms.

To the extent that parental influences are seen as critical in psychosocial development, and to the extent that lesbians and/or gay men may provide different kinds of influences than heterosexual parents, then the children of gay men and lesbians can be expected to develop in ways that are different from children of heterosexual parents. Whether any such differences are expected to be beneficial, detrimental, or nonexistent depends, of course, on the viewpoint from which the phenomena are observed. For instance, some feminist theorists have imagined benefits that might accrue to children growing up in an all-female world (e.g., Gilman, 1915/1979). Expectations based on many psychological theories are, however, more negative.

Theoretical Issues

Theories of psychological development have traditionally emphasized distinctive contributions of both mothers and fathers to the healthy personal and social development of their children. As a result, many theories predict negative outcomes for children who are raised in environments that do not provide these two kinds of inputs (Nungesser, 1980). An important theoretical question thus concerns the extent to which such predictions are sustained by results of research on children of gay and/or lesbian parents.

Psychoanalytic and social learning theories of personal and social development during childhood emphasize the importance of children having both heterosexual male and heterosexual female parents (Bronfenbrenner, 1960; Chodorow, 1978; Dinnerstein, 1976; Huston, 1983); as a result, they predict negative outcomes for children whose parents do not exemplify these qualities. Although cognitive developmental theory (e.g., Kohlberg, 1966) and gender schema theory (e.g., Bem, 1983) do not require such assumptions, proponents of these views have not challenged them. As a result, prominent perspectives on individual differences in personal and social development are commonly believed to predict difficulties in development among children of lesbian and gay parents.

Empirical research with children of gay and lesbian parents thus provides an opportunity to evaluate anew theoretical assumptions that are often taken for granted. Most prominent among these is the view that parental sexual orientation has a significant impact on children's development. By evaluating this and related assumptions, research with children of lesbian and gay parents may also stimulate conceptual innovations in the understanding of human development.

Legal and Public Policy Issues

The legal system in the United States has long been hostile to gay men and to lesbians who are or who wish to become parents (Basile, 1974; Hitchens, 1979/80; Hitchens & Kirkpatrick, 1985; Kleber, Howell, & Tibbits-Kleber, 1986; Polikoff, 1986, 1990). Because of judicial and legislative assumptions about adverse effects of parental homosexuality on children, lesbian mothers and gay fathers have often been denied custody and/or visitation with their children following divorce (Basile, 1974; Editors of the Harvard Law Review, 1990; Falk, 1989). Although some states now have laws stipulating that sexual orientation is indeterminative of parental fitness in custody disputes, in other states parents who identify themselves as gay or lesbian are presumed to be unfit as parents (Editors of the Harvard Law Review, 1990). In addition, regulations governing foster care and adoption in many states have made it difficult for lesbians and gay men to adopt children or to serve as foster parents (Ricketts & Achtenberg, 1990).

One issue underlying both judicial decision making in custody litigation and public policies governing foster care and adoption has been questions concerning the fitness of lesbians and gay men to be parents (Hitchens & Kirkpatrick, 1985). Courts have sometimes assumed that gay men and lesbians are mentally ill and hence not fit to be parents, that lesbians are less maternal than heterosexual women and hence do not make good mothers, and that lesbians' and gay men's relationships with sexual partners leave little time for ongoing parent-child interactions (Editors of the Harvard Law Review, 1990).

Although systematic empirical study of these issues is just beginning, results of research to date have failed to confirm any of these fears. The idea that homosexuality constitutes a mental illness or disorder has long been repudiated both by the American Psychological Association and by the American Psychiatric Association (Blumenfeld & Raymond, 1988). Lesbians and heterosexual women have been found not to differ markedly either in their overall mental health or in their approaches to child rearing (Kweskin & Cook, 1982; Lyons, 1983; Miller, Jacobsen, & Bigner, 1981; Mucklow & Phelan, 1979; Pagelow, 1980; Rand, Graham, & Rawlings, 1982; Thompson, McCandless, & Strickland, 1971), nor have lesbians' romantic and sexual relationships with other women been found to detract from their ability to care for their children (Pagelow, 1980). Research on gay fathers has been similarly unable to unearth any reasons to believe them unfit as parents (Barret & Robinson, 1990; Bozett, 1980, 1989). Studies in this area are still rather scarce, and more information would be helpful. On the basis of research to date, though, negative assumptions about gay and lesbian adults' fitness as parents appear to be without foundation (Cramer, 1986; Falk, 1989; Gibbs, 1988; Levy, 1989).

In addition to judicial concerns about gay and lesbian parents themselves, three major categories of fears about effects of lesbian or gay parents on children are reflected in judicial decision making about child custody and in public policies. The first is that children brought up by gay fathers or lesbian mothers will show disturbances in sexual identity (Falk, 1989; Hitchens & Kirkpatrick, 1985; Kleber et al., 1986). For instance, it is feared that children brought up by lesbian mothers or gay fathers will themselves become gay or lesbian (Falk, 1989; Green et al., 1986; Kleber et al., 1986), an outcome that the courts view as undesirable. A second category of fears is that these children will be less psychologically healthy than children growing up in homes with heterosexual parents (Falk, 1989; Editors of the Harvard Law Review, 1990; Kleber et al., 1986). Courts have expressed concern that children in the custody of gay or lesbian parents will be more vulnerable to mental breakdown, and/or that they will exhibit more adjustment difficulties and behavior problems. A third category of fears is that children of lesbian and gay parents may experience difficulties in social relationships (Editors of the Harvard Law Review, 1990; Falk, 1989; Hitchens & Kirkpatrick, 1985). For example, judges have expressed concern that children living with lesbian mothers may be stigmatized, teased, or otherwise traumatized by peers. Another common fear is that children living with gay or lesbian parents may be more likely to be sexually abused by the parent and/or by the parent's friends or acquaintances.

Because such negative assumptions have often been explicit in judicial determinations when child custody has been denied to lesbian and gay parents or when visitation with gay or lesbian parents has been curtailed (Basile, 1974; Polikoff, 1990), and because such assumptions are open to empirical test, they provide an important impetus for research. In the next section, I review the available research findings regarding these three categories of fears.

COMPARISONS BETWEEN CHILDREN OF GAY AND LESBIAN
PARENTS AND CHILDREN OF HETEROSEXUAL PARENTS

Systematic research comparing children of gay and lesbian parents with those of heterosexual parents is a phenomenon of the last 15 years. Case reports began to appear in the psychiatric literature in the early 1970s (e.g., Agbayewa, 1984; Osman, 1972; Weeks, Derdeyn, & Langman, 1975). Beginning with the pioneering work of Martin and Lyon (1972), first person and fictionalized descriptions of life in lesbian mother families have also become available (e.g., Alpert, 1988; Clausen, 1985; Jullion, 1985; Mager, 1975; Perreault, 1975; Pollack & Vaughn, 1987; Rafkin, 1990). Systematic research on the children of lesbian and gay parents did not, however, begin to appear in major professional journals until 1978, and most of the available research has been published more recently.

Despite the diversity of gay and lesbian communities, both in the United States and abroad, samples of children studied to date have been relatively homogeneous. With two exceptions (Golombok, Spencer, & Rutter, 1983; Miller, 1979), all of the research has been conducted in the United States. Samples for which demographic information was reported have been described as predominantly Caucasian, well-educated, and middle to upper middle class.

Although both lesbians and gay men may become parents in any of a variety of ways, the preponderance of research to date has focused on children who were born in the context of heterosexual marriages, whose parents divorced, and whose mothers have identified themselves as lesbians. Some research is available on children who have been born in the context of heterosexual relationships and whose fathers have identified themselves as gay (Barret & Robinson, 1990; Bozett, 1980, 1987, 1989; Miller, 1979; Paul, 1986). Two reports (McCandlish, 1987; Steckel, 1987) have focused on children born to lesbians in the context of ongoing lesbian relationships. Of the many other ways in which children might come to be brought up by lesbian or gay parents (e.g., through foster parenting, adoptive parenting, coparenting, or multiple parenting arrangements), no systematic research has yet appeared.

Reflecting issues relevant in the largest number of custody disputes, most of the research compares development of children with custodial lesbian mothers to that of children with custodial heterosexual mothers. Since many children living in lesbian mother-headed families have undergone the experience of parental separation and divorce, it has been widely believed that children living in families headed by divorced but heterosexual mothers provide the best comparison group. Although some studies focus exclusively on children of gay men or lesbians (e.g., Green, 1978; Paul, 1986), most compare children in divorced lesbian mother-headed families with children in divorced heterosexual mother-headed families.

Research has also focused mainly on age groups and topics relevant to the largest numbers of custody disputes. There is a greater volume of research on children and youth than on infants or on adult children of gay or lesbian parents. Areas of research have also grown up around concerns of the courts like those described above. In the next section, I review the existing research, much of which was designed to evaluate such judicial concerns.

Sexual Identity

Following Money (e.g., Money & Ehrhardt, 1972), I consider research on three aspects of sexual identity here. Gender identity concerns a person's self-identification as male or female. Gender-role behavior concerns the extent to which a person's activities, occupations, and the like are regarded by the culture as masculine, feminine, or both. Sexual orientation refers to a person's choice of sexual partners—for example, heterosexual, homosexual, or bisexual.

Gender identity. Gender identity among children of lesbian mothers has been assessed by several investigators using projective techniques. In this work, no evidence of special difficulties in gender identity among children of lesbian mothers has emerged. For instance, Kirkpatrick and her colleagues (Kirkpatrick, Smith, & Roy, 1981) compared development among 20 5–12-year-old children of lesbian mothers with that among 20 same-aged children of single heterosexual mothers. In the projective testing, 16 of the 20 children in each of the two groups drew a same-sex figure first, a finding that fell within expected norms. Of the eight children who drew an opposite-sex figure first, only three (one girl with a lesbian mother, and two boys with heterosexual mothers) showed concern about gender issues in clinical interviews. In studies of children ranging in age from 5 to 14, results of projective testing and related interview procedures have revealed normal development of gender identity among children of lesbian mothers (Green, 1978; Green, Mandel, Hotvedt, Gray, & Smith, 1986; Kirkpatrick et al., 1981). Similarly, Golombok et al. (1983) also studied gender identity among 37 5–17-year-old children (average age 9–10 years) of lesbian and 38 same-aged children of single heterosexual mothers. All children in this study reported that they were happy with the sex to which they belonged, and that they had no wish to be a member of the opposite sex.

Gender-role behavior. A number of studies have examined gender-role behavior among children of lesbian mothers. In the earliest such study, Green (1978) reported that 20 of 21 children of lesbian mothers in his sample named a favorite toy consistent with conventional sex-typed toy preferences, and that all 21 children reported vocational choices within typical limits for conventional sex roles. Kirkpatrick and her colleagues (1981) also found no differences between children of lesbian versus heterosexual mothers in toy preferences, activities, interests, or occupational choices relevant to sex-role conventions. Similarly, Hoeffer (1981) studied toy and activity preferences among 20 6–9-year-old children of lesbian mothers and 20 same-aged children of single heterosexual mothers, and reported no significant differences in toy choices or activity preferences. Interestingly, Hoeffer (1981) also reported that most mothers in her study said that they believed the principal influence on their children's toy and activity choices at this age was not parents or siblings, but the child's peers.

In Golombok and her colleagues' study (1983), children's sex-role behavior was assessed in interviews with children and with their mothers. Both children and mothers agreed that children's interests and activities varied substantially as a function of sex. Results for both children of lesbian and heterosexual mothers were closely in accord with those for the general population, and there were no differences between children of lesbian and heterosexual mothers.

Sex-role behavior of lesbian and heterosexual mothers' children was also assessed by Green and his colleagues (1986). In interviews with the children, no differences between 56 children of lesbian and 48 children of heterosexual mothers were found with respect to favorite television programs, favorite television characters, or favorite games or toys. There was some indication in interviews with children themselves that the offspring of lesbian mothers had less sex-typed preferences for activities at school and in their neighborhoods than did children of heterosexual mothers. Consistent with this result, lesbian mothers were also more likely than heterosexual mothers to report that their daughters often participated in rough-and-tumble play or occasionally played with "masculine" toys such as trucks or guns; however, they reported no differences in these areas for sons. Lesbian mothers were no more or less likely than heterosexual mothers to report that their children often played with "feminine" toys such as dolls. In both family types, however, children's sex-role behavior was seen as falling within normal limits.

Rees (1979) administered the Bem Sex Role Inventory to 12 children of lesbian mothers and 12 children of single heterosexual mothers. The children ranged in age from 10 to 20 years, with an average age of about 14 years. Children of lesbian and heterosexual mothers did not differ on masculinity or on androgyny, but children of lesbian mothers reported greater psychological femininity than those of heterosexual mothers. This result would seem to run counter to expectations based on stereotypes of lesbians as lacking in femininity, both in their own demeanor and in their likely influences on children. Although provocative, it should probably be interpreted with caution pending replication.

A study of 35 adult daughters of lesbian mothers was conducted by Gottman (1990), who compared their gender role preferences to those of 35 adult daughters of heterosexual mothers who had divorced and remarried and to those of 35 adult daughters of heterosexual mothers who had divorced but not remarried. The adult daughters ranged in age from 18 to 44 years, with a mean age of 24 years.

tman reported no significant differences in gender role preferences of women in the three groups.

Sexual orientation. A number of investigators have also studied a third component of sexual identity, sexual orientation. In an early study, Green (1978) assessed the erotic fantasies of pubertal and postpubertal offspring of lesbian mothers. In his sample, there were four children who were 11 years old or older, and all four reported fantasies that were exclusively heterosexual in their content. The adolescents in Rees's (1979) study were also asked about sexual orientation, and all described themselves as having a "heterosexual orientation with no inclination toward homosexuality" (Rees, 1979, p. 87).

Golombok and her colleagues (1983) also assessed the heterosexual versus homosexual interests of older children in their sample. Although precise ages of the older children were not reported, there were nine children of lesbian mothers and 11 children of heterosexual mothers for whom this assessment was done. Many children reported definite heterosexual interests, and there were no significant differences between children of lesbian and heterosexual mothers.

Huggins (1989) interviewed 36 youngsters, who were 13 to 19 years of age; 18 were offspring of lesbian mothers and 18 had mothers who were heterosexual in their orientation. No child of a lesbian mother identified as lesbian or gay, but one child of a heterosexual mother did; this difference was not statistically significant.

Miller (1979) studied a group of gay fathers, who had a total of 48 adult offspring. The ages of the adult sons and daughters ranged from 24 to 64 years; there were 27 adult daughters and 21 adult sons. According to fathers' reports, one son was gay and three daughters were lesbian. Thus, about 8% of the offspring of this group of gay fathers were themselves gay or lesbian in orientation, a figure which is within expected percentages in the population at large.

A study involving interviews with the young adult sons and daughters of lesbian, gay, or bisexual parents was reported by Paul (1986). In the interview, respondents (aged 18–28 years) were asked to report on their own sexual orientation. Of the 34 respondents, two identified themselves as bisexual, three identified themselves as lesbians, and two as gay men. Thus, about 15% of the sample identified themselves as gay or lesbian. Again, this figure was within the normal range of variability in the population.

In her study of adult daughters of lesbian and heterosexual mothers, Gottman (1990) reported figures similar to those of Paul (1986). About 16% of daughters in Gottman's study self-identified as lesbian. The percentages of lesbian daughters did not vary as a function of mothers' sexual orientation.

In two studies, Bozett (1980, 1982, 1987, 1989) investigated sexual preference among the sons and daughters of gay fathers. In one study (Bozett, 1980, 1982), 18 gay fathers were asked about the sexual orientation of their 25 children. Although some children had not yet reached puberty, no father reported having a gay son or lesbian daughter. In another study of 19 children of gay fathers, Bozett (1987, 1989) reported that two sons described themselves as gay and one daughter described herself as bisexual; the other 17 offspring described themselves as heterosexual. Thus, in neither study did the proportion of lesbian or gay offspring exceed that believed to characterize the population at large.

Overall, then, development of gender identity, of gender role behavior, and of sexual preference among offspring of gay and lesbian parents was found in every study to fall within normal bounds. Although studies have assessed over 300 offspring of gay or lesbian parents in 12 different samples, no evidence has been found for significant disturbances of any kind in the development of sexual identity among these individuals.

There is always a possibility that critical methodological problems will be identified and that future work will uncover hitherto unrecognized problems. For instance, many lesbian women do not self-identify as lesbians until adulthood (see, e.g., Golombok at al., 1983); for this reason, studies of sexual orientation among adolescents may count as heterosexual some individuals who will come out as lesbian later in life. Future research on sexual identity among offspring of lesbian and gay parents should certainly take account of methodological advances in the assessment of sexual identity (Bem, 1983; Yekel, Bigler, & Liben, 1991).

Other Aspects of Personal Development

Studies of other aspects of personal development among children of gay and lesbian parents have assessed a broad array of characteristics. Among these have been separation-individuation, psychiatric evaluations, assessments of behavior problems, personality, self-concept, locus of control, moral judgment, and intelligence. To explore the possibility that children of lesbian or gay parents experience difficulties in personal development, I review existing research on each topic in turn.

In the only systematic study of children born to lesbians, Steckel (1985, 1987) compared the progress of separation-individuation among 11 preschool children born via DI to lesbian couples with that among 11 same-aged children of heterosexual couples. Using parent interviews, parent and teacher Q sorts, and structured doll play techniques, Steckel compared independence, ego functions, and object relations among children in the two types of families. The main results documented impressive similarity in development among children in the two groups. Similar findings, based on clinical experience with seven children born to lesbian mothers, were also reported by McCandlish (1987).

Steckel (1985, 1987) did, however, report some suggestive differences between groups. Children of heterosexual parents saw themselves as somewhat more aggressive than did children of lesbians, and they were seen by both parents and teachers as more bossy, domineering, and negativistic. Children of lesbian parents, on the other hand, saw themselves as more lovable and were seen by parents and teachers as more affectionate, more responsive, and more protective toward younger children. In view of the small sample size, and the large number of statistical tests performed, these results must be considered suggestive rather than definitive. Steckel's study (1985, 1987) is, however, worthy of special attention in that it is the first to make systematic comparisons of development among children born to lesbian and to heterosexual couples.

As in the literature on sexual identity, most studies compare development among children of divorced lesbian mothers with that among the offspring of divorced heterosexual mothers. For instance, severity of psychiatric disturbance was examined by Kirkpatrick and her colleagues (1981), and by Golombok and her colleagues (1983). In these studies, ratings for children of lesbian mothers were compared to those for children of heterosexual mothers; in both studies, raters were blind to mothers' sexual orientation. In neither study was there any significant difference in rated psychiatric disturbance between children of heterosexual and lesbian mothers.

Golombok et al. (1983) also collected ratings of children on a wide array of behavioral and emotional problems. The scales included problems such as hyperactivity, unsociability, emotional difficulty, and conduct problems. None of the comparisons between children of lesbian and heterosexual mothers was statistically significant.

Gottman (1990) examined personality characteristics among adult daughters of lesbian and heterosexual mothers, using the California Psychological Inventory. Comparisons for 17 of 18 scales employed were nonsignificant. On one scale, called Well-Being, daughters of lesbians scored more favorably than did daughters of heterosexual mothers. Given the number of comparisons that were made, however, the possibility of a chance result in this case must be considered, and caution should be exercised in its interpretation.

Two different investigators have studied self-concepts of children of lesbian mothers. Puryear (1983) studied self-concepts among 15 elementary school aged children of lesbians and 15 children of heterosexual women. More recently, Huggins (1989) studied self-concept among adolescent offspring of lesbian versus heterosexual mothers. Self-concepts were within the normal range in both studies, and neither study reported any significant differences between the two groups in any aspect of self-concept.

Locus of control has also been a focus of research (Puryear, 1983; Rees, 1979). As assessed in these studies, the concept of internal versus external locus of control concerns the extent to which a person believes important events to be under his or her own control or subject to chance or to the control of others. Again, results were within the normal range for both samples. Neither among the elementary school children that Puryear (1983) tested nor among the teenagers that Rees (1979) studied was there any evidence for differences in locus of control between children of lesbian and heterosexual mothers.

The development of moral judgment among teenaged offspring of lesbian and heterosexual mothers was studied by Rees (1979). Using techniques developed by Kohlberg (1964, 1966), Rees assessed maturity of moral judgment using the adolescents' responses to hypothetical moral dilemmas. There were no differences in moral maturity between the children of lesbian versus heterosexual mothers.

Green and his colleagues (1986) assessed intelligence among children of heterosexual and lesbian mothers. Using standardized individual tests of intelligence, Green et al. reported that all of the children they tested had scores within a normal range. There were no differences in intelligence between children of lesbian and heterosexual mothers.

In summary, concerns about difficulties in personal development among children of gay and lesbian parents are not sustained by results of existing research. As was true for sexual identity, studies of other aspects of personal development—such as self-concept, locus of control, moral judgment, and intelligence—revealed no significant differences between children of lesbian or gay parents and children of heterosexual parents. It is always possible that future studies will identify hitherto overlooked difficulties. On the basis of existing evidence, though, fears that children of gay and lesbian parents suffer deficits in personal development appear to be without empirical foundation.

Social Relationships

Studies assessing potential differences between children of gay and lesbian versus heterosexual parents have sometimes included assessments of children's social relationships. Because of fears that children of gay fathers and/or lesbian mothers might encounter difficulties among their peers, the most common focus of attention has been on peer relations, but some information on children's relationships with adults is also available. To evaluate fears about disrupted social relationships among children of lesbian and gay parents, I describe relevant findings in this area. In light of concerns that children of gay and lesbian parents may be at greater risk for sexual abuse, I also outline research findings that address this issue.

The earliest study to assess peer relations among children of lesbian mothers was that of Green (1978). In an interview, children were asked to name their friends. As would be expected for this group of elementary school aged children, 19 of 21 children named a predominantly same-sex group of peer friends. Although this study did not include a comparison group of children with heterosexual mothers, the result was considered to be normal for this age group.

Golombok et al. (1983) also reported that most children in their study named a predominantly same-sex peer group. In addition, the overall quality of children's peer relations was rated by the investigators as good in most cases. This study included a comparison group of children with heterosexual mothers; there were, however, no significant differences between children of lesbian and heterosexual mothers in any of the outcomes.

Green and his colleagues (1986) asked children to rate their own popularity among same-sex and among opposite-sex peers, and they also asked mothers to rate their children's social skills and popularity among peers. Results showed that most mothers rated their children's social skills in a positive manner, and there were no differences between reports about their children given by lesbian and heterosexual mothers. In addition, self-reports of children of lesbian mothers did not differ from those of the offspring of heterosexual mothers.

Kirkpatrick and her colleagues (1981) were the first to investigate children's contacts with adult men in lesbian mother versus heterosexual mother homes. They reported that lesbian mothers in their sample were more concerned than heterosexual mothers that their children have opportunities for good relationships with adult men. Referring to further findings from this study, Kirkpatrick (1987) also indicated that lesbian mothers had more adult male family friends and included male relatives more often in their children's activities than did heterosexual mothers. She also described these findings as especially true of lesbian mothers who were living in committed relationships with partners (Kirkpatrick, 1987).

Golombok and her co-workers (1983) administered assessments of children's social relationships with their fathers. They found that children of lesbian mothers were more likely than children of heterosexual mothers to have contact with their fathers at least once a week. Specifically, 12 of 37 children of lesbian mothers, but only two of 38 children of heterosexual mothers, were reported as having contact with their fathers at least once a week. Children of lesbian mothers were also less likely to have had no contact with their fathers during the preceding year (15 of 37) than children of heterosexual mothers (22 of 38). In short, Golombok and her colleagues (1983) reported that most children of lesbian mothers in their sample had at least some contact with their fathers, whereas most children of heterosexual mothers did not.

Harris and Turner (1985/86) studied 10 gay fathers, 13 lesbian mothers, two heterosexual single fathers, and 14 heterosexual single mothers, most of whom had custody of their children. In all, the respondents had 39 children, who ranged in age from 5 to 31 years. Parents described their relationships with their children in generally positive terms, and there were no differences between gay, lesbian, and heterosexual parents in this regard. The majority of gay and lesbian parents reported that they did not feel that their homosexuality had created social problems for their children. Many parents also cited advantages of their homosexuality for their children, such as facilitating acceptance of their own sexuality, augmenting tolerance and empathy for others, and increasing exposure to new viewpoints. One significant difference between homosexual and heterosexual parents was that heterosexual parents were more likely to say that their children's visits with the other parent presented problems for them.

In the Golombok et al. (1983) study, children's contacts with adult friends of their lesbian mothers were also assessed. All of the children were reported to have contact with adult friends of their mothers. One-third of the mothers reported that their friends were predominantly women, and two-thirds of the mothers reported that their friends included substantial proportions of both men and women. Two-thirds of the lesbian mothers also reported that their adult friends were a mixture of homosexual and heterosexual adults.

Concerns that children of gay or lesbian parents are more likely than children of heterosexual parents to be sexually abused have been addressed in the research literature on abuse. Results of work in this area show that the great majority of adults who perpetrate sexual abuse are male; sexual abuse of children by adult women is extremely rare (Finkelhor & Russell, 1984; Jones & MacFarlane, 1980; Sarafino, 1979). Lesbian mothers are thus at very low risk for sexual abuse of their children. Moreover, the overwhelming majority of child sexual abuse cases can be characterized as heterosexual in nature, with an adult male abusing a young female (Jones & MacFarlane, 1980). Available evidence reveals that gay men are no more likely than heterosexual men to perpetrate child sexual abuse (Groth & Birnbaum, 1978; Sarafino, 1979). Fears that children in custody of gay or lesbian parents might be at heightened risk for sexual abuse are thus without empirical foundation.

Overall, then, results of research to date suggest that children of lesbian and gay parents have normal relationships with peers and that their relationships with adults of both sexes are also satisfactory. In fact, the findings suggest that children in custody of divorced lesbian mothers have more frequent contact with their fathers than do children in custody of divorced heterosexual mothers. There is no evidence to suggest that children of lesbian or gay parents are at greater risk of sexual abuse than other children. The picture of lesbian mothers' children that emerges from results of existing research is thus one of general engagement in social life with peers, with fathers, and with mothers' adult friends—both female and male, both homosexual and heterosexual.

RESEARCH ON DIVERSITY AMONG CHILDREN OF GAY AND LESBIAN PARENTS

Despite the diversity evident within gay and lesbian communities (Blumenfeld & Raymond, 1988), research on variations among lesbian and gay families with children is as yet quite sparse. In addition to documenting differences that exist among these families, such research can also describe conditions, interactions, and relationships that are associated with favorable or unfavorable outcomes for children of lesbian and gay parents. In this section, I first describe research findings on the impact of parental psychological and relationship status, and then examine research on the influence of other stresses and supports.

One dimension of difference among gay and lesbian families concerns whether or not the custodial parent is involved in a couple relationship, and if so, what implications this may have for children. Golombok et al. (1983), Kirkpatrick et al. (1981), and Pagelow (1980) all reported that, in their samples, divorced lesbian mothers were more likely than divorced heterosexual mothers to be living with a romantic partner; however, none of these investigators examined connections between this variable and children's adjustment or development in lesbian mother families.

Huggins (1989) reported that self-esteem among daughters of lesbian mothers whose lesbian partners lived with them was higher than that among daughters of lesbian mothers who did not live with a partner. Because of the small sample size and absence of statistical tests, this finding should be seen as a preliminary one. If replicated in future research, however, the finding suggests the possibility that judicial inclinations to award custody to lesbian mothers only with the stipulation that they not live with lesbian partners may be detrimental to the best interests of children in these families. On the basis of impressions from her own work, Kirkpatrick has also stated her view that "contrary to the fears expressed in court, children in households that included the mother's lesbian lover had a richer, more open and stable family life" than did those in single-parent lesbian mother households (Kirkpatrick, 1987, p. 204).

Another aspect of diversity among lesbian families relates to the psychological status and well-being of the mother. Research on parent-child relations in heterosexual families has consistently revealed that children's adjustment is often related to indexes of maternal mental health (Rutter, Izard, & Read, 1986; Sameroff & Chandler, 1975). Therefore, one might expect factors that enhance mental health among lesbian mothers also to benefit the children of these women.

It is worth noting in this regard that Rand, Graham, and Rawlings (1982) found that lesbian mothers' sense of psychological well-being was correlated with the extent to which they were open about their lesbian identity with employers, ex-husbands, and children. Mothers who felt more able to disclose their lesbian identity were more likely to express a positive sense of well-being. Unfortunately, no information about the relations of these findings to adjustment or development among children of these women has been reported to date.

Another area of diversity among families with a gay or lesbian parent involves the degree to which a parent's gay or lesbian identity is accepted by other significant people in children's lives. Huggins (1989) found a tendency for children whose fathers were rejecting of maternal lesbianism to report lower self-esteem than those whose fathers were neutral or positive. Due to small sample size and absence of significance tests, this finding should be regarded as suggestive rather than definitive. Huggins's (1989) finding does, however, raise questions about the extent to which reactions of important adults in a child's environment can influence responses to discovery of a parent's gay or lesbian identity.

Effects of the age at which children learn of parental homosexuality have also been a topic of study. Paul (1986) found that offspring who were told of parental gay, lesbian, or bisexual identity either in childhood or in late adolescence found the news easier to cope with than those who first learned of it during early to middle adolescence. Huggins (1989) also reported that those who learned of maternal lesbianism in childhood had higher self-esteem than did those who were not informed of it until they were adolescents. From a clinical perspective, it is widely agreed that early adolescence is a particularly difficult time for children to learn that a father is gay or that a mother is lesbian (Bozett, 1980; Pennington, 1987; Schulenberg, 1985).

Some investigators have also raised questions about the potential role of peer support in helping children to deal with issues raised by having a gay or lesbian parent. Lewis (1980) was the first to suggest that children's silence on the topic of parental sexual orientation with peers and siblings might add to their feelings of isolation from other children. Paul (1986) found that 29% of his young adult respondents had never known anyone else with a gay, lesbian, or bisexual parent, suggesting that the possibility of isolation is very real for some young people. Potentially negative effects of isolation have not, however, been documented to date. Lewis (1980) suggested that children would benefit from support groups consisting of other children of gay or lesbian parents, but systematic evaluations of such groups have not been reported.

In summary, research on diversity among families with gay and lesbian parents and on the potential effects of such diversity on children is only beginning (Freiberg, 1990; Martin, 1989). Existing data suggest that children may fare better when mothers are in good psychological health and living with a lesbian partner. There are indications that children find it easier to deal with issues raised by having lesbian or gay parents if they learn of parental sexual orientation during childhood rather than during adolescence. Existing data also suggest the value of a supportive milieu, in which parental sexual orientation is accepted by other significant adults, and in which children have contact with peers in similar circumstances. The existing data are, however, still very sparse. It is clear that much remains to be learned about differences among gay and lesbian families and about the impact of such differences on children growing up in these homes.

CONCLUSIONS

There is no evidence to suggest that psychosocial development among children of gay men or lesbians is compromised in any respect relative to that among off-spring of heterosexual parents. Despite long-standing legal presumptions against gay and lesbian parents in many states, despite dire predictions about their children based on well-known theories of psychosocial development, and despite the accumulation of a substantial body of research investigating these issues, not a single study has found children of gay or lesbian parents to be disadvantaged in any significant respect relative to children of heterosexual parents. Indeed, the evidence to date suggests that home environments provided by gay and lesbian parents are as likely as those provided by heterosexual parents to support and enable children's psychosocial growth.

Without denying the convergence of results to date, it is important also to acknowledge that research comparing children of gay or lesbian parents with those of heterosexual parents has presented a variety of methodological challenges, not all of which have been surmounted in every case. For instance, questions can be raised with regard to individual studies about sampling issues, assessment techniques, statistical power, and other technical matters; no individual study would be entirely invincible to such criticism. A particularly notable weakness of existing research has been the tendency in most studies to compare development among children of a group of divorced lesbian mothers, many of whom are living with lesbian partners, to that among children of a group of divorced heterosexual mothers who are not currently living with heterosexual partners. It will be important for future research to separate the potential significance of maternal sexual orientation from that of mothers' partner status.

Despite shortcomings, however, results of existing research comparing children of gay or lesbian parents with those of heterosexual parents are extraordinarily clear, and they merit attention from a number of perspectives. In addition to its role in the empowerment of lesbian and gay parents, evidence from this research also has important implications for well-known, psychological theories of psychosocial development. If, as McCandlish (1987) and Steckel (1987) have reported, the development of children born into lesbian mother homes is normal, then traditional emphases on the importance of heterosexual male and female parents for children's psychosocial development may need to be reconsidered.

A number of different approaches might be examined. It might be argued that certain kinds of family interactions, processes, and relationships are beneficial for children's development, but that parents need not be heterosexual to provide them. In other words, variables related to family processes (e.g., qualities of relationships) may be more important predictors of child adjustment than are variables related to family structure (e.g., sexual orientation, number of parents in the home).

A useful analogy in this regard is provided by research on the impact of parental divorce on children. While early studies of children's reactions to divorce focused on variables related to household composition and family structure (e.g., divorced vs. nondivorced families), more recent research has highlighted the important contributions of variables related to family processes and interactions (e.g., conflict, warmth). For instance, a number of investigators (e.g., Emery, 1982; O'Leary & Emery, 1984) have argued that child behavior problems associated with parental divorce are best understood as the result of interparental conflict rather than changes in household composition or structure as such. Research on divorcing families has thus suggested the preeminence of process over structure in mediating outcomes for children.

Applied to the present concerns, this perspective implies the hypothesis that structural variables such as parental sexual orientation may be less important in mediating child outcomes in lesbian and gay families than qualities of family interactions, relationships, and processes. Many theoretical perspectives are compatible with an emphasis on function. For instance, attachment theory (Ainsworth, 1985a, 1985b; Bowlby, 1988) emphasizes the functional significance of sensitive parenting in creating secure relationships, but does not stipulate the necessity of any particular family constellation or structure. Similarly, self psychology (Kohut, 1971, 1974, 1984) describes the significance of mirroring and idealizing processes in human development, but does not insist on their occurrence in the context of any specific family structure. Theoretical perspectives such as attachment theory and self psychology would seem to be compatible with an emphasis on functional rather than structural aspects of family life, and hence to provide promising interpretive frameworks within which to conceptualize further research in these directions.

To evaluate the impact of both process and structural variables on child outcomes in lesbian, gay, and heterosexual families, research would need to assess variables of both types. Research with other kinds of nontraditional families (Eiduson & Weisner, 1978; Weisner & Wilson-Mitchell, 1990) has demonstrated the potential utility of this approach. Most research on lesbian and gay families, however, has focused on structural rather than process variables (e.g., on comparisons between children of lesbian and heterosexual mothers rather than on the qualities of interactions and relationships within these families). An adequate evaluation of the significance of process versus structure in lesbian and gay families therefore awaits the results of future research.

An alternative theoretical response might be to broaden the focus of attention to include influences other than those from parents on children's development. Important forms of learning (e.g., about behavior considered appropriate for members of each sex) may be less dependent on parental input than traditionally believed (Maccoby, 1990). Other social influences, such as those of peers, should also be considered. It will also be important to identify and acknowledge contributions of genetic influences (Dunn & Plomin, 1990). By investigating the impact of new family forms on the development of children who are growing up in them, it seems likely that research on children of lesbian and gay parents will test existing theoretical positions, and in so doing, open up opportunities for conceptual innovation.

Results of research reviewed here also have significant implications for public policies governing child custody, foster care, and adoption in the United States (Falk, 1989; Green, 1982; Polikoff, 1986, 1990). Existing research evidence provides no justification for denial of parental rights and responsibilities to lesbians and gay men on the basis of their sexual orientation (Editors of the Harvard Law Review, 1990; Green, 1982; Ricketts & Achtenberg, 1990). Indeed, protection of the best interests of children in lesbian and gay families increasingly demands that courts and legislative bodies acknowledge realities of life in nontraditional families (Falk, 1989; Green, 1982; Polikoff, 1990).

Consider, for example, a family created by a lesbian couple who undertake the conception, birth, and upbringing of their child together. Should this couple separate, it is reasonable to expect that the best interests of the child will be served by preserving the continuity and stability of the child's relationships with both parents. In law, however, it is only the biological mother who is recognized as having parental rights and responsibilities. When courts and legislatures fail to acknowledge facts of children's lives in nontraditional families, they experience great difficulty in serving the best interests of children in these families (Polikoff, 1990).

A number of approaches to rectifying this situation have been proposed. For instance, a small number of families have obtained second-parent adoptions (Ricketts & Achtenberg, 1990), in which a nonbiological parent legally adopts a child without the biological parent giving up his or her legal rights and responsibilities; this avenue is not, however, widely available. Others (e.g., Polikoff, 1990) have advocated legislative reform, including changes in the standards for legal designation as a parent. As the numbers of lesbian and gay families with children increase, pressures for legal and judicial reform seem likely to mount.

Existing research has focused primarily on comparisons between children of gay or lesbian parents and those of heterosexual parents. This approach reflects a concern with addressing what can be considered heterosexist and/or homophobic questions. Heterosexism reflects the belief that everyone is or ought to be heterosexual. Homophobic questions are those which are based on prejudice against lesbians and gay men, and which are designed to raise the expectation that various negative outcomes will befall children of gay or lesbian parents as compared to children of heterosexual parents. Examples of such questions that were considered above include: Won't the children of lesbians and gay men have difficulty with sexual identity? Won't they be more vulnerable to psychiatric problems? Won't they be sexually abused? Now that research has addressed such heterosexist and/or homophobic questions, it would appear that the time has come for child development researchers to address a broader range of issues in this area.

Many important research questions can stem from an interest in the children of gay and lesbian parents. Such questions may raise the possibility of various desirable outcomes for these children. For instance, won't these children grow up with increased tolerance for viewpoints other than their own? Won't they be more at home in the multicultural environments that Americans increasingly inhabit? Children of lesbian mothers have described an increased tolerance for divergent viewpoints as a benefit of growing up in lesbian mother families (Rafkin, 1990), but systematic research in this area is still needed.

Alternatively, other approaches may involve study of the great diversity among gay and lesbian families. For example, researchers may ask how the experience of growing up with multiple gay and lesbian parents differs from that of growing up with a single parent or with two parents who are a gay or lesbian couple. Future research should explore ways in which family processes are related to child outcomes in different kinds of lesbian and gay families.

A few studies that provide information relevant to issues of diversity among children of gay and lesbian parents have already been reported. Results of work with families headed by divorced lesbian mothers suggest that children are better off when their mothers have high self-esteem and are currently living with a lesbian partner (Huggins, 1989; Kirkpatrick, 1987). Children in such families also appear to show more favorable adjustment when their fathers and/or other important adults accept their mothers' lesbian identities, and perhaps also when they have contact with other children of lesbians and gay men (Huggins, 1989; Lewis, 1980). In addition, there are indications that those who learn as children that they have a gay or lesbian parent experience less difficulty in adapting to this reality than do those who are not told until adolescence (Paul, 1986). These findings are best regarded as preliminary glimpses of a territory in need of future exploration.

Much remains to be done to understand differences between and among gay and lesbian families, and to comprehend the impact of such differences on children and youth (Martin, 1989; Pollack, in press; Riley, 1988). Information is needed about the economic, religious, racial, ethnic, and cultural diversity in gay and lesbian families, and about the ways in which parents and children in such families manage the multiple identities available to them. Almost no research has studied families in which gay men and lesbians have had or have adopted children after coming out. We need to know more about different kinds of parenting experiences—such as noncustodial parenting, nonbiological parenting, coparenting, multiple parenting, adoption, and foster care—and about their likely influences on the children involved. We also need to know more about the nature of stresses and supports encountered by children of lesbian and gay parents —in the parents' families of origin (e.g., with grandparents and other relatives), among parents' and children's friends, and in their larger communities. Research is needed to explore the pains and pleasures of growing up in gay and lesbian families, and also to identify the costs and benefits of court-ordered separations between children and their gay and lesbian parents. We need to know more about the ways in which effects of heterosexism and homophobia are felt by parents and children in lesbian and gay families, and about the ways in which they cope with ignorance and prejudice that they encounter.

To address these issues more effectively, future research should maintain an ecological perspective and should, where possible, employ longitudinal designs. Longitudinal studies of development, especially during middle and later childhood and adolescence, are badly needed. Such studies should seek to assess not only child adjustment over time, but also the family processes, relationships, and interactions to which child adjustment may be linked. Family processes, in turn, should be viewed in context of the surrounding ecological conditions of family life.

In conclusion, it would seem that research on children of gay and lesbian parents has reached a significant turning point. Having addressed heterosexist and homophobic concerns represented in psychological theory, judicial opinion, and popular prejudice, child development researchers are now in a position also to explore a broader range of issues raised by the emergence of different kinds of lesbian and gay families. Results of future research on such issues have the potential to increase our knowledge about nontraditional family forms and about their impact on children, stimulate innovations in theoretical understanding of human development, and inform legal rulings and public policies relevant to children of gay and lesbian parents.

REFERENCES

Adam, B. D. (1987). *The rise of a gay and lesbian movement.* Boston: Twayne.

Agbayewa, M. O. (1984). Fathers in the newer family forms: Male or female? *Canadian Journal of Psychiatry, 29,* 402–406.

Ainsworth, M. D. S. (1985a). Patterns of infant-mother attachments: Antecedents and effects on development. *Bulletin of the New York Academy of Medicine, 61,* 771–791.

Ainsworth, M. D. S. (1985b). Attachments across the life span. *Bulletin of the New York Academy of Medicine, 61,* 792–812.

Alpert, H. (1988). *We are everywhere: Writings by and about lesbian parents.* Freedom, CA: Crossing Press.

Baptiste, D. A. (1987). Psychotherapy with gay/lesbian couples and their children in "step-families": A challenge for marriage and family therapists. In E. Coleman (Ed.), *Integrated identity for gay men and lesbians: Psychotherapeutic approaches for emotional well-being* (pp. 223–238). New York: Harrington Park.

Barret, R. L., & Robinson, B. E. (1990). *Gay fathers.* Lexington, MA: Lexington Books.

Basile, R. A. (1974). Lesbian mothers: I. *Women's Rights Law Reporter, 2,* 3–25.

Bell, A. P., & Weinberg, M. S. (1978). *Homosexualities: A study of diversity among men and women.* New York: Simon & Schuster.

Bem, S. L. (1983). Gender schema theory and its implications for child development: Raising gender-aschematic children in a gender-schematic society. *Signs: Journal of Women in Culture and Society, 8,* 598–616.

Bigner, J. J., & Bozett, F. W. (1990). Parenting by gay fathers. In F. W. Bozett & M. B. Sussman (Eds.), *Homosexuality and family relations* (pp. 155–176). New York: Harrington Park.

Blumenfeld, W. J., & Raymond, D. (1988). *Looking at gay and lesbian life.* Boston: Beacon.

Boswell, J. (1980). *Christianity, social tolerance, and homosexuality: Gay people in Western Europe from the beginning of the Christian era to the fourteenth century.* Chicago: University of Chicago Press.

Bowlby, J. (1988). *A secure base: Parent-child attachment and healthy human development.* New York: Basic.

Bozett, F. W. (1980). Gay fathers: How and why they disclose their homosexuality to their children. *Family Relations, 29,* 173–179.

Bozett, F. W. (1982). Heterogeneous couples in heterosexual marriages: Gay men and straight women. *Journal of Marital and Family Therapy, 8,* 81–89.

Bozett, F. W. (1987). Children of gay fathers. In F. W. Bozett (Ed.), *Gay and lesbian parents* (pp. 39–57). New York: Praeger.

Bozett, F. W. (1989). Gay fathers: A review of the literature. In F. W. Bozett (Ed.), *Homosexuality and the family* (pp. 137–162). New York: Harrington Park.

Bozett, F. W., & Sussman, M. B. (Eds.). (1990). *Homosexuality and family relations.* New York: Harrington Park.

Bronfenbrenner, U. (1960). Freudian theories of identification and their derivatives. *Child Development, 31,* 15–40.

Chodorow, N. (1978). *The reproduction of mothering: Psychoanalysis and the sociology of gender.* Berkeley: University of California Press.

Clausen, J. (1985). *Sinking stealing.* Trumansburg, NY: Crossing Press.

Cole, M. (1988). Cross-cultural research in the sociohistorical tradition. *Human Development, 31,* 137–157.

Cramer, D. (1986). Gay parents and their children: A review of research and practical implications. *Journal of Counseling and Development, 64,* 504–507.

D'Emilio, J. (1983). *Sexual politics, sexual communities: The makings of a homosexual minority in the United States, 1940–1970.* Chicago: University of Chicago Press.

Dinnerstein, D. (1976). *The mermaid and the minotaur: Sexual arrangements and human malaise.* New York: Harper & Row.

Dunn, J., & Plomin, R. (1990). *Separate lives: Why siblings are so different.* New York: Basic.

Dunne, E. J. (1987). Helping gay fathers come out to their children. *Journal of Homosexuality, 13,* 213–222.

Editors of the Harvard Law Review. (1990). *Sexual orientation and the law.* Cambridge, MA: Harvard University Press.

Eiduson, B. T., & Weisner, T. S. (1978). Alternative family styles: Effects on young children. In J. H. Stevens & M. Mathews (Eds.), *Mother/child father/child relationships* (pp. 197–221). Washington, DC: National Association for the Education of Young Children.

Elder, G. H., Jr. (1986). Military timing and turning points in men's lives. *Developmental Psychology, 22,* 233–245.

Emery, R. E. (1982). Interparental conflict and the children of discord and divorce. *Psychological Bulletin, 92,* 310–330.

Faderman, L. (1981). *Surpassing the love of men.* New York: William Morrow.

Faderman, L. (1991). *Odd girls and twilight lovers: A history of lesbian life in twentieth-century America.* New York: Columbia University Press.

Falk, P. J. (1989). Lesbian mothers: Psychosocial assumptions in family law. *American Psychologist, 44,* 941–947.

Finkelhor, D., & Russell, D. (1984). Women as perpetrators: Review of the evidence. In D. Finkelhor (Ed.), *Child sexual abuse: New theory and research* (pp. 171–187). New York: Free Press.

Freiberg, P. (1990). Lesbian moms can give kids empowering models. *APA Monitor, 21,* 33.

Gibbs, E. D. (1988). Psychosocial development of children raised by lesbian mothers: A review of research. *Women and Therapy, 8,* 55–75.

Gilman, C. P. (1979). *Herland.* New York: Pantheon. (Originally published 1915.)

Golombok, S., Spencer, A., & Rutter, M. (1983). Children in lesbian and single-parent households: Psychosexual and psychiatric appraisal. *Journal of Child Psychology and Psychiatry, 24,* 551–572.

Gottman, J. S. (1990). Children of gay and lesbian parents. In F. W. Bozett & M. B. Sussman (Eds.), *Homosexuality and family relations* (pp. 177–196). New York: Harrington Park.

Green, R. (1978). Sexual identity of 37 children raised by homosexual or transsexual parents. *American Journal of Psychiatry, 135,* 692–697.

Green, R. (1982). The best interests of the child with a lesbian mother. *Bulletin of the American Association for Psychiatry and Law, 10,* 7–15.

Green, R., Mandel, J. B., Hotvedt, M. E., Gray, J., & Smith, L. (1986). Lesbian mothers and their children: A comparison with solo parent heterosexual mothers and their children. *Archives of Sexual Behavior, 15,* 167–184.

Groth, A. N., & Birnbaum, H. J. (1978). Adult sexual orientation and attraction to under-age persons. *Archives of Sexual Behavior, 7,* 175–181.

Harris, M. B., & Turner, P. H. (1985/86). Gay and lesbian parents. *Journal of Homosexuality, 12,* 101–113.

Harrison, A. O., Wilson, M. N., Pine, C. J., Chan, S. Q., & Buriel, R. (1990). Family ecologies of ethnic minority children. *Child Development, 61,* 347–362.

Hernandez, D. J. (1988). Demographic trends and the living arrangements of children. In E. M. Hetherington & J. D. Arasteh (Eds.), *Impact of divorce, single parenting, and stepparenting on children* (pp. 3–22). Hillsdale, NJ: Erlbaum.

Hetherington, E. M., & Arasteh, J. D. (Eds.). (1988). *Impact of divorce, single parenting, and stepparenting on children.* Hillsdale, NJ: Erlbaum.

Hitchens, D. J. (1979/80). Social attitudes, legal standards, and personal trauma in child custody cases. *Journal of Homosexuality, 5,* 1–20, 89–95.

Hitchens, D. J., & Kirkpatrick, M. J. (1985). Lesbian mothers/gay fathers. In D. H. Schetky & E. P. Benedek (Eds.), *Emerging issues in child psychiatry and the law* (pp. 115–125). New York: Brunner/Mazel.

Hoeffer, B. (1981). Children's acquisition of sex-role behavior in lesbian-mother families. *American Journal of Orthopsychiatry, 5,* 536–544.

Hoffman, L. W. (1984). Work, family, and socialization of the child. In R. D. Parke (Ed.), *Review of child development research: Vol. 7. The family* (pp. 223–282). Chicago: University of Chicago Press.

Huggins, S. L. (1989). A comparative study of self-esteem of adolescent children of divorced lesbian mothers and divorced heterosexual mothers. In F. W. Bozett (Ed.), *Homosexuality and the family* (pp. 123–135). New York: Harrington Park.

Huston, A. (1983). Sex typing. In E. M. Hetherington (Ed.), P. H. Mussen (Series Ed.), *Handbook of child psychology: Vol. 4. Socialization, personality, and social development* (pp. 387–487). New York: Wiley.

Jacob, T. (Ed.). (1987). *Family interaction and psychopathology: Theories, methods, and findings.* New York: Plenum.

Jones, B. M., & MacFarlane, K. (Eds.). (1980). *Sexual abuse of children: Selected readings.* Washington, DC: National Center on Child Abuse and Neglect.

Jullion, J. (1985). *Long way home: The odyssey of a lesbian mother and her children.* San Francisco: Cleis.

Kinsey, A. C., Pomeroy, W. B., & Martin, C. E. (1948). *Sexual behavior in the human male.* Philadelphia: Saunders.

Kirkpatrick, M. (1987). Clinical implications of lesbian mother studies. *Journal of Homosexuality, 13,* 201–211.

Kirkpatrick, M., Smith, C., & Roy, R. (1981). Lesbian mothers and their children: A comparative survey. *American Journal of Orthopsychiatry, 51,* 545–551.

Kleber, D. J., Howell, R. J., & Tibbits-Kleber, A. L. (1986). The impact of parental homosexuality in child custody cases: A review of the literature. *Bulletin of the American Academy of Psychiatry and Law, 14,* 81–87.

Kohlberg, L. (1964). Development of moral character and moral ideology. In M. L.

Hoffman & L. W. Hoffman (Eds.), *Review of child development research* (pp. 383–431). New York: Russell Sage.

Kohlberg, L. (1966). A cognitive-developmental analysis of children's sex-role concepts and attitudes. In E. E. Maccoby (Ed.), *The development of sex differences* (pp. 82–173). Stanford, CA: Stanford University Press.

Kohut, H. (1971). *The analysis of the self.* Madison, CT: International Universities Press.

Kohut, H. (1977). *The restoration of the self.* Madison, CT: International Universities Press.

Kohut, H. (1984). *How does analysis cure?* Chicago: University of Chicago Press.

Kweskin, S. L., & Cook, A. S. (1982). Heterosexual and homosexual mothers' self-described sex role behavior and ideal sex role behavior in children. *Sex roles, 8,* 967–975.

Lamb, M. E. (Ed.). (1982). *Nontraditional families: Parenting and child development.* Hillsdale, NJ: Erlbaum.

Laosa, L. M. (1988). Ethnicity and single parenting in the United States. In E. M. Hetherington & J. D. Arasteh (Eds.), *Impact of divorce, single parenting, and stepparenting on children* (pp. 23–49). Hillsdale, NJ: Erlbaum.

Lauritsen, J., & Thorstad, D. (1974). *The early homosexual rights movement (1864–1935).* New York: Times Change Press.

Levy, E. F. (1989). Lesbian motherhood: Identity and social support. *Affilia, 4,* 40–53.

Lewis, K. G. (1980). Children of lesbians: Their point of view. *Social Work, 25,* 198–203.

Lyons, T. A. (1983). Lesbian mothers' custody fears. *Women and Therapy, 2,* 231–240.

Maccoby, E. E. (1990). Gender and relationships: A developmental account. *American Psychologist, 45,* 513–520.

MacPike, L. (Ed.). (1989). *There's something I've been meaning to tell you.* Tallahassee, FL: Naiad Press.

Mager, D. (1975). Faggot father. In K. Jay & A. Young (Eds.), *After you're out* (pp. 128–134). New York: Links Books.

Martin, A. (1989). The planned lesbian and gay family: Parenthood and children. *Newsletter of the Society for the Psychological Study of Lesbian and Gay Issues, 5,* 6, 16–17.

Martin, D., & Lyon, P. (1972). *Lesbian/woman.* San Francisco: Glide Publications.

McCandlish, B. (1987). Against all odds: Lesbian mother family dynamics. In F. Bozett (Ed.), *Gay and lesbian parents* (pp. 23–38). New York: Praeger.

McLoyd, V. (1990). The impact of economic hardship on black families and children: Psychological distress, parenting, and socioemotional development. *Child Development, 61,* 311–346.

Miller, B. (1979). Gay fathers and their children. *Family Coordinator, 28,* 544–552.

Miller, J. A., Jacobsen, R. B., & Bigner, J. J. (1981). The child's home environment for lesbian vs. heterosexual mothers: A neglected area of research. *Journal of Homosexuality, 7,* 49–56.

Money, J., & Ehrhardt, A. A. (1972). *Man and woman, boy and girl: The differentiation and dimorphism of gender identity from conception to maturity.* Baltimore: Johns Hopkins University Press.

Mucklow, B. M., & Phelan, G. K. (1979). Lesbian and traditional mothers' responses to adult responses to child behavior and self concept. *Psychological Reports, 44,* 880–882.

Noble, E. (1987). *Having your baby by donor insemination.* Boston: Houghton Mifflin.

Nungesser, L. G. (1980). Theoretical basis for research on the acquisition of social sex roles by children of lesbian mothers. *Journal of Homosexuality, 5,* 177–188.

O'Leary, K. D., & Emery, R. E. (1984). Marital discord and child behavior problems. In M. D. Levine & P. Satz (Eds.), *Middle childhood: Development and dysfunction* (pp. 345–364). Baltimore: University Park Press.

Osman, S. (1972). My stepfather is a she. *Family Process, 11,* 209–218.

Pagelow, M. D. (1980). Heterosexual and lesbian single mothers: A comparison of problems, coping and solutions. *Journal of Homosexuality, 5,* 198–204.

Parke, R. D. (Ed.). (1984). *Review of child development research: Vol. 7. The family.* Chicago: University of Chicago Press.

Paul, J. P. (1986). *Growing up with a gay, lesbian, or bisexual parent: An exploratory study of experiences and perceptions.* Unpublished doctoral dissertation, University of California at Berkeley, Berkeley, CA.

Pennington, S. (1987). Children of lesbian mothers. In F. W. Bozett (Ed.), *Gay and lesbian parents* (pp. 58–74). New York: Praeger.

Perreault, J. (1975). Lesbian mother. In K. Jay & A. Young (Eds.), *After you're out* (pp. 125–127). New York: Links Books.

Peterson, N. (1984, April). Coming to terms with gay parents. *USA Today,* p. 30.

Pies, C. (1985). *Considering parenthood.* San Francisco: Spinsters/Aunt Lute.

Pies, C. (1990). Lesbians and the choice to parent. In F. W. Bozett & M. B. Sussman (Eds.), *Homosexuality and family relations* (pp. 137–154). New York: Harrington Park.

Polikoff, N. (1986). Lesbian mothers, lesbian families, legal obstacles, legal challenges. *Review of Law and Social Change, 14,* 907–914.

Polikoff, N. (1990). This child does have two mothers: Redefining parenthood to meet the needs of children in lesbian mother and other nontraditional families. *Georgetown Law Journal, 78,* 459–575.

Pollack, S. (in press). Lesbian parents: Claiming our visibility. *Women and Therapy.*

Pollack, S., & Vaughn, J. (1987). *Politics of the heart: A lesbian parenting anthology.* Ithaca, NY: Firebrand.

Puryear, D. (1983). *A comparison between the children of lesbian mothers and the children of heterosexual mothers.* Unpublished doctoral dissertation, California School of Professional Psychology, Berkeley, CA.

Rafkin, L. (Ed.). (1990). *Different mothers: Sons and daughters of lesbians talk about their lives.* Pittsburgh: Cleis.

Rand, C., Graham, D. L. R., & Rawlings, E. I. (1982). Psychological health and factors the court seeks to control in lesbian mother custody trials. *Journal of Homosexuality, 8*, 27–39.

Rees, R. L. (1979). *A comparison of children of lesbian and single heterosexual mothers on three measures of socialization*. Unpublished doctoral dissertation, California School of Professional Psychology, Berkeley, CA.

Ricketts, W., & Achtenberg, R. (1990). Adoption and foster parenting for lesbians and gay men: Creating new traditions in family. In F. W. Bozett & M. B. Sussman (Eds.), *Homosexuality and family relations* (pp. 83–118). New York: Harrington Park.

Riley, C. (1988). American kinship: A lesbian account. *Feminist Issues, 8*, 75–94.

Robinson, B. E., & Barret, R. L. (1986). Gay fathers. In B. E. Robinson & R. L. Barret (Eds.), *The developing father: Emerging roles in contemporary society* (pp. 145–168). New York: Guilford.

Rogoff, B. (1990). *Apprenticeship in thinking*. New York: Oxford University Press.

Rohrbaugh, J. B. (1988). Choosing children: Psychological issues in lesbian parenting. *Women and Therapy, 8*, 51–63.

Rutter, M., Izard, C. E., & Read, P. B. (Eds.). (1986). *Depression in young people: Developmental and clinical perspectives*. New York: Guilford.

Saghir, M. T., & Robins, E. (1973). *Male and female homosexuality: A comprehensive investigation*. Baltimore: Williams & Wilkins.

Sameroff, A. J., & Chandler, M. (1975). Reproductive risk and the continuum of caretaking casualty. In F. D. Horowitz (Ed.), *Review of child development research* (Vol. 4). Chicago: University of Chicago Press.

Sarafino, E. P. (1979). An estimate of nationwide incidence of sexual offenses against children. *Child Welfare, 58*, 127–134.

Schulenberg, J. (1985). *Gay parenting: A complete guide for gay men and lesbians with children*. New York: Anchor.

Seligmann, J. (1990). Variations on a theme. *Newsweek* (Special Ed.: "The 21st Century Family," Winter/Spring 1990), pp. 38–46.

Spencer, M. B., Brookins, G. K., & Allen, W. R. (Eds.). *Beginnings: The social and affective development of black children*. Hillsdale, NJ: Erlbaum.

Steckel, A. (1985). *Separation-individuation in children of lesbian and heterosexual couples*. Unpublished doctoral dissertation, the Wright Institute Graduate School, Berkeley, CA.

Steckel, A. (1987). Psychosocial development of children of lesbian mothers. In F. W. Bozett (Ed.), *Gay and lesbian parents* (pp. 75–85). New York: Praeger.

Thompson, N., McCandless, B., & Strickland, B. (1971). Personal adjustment of male and female homosexuals and heterosexuals. *Journal of Abnormal Psychology, 78*, 237–240.

Van Gelder, L. (1988). Gay gothic. *Plain Brown Rapper, 2*, 5–12.

Weeks, R. B., Derdeyn, A. P., & Langman, M. (1975). Two cases of children of homosexuals. *Child Psychiatry and Human Development, 6*, 26–32.

Weisner, T. S., & Wilson-Mitchell, J. E. (1990). Nonconventional family life-styles and sex typing in six-year-olds. *Child Development, 61*, 1915–1933.

Wolf, M. (1990). Checking out the sperm bank. *Gaybook*, Winter (Book 9), 8–13.

Yekel, C. A., Bigler, R. S., & Liben, L. S. (1991). *Children's gender schemata: Occupation, activity, and trait attributions for self and others.* Paper presented at the biennial meeting of the Society for Research in Child Development, Seattle.

3

Children's Reactions in the Early Months After the Death of a Parent

Phyllis R. Silverman

Massachusetts General Hospital, Boston

J. William Worden

Harvard Medical School, Boston

The reactions of a nonclinical group of 125 dependent children aged 6–17 years were examined within four months of the death of a parent. Focus was on normative behavior in the domains of the children's reactions to the death itself, their affective experience, their efforts at remaining connected to the deceased, their social network and support system, and changes in their families resulting from the death.

The death of a parent is not something a dependent child expects to experience, yet it is not uncommon. Approximately 1.5 million children in the United States live in single-parent families because the other parent is dead *(U.S. Bureau of the Census, 1989)*. Bowlby's *(1980)* study of young children in post–World War II Europe implicated the loss of a parent by separation or death as a causal factor in childhood depression and other types of problem behavior. Other research has supported Bowlby's findings *(Elizur & Kaffman, 1983; Furman, 1974)*. Although Brown, Harris, and Bifulco *(1986)* found that the death of a mother in childhood was associated with depression in adult women, some studies *(Osterweis, Solomon, & Greene, 1984; Van Eerdewegh, Biere, Parilla, & Clayton, 1982)* have not supported the hypothesis that the death of a parent in childhood leads to an increased risk of subsequent psychological problems. In a review of the research literature, Berlinsky and Biller *(1982)* observed that this lack of consistent find-

Reprinted with permission from *American Journal of Orthopsychiatry*, 1992, Vol. 62(1), 93–104. Copyright © 1992 American Orthopsychiatric Association.

A revised version of a paper submitted to the Journal in September 1990. Work was funded by grants from the National Institute of Mental Health (MH 41791), from the National Funeral Directors Association, and from the Hillenbrand Corporation.

ings may be due to an oversimplification of the issues associated with the death of a parent. The outcome measures used in most studies focused primarily on the presence or absence of psychiatric symptoms and often obscured the complexity of the situation.

The death of a parent should not be viewed as a single stressful event, but as a series of events that occurred before and after the death *(Berlinsky & Biller, 1982; Norris & Murrell, 1987)*. Thus, factors other than the loss need to be in place before a bereaved child can be considered at risk *(Brown et al., 1986; Elizur & Kaffman, 1983)*. The way the surviving parent responds to the child, the availability of social support, and subsequent life circumstances make a difference in whether a child develops problems. Reese *(1982)* noted that the increased risk of developing behavioral problems was associated with lack of continuity in the child's daily life after the death, that is, the surviving parent's inability to provide a stable home for the child. Therefore, it is necessary to understand the context in which the stress of bereavement is experienced. Bereavement outcomes need to be conceptualized in dynamic terms that emphasize change and adaptation, rather than merely the presence or absence of symptoms or signs of psychological disturbance. Silverman *(1987)* reported that women in college, reflecting on the death of a parent when they were younger, were changed by the death, but their lives were not necessarily more difficult.

The death of a loved one invariably leads to psychological and social stress, but not necessarily to psychiatric symptoms. In the face of this stress, children need to adapt to many changes in their lives. But what influences this ability to deal with change? The authors suggest that the answer lies in understanding the interaction among the social context, the family system, and the personal characteristics of those involved.

A limitation of many studies *(Furman, 1974; Kliman, 1968; Raphael, 1982)* is that they have involved small samples of children who were in psychiatric treatment. In other studies *(Elizur & Kaffman, 1983; Van Eerdewegh et al., 1982)*, the surviving parent was the informant for the family. To better understand the impact of parental death on children, researchers need not only to look at the context in which the death has occurred, but to learn more about how the death is experienced by a nonclinical sample of bereaved children who can speak for themselves *(Berlinsky & Biller, 1982; Osterweis et al., 1984; Vida & Grizenko, 1989)*.

Using data gathered by the Child Bereavement Study, Massachusetts General Hospital, Boston, from a community sample of 125 bereaved dependent children, this article reports on how these children responded to the death of one of their parents. The purpose of the article is to describe the normative responses of these children and the family context that framed their reactions shortly after the death.

METHOD

Study Population

Bereaved families, representing a range of socioeconomic, religious, and ethnic backgrounds, were recruited from communities in the greater Boston area. These families were invited to participate by the funeral directors who served them. Criteria for inclusion in the study were that the parents were living together at the time of the death and that the surviving children in the family were aged 6–17. All but a few bereaved families in the selected target communities were identified, and 51% agreed to participate. There were no significant differences between those who accepted and those who refused in the gender and age of the deceased, the suddenness and cause of the death, the religion of the families, and the number of children. From a demographic point of view, the study population seems to be a representative sample of bereaved families in these communities, although it should be noted that the Afro-American families in which deaths had occurred did not have children in the eligible range. Factors other than demographics may influence people's decision to participate. For example, those who accept are likely to be those who see value in talking about their situation *(Stroebe & Stroebe, 1989)*.

The sample consisted of 70 families with 125 children (65 boys and 60 girls) aged 6–17 (mean = 11.6 years; *SD* = 3.08), who were attending the first through twelfth grades (see Table 1). Seventy-four percent of the children had lost a father and 26% had lost a mother.

The average age of the surviving parent was 41 years, with a range of 30–57 years for the surviving mothers and of 33–50 for the surviving fathers. For most of the couples (91%), this was their only marriage (mean length of 17 years). The number of children in the families ranged from 1 to 5 with a mean of 2.56

TABLE 1
Child Demography (*N* = 125)[a]

CHARACTERISTIC	BOYS		GIRLS		TOTAL	
	N	%	N	%	N	%
Age at Time 1						
6–11 yrs	30	24.0	32	25.6	62	49.6
12–16 yrs	35	28.0	28	22.4	63	50.4
Parent Who Died						
Father	48	38.4	44	35.2	92	73.6
Mother	17	13.6	16	12.8	33	26.4
Warning of Death						
Expected	34	27.2	38	30.4	72	57.6
>1 week	7	5.6	6	4.8	13	10.4
>1 day	24	19.2	16	12.8	40	32.0

[a] 65 boys (52%), 60 girls (48%).

TABLE 2
Family Demography (*N* = 70)[a]

	SURVIVING PARENTS					
	MALE		FEMALE		TOTAL	
CHARACTERISTIC	*N*	%	*N*	%	*N*	%
Parents' Age at Time 1						
30–34 yrs	2	2.9	1	1.4	3	4.3
35–39 yrs	5	7.1	13	18.6	18	25.7
40–44 yrs	7	10.0	19	27.1	26	37.1
45–49 yrs	4	5.7	13	18.6	17	24.3
50–54 yrs	2	2.9	2	2.9	4	5.7
Over 55 yrs			2	2.9	2	2.9
Family Religion						
Protestant	3	4.3	13	18.6	16	22.9
Catholic	17	24.3	32	45.7	49	70.0
Jewish			4	5.7	4	5.7
Other			1	1.4	1	1.4
Type of Death						
Natural	18	25.7	44	62.9	62	88.6
Accidental	1	1.4	4	5.7	5	7.1
Suicidal	1	1.4	1	1.4	2	2.9
Homicidal			1	1.4	1	1.4
Warning of Death						
Prolonged illness	13	18.6	29	41.4	42	60.0
>1 day	2	2.9	2	2.9	4	5.7
<1 day	5	7.1	19	27.1	24	34.3
Income Level at Time 1						
>$10,000	3	4.5	2	3.0	5	7.5
$10,000–$19,000	2	3.0	13	19.4	15	22.4
$20,000–$29,000	3	4.5	15	22.4	18	26.9
$30,000–$39,000	3	4.5	8	11.9	11	16.4
$40,000–$49,000	5	7.5	4	6.0	9	13.4
<$50,000	4	6.0	5	7.5	9	13.4
Children in Family (*N*)						
1	2	2.9	7	10.0	9	12.9
2	9	12.9	21	30.0	30	42.9
3	5	7.1	14	20.0	19	27.1
4	1	1.4	6	8.6	7	10.0
5	3	4.3	2	2.9	5	7.1

[a] 20 surviving fathers (28.6%), 50 surviving mothers (71.4%).

(*SD* = 1.07). Nine children had no siblings. Sixty-nine percent of the families had at least one child under age 12. The religious affiliation of this population reflects the large concentration of Catholics (70%) in the greater Boston area (see Table 2).

Most of the deaths (89%) were from natural causes. The spouses of an almost equal percentage of the men (65%, *N* = 13) and women (59%, *N* = 29) had been ill for some time before the death. Of those who died after a long illness, 25% (*N* = 18) had been ill for over a year.

From a socioeconomic point of view, these families represented a cross-section of the community. Eighty percent of the fathers worked full-time outside the home, while the mothers were more likely to work part-time outside the home or to be full-time homemakers (*N* = 70) (χ^2 = 12.68, *df* = 4, *p*<.01). The families' socioeconomic status (SES), based on the fathers' education and occupation

(Hollingshead & Redlich, 1958) was as follows: Level I (unskilled laborer), 9%; Level II (semiskilled laborer), 29%; Level III (skilled craftsperson, clerical worker), 14%; Level IV (medium business, minor professional), 43%; and Level V (major business or professional), 6%.

Study Design

Interviews. Interviews with the children and their surviving parents were conducted by the same interviewer in the family home four months following the death and at the first and second anniversaries of the death. Family members were interviewed separately, and each of the interviews was audiotaped.

The children were asked, in a semistructured interview, questions about their *1)* pre-death status, *2)* experiences with the death, *3)* life changes since the death, *4)* functioning in school, *5)* health status, *6)* relationships with peers, and *7)* attitudes and behavior related to the loss.

Interviews with the surviving parents covered *1)* family demography, *2)* their pre-death status, *3)* circumstances of the death, *4)* their mourning behavior, *5)* their current support, *6)* an appraisal of stress and coping, *7)* concerns about the children, *8)* family activities, and *9)* family responses to the death.

Measures. In addition to interviews, both parents and children responded to several standardized measures. The measures included in this article are as follows: *Child Behavior Checklist (CBC) (Achenbach, 1983).* Reports of each child's emotional and behavioral problems were obtained from the surviving parent using this inventory of 118 behavioral problems rated "not true" "somewhat or sometimes true," or "very true or often true." Normalized *t*-scores, based on Achenbac's sample of clinical and nonclinical children, were used for both the broad-band and narrow-band clinical scales.

Perceived Competence Scale for Children (PCSC) (Harter, 1985). Six areas of perceived competence are assessed on this self-report scale: *1)* scholastic competence, *2)* social acceptance, *3)* athletic competence, *4)* physical appearance, *5)* behavioral conduct, and *6)* global self-worth. The test consists of 28 pairs of statements describing two opposite ends of a specific behavior; children select the place on the continuum that is "true" or "sort of true" for themselves. Internal consistency values range from .73 to .83.

Locus of Control Scale (LCS) (Nowicki & Strickland, 1973). This 40-item paper-and-pencil test measures generalized expectancies for internal versus external control of reinforcement among children. It has been used with children from third grade through college, and norms are available for various age groups in that range. The scale has both internal and temporal consistency.

In the following analysis, data are taken from the children's responses to questions in the first interview. When indicated, data from the parents' interview are presented as well. Although these observations of the children may not be totally independent, recent research has suggested *(Dunn & Plomin, 1990)* that there is wide variation between children raised in the same family. These findings support the authors' treatment of these children as individuals, each experiencing the death in his or her own way. This article is intended to be descriptive, and the statistics used were chosen with this aim in mind.

FINDINGS

Five areas related to the children's concerns, experiences, and reactions in the early months following the death of their parents will be discussed: *1)* their reactions to the death, *2)* their affective experience, *3)* their efforts to maintain a connection to their deceased parents, *4)* their social networks and support systems, and *5)* changes in their families' routine since the death. Of particular interest were the children's gender and age, the suddenness of the death, and the gender of the parent who died, since these factors affected the children's reactions in these five domains. Gender and age of the child are key factors in understanding children's behavior *(Hartup, 1989; Jacklin, 1989; Selman, 1980; Youniss, 1980)*. Differences have been identified in the ways boys and girls mobilize social support *(Belle, 1989)*, in the roles they play in the family *(Carter, Scott, & Martyna, 1976; Lynn, 1974)*, and in their responses to bereavement *(Silverman, 1988; Stroebe & Stroebe, 1983)*. The suddenness of the death may have an impact on the nature of the stress experienced by the family *(Antonovsky, 1987)*.

Death and the Funeral

The children's participation in the funeral had repercussions for how they understood the death and how they saw themselves as participants in the family drama. The ways in which the surviving parents dealt with the fact of the impending death and of the death itself had repercussions for how the family maintained itself as a functioning system.

Three-fourths of the children were told of the death by their surviving parents (see Table 3). Fifteen children were present at the death (the children were more likely to be present at the death if the mother was the surviving parent). In families in which the fathers died, the mothers were more likely to plan financially with their husbands in advance of the death $(N = 44)$ $(\chi^2 = 5.98, df = 2, p<.05)$. The women were also more likely to stop working when their husbands were very ill, whereas the men with sick wives continued to work. The mothers seemed to be more in touch with the family's changing needs in light of an impending death and more available to the children during this period.

When told of the death, the children often seemed contained and more subdued

TABLE 3
Characteristics of the Death Event for the Children ($N = 125$)

CHARACTERISTIC	BOYS		GIRLS		TOTAL	
	N	%	N	%	N	%
Who Told Child of Death						
Surviving parent	50	40.0	43	34.4	93	74.4
Sibling	2	1.6	3	2.4	5	4.0
Other family member	3	2.4	5	4.0	8	6.4
Hospital personnel	1	.8	1	.8	2	1.6
Present at death	9	7.2	6	4.8	15	12.0
Other			2	1.6	2	1.6
Child Cried Right Away						
No or unsure	23	18.4	20	16.0	43	34.4
Yes	42	33.6	40	32.0	82	65.6
Child Cried Later On						
No	9	7.3	2	1.6	11	8.9
Yes	56	45.5	56	45.5	112	91.1
Behavioral Expectation						
No	29	23.2	33	26.4	62	49.6
Unsure	6	4.8	4	3.2	10	8.0
Yes	30	24.0	23	18.4	53	42.4
Mourning Ritual Was Observed						
No	3	2.4	2	1.6	5	4.1
Yes	61	49.6	57	46.3	118	95.9
Child Attended the Funeral						
No	5	4.0	1	.8	6	4.8
Yes	60	48.0	59	47.2	119	95.2
Child Remembers What Was Said at the Funeral						
No	19	16.2	21	17.9	40	34.2
Yes	41	35.0	36	30.8	77	65.8
Child Saw Body of Parent						
No	13	10.4	15	12.0	28	22.4
Yes	52	41.6	45	36.0	97	77.6
Child Went to the Cemetery						
No	9	7.3	5	4.0	14	11.3
Yes	54	43.5	52	41.9	106	85.5
NA	1	.8	3	2.4	4	3.2

than might have been anticipated. When the death was sudden (no warning), the children described their reactions with such words as "shocked," "stunned," and "I couldn't believe it." One teenager, who was told by his cousin, at first thought it was a cruel joke and then said he was "very confused about how to react." Few children expressed any immediate anger (7%, $N = 9$) or relief (4%, $N = 5$) when there had been a prolonged illness with considerable suffering. Most children (44%, $N = 55$) talked of feeling sad or confused on hearing the news, even when the death was expected. They also talked of not being sure how to respond. Children chose different ways to deal with their feelings; some turned to other family members for comfort, while others withdrew. A few children reported needing to be alone and retreating to their rooms, going out for a walk, or riding their bicycles. Still others went in search of a friend.

At some point during the day, the majority of children (91%) broke down in tears. When there had been a long illness, the children were less likely to cry immediately upon hearing the news than they were to cry later ($N = 125$) ($\chi^2 = 10.14$, $df = 2$, $p<.01$). There were no significant differences in boys' and girls' immediate responses based on either the children's or the dead parents' gender.

Ninety-five percent of the children attended the funeral. Their age and the gender of the deceased parents were factors in deciding whether to include them in the funeral ritual. Younger children were less likely to attend, as were those whose mothers had died.

Affective Responses

The children's inner feelings about the death and their associated behavior included crying, insomnia, learning difficulties, and early health problems that reflected the somatization of feelings. Four months after the death, 62% ($N = 77$) of the children were no longer crying at frequent intervals or with any regularity; only 8% ($N = 10$) reported crying daily. Those who cried frequently at four months were more likely to be younger ($r = .17$, $p.<.03$). There were no significant gender differences in crying behavior at this time, nor were there differences depending on which parent died.

Most children (70%, $N = 87$) slept well; the third who had sleep problems had difficulty falling asleep or awoke early in the morning—problems that they attributed to their parents' death. Other problems included headaches, experienced by 74% ($N = 92$) of the children, difficulty concentrating in school, experienced by 19% ($N = 24$), and uneasiness at the absence of their dead parent from the dinner table, experienced by 18% ($N = 23$).

When this information on the children's distress was submitted to a principal component factor analysis, the first principal factor accounted for 40% of the variance and can be identified as "emotional distress." Children with the highest distress scores were doing poorly in school ($r = .26$, $p<.01$), experienced more hassling by peers for having a dead parent ($r = .26$, $p<.01$), were more preoccupied with thoughts of their dead parent ($r = -.24$, $p<.05$), and suffered from more health problems ($r = .20$, $p<.05$). There was no correlation between this distress score and the children's age or gender. Nor was there a correlation with the score on the LCS *(Nowicki & Strickland, 1973)*.

To identify the parents' perceptions of the children's emotional and behavioral problems, the authors assessed each child on the CBC *(Achenbach, 1983)* at each interview. The 118 identified types of behavior can be scored as a series of narrow-band clinical scales that note the presence of problem behavior. Most bereaved children scored in the low to normal range on these scales, which indicates few serious behavioral problems during this early period after the parent's death. A small percentage of bereaved children did score high, above 70 Standard Score on one or more of the various clinical scales. Elevated clinical scores ranged in frequency from a low of 2% of the children on Delinquent Behaviors to a high of 13% on Somatic Behaviors. The percentage of children scoring above 70 for the remaining clinical scales ranged from 6% to 7%, depending on the scale.

In addition to the narrow-band clinical scales normed for subgroups by age and gender, there are three broad-band CBC scales that enable one to compare behavioral profiles across age-gender quadrants (boys, girls, younger, older). These broad-band scales measure total behavioral problems; internalized behavior, such as anxiety and depression; and externalized behavior, such as delinquency and acting out. The highest total CBC scores were found for the younger girls (mean = 55.26, SD = 11.18), and the lowest scores were found for the younger boys (mean = 52.97, SD = 11.03); the scores of the older boys (mean = 53.81, SD = 11.75) and the older girls (mean = 53.44, SD = 10.10) fell in between. A t-score of 65 or greater (above 1.5 SD) was used to identify the 21 children (17%) who were most distressed at four months.

Children with the highest CBC Total Scores had the poorest peer support (r = .19, $p<.05$); felt they had less control over the things happening to them (r = .30, $p<.01$) as measured by the LCS *(Norwicki-Strickland, 1973)*; and had lower levels of self-esteem (r = .25, $p<.05$), measured by the PCSC scale *(Harter, 1985)*. The age and gender of the child, gender of the dead parent, and the suddenness of the death were not significantly related to the level of problems on the CBC. The children with the most disturbed behavior, as reflected by high scores on the broad-band CBC scales, had lower self-esteem and felt less in control of their lives, regardless of their age.

Health

Health problems have often been reported as important consequences of bereavement in children. The clinical CBC scale with the highest percentage of scores exceeding a t-value of 70 (2 SD above the norming mean) was the somatic scale. Although only five children (4%) reported a serious illness after the death, 76 (61%) reported some form of illness during this four-month period; only 35% (N = 44) reported no health problems. Children with the most health problems were younger (r = $-.18$, $p<.05$), had lost a mother (r = .18, $p<.05$), and were fearful for the surviving parent's safety (r = .18, $p<.05$).

School Performance

When the mother died after a long illness, children were more likely to be sent back to school the day after the funeral ($r = -.26$, $p<.01$). Only 22% ($N = 27$) of the children thought that their school performance had changed for the worse since the death, and 18% ($N = 22$, 11 boys and 11 girls) thought that their work improved. Some children, mostly teenagers, resolved to do better in school in light of the loss. The inability to function in school was one area in which the impact of the death could be seen concretely. Children who reported that they had no difficulties in school had locus-of-control scores that reflected a strong sense of control over their environment, and this sense of agency included their school-work, as measured by the Nowicki-Strickland Locus of Control Scale ($r = -.28$, $p<.01$). In spite of the loss, most (71%, $N = 89$) of the children reported that they retained an ability to deal effectively with school.

Connection to the Deceased

Many of the children devoted considerable energy to staying connected with their deceased parents in some way. They did so through dreams, by talking to or frequently thinking about their deceased parents, by believing that their dead parents were watching them, by keeping things that had belonged to their dead parents, and by visiting their parents' graves. Such behavior could be interpreted as an attempt either to keep the deceased parents alive or to make the loss real.

When asked what they believed happened after the death, most of the children (74%, $N = 92$) believed that their parents had gone to a specific place, and they usually talked about Heaven. Fifty-seven percent ($N = 71$) reported speaking to the deceased parent; of these, 43% ($N = 29$), who tended to be younger children, felt they received an answer ($r = -.31$, $p<.01$). Eighty-one percent ($N = 101$) thought that their dead parents were watching them; this frightened 57% ($N = 71$) of them, and their uneasiness was related to a fear that their dead parents might not approve of what they were doing. Those who felt watched but were not scared (24%, $N = 30$) were more likely to perceive the watching as protective. The deceased parents continued to be a real presence for many of the children, who carried on a relationship similar to the one prevailing before the death (e.g., protector or disciplinarian).

Most children (55%, $N = 69$) also dreamed about their dead parents, and for the majority who dreamed, their parents appeared alive in the dreams (50%, $N = 63$). Some children ($N = 12$) were frightened by these dreams, some ($N = 10$) were saddened by them, and some ($N = 25$) found the dreams reassuring.

At the time of the first interview, 79% ($N = 99$) of the children were still thinking about their dead parents at least several times a week. When asked what they thought about, most (54%, $N = 67$) remembered in fairly literal and concrete terms what they used to do with their parents. A few children (3%, $N = 4$) reported that they still could not believe the death was real, and a few (4%, $N = 4$) reported forgetting at times that their parents were dead. Others wished that their dead parents would come back or thought about how hard it was to get along without them (16%, $N = 20$). Children whose mothers had died were likely to think about them more frequently than were those whose fathers had died ($r = .20$, $p<.05$)/

Seventy-six percent ($N = 95$) of the children kept something personal that belonged to their dead parents either on their person or in their rooms. These objects often had the quality of a linking object, described by Winnicott *(1953)* to provide, through a concrete object, a symbolic connection to their lost parents. According to their surviving parents, 22% ($N = 27$) of the children idealized the deceased; this was more likely to happen if the parents died after a long illness. When the children were asked to identify the parent that they most resembled, many (46%, $N = 58$) selected the deceased parent.

Social Network and Context

These variables reflect the context of the child's life, which determines how the child will express his or her grief and make meaning out of the loss. Such a network can provide children with a feeling of being supported and cared about and make resources available that facilitate coping. The nature of the exchange of feelings and information are part of the network's activity that facilitates this coping. A child's network includes people with whom the child interacts, such as siblings, teachers, and friends.

School support. Teachers uniformly knew about the death, but only about half of them shared this information with the child's classmates. They were more likely to do so in the lower grades (where children had one teacher for the entire school day) and at a time when the bereaved child was not in school (thus, the child learned about it from friends in the class). There was little conversation about the death in the classroom in which the bereaved child was involved. When a child attended a Catholic school, his or her classmates typically came to the funeral mass held at the church.

Peer support. All the children reported having at least one close friend, and half had four or more friends. Sixty-six percent ($N = 82$) of these children saw their friends at least every day, since they usually attended school with them. Only 54% ($N = 67$) reported that they talked with their friends about their dead parents; the remaining 46% ($N = 58$) did not wish to do so, although most of them thought that at least one friend would listen if they wanted to talk. Boys were less likely than girls to talk to their friends about the death ($r = .18$, $p<.05$). Fourteen percent ($N = 18$) of the children (especially the younger girls) felt that there were children in their neighborhood or in school who gave them a hard time because they had only one parent.

Family support. Around the time of the death and the funeral, 42% ($N = 53$) of the children thought that their behavior should be restrained so as not to make problems for their surviving parent; three-quarters of them ($N = 40$) complied. This feeling was especially present in families in which the death had been expected. Children over age 12 were more likely to be told specifically that they had to be more grown up now ($N = 125$) ($\chi^2 = 5.66$, $df = 1$, $p<.02$), and this message was more likely to be sent to older boys ($N = 125$) ($\chi^2 = 4.26.66$, $df = 1$, $p<.05$).

When asked to identify the person to whom they felt closest in their family, 15 children did not answer the question. Most of the children (43%, $N = 54$) indicated that they felt closest to their surviving parent; 14% ($N = 18$), an older sibling; 6% ($N = 6$), a younger sibling; and 18% ($N = 20$) a grandparent or other relative. Twelve children (10%) reported that they were not close to anyone; four of these children were from two families in which the mother had died. Most children (66%, $N = 83$) reported that they could talk about the death and their feelings with this identified family member. Even when they did not feel close to them, the children (including 3 of the 4 who did not feel close to anyone) felt that they could talk with their surviving parent if they needed to. Girls were much more likely to share their feelings with their identified family member than were boys ($N = 125$) ($\chi^2 = 5.55$, $df = 1$, $p<.01$). The children did not feel that family communication was any more or less hampered if their mothers died, but they did report a greater reluctance to share dreams of their deceased mothers with their surviving fathers.

Changes in Daily Life

Many children experienced changes in their daily lives during these early months after the death, but not to the degree that one might expect. The change experienced by the largest number (44%, $N = 55$) was an increase in the household tasks and chores they were required to do; such changes occurred more frequently after the death of a mother ($r = .16$, $p<.05$). Changes in mealtimes were also noted by 35% of the children, again most often by those who had lost their mothers ($r = .29$, $p<.01$). When their fathers died, older children experienced more changes in their allowance or in their employment (28%, $N = 35$). Other postdeath changes for the children were changes in their rooms (40%, $N = 50$) and in their bedtime (27%, $N = 34$). When mothers of children under age 12 died, the children were more likely to experience a change in who took care of them when they were sick; they either took care of themselves or were cared for by a relative. Most children (67%, $N = 84$) felt that there was little change in the time they spent outside their homes with their friends since the death.

When a composite change score was created by combining change scores from each of the areas just discussed, children with the greatest number of changes following a parental death were those who had lost a mother ($r = .17, p<.05$), who suffered more health problems during these early months ($r = .21, p<.01$), who kept an object from the deceased parent close at hand ($r = .22, p<.01$), and who felt most uneasy about coming to the dinner table ($r = .20, p<.05$). Since these correlations represent a small percentage of the variance in a population of this size, they should be seen as suggestive of a trend, rather than definitive. The death of mothers, rather than of fathers, caused the greatest discontinuity in the lives of these children after the death occurred, and such changes can be seen as concomitant losses for them.

DISCUSSION

Understanding a child's responses to the death of a parent requires a focus on many interacting variables. For the children in the study, the event itself was stressful and, in addition, its impact pervaded most aspects of the child's life. It reached to the inner workings of the child's meaning-making system and to the way his or her world was structured. The stresses did not seem to overwhelm most of the children during this early period. There was little, if any, indication of serious dysfunctional behavior in most of them. Some of the children were sad and somewhat confused, most were carrying on by going to school and by maintaining relationships with their friends and family members. It was clear that these children were grieving, but they did not express their grief in prolonged periods of crying, aggression, or withdrawal, as has been traditionally thought.

These children were dealing not only with the death of a person, but with the death of a way of life. With one or two exceptions, the mothers seemed to be the parents who dealt with the affective life of the family and upon whom the stability of daily routines was dependent. This situation seemed to be true before the death, as reflected in differences in how mothers and fathers handled the impending death and the death scene. When a father was left in charge, the children were less likely to talk with him about their feelings or their dreams, and they experienced many more changes in their daily lives. The finding that children talked less to their fathers may have been compounded by the fact that the fathers not only had cared for the mothers, but had continued to work and care for the children as well. Fathers added roles to their lives that they were not necessarily prepared for. They also sent the children back to school almost immediately; this may have reflected the children's wish to return to a normal routine as soon as possible, and it may also have reflected the fathers' need to return to work or their inexperience in knowing what to do with the children. The parents' ability to assume a new role and to adapt to a single-parent household became an important factor in the children's overall adaptation to change.

Boys, especially the older ones, were less comfortable with their feelings and were more likely to get reinforcement from their support network to contain their feelings. This finding raises the question of whether these boys were already being socialized, at this early age, to perpetuate the pattern of the larger society in which women deal with feelings in the family *(Belle, 1989; Miller, 1986)*. The study looked not only at gender-specific roles to which these children and their parents have been or are being socialized, but at how these children were learning the roles of bereaved child and of a child with only one parent. An analysis of the longitudinal data will reveal if and how gender affects this learning and the roles that children assume in the family.

The most interesting findings were those related to the children's efforts to maintain a connection to the deceased. Such behavior has frequently been labeled in the psychiatric literature as "preoccupation with the deceased." This term may be construed to imply symptomatic behavior found early in the bereavement process that should come to an end. Furman *(1974)*, Volkan *(1981)*, and other psychoanalytic writers *(Dietrich & Shabad, 1989; Miller, 1971)* have described similar behavior in clinical samples and reported that this behavior caused problems for the bereaved children. These authors focused on the need to disengage from the deceased. However, little is known about the meaning and function of maintaining a connection to the deceased in a nonclinical population of bereaved children. In a study by Silverman and Silverman *(1979)*, children found that it was easier to accept the finality of the loss if the bereaved child had an appropriate way to maintain a sense of the deceased in his or her current life. A retrospective study of college-age women who had lost a parent to death found that as these women got older, they were constantly renegotiating their relationship to their dead parents *(Silverman, 1987)*. The parent was dead, but the relationship did not die *(Anderson, 1974; Silverman & Silverman, 1979)*. Both Klass *(1988)* and Rubin *(1985)* identified similar behavior among parents after the death of a child. These early connections to the deceased may, in the long run, help these children accept a new reality, a task identified by Worden *(1991)* as critical to the bereavement process.

The children in the present study were trying to make the loss real, testing its parameters, and trying to find out what really happened to their parents. The activities they shared with their dead parents and the things the parents had done for them were very much a part of the children's thoughts four months after the death. One task for the surviving parents in this early phase of bereavement was to help the children develop a language that allowed them to talk about their dead parent and to maintain a place for that parent in their lives *(Klass, 1988; Rubin,*

1985; Silverman & Silverman, 1979; Worden, 1991). Most of the surviving parents did not focus sufficiently on what their children were doing to maintain this connection. They often expressed concern that their children were not talking about their feelings, an activity they viewed as the primary way for their children to express their grief. They did not sufficiently appreciate the value in this respect of the children's conversations about the dead parent, which often involved simply reminiscing about things the children had done with the deceased. Both parents and children need help in learning that this kind of reflecting and remembering is also a critical part of the bereavement process. How well children and their surviving parents learn this may hold the key to the kind of accommodation the family makes to the loss over time. Future analysis of the longitudinal data from this study may help answer this question.

The early analysis of these data points to the importance of looking at the child in the context of his or her social and family system. Thus, one should keep in mind that, in contrast to the 17% of the children who displayed significant problem behavior within the first months after the death, 83% of the children carried on, and their efforts to cope seemed to be effective. The behavior that the majority of the children exhibited must be seen as part of the range of appropriate responses that children develop at such a time. We need to respect the resilience they may display *(Garmezy, 1987).* To understand this ability to carry on, subsequent analyses will focus on how children cope and adapt and on the relationship of family context to such coping and adaptation.

REFERENCES

Achenbach, T.M. (1983). *Developmental psychopathology* (2nd ed). New York: John Wiley.

Anderson, R. (1974). Notes of a survivor. In S.B. Troop & W.A. Green (Eds.), *The patient, death and the family.* New York: Scribner's.

Antonovsky, A. (1987). *Unraveling the mystery of health: How people manage stress and stay well.* San Francisco: Jossey-Bass.

Belle, D. (1988). Gender differences in the social moderators of stress. In R.C. Barnett, L. Beiner, & G.K. Baruch (Eds.), *Gender and stress* (pp. 257–277). New York: Free Press.

Belle, D. (Ed.). (1989). *Children's social networks and social supports.* New York: John Wiley.

Berlinsky, E.B., & Biller, H.B. (1982). *Parental death and psychological development.* Lexington, MA: D.C. Heath.

Bowlby, J. (1980). *Attachment and loss: Vol. 3. Loss, sadness, and depression.* New York: Basic Books.

Brown, G.W., Harris, T.O., & Bifulco, A. (1986). Long term effects of early loss of parent. In M. Rutter, C.E. Izard, & P. Read (Eds.), *Depression in young people: Developmental and clinical perspectives* (pp. 251–297). New York: Guilford Press.

Carter, L.A., Scott, A.F., & Martyna, W. (1976). *Women & men: Changing roles relationship and perceptions.* New York: Aspen Institute for Humanistic Studies.

Dietrich, D.R., & Shabad, P.C. (1989). *The problem of loss and mourning.* Madison, CT: International Universities Press.

Dunn, J., & Plomin, R. (1990). *Separate lives: Why siblings are so different.* New York: Basic Books.

Elizur, E., & Kaffman, M. (1983). Factors influencing the severity of childhood bereavement reactions. *American Journal of Orthopsychiatry, 53,* 668–676.

Furman, E. (1974). *A child's parent dies: Studies in childhood bereavement.* New Haven, CT: Yale University Press.

Garmezy, N. (1987). Stress, competence, and development: Continuities in the study of schizophrenic adults, children vulnerable to psychopathology, and the search for stress-resistant children. *American Journal of Orthopsychiatry, 57,* 159–185.

Harter, S. (1985). Processes underlying the construction, maintenance, and enhancement of the self concept in children. In J. Sulo & A. Greenwall (Eds.), *Psychological perspectives on the self* (pp. 138–181). Hillsdale, NJ: Lawrence Erlbaum.

Hartup, W.W. (1989). Social relations and their developmental significance. *American Psychologist* [Special issue], *44*(2), 120–126.

Hollingshead, A.B., & Redlich, F.C. (1958). *Social class and mental illness.* New York: John Wiley.

Jacklin, S.N. (1989). Female and male: Issues of gender. *American Psychologist* [Special issue], *44*(2), 127–133.

Klass, D. (1988). *Parental grief: Solace and resolution.* New York: Springer.

Kliman, G. (1968). *Psychological emergencies of childhood.* New York: Grune & Stratton.

Lynn, D.B. (1974). *The father: His role in child development.* Monterey, CA: Brooks/Cole.

Miller, J.B.M. (1971). Children's reactions to the death of a parent: A review of the psychoanalytic literature. *Journal of the American Psychoanalytic Association, 19,* 697–719.

Miller, J.B. (1986). *Toward a new psychology of women* (2nd ed.). Boston: Beacon Press.

Norris, F.H., & Murrell, S.A. (1987). Older adult family stress and adaptation before and after bereavement. *Journal of Gerontology, 42,* 606–612.

Nowicki, S., & Strickland, B.R. (1973). A Locus of Control Scale for Children. *Journal of Consulting Psychology, 40,* 148–154.

Osterweis, M., Solomon, F., & Greene, M. (Eds.). (1984). *Bereavement: reactions, consequences, and care.* Washington, DC: National Academy Press.

Raphael, B. (1982). The young child and the death of a parent. In C.M. Parkes & J. Stevenson-Hinde (Eds.), *The place of attachment in human behavior* (pp. 131–150). New York: Tavistock Publications.

Reese, M.F. (1982). Growing up: The impact of loss and change. In D. Belle (Ed.), *Lives in stress: Women and depression* (pp. 65–88). Beverly Hills, CA: Sage.

Rubin, S.S. (1985). The resolution of bereavement: A clinical focus on the relationship to the deceased. *Psychotherapy: Theory, Research, Training and Practice, 22*, 231–235.

Selman, R.L. (1980). *The growth of interpersonal understanding.* New York: Academic Press.

Silverman, P.R. (1987). The impact of parental death on college-age women. *Psychiatric Clinics of North America, 10*, 387–404.

Silverman, P.R. (1988). In search of new selves: Accommodating to widowhood. In L.A. Bond (Ed.), *Families in transition: Primary prevention programs that work* (pp. 200–220). Beverly Hills, CA: Sage.

Silverman, S.M., & Silverman, P.R. (1979). Parent-child communication in widowed families. *American Journal of Psychotherapy, 33*, 428–441.

Stroebe, M.S., & Stroebe, W. (1989). Who participates in bereavement research? A review and empirical study. *Omega, 20*(1), 1–29.

U.S. Bureau of the Census. (1989). *Marital status and living arrangements: March 1989* (Series P-20, No. 445). Washington, DC: U.S. Government Printing Office.

Van Eerdewehg, M., Bieri, M.D., Parilla, R.H., & Clayton, P.J. (1982). The bereaved child. *British Journal of Psychiatry, 140*, 23–29.

Vida, S., & Grizenko, N. (1989). DSM-III-R and the phenomenology of childhood bereavement: A review. *Canadian Journal of Psychiatry, 34*, 148–154.

Volkan. V.D. (1981). *Linking objects and linking phenomena.* New York: International Universities Press.

Winnicott, D.W. (1953). Transitional objects and transitional phenomena. *International Journal of Psycho-Analysis, 34*, 89–97.

Worden, J.W. (1991). *Grief counseling and grief therapy: A handbook for the mental health practitioner* (2nd ed.). New York: Springer.

Youniss, J. (1980. *Parents and peers in social development: A Piagetian-Sullivan perspective.* Chicago: University of Chicago Press.

4

Psychophysiology in Attachment Interviews: Converging Evidence for Deactivating Strategies

Mary Dozier

Trinity University, San Antonio, Texas

R. Rogers Kobak

University of Delaware, Newark

By asking the subject to consider a host of potentially threatening attachment-related issues, the Adult Attachment Interview (AAI) allows an assessment of different strategies for regulating the attachment system. These strategies can be assessed along the 2 dimensions of security/anxiety and deactivation/hyperactivation. The greatest inferential leaps may be in characterizing strategies as deactivating. For example, individuals using deactivating strategies often report extremely positive relationships with parents, display restricted recall of attachment memories, and play down the significance of early attachment experiences. If these descriptive features are guided by a strategy that requires diverting attention from attachment information, subjects employing this strategy should experience conflict or inhibition during the Attachment Interview. In the present study, skin conductance levels were monitored for 50 college students during a baseline period and throughout the Attachment Interview. Subjects

Reprinted with permission from *Child Development*, 1992, Vol. 63, 1473–1480. Copyright © 1992 by the Society for Research in Child Development, Inc.

Preparation of this manuscript was supported by an NIMH FIRST Award (MH44691) to the first author. Portions of these results were presented at the biennial meetings of the Society for Research in Child Development held in Kansas City, April 1989, and in Seattle, April 1991. We are especially grateful to Lori Bast Thompson for coordinating research activities. Also, we thank Jenine Meston and Neisha Nelson for coding interviews, and Robert Pianta and Carol George for helpful comments on an earlier version of this paper. Correspondence concerning this article should be addressed to Mary Dozier, Department of Psychology, Trinity University, San Antonio, TX 78212.

> *employing deactivating strategies showed marked increases in skin conductance levels from baseline to questions asking them to recall experiences of separation, rejection, and threat from parents. This finding supports the notion that individuals employing deactivating attachment strategies experience conflict or inhibition during the Attachment Interview.*

Attachment theory and research have provided developmental and clinical psychologists with an invaluable account of the way that children adapt to different types of caregiving (Ainsworth, Blehar, Waters, & Wall, 1978; Bowlby, 1969, 1973, 1980). For example, Ainsworth's patterns of attachment can be viewed as strategies that allow the child to maintain access to parents with different types of responsiveness. Once developed, these strategies regulate attachment behavior and provide rules that guide the individual in appraising and processing information relevant to attachment. The importance of information processing is particularly apparent in George, Kaplan, and Main's Adult Attachment Interview (1984). By directing subjects' attention to attachment-related topics, the interview creates a context that tests subjects' abilities to process and integrate attachment-related thoughts, feelings, and memories. Main and Goldwyn (in press) describe different information-processing styles in the interview as "states of mind" about attachment. In this paper, we will consider how strategies for regulating the attachment system lead to different rules for processing information in the Attachment Interview. We then test this conceptualization by examining the link between deactivating strategies during the Attachment Interview and concurrent changes in skin conductance.

Attachment Strategies and Information Processing

A secure strategy is guided by expectations that the individual can effectively gain support and comfort from attachment figures. As a result, information about the attachment figure can be integrated and coordinated to regulate access to attachment figures. Main (1990) views this as a "primary" strategy because it is consistent with allowing the biologically based attachment system to achieve its predictable outcome of protection. In the Strange Situation, a secure strategy is inferred from the child's use of the attachment figure as a secure base and safe haven (Ainsworth et al., 1978). Security in the Adult Attachment Interview is inferred when subjects are "free to evaluate" attachment information. These subjects demonstrate an ability to cooperate with the interviewer by flexibly directing attention toward interview topics. Main and Goldwyn (in press) developed formal criteria for secure information processing in terms of the *coherency* of subjects' discourse. Discourse is considered coherent when subjects provide relevant supporting memories for their generalizations, give adequate but not excessive information, respond with relevant information to interview questions, and develop their answers in a clear and well-organized manner.

When a secure strategy fails to produce positive outcomes, *secondary* strategies must be developed to regulate the attachment system (Main, 1990). Deactivation of the attachment system may be a useful secondary strategy for infants classified as avoidant in the Strange Situation. These infants show an apparent *absence* of attachment behavior in a situation in which such behavior would normally be elicited. Instead of actively seeking access to their parents, these children display little distress on separation and ignore or turn away from attachment figures during reunion. Ainsworth's extensive home observations of avoidant babies indicated that these children often experienced insensitive or rejecting responses from parents in response to their attachment signals (Ainsworth et al., 1978). As a result, the primary strategy of actively seeking contact with the parent would lead to further rejection and cause painful conflict (Main, 1981). To reduce conflict, the child develops a "secondary conditional strategy" that involves "overriding or manipulating of the otherwise naturally occurring behavioral output of the attachment behavioral system" (Main, 1990, p. 57). Avoidance is conceived as a behavioral mechanism that permits the infant to shift attention away from conditions normally eliciting attachment behavior (Main, 1990).

A deactivating strategy also accounts for many of the features of the dismissing pattern of thought described by Main and Goldwyn in the Attachment Interview (Kobak, Cole, Ferenz-Gillies, Fleming, & Gamble, in press). These subjects devalue the importance of relationships, report extremely positive relationships with their parents (even "perfect relationships"), and downplay the influence of childhood experiences (Main & Goldwyn, in press). These features of the interview are consistent with the notion that dismissing subjects employ a strategy of deactivating the attachment system by excluding attachment-related information (Bowlby, 1980). Rules consistent with such a strategy restrict subjects' awareness and acknowledgment of negative affect, limit recall of distressing or attachment-related memories, and lead to general or vague descriptions of parents that are not based on actual memories.

Kobak et al. (in press) have suggested that the three major "states of mind" can be conceived in terms of two continuous dimensions describing primary secure/anxious and secondary deactivating/hyperactivating strategies. These primary and secondary dimensions are conceived as coactive. Thus, a primary secure strategy could dominate performance in the AAI, while some secondary tendencies involving either deactivation or hyperactivation are present. For instance, subjects classified as F4 or F5 in Main and Goldwyn's system can be viewed as secure with hyperactivating tendencies, while those classified as F1 or F2 can be viewed as secure with deactivating tendencies. Insecure subjects, from this perspective, have secondary deactivating or hyperactivating tendencies that dominate performance over primary secure tendencies. However, even among subjects classified as insecure, differences may be present in the extent to which secondary strategies are evident in interview discourse. For instance, a subject employing a strategy of idealizing parents may recall a memory of clear rejection that would be consistent with a secure or coherent interview strategy. Yet, if the secondary strategy dominates interview discourse, such a memory will not be integrated with the overall depiction of parents.

To assess primary and secondary strategies as continuous variables, Kobak (1989) developed Q-items that describe different aspects of interview transcripts including information-processing features, emotion regulation, and working models of self and parents. Raters using the Q-sort system focus on descriptive detail in interview transcripts. Guided by a control theory analysis of primary and secondary attachment strategies, criterion sorts were developed (Kobak et al., in press). The first criterion identifies the extent that a primary secure strategy organizes a subject's discourse in the interview. The second criterion, deactivation/hyperactivation, assesses the strength of secondary strategies designed to alter the output of the attachment system. Continuous scores are then derived by correlating interview descriptions with criterion sorts. Initial studies with the Q-sort system (Kobak et al., in press) suggest that the security/anxiety dimension differentiates Main and Goldwyn's "free to evaluate attachment" group from those who are insecure. The deactivation/hyperactivation dimension differentiates between the two insecure classifications, dismissing of attachment and preoccupied with attachment.

Physiological Indicators of Deactivation in the Attachment Interview

Our view of the attachment strategies suggests that individuals who employ deactivating strategies should experience conflict or inhibition during the Attachment Interview. While normally attempting to avoid situations that elicit attachment thoughts or responses, in the interview they are asked to recall and think about attachment-related experiences. The demands of the interview thus conflict with a deactivating strategy for excluding attachment information from awareness. If this interpretation is correct, subjects who employ deactivating strategies should show subtle signs of conflict or inhibition during the Attachment Interview. Concurrent measures of skin conductance offer a promising means to test this interpretation.

Gray (1975) has posited a two-factor learning theory, in which behavioral activation and behavioral inhibition are two antagonistic components of the arousal system. Extending Gray's work, Fowles (1980) argued that behavioral activation is associated with cardiovascular activity (heart rate), and behavioral inhibition is associated with electrodermal activity (skin conductance). Work by Pennebaker and his colleagues (Pennebaker & Chew, 1985; Pennebaker, Hughes, & O'Heeron, 1987) provides compelling evidence for the *specific* relation between inhibition and skin conductance activity. For example, Pennebaker and Chew (1985) found that deception was associated with increases in skin conductance activity, but was not related to other autonomic nervous system activity. Both as induced in the laboratory (Pennebaker & Chew, 1985; Wegner, Shortt, Blake, & Page, 1990) and as observed naturalistically (Waid & Orne, 1982; Weinberger, Schwartz, & Davidson, 1979), inhibition has been associated with heightened skin conductance activity. In the laboratory, subjects asked to inhibit emotionally charged thoughts, for example, thoughts of sex (Wegner et al., 1990), or to react with detachment to disturbing movie clips that depicted amputations (Koriat, Melkman, Averill, & Lazarus, 1972), showed elevated levels of skin conductance activity.

In this paper, we adopted a Q-sort approach to assessing primary and secondary attachment strategies in the Attachment Interview. Our central hypothesis was that subjects employing deactivating secondary strategies experience greater inhibition in the Attachment Interview than subjects employing other strategies. By assessing strategies as continuous variables, we hoped to lend some specificity to our hypothesis. First, we were not expecting skin conductance to be linked to general insecurity or incoherence in the Attachment Interview. Only one type of incoherence, organized by a deactivating as contrasted with a hyperactivating strategy, should be associated with inhibition during the interview. Since some degree of deactivating tendencies can coexist with secure tendencies in the secure group, our continuous measure of deactivation/hyperactivation should provide a strong test of our central hypothesis. If we relied on classificatory methods, our analysis of deactivating tendencies would be restricted to subjects in the dismissing group. We proposed to test this hypothesis with concurrent measures of skin conductance. Subjects who relied on deactivating strategies in the Attachment Interview were expected to show the greatest increases in skin conductance activity.

METHOD

Overview

Skin conductance levels were monitored while subjects were administered the Adult Attachment Interview (George et al., 1985). During a 5-min baseline period prior to the interview and throughout the interview, means for skin conductance levels were recorded for every 30-sec period. An experimenter recorded the time when each interview question was asked, thus allowing rises or falls in skin conductance level to be linked with specific interview questions.

Subjects

Subjects were 50 Trinity University undergraduates (39 females and 11 males), all between the ages of 18 and 21. All students who agreed to participate completed the interview. Students received extra credit in their psychology classes in exchange for their participation.

Adult Attachment Interview

The Attachment Interview (George et al., 1984) allows an assessment of the regulation of the attachment system by providing a context for activating the attachment system. Subjects are asked in the interview to remember incidences of separation and threatened separation from parents, to provide specific support for global impressions of attachment figures, and to conceptualize relationship influences, among other things. In this semistructured interview, questions are asked in a predetermined order, but flexibility is allowed in following up responses. The time required for the interview varies from about 45 to 70 min.

Rating of interviews. —The Attachment Interview Q-set (Kobak, 1989) was used for the rating of interviews. Q-items were derived from descriptions used in Main and Goldwyn's classification system (in press). Two raters listened to an audiorecording of each interview. They then placed the 100 Q-set items in one of nine categories, ranging from least characteristic of the subject to most characteristic of the subject. There was a forced distribution of items, with fewer descriptors placed in more extreme categories (5, 8, 12, 16, 18, 16, 12, 8, and 5, descriptors in the nine categories, respectively). A criterion of .60 was used as the minimum acceptable level of composite interrater reliability met this criterion level. For the remaining 22%, a third rater was used, with agreement between raters reaching criterion for all subjects. Raters' Q-sorts were composited to provide a more reliable description of each subject. Resulting composite reliability ranged from .60 to .91, with a mean of .73 (Spearman-Brown formula).

Composited interview Q-sorts were corrrelated with the two criterion prototypes that had been generated for secure (as contrasted with anxious) strategies, and for deactivating (as contrasted with hyperactivating) strategies. These prototypes were generated by raters using conceptual criteria derived from a control theory analysis of attachment functioning (Kobak et al., in press). Items central to the security prototype describe subjects' coherency and cooperation in the interview and working models of self as efficacious and parents as available. Items central to the deactivating/hyperactivating dimension describe access to memory, with deactivating strategies associated with restricted access and hyperactivating strategies associated with excessive detail. Also central are items regarding models of the self and parents, with deactivating strategies associated with the devaluing of attachment and hyperactivating strategies associated with negative involvement.

Skin Conductance Measurement

The procedure developed by Fowles et al. (1981) for measuring skin conductance levels (SCL) was followed. Each subject's fingers were scrubbed with alcohol, and electrode conductivity gel was applied. The Ag/AgCl electrodes were fastened to the second phalange of the ring finger and forefinger of the dominant hand. The electrodes were attached to a J & J Enterprises IG-3 Preamp and Model T-68 for digital readout of skin conductance levels.

Mean skin conductance levels were recorded for each 30-sec period during a 5-min baseline period and throughout the Attachment Interview. A research assistant in an adjoining room could hear the interview through an intercom; she recorded when each interview question was asked by pressing a key corresponding to that question on the computer that recorded skin conductance levels.

Procedure

Subjects were brought individually into a 15 x 18-foot interview room. Drapes covered one-way mirrors on two of the walls, and the floor was carpeted. An indirect ceiling light provided soft light. Two comfortable living room chairs were placed 3 feet apart, facing one another.

The experimenter asked subjects to sit in whichever chair allowed the dominant hand to be on the side of the skin conductance monitors, and she sat in the other chair. Procedures were then explained. Subjects were told that they would be interviewed while skin conductance levels were monitored. In the interview, they would be asked about their family while they were growing up. They were told that the interview would be taped to allow for later coding. The interviewer explained that a research assistant would be able to hear the interview through an intercom in an adjoining laboratory room, thus allowing the recording of the timing of various interview questions. Subjects were invited to ask questions about the procedures and to read and sign a consent form.

The experimenter connected subjects to the physiological monitors, explaining each step of the process in nontechnical language. She then explained that she would leave the room for 5 min to allow the establishment of a baseline period for skin conductance activity.

After 5 min, the experimenter knocked quietly and returned. She informed subjects that she was turning the tape recorder on, and began the Attachment Interview (George et al., 1984). The interview began with a general background question, intended both to provide the interviewer with background material and to help the subject relax. Then the interviewer asked the subject to describe early relationships with parents, generate adjectives describing each parent, and to provide memories supporting these adjectives. Subjects were then asked to recall incidences of distress as a child, including being upset, separated from parents, rejected by parents, and threatened by parental separation. Subjects were then asked to consider the effects of their upbringing on their personality, and to consider why their parents had behaved as they had. The interviewer then asked subjects to recall experiences of early and later loss. Finally, subjects were asked to consider changes in, as well as the current status of, their relationships with parents, and to think about the most important thing learned from attachment experiences.

At the completion of the interview, the experimenter turned the tape recorder off and removed physiological monitors. The experimenter then debriefed subjects and answered any questions. Several subjects indicated that the interview had raised concerns for them for which they might like additional help. The experimenter discussed options of getting help from the campus counseling center or from private therapists in the area. She offered to make specific referrals if desired. In addition, all subjects were told that, if they found that they had later concerns about the interview, they could contact the interviewer.

RESULTS

Scores for the two attachment dimensions (security/anxiety and deactivation/hyperactivation) were derived for each subject. These scores were correlated with rises or falls in skin conductance from baseline.

Attachment Organization

Correlations between subjects' Q-sorts and the security/anxiety prototype ranged from −.76 to .84, with a mean of .22. Correlations with the deactivation/hyperactivation prototype ranged from −.51 to .45, with a mean of −.08. These correlations were transformed to % scores (Edwards, 1967).

Skin Conductance

For each subject, a mean was calculated across the last 3 min of the baseline period which preceded the interview. This baseline level was then subtracted from the skin conductance level recorded for each question of interest, yielding a drop or rise in skin conductance. The mean baseline skin conductance level was 8.8, ranging from 4.2 to 24.9, with a standard deviation of 4.0. The mean rise in skin conductance from baseline to the parental rejection question (midway through the interview) was 4.6, ranging from −.7 to 14.3, with a standard deviation of 3.2. The mean rise from baseline to the final interview question was 5.4, ranging from −1.0 to 17.9, with a standard deviation of 4.0.

Relationship Between Attachment Organization and Skin Conductance

The variables included in analyses were first examined to assess the fit between their distributions and the assumptions of multivariate analysis. The assumptions were not violated, thus making the further transformation of data unnecessary. There were no univariate outliers with extremely high or low % scores ($p > .001$), and no multivariate outliers with Mahalanobis distance with $p < .001$. Therefore, no cases were deleted or transformed.

Scores for the two attachment dimensions were correlated with rises in skin conductance from baseline for each of the principal interview questions. Table 1 presents correlations between attachment dimensions and rises in skin conductance for interview questions in the order in which questions were asked.

As predicted, scores on the deactivation/hyperactivation dimension correlated positively with skin conductance rises for questions regarding separation or threat-

TABLE 1
Correlations Between Attachment Dimensions and Rises in Skin
Conductance on Adult Attachment Interview

| | ATTACHMENT DIMENSIONS | |
INTERVIEW QUESTION	Security/ Anxiety	Deactivation/ Hyperactivation
1. Background	.11	−.07
2. Describe relationships	−.09	.15
3. Describe mom	−.15	.24
4. Memories for mom adjectives	−.09	.19
5. Describe dad	−.17	.29*
6. Memories for dad adjectives	−.10	.20
7. Upset	−.18	.28
8. Separated	−.27	.43**
9. Rejected	−.18	.34*
10. Threatened	−.28	.39**
11. How affected by upbringing	−.16	.29*
12. Why parents parented as they did	−.24	.30*
13. Loss	−.21	.28
14. Changes in relationship	−.23	.39**
15. Relationship with parents now	−.07	.22
16. One thing learned	−.12	.26

* $p < .05$.
** $p < .01$.

ened separation from caregivers. In particular, greater reliance on deactivating strategies (as rated from Attachment Interview responses) was associated with greater rises in skin conductance for questions regarding separation from parents, rejection by parents, and threatened separation from parents. Significant positive correlations between deactivation/hyperactivation and rises in skin conductance also emerged for questions regarding how subjects were affected by the way they were raised, why their parents had raised them in the way they did, and changes in relationships with parents. Again, greater deactivation was associated with larger rises in skin conductance. Finally, subjects who employed deactivating strategies showed greater rises in skin conductance from baseline when they were asked to generate several adjectives to describe childhood relationships with their fathers. Correlations between the security/anxiety dimension and skin conductance rises were not significant.

DISCUSSION

A deactivating strategy is maintained by diverting attention from attachment-related thoughts, memories, and feelings. The Attachment Interview challenges this strategy by asking the subject to direct attention to a host of attachment-related issues. However, even in a context that requires attending to attachment-related issues, subjects using deactivating strategies often present themselves as unperturbed. For example, they may respond with little apparent emotion that they had no difficulties with parents or were not bothered by separations or rejections from parents. If our interpretation is correct, there should be subtle signs of conflict for these individuals, particularly in a context in which the interviewer continually directs attention to attachment topics. To test this interpretation, converging evidence must be provided so that we are not merely *inferring* that these individuals are disturbed by the issues raised. The findings of differential physiological reactivity among college students during the Attachment Interview provide such converging evidence, supporting the hypothesis that deactivating strategies reflect attempts to divert attention from attachment-related issues.

As expected, subjects who used deactivating strategies showed larger rises in skin conductance for the three interview questions that ask them to consider real and threatened separations or rejections from their parents. These questions direct attention to memories in which the attachment system would normally be activated by fears about the availability of parents, thus making it particularly difficult to maintain a deactivating strategy. Significant correlations between deactivation and rises in skin conductance emerged for questions regarding the conceptualization of relationship influences and relationship changes as well. We speculate that such questions ask subjects to *reflect* upon relationships with attachment figures in ways that conflict with a deactivating strategy. Indeed, on the initial background question, which requires very little reflection, the correlation between deactivation/hyperactivation and skin conductance rises is negligible. On the other hand, questions about how the current personality has been influenced by early relationships with parents require that subjects not only access early attachment experiences but make those experiences relevant to the self. Two central premises of a deactivating strategy, restricting access to attachment information and minimizing the personal significance of relevance of attachment information, are thus violated.

At a more speculative level, our findings point to an important limitation of deactivating strategies. Although these strategies may serve to divert attention from attachment issues, such attempts cannot be seen as fully effective. The elevation in skin conductance levels associated with avoidance indicates that the subject is effortfully engaged in diversionary activities, rather than having fully deactivated the attachment system. These findings are consistent with Main's position that deactivation of the attachment system represents a secondary strategy that is "enacted in conjunction with an incomplete overriding of [the] primary strategy" (p. 49). The complete overriding of the primary strategy is impossible, according to Main, but "will necessarily be incomplete and partial" (p. 57). Sroufe and Waters's investigation of heart-rate variability among infants separated from their parents (Sroufe & Waters, 1977; Waters, Matas, & Sroufe, 1975) provides parallel support for the incomplete overriding of the attachment system in infancy. Despite *looking* as if engaged with a toy upon the caregiver's return, avoidant infants' accelerated heart rate suggested that they were not actually engaged with the toy, but only trying (somewhat unsuccessfully) to distract themselves.

Conceivably, the conflict experienced in processing attachment-related information for those using deactivating strategies might motivate them to avoid tasks in which their attachment systems would be activated. For example, they might avoid insight-oriented psychotherapy or other intimate relationships in which attention is directed to attachment experiences. Scarr and McCartney (1983) refer to this selection of comfortable environments, and avoidance of uncomfortable environments, as niche-picking. Despite attempts to select comfortable environments, however, individuals may sometimes find themselves in uncomfortable environments either because they did not anticipate task demands correctly or because their choices were limited. For example, subjects employing deactivating strategies may not have anticipated that they would be asked to talk about separations from parents during the Attachment Interview.

The self-perpetuating qualities of such avoidance behavior have been well documented (Mowrer, 1947), perhaps leaving it unclear what would lead to change for individuals using deactivating strategies. However, although attachment organization appears to be relatively stable, a reorganization of the attachment system is certainly possible. Main (1990) suggested that on some level, "the attachment system remains 'aware' of the 'real' status of environmental conditions" (p. 58). Thus, the individual who employs deactivating strategies may have some awareness of the strategic nature of his or her presentation of the self as invulnerable and the family as ideal. In the context of a safe, trusting relationship, it may be most likely that this individual would be able to acknowledge the "countertendencies" between the primary and secondary strategies. Indeed, some evidence exists to suggest that reorganization is most likely in the context of a "safe" relationship (Egeland, Jacobvitz, & Sroufe, 1988) or relationships (Pianta, Sroufe, & Egeland, 1989) which allow the individual to relinquish deactivating strategies.

REFERENCES

Ainsworth, M. D. S., Blehar, M. C., Waters, E., & Wall, S. (1978). *Patterns of attachment: A psychological study of the strange situation.* Hillsdale, NJ: Erlbaum.

Bowlby, J. (1969). *Attachment and loss: Vol. 1. Attachment.* New York: Basic.

Bowlby, J. (1973). *Attachment and loss: Vol. 2. Separation.* New York: Basic.

Bowlby, J. (1980). *Attachment and loss: Vol. 3. Loss, sadness, and depression.* New York: Basic.

Edwards, A. L. (1967). *Statistical methods* (2d ed.). New York: Holt, Rinehart & Winston.

Egeland, B., Jacobvitz, D., & Sroufe, L. A. (1988). Breaking the cycle of abuse. *Child Development, 59,* 1080–1088.

Fowles, D. C. (1980). The three arousal model: Implications of Gray's two-factor learning theory for heart rate, electrodermal activity, and psychopathy. *Psychophysiology, 17,* 87–104.

Fowles, D. C., Christie, M. J., Edelberg, R., Grings, W. W., Lykken, D. T., & Venables, P. H. (1981). Publication recommendations for electrodermal measurements. *Psychophysiology, 18,* 232–239.

George, C., Kaplan, N., & Main, M. (1984). *Attachment Interview for Adults.* Unpublished document, University of California, Berkeley.

Gray, J. A. (1975). *Elements of a two-process theory of learning.* New York: Academic Press.

Kobak, R. R. (1989). *The Attachment Interview Q-Set.* Unpublished document, University of Delaware.

Kobak, R. R., Cole, H. E., Ferenz-Gillies, R., Fleming, W., & Gamble, W. (in press). Attachment and emotion regulation during mother-teen problem solving: A control theory analysis. *Child Development.*

Koriat, A., Melkman, R., Averill, J. R., & Lazarus, R. S. (1972). The self-control of emotional reactions to a stressful film. *Journal of Personality, 40,* 601–619.

Main, M. (1990). Cross-cultural studies of attachment organization: Recent studies, changing methodologies, and the concept of conditional strategies. *Human Development, 33,* 48–61.

Main, M. (1981). Avoidance in the service of proximity: A working paper. In K. Immelmann, G. Barlow, L. Petrinovitch, & M. Main (Eds.), *Behavioral development: The Bielefeld Interdisciplinary Project* (pp. 651–693). New York: Cambridge University Press.

Main, M., & Goldwyn, R. (in press). Adult attachment classification system. In M. Main (Ed.), *Behavior and the development of representational models of attachment: Five methods of assessment.* Cambridge: Cambridge University Press.

Mowrer, O. H. (1947). On the dual nature of learning—a reinterpretation of "conditioning" and "problem solving." *Harvard Educational Review, 17,* 102–148.

Pennebaker, J. W., & Chew, C. H. (1985). Deception, electrodermal activity, and the inhibition of behavior. *Journal of Personality and Social Psychology, 49,* 1427–1433.

Pennebaker, J. W., Hughes, C. F., & O'Heeron, R. C. (1987). The psychophysiology of confession: Linking inhibitory and psychosomatic processes. *Journal of Personality and Social Psychology, 52,* 781–793.

Pianta, R. C., Sroufe, L. A., & Egeland, B. (1989). Continuity and discontinuity in maternal sensitivity at 6, 24, and 42 months in a high-risk sample. *Child Development, 60,* 481–487.

Scarr, S., & McCartney, K. (1983). How people make their own environments: A theory of genotype-environment effects. *Child Development, 54,* 424–435.

Sroufe, L. A., & Waters, E. (1977). Heart rate as a convergent measure in clinical and developmental research. *Merrill-Palmer Quarterly, 23,* 3–27.

Waid, W. M., & Orne, M. T. (1982). Reduced electrodermal response to conflict, failure to inhibit dominant behaviors, and delinquent proneness. *Journal of Personality and Social Psychology, 43,* 769–774.

Waters, E., Matas, L., & Sroufe, L. A. (1975). Infants' reactions to an approaching stranger: Description, validation, and functional significance of wariness. *Child Development, 46,* 384–356.

Wegner, D. M., Shortt, J. W., Blake, A. W., & Page, M. S. (1990). The suppression of exciting thoughts. *Journal of Personality and Social Psychology, 58,* 404–418.

Weinberger, D. A., Schwartz, G. E., & Davidson, R. J. (1979). Low-anxious, high-anxious, and repressive coping styles: Psychometric patterns and behavioral and physiological responses to stress. *Journal of Abnormal Psychology, 88,* 369–380.

Part II
METHODOLOGICAL ISSUES

This section presents three measures: two are new and one is a revision of a well-established measure. The first paper deals with the early prediction of autism. Baron-Cohen, Allen, and Gillberg present a brief questionnaire, the Checklist for Autism in Toddlers (CHAT), that has potential use in a pediatric setting to screen for autistic and developmental disorders at an age earlier than most children are brought to the attention of mental health professionals. Early intervention is critical, yet most autistic children are not discernibly different to families until 24 to 36 months, when parents notice language is not progressing. The CHAT emphasizes two main areas that can differentiate autistic infants from normally developing infants at 18 months of age. Pretend play and joint-attention behavior (such as pointing and showing) are usually present in 15-month-olds, thus the absence of such behaviors at 18 months constitute red flags.

The authors assessed 50 18-month-olds receiving a routine health visit and 41 children-at-risk for autism (younger siblings of autistic children). The checklist consists of nine items, answered yes or no by parents. Each question focuses on a different area of development. Four of the nine areas are present in autistic and normally developing children and five are not. Four cases of autism were present by 30 months. All of the children were lacking two or more of the five key items at 18 months: pretend play, protodeclarative pointing, social interest, social play, and joint-attention. Despite the methodological difficulties inherent in trying to predict a low-frequency disorder, this is an interesting attempt to provide a very simple screening tool that can be used among persons not trained to recognize children with autism.

The second paper presents a new measure: the Preschool Socioaffective Profile (PSP). It is an interesting measure that assesses both competence and pathology. The PSP was designed to obtain information about preschoolers' patterns of affective expression, social competence, and maladjustment as observed and rated by their preschool teachers. The 80-item scale (rated on 6-point Likert scales) yielded three factors representing internalizing (anxious-withdrawn) and externalizing (angry-aggressive) behavior problems and social competence.

Authors La Frenière, Dumas, Capuano, and Dubeau present a series of validation studies using multiple methodologies: teacher report, peer sociometric, classroom interactions, and parent-child interaction data. Findings revealed consistency of behavior patterns across family and school settings. For example, children rated by their teachers on the PSP as anxious-withdrawn were observed to be the least interactive with peers and expressed more negative affect with their mothers during a problem-solving task than the children in all other groups. Although the authors continue to refine the PSP, this is an important introduction to a measure based on developmental theory that assesses individual differences in competence.

The third paper in this section presents a "common-language" version of the California Child Q-set. This paper also presents the rationale and advantages of using Q-methodology. The California Child Q-set, originally developed by Jack and Jeanne Block in 1969, focuses on the wide variation in children's personalities and distinctive styles of coping. It does not assess behavior problems as do many instruments developed for child assessment. The Q-sort is unique in a variety of ways. It can be completed by parents, teachers, clinicians, and researchers—any person who is familiar with a child's behavior. By having sorters place cards into a fixed distribution, it reduces response bias (e.g., halo effect). It provides an ipsative (person-centered) description; the sorter compares each attribute with other attributes within the individual. Once the Q-sort data is obtained, a variety of constructs can be created (e.g., ego resiliency, ego control, self-esteem, social competence).

Despite the appeal of the Child Q-set, it has been difficult to use in many studies of children-at-risk because it required a reading level of Grade 11. The revised version presented here has an overall reading level of Grade 4.8, thus enabling it to be used with less educated populations. This paper also presents validity data by using the Q-sort in the context of a population screened for delinquency and psychiatric symptoms. Q-items significantly discriminated between boys with and without DSM-III-R disruptive disorders and self-reported delinquency. The items also revealed similarities and differences in the functioning of children presenting with internalizing and externalizing problems. For example, both groups experienced difficulty forming close friendships and tended to "freeze up" under stress. They differed on dimensions such as feeling unworthy or shy. The modified Child Q-set may be a useful measure for assessing personality changes over the course of treatment.

5

Can Autism Be Detected at 18 Months? The Needle, the Haystack, and the CHAT

Simon Baron-Cohen
University of London
Jane Allen
Wimbledon Village Practice, London
Christopher Gillberg
University of Gothenburg, Gothenburg, Sweden

Autism is currently detected only at about three years of age. This study aimed to establish if detection of autism was possible at 18 months of age. We screened 41 18-month-old toddlers who were at high genetic risk for developing autism, and 50 randomly selected 18-month-olds, using a new instrument, the CHAT, administered by GPs or health visitors. More than 80% of the randomly selected 18-month-old toddlers passed on all items, and none failed on more than one of the pretend play, protodeclarative pointing, joint-attention, social interest, and social play. Four children in the high-risk group failed on two or more of these five key types of behaviour. At follow-up at 30 months of age, the 87 children who had passed four or more of these key types of behaviour at 18 months of age had continued to develop normally. The 4 toddlers who had failed on two or more of these key types of behaviour at 18 months received a diagnosis of autism by 30 months.

Autism is widely regarded as the most severe of childhood psychiatric disorders, yet detection of autism is unacceptably late. Thus, even specialist clinicians are rarely referred a child with suspected autism much before three years old (specialist centres are beginning to have referrals of two-year-olds, but this is still

Reprinted with permission from *British Journal of Psychiatry*, 1992, Vol. 161, 839–843. Copyright © 1992 by the Royal College of Psychiatrists.

exceptional), despite the consensus among researchers that the disorder almost always has prenatal onset (Volkmar *et al*, 1985).

This relatively late age of detection is not surprising, since (a) primary health practitioners are not specifically trained to detect autism early, (b) nothing in the current routine developmental screening would alert a general practitioner (GP) or health visitor to a possible case of autism since in most countries they only screen motor, intellectual, and perceptual development, all of which may appear normal in autism (Frith & Baron-Cohen, 1987), (c) the disorder is quite rare, and (d) most sets of criteria for autism (American Psychiatric Association, 1987; World Health Organization, 1987) emphasise abnormalities in social and communicative development, both of which are difficult to assess in the pre-school period.

To date, most researchers have recognised the importance of early detection but have not attempted this, simply because the odds of finding autism at such a young age were not dissimilar to those of finding the proverbial needle in a haystack: only 4–8 per 10,000 infants develop autism (Gillberg *et al*, 1991). Given its rarity, it appears uneconomical to attempt early detection in a random sample.

A basic tenet of the present study is that the early detection of autism is both possible and economic. It is possible because findings from experimental psychology have shown us what to look for in toddlers if we want to detect autism early. Firstly, *pretend play* (in which objects are used as if they have other properties or identities and which is normally present by 12–15 months) is absent or abnormal in autism (Wing & Gould, 1979; Baron-Cohen, 1987). This deficit seems to be highly specific—there is not a general absence of play *per se*. For example, children with autism do show functional play (using toys as they were intended to be used) and sensorimotor play (exploring the physical properties of objects only, with no regard to their function, e.g., banging, waving, sucking, throwing, etc.) (Baron-Cohen, 1987).

Secondly, *joint-attention* behaviour (normally present by 9–14 months old) is also absent or rare in autism (Sigman *et al*, 1986). Again, this is a strikingly specific deficit. For example, while the joint-attention behaviour of protodeclarative pointing is absent or rare in autism (Baron-Cohen, 1989), pointing for 'non-social' purposes is present. Thus, they do show protoimperative pointing (Baron-Cohen, 1989), and pointing for naming (Goodhart & Baron-Cohen, 1992). (Joint-attention behaviour includes pointing, showing, and gaze monitoring, and is defined as attempts to monitor or direct the attention of another person to an object or event: protodeclarative pointing is the use of the index finger to indicate to another person an object of interest, as an end in itself; protoimperative pointing is the use of the index finger simply to attempt to obtain an object; pointing for naming is to pick out an object within an array while naming it, and this can be non-social.) Other deficits in joint-attention in autism include a relative lack of showing objects to others, and of gaze monitoring—directing one's gaze where someone else is looking (Sigman *et al*, 1986).

Since both pretend play and joint-attention behaviour, especially protodeclarative pointing, are universal development achievements (Butterworth, 1991; Leslie, 1991), normally present in simple forms by 15 months, their absence at the routine 18-month screening could be clear, specific indicators of autism or related disorders. Yet neither of these two psychological markers are currently checked.

But what about the economics of early detection? Screening even 10,000 randomly selected children would find few children with autism. Our alternative was to screen 18-month-old children who were at high risk for autism—younger siblings of children with diagnosed autism, 2–3% of whom on genetic grounds would also develop autism (Folstein & Rutter, 1987). We reasoned that if we could demonstrate the value of a screening instrument on a high-risk sample, then it would be safer to use such an instrument on a random population later.

METHOD

We tested two groups of subjects. Firstly, 50 randomly selected 18-month-olds (group 1) attending a London health centre for their routine 18-month check-up were tested, in order to collect normative data. The mean age of this group was 18.3 months (range 17–20 months, s.d. 1.04 months). They comprised 28 boys and 22 girls. Secondly, we tested 41 younger siblings of children with autism (group 2), identified with the help of the National Autistic Society (UK) and the Statewide Diagnostic Autism Register, kept at the Child Neuropsychiatric Clinic in Gothenburg. Group 2 was our high-risk group. The older siblings of this group all had a diagnosis of autism that met accepted criteria (Rutter, 1978; American Psychiatric Association, 1987). The mean age of subjects in group 2 was 19.3 months (range 17–21 months, s.d. 1.6 months). The difference in age between groups 1 and 2 was not significant ($t = 1.78$, d.f. $= 89$, $P > 0.05$).

Both groups were tested using our newly developed instrument, the Checklist for Autism in Toddlers (the CHAT). Subjects were tested by their GP or health visitor. GP cooperation for group 2 was obtained by explaining to them that the CHAT would only take about 15 minutes to complete, that it could be fitted into the routine 18-month check-up, that there was only one child among their patients who needed to be tested in this way, and that this would aid research. In the case of GP refusal ($n = 10$ in group 2), subjects were tested by a parent on Section A only (see below).

Subjects in both groups were followed up 12 months later (at age 30 months), with a letter to the parent (in the case of group 2) or the GP (in the case of group 1), asking if the child had developed any psychiatric problems.

The CHAT was initially constructed by including several questions in each of six areas of development reported in the literature to be abnormal in autism: social play, social interest, pretend play, joint-attention, protodeclarative pointing, and imitation. In addition, we also included several items in each of four areas of development reported to be normal in autism: functional play, protoimperative pointing, motor development, and rough and tumble play. This made a total of 10 areas of development. This rather long version of the CHAT was only given to group 1. It had two sections: section A comprised questions for the parent, while section B comprised attempts to elicit some of these types of behaviour by the clinician.

In an effort to ensure the CHAT was both easy and quick to use by busy clinicians, and only included questions that normal 18-month-olds easily passed, the CHAT was then shortened. Firstly, those items that were failed by more than 20% of group 1 were dropped (20% was chosen as an arbitrary index that this behaviour was not reliably present in normal 18-month-olds). This resulted in dropping imitation. Secondly, within each of the nine remaining areas of development, the question that was passed by the largest number of children in group 1 was kept, but the other questions were dropped. These two modifications produced the short CHAT (see Appendix).

Section A of the resulting check-list therefore assessed each of nine areas of development, with one question for each: rough and tumble play; social interest; motor development; social play; pretend play; protoimperative pointing; protodeclarative pointing; functional play; joint-attention. The order of questions was designed to avoid a yes or a no bias, by interspersing the predicted areas of abnormality with the predicted areas of normality in children with autism.

Section B was included for the clinician to check the child's actual behaviour against the parental report given in section A. Thus, item Biii checked for pretend play and corresponded to question A5. Item Biv checked for protodeclarative pointing and corresponded to question A7. Items Bi and Bii recorded actual social interaction, but were not intended to correspond to particular questions in section A, and Bv was a check for mental handicap.

Predictions

Following Folstein & Rutter (1987), we predicted we should find approximately 3% of group 2 would develop autism. Since group 2 contained only 41 subjects (this being the total number of 18-month-olds who were siblings of already diagnosed children with autism that we could locate in the whole of the UK and Sweden), this meant we could expect only 1.2 cases of autism. The question was, would the CHAT identify these one or two cases at 18 months? We predicted that these cases should fail questions A2, 4, 5, 7, and 9, but pass A1, 3, 6, and 8. We knew that more than 80% of children in group 1 were able to pass all items in the CHAT, as the instrument had been constructed on this basis.

RESULTS

Table 1 shows the percentage of subjects in each group passing (i.e. recording a 'yes') on each item in section A. Groups 1 and 2 did not differ statistically on any question. While a small percentage of the toddlers in group 1 still lacked protodeclarative pointing (8%), social interest (6%), joint-attention (6%), and pretend play (14%), as measured by section A (7, 2, 9, and 5, respectively), none lacked more than one of these four types of behaviour. The fifth behaviour of interest, social play (A4), was present in all of group 1. This pattern was also true of the toddlers in group 2, with the exception of four subjects (9.75% of group 2) who lacked two or more of these five key types of behaviour. Questions A3 and A8 demonstrated that none of the groups showed gross motor or intellectual delay, and nor were parents prone to a 'no' bias.

Validation of the CHAT: Follow-up Data

At follow-up at 2.5 years old, none of group 1 were reported to have developed any psychiatric problems, and certainly there were no cases of autism. In group 2, 37 out of 41 were reported to be free of psychiatric problems, but four had been

TABLE 1
Percentage of Each Group 'Passing' Each Item on the CHAT

	Group 1 (n = 50)	Group 2 (n = 41)
Section A questions		
1	90	92.7
2	94	97.5
3	100	95.0
4	100	95.1
5	86	82.9
6	98	87.8
7	92	87.8
8	100	100
9	94	92.7
Section B items[1]		
i	100	96.8
ii	98	90.3
iii	82	74.2
iv	88	80.6

Note N = 31. balance of line one.
was given by parents.

diagnosed (between 24 and 30 months old) as having autism, by two independent psychiatrists, using DSM-III-R criteria (American Psychiatric Association, 1987). These subjects were the only ones in group 2 to have lacked two or more of the five key types of behaviour. Two of these cases were in the British sample, and two were in the Swedish sample. This shows that the CHAT correctly predicted at 18 months old which children were developing normally versus which children were developing autism.

Reliability of the CHAT

Items Biii and Biv were included as a test of whether parents might be either under- or overestimating their child's ability, as they had reported it to the clinician on questions A5 and A7. In group 1 (who were all tested by a clinician), each of the two section A questions was passed by 92% of the children passing the corresponding section B item, as can be seen in Table 1. That is, most children who passed an item in section A were also scored as showing the relevant behaviour in section B. The four children (out of 50) who passed a question in section A but who did not show the relevant behaviour in section B were all accounted for by the clinician's notes. In three of these cases the clinician noted this was because of the child's shyness, and the other child's native language was not English. The opposite pattern (failing an item in section A but showing the relevant behaviour in section B) never occurred.

The final aspect of reliability that was tested concerned the ten subjects in group 2 who were assessed by their parents, because of GP refusal. The predictive accuracy from their assessment was just as reliable as that from the GP assessment.

DISCUSSION

This first study using the CHAT revealed that key psychological predictors of autism at 30 months are showing two or more of the following at 18 months: (a) lack of pretend play, (b) lack of protodeclarative pointing, (c) lack of social interest, (d) lack of social play, and (e) lack of joint-attention. The CHAT detected all four cases of autism in a total sample of 91 18-month-olds. Partly this must reflect that we chose the right measurements and the right high-risk group, although in part we were 'lucky,' in that statistically a sample of only 41 high-risk children could have contained no cases of incipient autism (Folstein & Rutter, 1987). This predictive success provides a preliminary test of the validity of the CHAT. We therefore recommend that if any child lacks any combination of these key types of behaviour on examination at 18 months, it makes good clinical sense to refer him/her for a specialist assessment for autism.

We are currently extending this research into an epidemiological study of 20,000 randomly selected 18-month-olds in the South East Thames Region of England, as a necessary next step towards further validation of this instrument. This will help establish the rate of false negatives, such as cases of mental handicap. We expect that most children with general and severe mental handicap will fail questions A3 and A8, and thus not be confused with early cases of autism. In addition, we recommend adding a further item to the CHAT (see Appendix item Bv) to help differentiate severe mental handicap without autism from autism itself. This item is already widely used in routine check-ups. Whether children with other kinds of disorders (e.g. Asperger's syndrome, language disorder, etc.) show a different pattern of failure on the CHAT will be an important question to answer.

Finally, it is of considerable theoretical interest that three of the items that predicted which children would receive a diagnosis of autism are those that have been postulated to stand in a precursor relationship to the impaired 'theory of mind' found later in autism: pretend play, protodeclarative pointing, and joint-attention (Baron-Cohen, 1991; Leslie, 1991). Our epidemiological study, being prospective, will allow a stronger test of this precursor relationship. It is hoped that research with the CHAT will lead to improvements in the early diagnosis of autism.

APPENDIX: THE CHAT

To be used by GPs or health visitors during the 18-month developmental check-up.

Child's name
Date of birth
Age
Child's address
Phone number

Section A. Ask parent:

1.	Does your child enjoy being swung, bounced on your knee, etc?	Yes	No
2.	Does your child take an interest in other children?	Yes	No
3.	Does your child like climbing on things, such as up stairs?	Yes	No
4.	Does your child enjoy playing peek-a-boo/hide-and-seek?	Yes	No
5.	Does your child ever pretend, for example, to make a cup of tea using a toy cup and teapot, or pretend other things?	Yes	No

6. Does your child ever use his/her index finger to point, to   Yes   No
    ask for something?
7. Does your child ever use his/her index finger to point, to   Yes   No
    indicate interest in something?
8. Can your child play properly with small toys (e.g. cars or   Yes   No
    bricks) without just mouthing, fiddling, or dropping
    them?
9. Does your child ever bring objects over to you (parent), to   Yes   No
    show you something?

Section B. GP's or Health Visitor's Observation:

i.   During the appointment, has the child made eye contact   Yes   No
      with you?
ii.   Get child's attention, then point across the room at an inter-
      esting object and say "Oh look! There's a [name a toy]!"
      Watch child's face. Does the child look across to see what   Yes[1]   No
      you are pointing at?
iii. Get the child's attention, then give child a miniature toy cup
      and teapot and say "Can you make a cup of tea?" Does   Yes[2]   No
      the child pretend to pour out tea, drink it, etc.?
iv.   Say to the child "Where's the light", or "Show me the
      light". Does the child point with his/her index finger at   Yes[3]   No
      the light?
v.   Can the child build a tower of bricks? (If so, how many?)   Yes   No
      (Number of bricks . . .)

1. To record yes on this item, ensure the child has not simply looked at your hand,
but has actually looked at the object you are pointing at.
2. If you can elicit an example of pretending in some other game, score a yes on
this item.
3. Repeat this with "Where's the teddy?" or some other unreachable object, if
child does not understand the word "light." To record yes on this item, the child
must have looked up at your face around the time of pointing.

REFERENCES

American Psychiatric Association (1987) *Diagnostic and Statistical Manual of Mental
    Disorders* (3rd ed., revised) (DSM-III-R). Washington, DC: APA.
Baron-Cohen, S. (1987) Autism and symbolic play. *British Journal of Developmental
    Psychology, 5*, 139–148.

————(1989) Perceptual role-taking and protodeclarative pointing in autism. *British Journal of Developmental Psychology, 7,* 113–127.

————(1991) Precursors to a theory of mind: understanding attention in others. In *Natural Theories of Mind* (ed. A. Whiten). Oxford: Basil Blackwell.

Butterworth, G. (1991) The ontogeny and phylogeny of joint visual attention. In *Natural Theories of Mind* (ed. A. Whiten). Oxford: Basil Blackwell.

Goodhart, F. & Baron-Cohen, S. (1992) How many ways can the point be made? Evidence from children with and without autism. Unpublished ms, Institute of Psychiatry, University of London.

Folstein, S. & Rutter, M. (1987) Autism: familial aggregation and genetic implications. *Journal of Autism and Developmental Disorders, 18,* 3–30.

Frith, U. & Baron-Cohen, S. (1987) Perception in autistic children. In *Handbook of Autism and Pervasive Developmental Disorders* (eds D. Cohen, A. Donnellan & R. Paul). New York: Wiley.

Gillberg, C., Steffenburg, S. & Schaumann, H. (1991) Is autism more common now than 10 years ago? *British Journal of Psychiatry, 158,* 403–409.

Leslie, A. M. (1991) The theory of mind deficit in autism: evidence for a modular mechanism of development. In *Natural Theories of Mind* (ed. A. Whiten). Oxford: Basil Blackwell.

Rutter, M. (1978) Diagnosis and definition. In *Autism: A Reappraisal of Concepts and Treatment* (eds M. Rutter & E. Schopler). New York: Plenum.

Sigman, M., Mundy, P., Ungerer, J., *et al* (1986) Social interactions of autistic, mentally retarded, and normal children and their caregivers. *Journal of Child Psychology and Psychiatry, 27,* 647–656.

Volkmar, F., Stier, D. & Cohen, D. (1985) Age of recognition of pervasive developmental disorders. *American Journal of Psychiatry, 142,* 1450–1452.

Wing, L. & Gould, J. (1979) Severe impairments of social interaction and associated abnormalities in children: epidemiology and classification. *Journal of Autism and Developmental Disorders, 9,* 11–29.

6

Development and Validation of the Preschool Socioaffective Profile

Peter J. La Frenière

University of Montréal

Montréal, Québec, Canada

Jean E. Dumas

Purdue University

West Lafayette, Indiana

France Capuano and Diane Dubeau

University of Montréal

Montréal, Québec, Canada

An analysis of the Preschool Socioaffective Profile (PSP) using a sample of 608 preschoolers revealed high internal consistency, interrater reliability, and stability for the 8 10-item scales and identified 3 coherent factors representing externalizing and internalizing behavior problems and social competence. Boys scored higher than girls on externalizing measures, but not on internalizing measures, which were largely orthogonal. PSP scores were correlated with Child Behavior Check List teacher ratings, and each scale was found to differentiate a clinical sample from the complete sample. Using a typological approach, the anxious-withdrawn group was found to be the

Reprinted with permission from *Psychological Assessment*, 1992, Vol. 4, 442–450. Copyright © 1992 by the American Psychological Association, Inc.

Funding was provided by the Social Sciences and Humanities Research Council of Canada, Grant 498-89-0028 and Fonds Pour la Formation de Chercheurs et l'Aide à la Recherche du Québec, Grant 90-ER-0168 to Peter J. La Frenière and Jean E. Dumas.

We thank our research assistants—in particular, Louise Beaudin, Catherine Gosselin, and Pierrette Verlaan—and the many devoted preschool teachers without whom this study would not have been possible.

A previous version of this article was presented at the Society for Research in Child Development Conference in April 1991.

least interactive with peers; the angry-aggressive group, the most interactive and most rejected; and the competent group, highest in sociometric status. Finally, substantial coherence was reported between laboratory observations of mother-child interaction and PSP classification.

The Preschool Socioaffective Profile (PSP) assesses characteristic patterns of affective expression, social competence, and adjustment difficulties of preschool children in interaction with peers and adults. The PSP was designed expressly for preschool teachers to enhance their understanding of the emotional and behavioral signals of adjustment difficulties to preschool life. Because many behavioral-emotional problems of early childhood are not often directly observed by psychiatrists or psychologists, it is important to obtain information from those people who observe children under conditions in which problems typically occur.

Our decision to create a new instrument was based on both clinical and research imperatives. From the standpoint of research potential, the PSP is intended to address an important issue in prospective longitudinal research of children at risk for later disorders. As research goals become more precise and investigators seek to understand both differential etiologies and sequelae of developmental disorders, greater precision, reliability, and discriminant validity will be required of measures used to evaluate various problem behaviors at various ages. Scales produced through factor-analytic techniques have inevitably yielded variables comprising unequal numbers of items, and quite different psychometric characteristics. Typically, a large first factor representing conduct disorder is found to be more internally consistent, reliable, and stable than a much smaller factor representing emotional disorder or anxiety (e.g., Behar & Stringfield, 1974; Hogan, Quay, Vaughn, & Shapiro, 1989). Subsequent comparisons demonstrating differences between scales in terms of etiological factors, temporal stability, or external correlates may be attributed to the initial differences in the psychometric characteristics of the scales rather than substantive differences in the phenomenon under investigation.

Our clinical objective is to describe behavioral tendencies for the purpose of socialization and education rather than classify children within diagnostic categories for the purpose of clinical intervention. One consequence of this orientation is our emphasis on assessing the overall quality of the child's adaptation, including social competence, allowing teachers to orient classroom intervention efforts toward the child's strengths as well as weaknesses. Second, this emphasis allows for a more refined description of developmental deviance by focusing on the presence or absence of positive behavior as well as problem behavior. Finally, this focus may also enhance prediction of later disorders because early investigators have reported better prediction from "indices of competence and ego maturity rather than the absence of problems and symptoms as such" (Kohlberg, LaCrosse, & Ricks, 1972, p. 1274).

In summary, the PSP was designed to meet the following criteria: (a) It should provide a standardized description of behavior in context that is reliable, valid, and useful for preschool teachers; (b) it should attempt to differentiate specific types of problems, in addition to global assessments; (c) it should provide an assessment of children's positive social adaptation or competence; (d) the measures derived from the instrument should yield variables of approximately equivalent internal consistency, reliability, and stability; and (e) measures should be sufficiently sensitive to behavioral change over time to evaluate short-term treatment outcomes.

CONCEPTUAL BASIS, STRUCTURE, AND ITEM SELECTION

We approached the task of constructing the PSP from a developmental-adaptational perspective, significantly influenced by ethologists and other social scientists who have emphasized the functional significance of affect in regulating social exchange (Bowlby, 1980; Ekman, 1984; Izard, 1977; Plutchik, 1980). From this perspective, emotions signal needs, attitudes, anticipations, and impulses toward action. Discrete, primary emotions, such as joy, love, anger, fear, and sadness, are evident in infancy and generally shared across cultures. They are widely recognized, not just as common verbal labels for emotional experience, but as core species-specific motivational systems that shape or organize both behavior and development across the life span (Fischer, Shaver, & Carnochan, 1990; Sroufe, 1979). Among preschool children, the expression of positive affect is associated with peer acceptance, leadership, and positive evaluations of social competence by teachers (La Frenière & Sroufe, 1985). Although negative affective displays may also be adaptive as social signals (Sroufe, Schork, Motti, Lawroski, & La Frenière, 1984), generalized and chronic anger, hostility, sadness, or anxiety more often indicate a poor quality of adaptation.

On the basis of this previous research, the target behaviors for the new instrument included emotional expression in social interaction with peers and adults, as well as expressions of characteristic emotion in a nonsocial context. Eight dimensions were identified as central to the quality of the child's adaptation to the preschool or daycare environment. For each of these dimensions, 10 items were written, 5 describing successful adjustment and 5 describing adjustment difficulties. Within the realm of emotional expression, unrelated to a specific interpersonal context, three scales were developed, defined by positive and negative poles: Joyful-Depressive, Secure-Anxious, and Tolerant-Angry. Likewise, three scales were developed to describe peer relations: Integrated-Isolated, Calm-Aggressive, and Prosocial-Egotistical. Finally, two scales were developed for assessing teacher-child relations: Cooperative-Oppositional and Autonomous-Dependent.

An initial pool of 80 items was pretested on a sample of 140 preschool children who ranged in age from 30 to 66 months (La Frenière, Dubeau, Janosz, & Capuano, 1990). Teachers made full use of the 6-point Likert scale on most items, with the exception of the items reflecting more severe disturbances (e.g., *takes pleasure in harming others*). Teacher evaluations were normally distributed for social competence items and positively skewed for emotional-behavioral problems. Variation was approximately equivalent across all eight scales.

Each of the eight scales clearly differentiated clinical from nonclinical samples, which must be considered a low hurdle in the validation process because our objective was to create an instrument sensitive to individual differences and behavioral change over time in a normal population. Nevertheless, this analysis establishes the first and most fundamental claim of validity: identifying the developmentally deviant child. Although all eight scales differentiated the two groups, it is interesting to note that among the broadband measures, the clinical group could best be identified by noting the relative absence of age-appropriate behaviors in the competence domain. On the basis of this pilot study's results, items were selectively revised to increase the interrater reliability and internal consistency of the scales while keeping the initial structure of the instrument intact.

STUDY 1

Method

Subjects. The sample consisted of 608 preschool children (282 girls, 326 boys) of French-Canadian background, recruited from 60 different preschool classrooms from the Montréal metropolitan area. Children ranged in age from 28 to 76 months at the start of data collection: The mean age of the girls was 49.3 months ($SD = 10.7$); that of the boys was 49.9 months ($SD = 10.4$).

Teacher evaluations. The children were evaluated by their two classroom teachers near the end of the fall session using the Preschool Socioaffective Profile (PSP). All children whose parents consented to their participation (70%) and who had been enrolled in the daycare for at least 2 months were evaluated. To provide a basis for concurrent validation of the PSP, the Child Behavior Checklist (CBCL; Edelbrock & Achenbach, 1984) was completed by teachers of 177 of the original 608 children. In these cases, parents had agreed to participate in a more detailed study. The Teacher Report Form (TRF) of the CBCL was chosen because of its reliability, validity, and widespread usage in research with school children. It consists of 20 social competence items and 118 behavior problem items, evaluated according to a 3-point scale. Because of the nature of the competence items (e.g., related to sports, hobbies, and clubs), this portion of the questionnaire was not scored by the preschool teachers. The 118 behavior problem items were scored using the norms for 6- to 11-year-olds because we wished to compare instruments appropriate for use by teachers. (Norms for 4- to 5-year-olds are available for the parental version only.)

Results

The *Results* section is organized with respect to the following topics: (a) reliability, internal consistency, and stability of the PSP; (b) factor structure; (c) effects of age, sex, and socioeconomic status (SES); and (d) concurrent validation vis-à-vis the CBCL.

Reliability, consistency, and stability of the PSP. Interrater reliability was calculated for each of the eight PSP scales using Spearman-Brown estimates based on correlations averaged across all classrooms combined. These reliability estimates were uniformly high, ranging from .72 to .89 as shown in Table 1. In addition, the internal consistency of each scale was assessed by Cronbach's alpha. Again the scales were all highly consistent, with scores ranging from .79 to .91.

Data on test-retest reliability are based on a subsample of 29 subjects who were selected at random and reevaluated by their teachers 2 weeks after the initial evaluation. Pearson correlations for the eight scales ranged from .74 to .87, whereas the scores, which are based on a larger pool of items, were slightly higher, ranging from .78 to .93.

Factor structure. On the basis of their high internal consistency, item-clusters (clusters of 5 positive or negative items associated with each scale) were selected as variables for a principal-components analysis, using varimax rotation procedures. This analysis confirmed the underlying structure of the PSP, yielding three principal factors, which accounted for 67.1% of the total variance. As shown in

TABLE 1
Interrater Reliability, Internal Consistency, and Temporal
Stability of Preschool Socioaffective Profile Scales

Scales	Interrater reliability	Cronbach's alpha	2-week stability
Depressive–Joyful	.84	.87	.80
Anxious–Secure	.85	.84	.76
Angry–Tolerant	.85	.89	.74
Isolated–Integrated	.89	.91	.87
Aggressive–Calm	.82	.89	.87
Egotistical–Prosocial	.72	.84	.83
Oppositional–Cooperative	.73	.85	.85
Dependent–Autonomous	.82	.79	.78

TABLE 2
Factor Structure of the Preschool Socioaffective Profile

Item clusters	Factor 1	Factor 2	Factor 3
Factor 1			
Joyful	.71	—	−.53
Secure	.64	—	−.61
Integrated	.68	—	−.56
Autonomous	.58	—	−.60
Tolerant	.71	−.55	—
Calm	.77	−.49	—
Prosocial	.81	−.39	—
Cooperative	.77	−.43	—
Factor 2			
Angry	—	.86	—
Aggressive	—	.83	—
Egotistical	—	.89	—
Oppositional	—	.83	—
Factor 3			
Depressive	—	—	.82
Anxious	—	—	.84
Isolated	—	—	.75
Dependent	—	.32	.75

Table 2, the first factor, designated *Social Competence*, comprised the eight positive item-clusters, with factor loadings ranging from .58 to .81. The second factor, labeled *Externalizing Behavior* comprised four negative item-clusters (angry, aggressive, egotistical, oppositional), with loadings ranging from .83 to .89. Finally, the third factor, *Internalizing Behavior*, comprised the remaining four negative item-clusters (depressed, anxious, isolated, dependent), with loadings ranging from .75 to .84.

Effects of gender, age, and SES. Sex differences were assessed for the eight PSP scales and the three factors mentioned above, and for a global score comprising all 80 items, labeled *General Adaptation*. Because multiple *t* tests (12) were conducted, Bonferroni corrections were applied, shifting the alpha level from .05 to .004.

As shown in Table 3, boys were assessed more negatively than girls for Externalizing Behavior (and each of the four scales associated with this factor), Social Competence, and General Adaptation. Boys were also assessed as being more anxious than their female peers, though no significant differences were found for the Joyful-Depressive, Integrated-Isolated, or Autonomous-Dependent scales, nor for the Internalizing factor itself.

Pearson correlations between age and PSP measures were computed for the total sample and for boys and girls separately. No sex differences in these corre-

TABLE 3
Sex Differences in Preschool Socioaffective Profile Scales and Scores

Measure	Girls (n = 282)		Boys (n = 326)		
	M	SD	M	SD	t
Scales					
Depressive–Joyful	2.41	1.3	2.10	1.3	2.90
Anxious–Secure	2.33	1.2	1.96	1.3	3.56*
Isolated–Integrated	2.08	1.4	1.97	1.4	0.91
Dependent–Autonomous	1.56	1.3	1.32	1.4	2.21
Angry–Tolerant	1.26	1.6	0.72	1.6	4.08*
Aggressive–Calm	2.08	1.4	1.22	1.5	7.34*
Egotistical–Prosocial	1.21	1.4	0.53	1.3	6.11*
Oppositional–Cooperative	2.52	1.3	1.96	1.4	5.03*
Scores					
Externalizing Behavior	2.15	0.7	2.44	0.8	4.83*
Social Competence	4.04	0.6	3.76	0.7	5.33*
General Adaptation	1.93	1.0	1.48	1.0	5.50*

*$p<.001$

lations were evident. For the sample as a whole, correlations with age varied from .07 to .16 across the eight scales. As expected, age was most highly correlated with the social competence index ($r = .20$, $df = 604$, $p < .001$) but was unrelated to internalizing ($r = -.07$) or externalizing behavior ($r = .01$). Considering that age explained between 0 and 4% of the total variance of the different PSP variables, separate age norms for preschoolers were deemed unnecessary when the age limits (30 to 76 months) of the instrument are respected. As other investigators have noted, teachers tend to evaluate each child with reference to his or her age group, thus minimizing the impact of this variable in preschool groups of children of similar age (Behar & Stringfield, 1974).

A composite score of SES indicators was derived by averaging the standardized scores for family income, parental education, and occupational prestige. This SES variable was found to be modestly correlated with PSP assessments, with the exception of Externalizing Behavior problems. Significant negative correlations were obtained for both Internalizing Behavior problems and Social Competence, with correlations for boys slightly higher than those of girls, though the latter difference was not significant. As expected, children from disadvantaged families showed somewhat more adjustment problems and less social competence than did peers from more affluent families.

Concurrent validation: Comparison of the PSP with the CBCL. Pearson correlations were computed for groups of boys and girls separately in order to compare both narrow- and broadband indexes of the two instruments. A summary of these analyses is shown in Table 4. No significant sex differences in correlations were obtained. A slightly higher degree of convergence was expected and obtained for Externalizing Behaviors, though this difference was slight when considering broadband measures. Among the three comparable narrow-band measures, Anxiety was the least convergent and presumably the most difficult dimension to reliably assess by teacher evaluations. One important difference between the pairs of broadband indexes concerns the degree of association between the two conceptually distinct constructs. As assessed by the CBCL, Externalizing and Internalizing problems tended to co-occur to a considerable extent, as reflected by a .60 correlation between the two measures. This aspect of the CBCL hinders developmental research designed to address questions of specific etiologies or consequences of these broadband disorders. In contrast, PSP measures of Internalizing and Externalizing behaviors were more orthogonal, $r = .28$, a difference that is statistically significant ($z = 5.33$, $df = 174$, $p < .001$).

Discussion

In this study, data were reported concerning the reliability and concurrent validity of the PSP. These initial results, although preliminary, are promising in both respects. Because revision of the PSP pilot items was based on their contribution to the internal consistency of their corresponding scale, it is not surprising that

TABLE 4

Correlations Between Profile Socioaffective Profile (PSP) and Child Behavior Checklist (CBCL) Measures for Boys and Girls

PSP/CBCL	Anxiety	Withdrawal	Aggression	Internalizing	Externalizing
Anxious					
Boys	.48***	.48***	.01	.52***	.15
Girls	.40***	.37***	.10	.43***	.19*
Isolated					
Boys	.51***	.58***	−.11	.59***	.03
Girls	.30**	.53***	−.01	.47***	.09
Aggressive					
Boys	−.12	−.10	.53***	−.11	.49***
Girls	−.01	−.08	.63***	−.04	.61***
Internalizing Behavior					
Boys	.57***	.60***	.13	.63***	.27**
Girls	.50***	.45***	.20*	.53***	.29**
Externalizing Behavior					
Boys	.00	−.07	.68***	−.03	.64***
Girls	−.03	−.20*	.71***	.12	.66***

* $p < .05$.   ** $p < .01$.   *** $p < .001$.

all eight scales show high internal consistency. Scales were balanced for positive (competence) and negative (emotional or behavior problems) items and covered an extensive array of typical behaviors within a preschool setting. A factor analysis clearly identified three factors: Social Competence, Externalizing Behavior, and Internalizing Behavior. The Social Competence factor comprises a broad range of items designed to assess the positive qualities of the child's adaptation rather than specific behavioral competencies. As a developmental construct, social competence refers to behaviors that indicate a well-adjusted, flexible, emotionally mature, and generally prosocial pattern of adaptation. Such children score high on assessments of ego resiliency, are well liked and sought out by their peers, and are appreciated by their teachers (La Frenière & Sroufe, 1985; Waters & Sroufe, 1983). The four item-clusters composing the second factor may be considered the preschool equivalent of previous broadband syndromes labeled variously as *conduct disorder* (Peterson, 1961; Quay, 1983) or *externalizing symptoms* (Achenbach & Edelbrock, 1981) and comprised items measuring angry, aggressive, selfish, and oppositional behaviors. The third factor is also composed of four item-clusters, comprising items measuring anxious, depressed, isolated, and overly dependent behavior. It is similar to previous broadband indexes labeled *affective disorder* or *internalizing symptoms*. This initial division between two broad types of disorder has been extensively verified for children in early and middle childhood and adolescence (Achenbach & Edelbrock, 1981; Behar & Stringfield, 1974; Kohn & Rossman, 1972; Peterson, 1961; Quay, 1983).

The hierarchical organization of the eight scales and the positive and negative valences embedded within each provide a flexible range of scores. The level of analysis that is most appropriate to the purpose at hand may be selected from the narrow-band profile of eight 10-item scales to the broadband measures of Social Competence (40 items), Internalizing Problems (20 items), Externalizing Problems, (20 items), and a Global score reflecting the child's quality of adaptation to the preschool environment (all 80 items).

As predicted, sex differences were striking for all externalizing dimensions but not for internalizing problems—with one exception. Boys were rated as more anxious than their female peers by their preschool teachers. This result suggests future lines of inquiry into the factors underlying the emergence of externalizing behavior problems in boys during the preschool period. Rather than viewing anxiety as a narrow-band component of the internalizing syndrome, anxiety may be an underlying component of both externalizing and internalizing problems in young children. Our current longitudinal research addresses this question concerning the role of early anxiety in the etiology of sexually differentiated expressions of child psychopathology.

Concurrent validity for the PSP must also be established by a direct comparison with previously validated instruments. Moderate convergence between the PSP and the CBCL for narrow-band and broadband measures has been demonstrated. We view this as an optimal result because lower correlations would raise legitimate questions of potential validity, whereas a pattern of correlations that is too high would undermine the rationale for a new instrument. We also view the significantly greater orthogonality of the PSP assessments of externalizing and internalizing behaviors as optimal for current research in developmental psychopathology investigating specific etiologies and sequelae of early patterns of disorder.

STUDY 2

To further establish the construct validity of the PSP, additional validation criteria were studied using a typological approach. Two external criteria were selected to provide dependent variables: direct observation of social participation and peer sociometrics. Although the former is mute with respect to the quality of peer behavior, it was selected to provide an objective, quantitative index of social withdrawal, hypothesized to differentiate angry-aggressive and anxious-withdrawn groups. Because of its external correlates indicating positive adaptation and independence, solitary play was not included in the index of passive withdrawal. Peer sociometrics were chosen to provide an intersubjective, qualitative index. Peer acceptance was hypothesized to differentiate the competent group from all other groups, whereas peer rejection was hypothesized to differentiate the angry-aggressive group from all other groups.

Construct validity of the PSP was further investigated by laboratory assessments of mother-child interaction in a problem-solving situation. We hypothesized that anxiety and withdrawal would interfere with the development and deployment of metacognitive skills, including the planning, monitoring, and outcome-checking skills involved in joint problem-solving. Specifically, we hypothesized that mothers of competent children, but not anxious children, would be more supportive and encouraging of their child's efforts to solve the problem. We also hypothesized that anxious-withdrawn children would be less likely to persist and more easily frustrated in their problem-solving attempts, and would be more likely to display negative affect and behaviors than the average or competent groups.

Method

Subjects. A random-stratified sample of 107 children was drawn from an initial sample of 608 preschool children of French-Canadian background recruited from 60 different preschool classrooms from the Montréal metropolitan area. This sample was selected on the basis of PSP scores derived from teacher evaluations as described below. Children (57 girls, 49 boys) ranged in age from 31 to 73 months at the start of data collection: The mean age of the girls was 49.3 months ($SD =$ 10.9); that of the boys was 48.7 months ($SD = 9.9$).

Teacher evaluations. The children were evaluated by their two classroom teachers near the end of the fall session using the PSP. All children whose parents consented to their participation (70%) and who had been enrolled in the daycare for at least 2 months were evaluated. Children were selected for participation in the larger study on the basis of their PSP classification. Children were classified as socially competent (S-C), angry-aggressive (A-A), or anxious-withdrawn (A-W) using standardized (Z) scores calculated for boys and girls separately. These groups were formed using cutoff points of 1.0 SD for each of the three factors, with the further criterion of a minimal difference of 0.5 SD scores for A-A and A-W. Finally, children whose scores were within 0.5 SD of the mean on all three scales were designated average (AV).

Peer sociometrics. Near the end of the fall or winter sessions, each child was administered a picture-sociometric interview. The interviews were conducted by the two classroom observers at the conclusion of the 1-month observational period. Each child began the interview by naming all of the children's photographs and then making three positive nominations, followed by a maximum of three negative nominations. The number of positive and negative nominations received by each child was then divided by the number of potential nominators, correcting for variations in group size.

Direct observation. Children were observed by teams composed of two different observers using a modified version of Parten's classification of social participation. An average of 50 focal-child 1-min time samples were collected on the participating children during periods of free play over a 1-month period. The predominant behavior occurring during the 1-min observational period was coded by the observer, who observed the children in the group in rotation. For the purposes of the present study, categories of noninteraction (unoccupied, onlooker, and parallel play) were combined. Solitary play was not included in this global category of noninteraction, because of its generally positive external correlates (Provost & La Frenière, 1991; Roper & Hinde, 1978). A team of six observers was trained to a criterion of 80% agreement and periodically retested throughout the period of data collection. Because only one observer at a time was permitted to enter the classroom, only those observers who maintained a minimum of 80% agreement on videotaped free play were responsible for the data collection. Their reliability, as assessed by the average correlation between all pairs of observers across all teams, was .78, $p < .001$.

Laboratory procedure. The mother-child dyads were greeted by research assistants on arrival and escorted to the laboratory testing room, where the "grocery store task," a paradigm recently developed by Gauvin and Rogoff (1989) and adapted by us for use with preschool children, was explained to them. The task consists of planning an efficient route through a miniature grocery store laid out as a board game on a surface of 71 x 61 cm. In the grocery store, 57 items are arranged on shelves on each side of three rows and along the inside of the four outer walls. On these 10 shelves are arranged miniature grocery items grouped according to the following categories: vegetables (5 items), fruit (6 items), meats (7 items), milk products (9 items), candy (4 items), baked goods (7 items), toiletries (10 items), and small jars and canned goods (9 items). After explaining the task to the child and the mother, the child was given a practice list of three items and asked to move a toy shopper through the grocery store to pick up the items on the list using the shortest possible route. Following the practice session, the experimenter made any necessary corrections and offered further explanations as needed. After ensuring that the child (and mother) understood the game, the experimenter presented the child with a different list of five items each on five separate trials but made no further interventions except to verify the child's recognition of the five items drawn on cards composing each "shopping list." After each list was completed, the children checked out their groceries using a Fisher-Price toy register. Mothers were instructed to assist the child as needed in the completion of the game for the first three shopping lists. After three lists were completed (or in some cases, after 18 min, even if the lists were not completed), the mother was asked to complete a task on an adjacent computer. The child continued the grocery store task alone with the understanding that at any time the mother could assist the child or the child could ask for help as needed. In general, children found the task entertaining and shopped enthusiastically.

Laboratory observations. Mother-child interactions during the grocery store task were videotaped through a one-way mirror and later coded with the INTERACT coding system, a real-time microcomputer coding system (Dumas, 1987). The systems consist of five categories of codes (actor, behavior, setting, adverb, and valences) that are combined to form discrete observation strings. Following each observation, all raw data were stored on a desktop computer for later clean up, verification, and analysis.

For the purpose of this study, individual behavior codes were collapsed to form clusters of mother and child behaviors: (a) *positive* behavior, which consisted of laughter, helping, approving, and affectionate behavior; (b) *negative* behavior, which consisted of critical, punishing, disapproving, or aggressive behavior; (c) *controlling* behavior, which consisted of commands and physical intrusions; (d) *positive affect*, which consisted of the expression of positive emotions (e.g., loud or sarcastic tone of voice) that accompanied any coded behavior. Each cluster was then calculated separately for mother and child.

The reliability of the coding categories was assessed by requiring two graduate students to code 75% of the observations simultaneously but independently. Cohen's kappa was subsequently computed for each of the clusters described above. Results show that interobserver agreement (corrected for chance agreement) averaged .89 for behavior clusters and .70 for affective clusters.

Results

Using the PSP classification system, one-way analyses of variance (ANOVAs) for the four comparison groups (socially competent, average, angry-aggressive, and anxious-withdrawn) were computed for the dependent variables described above, with appropriate contrasts for group comparisons. These results are organized according to the following sets of dependent variables: (a) naturalistic observation of passive withdrawal, (b) sociometric assessments of peer acceptance and peer rejection; (c) laboratory observation of children's positive and negative affect and behavior; and (d) laboratory observation of mothers' positive and negative affect and behavior.

As predicted, the anxious-withdrawn (A-W) group spent the most time in noninteraction (34%) compared with 18% for the angry-aggressive group (A-A), a difference that was statistically significant, $F(3,97) = 4.79, p < .01$. In addition, the A-W group was significantly less interactive than both the SC (24%) and AV (25%) groups ($p < .05$).

The overall ANOVA for peer acceptance was not significant, $F(3,173) = 1.93$, $p = .128$. Only the a priori contrast between SC (60%) and A-A (38%) was significant ($p < .05$). One probable reason for the lack of discrimination for this variable is the relatively small size of the classroom groups. Because of the well-known tendency for young children to nominate same-sex classmates as preferred partners, most children received nominations from nearly all of their same-sex peers. In contrast, the average percentage of negative nominations received is less than half as great because, for ethical reasons, we did not insist on three negative nominations. As a result, the one-way ANOVA for peer rejection is more discriminating, $F(3,173 = 6.83, p < .001$, with A-A significantly higher (30%) and SC (13%) significantly lower than the two intermediate groups (A-W, 22%; AV, 23%).

As shown in Table 5, PSP classification was strongly predictive of the child's affective expression when collaborating with the mother on the grocery store task but less predictive of behavioral measures. Significant group differences were obtained for child positive and negative affect, and controlling behaviors. Subsequently, appropriate a priori contrasts were calculated. As expected, the S-C group expressed significantly more positive affect during the task than did all other groups ($p < .05$). The A-W group expressed significantly more negative affect than did all other groups ($p < .05$) and behaved in a more controlling fashion toward their mothers than did either the SC or AV groups ($p < .05$).

Similar analyses of maternal behavior revealed even more pronounced group

TABLE 5

Child Affect and Behavior in the Laboratory Situation as a Function of
Preschool Socioaffective Profile Classification

Behavior	PSP classification				$F(3, 103)$
	SC	AV	A-A	A-W	
Positive affect	.15	.03	.05	.02	6.42**
Positive behavior	.12	.16	.06	.08	2.49
Negative affect	.04	.02	.03	.13	5.07**
Negative behavior	.08	.08	.04	.10	0.86
Controlling behavior	.07	.08	.12	.18	2.89*

Note. SC = socially competent; AV = average; A-A = angry–aggressive; A-W = anxious–withdrawn.
* $p < .05$. ** $p < .01$.

differences, as shown in Table 6. Mothers of the SC group engaged in significantly more positive behaviors than did those in all other groups ($p < .05$) and were more expressive of positive affect than was the AV group ($p < .05$). In stark contrast, mothers of the A-W group expressed significantly more negative affect ($p < .05$) and were significantly more controlling of their child than were those in all other groups ($p < .05$). In addition, these mothers directed significantly more negative behaviors to their child than did the SC or AV groups ($p < .05$). It is not surprising that the expression of negative affect was relatively rare or completely absent during the grocery game for most mothers and children. However, A-W children and their mothers expressed four and six times more negative affect, respectively, than did those in all other groups.

TABLE 6

Maternal Affect and Behavior in the Laboratory Situation as a Function of
Child's Preschool Socioaffective Profile (PSP) Classification

Behavior	PSP classification				$F(3, 103)$
	SC	AV	A-A	A-W	
Positive affect	.15	.04	.10	.07	2.94*
Positive behavior	.15	.10	.10	.07	4.12**
Negative affect	.01	.02	.03	.12	6.93**
Negative Behavior	.01	.02	.02	.04	3.01**
Controlling behavior	.14	.20	.20	.33	8.93**

Note SC = socially competent this is line one
sive: A-W = anxious withdrawn.
* $p<.05$ ** $p<.01$

Discussion

In Study 2 the PSP was used to recruit a stratified random subsample of the initial sample for more extensive testing. Two well-known and methodologically independent assessments were chosen as validation criteria: observation of social participation and peer sociometrics. These external criteria provide further evidence of construct validity of the PSP; it is also important that they clearly differentiated the anxious-withdrawn and angry-aggressive groups. As predicted, the anxious-withdrawn group was observed to be significantly less interactive than all other groups, though not necessarily neglected or rejected by their peers. More than those in all other groups, they spent time in activities on the periphery of group life, such as onlooking and parallel play, and were also more prone to be alone and unoccupied. It is significant that their anxiety was not expressed through solitary play, which might be more aptly named *independent play*, because this behavior seems reflective of positive qualities distinct from social withdrawal (Roper & Hinde, 1978).

In contrast, the angry-aggressive group was the most interactive with peers and also the most rejected. These results correspond precisely with theoretical and empirical expectations. Because high aggression and hyperactivity co-occur in young children, particularly boys, factor-analytic studies often result in a single large factor, Aggressive-Hyperactive, rather than two distinct factors (e.g., Behar & Stringfield, 1974). In addition, aggression is one of the principal correlates of rejection in the preschool peer group (La Frenière & Sroufe, 1985).

The socially competent group received the most positive nominations and the least negative nominations, and was significantly higher in sociometric status (positive minus negative nominations) than all other groups. Because of its qualitative dimension, sociometric status is one of the most robust correlates of teacher ratings of social competence in preschoolers (La Frenière & Sroufe, 1985). Regarding sociometric status, the average group represented an intermediate point between the socially competent and the angry-aggressive groups. Together, this pattern of results provides a sound basis for continuing to refine the PSP and extending the validation process.

GENERAL DISCUSSION

These initial analyses of the PSP demonstrated high internal consistency, reliability, and stability of PSP scales and identified three coherent factors representing externalizing and internalizing behavior problems and social competence. Concurrent validation of the PSP is established by substantial correlations with CBCL-TRF ratings and the ability of each scale to differentiate a smaller clinical sample from the complete sample. Construct validity was further demonstrated with respect to classroom social participation and peer sociometrics using a typological approach. The anxious-withdrawn group was found to be the least interactive with peers, and the angry-aggressive group, the most interactive and most rejected; the socially competent group was highest in sociometric status. Moreover, the externalizing and internalizing dimensions were largely orthogonal, with boys scoring higher than girls on externalizing but not internalizing measures.

In addition to the issues of reliability and validity, substantive issues were addressed concerning the consistency of behavior problems in the family and daycare settings and the conjunction of mother-child and peer relations. In a dyadic problem-solving game situation, mothers of anxious-withdrawn children expressed more negative affect and behaved in a more negative, controlling manner than did mothers of all other groups. Reciprocally, anxious-withdrawn children expressed more negative affect and engaged their mothers in a battle for control of the game more often than did those in all other groups. In contrast, socially competent children were found to express more positive affect in the grocery store task and their mothers engaged in more positive, supportive behavior than did those in all other groups, expressing more positive affect than shown by the mothers of those in the normative group. From a developmental perspective, these results suggest that affective dimensions of early childhood are coherent between the child's life in the family and the daycare, and that unresolved issues of anxiety-security covary with difficulty in resolving issues of autonomy within the mother-child dyad and beyond it.

In conclusion, although these results do not terminate the validation process, they do serve to extend it, particularly with respect to measures of early anxiety and social competence. In future work we plan to continue this process of validation in reference to variables in the cognitive domain that are not hypothesized to relate to PSP variables and to expand the nomological network of social competence as a developmental construct. Longitudinal data that are at present being collected and analyzed will be used to respond to fundamental questions concerning the stability of early measures of competence and behavioral problems. Finally, we are currently exploring the validity and utility of a short form of the PSP for use with extensive samples. This work involves the application of the instrument to a sample of American children, for which separate norms will be developed if necessary.

Clinical Applications

The PSP is intended to assist teachers in their understanding of the strengths and weaknesses of a child's social adaptation to the preschool milieu and to empower them in their efforts to provide timely, developmentally sensitive care in their classroom. As with most instruments of this genre, at no time should the PSP be used as the sole basis for any clinical decision regarding intervention with the child. Rather, interpretations based on the profile should be viewed as hypotheses that require further corroboration from other data sources and the exercise of sound professional judgment. It is certainly not our intention that the PSP be used to label children or as the basis for their removal from their group. In our view, no instrument should serve this function at the preschool level.

Because of the level of behavioral specificity of the items and the greater number of scale points, teachers' descriptions rely on careful, accurate, and extensive observation of the child's behavior within the preschool setting. That the quality of the teacher's observation is the key to description and evaluation cannot be overstressed. It has been our practice to provide teachers with the list of items in order to become familiar with the relevant concepts and behavioral descriptors encoded within the instrument. This permits teachers to target specific behaviors of interest and to standardize to some extent the quality of observation across different teachers prior to evaluation. In addition, teachers should not attempt to use the instrument to describe the behavior of children who have recently arrived (less than 2 months) or who participate in the program on a very limited basis (2 days per week or less). These constraints are suggested for two reasons. First, most children need a period of time to adjust to a new setting or new group of peers. Research has shown that expressive and social behavior of preschool children undergoes significant change over the first month after entering a new group (McGrew, 1972). Second, our own research has shown that teachers need time to observe the child in a variety of situations before they begin to converge in their independent descriptions of an individual child. This is particularly true for teachers who begin the fall with a large group of new faces. In such instances we typically allow 3 months before asking teachers to provide a description based on the PSP. Finally, because of the complexity of computerized scoring of the PSP, as well as our own need to develop norms based on large numbers of children, we request that those who wish to make use of this instrument contact us for further information.

REFERENCES

Achenbach, T. M., & Edelbrock, C. S. (1981). Behavioral problems and competencies reported by parents of normal and disturbed children aged four through sixteen. *Monographs of the Society for Research in Child Development, 46*(no. 1).

Behar, L., & Stringfield, S. (1974). A behavior rating scale for the preschool child. *Developmental Psychology, 10*, 601–610.

Bowlby, J. (1980). *Attachment and loss. Vol. 3: Loss.* New York: Basic Books.

Dumas, J. E. (1987). Interact: A computer-based coding and data management system to assess family interactions. *Advances in Behavioral Assessment of Children and Families, 3*, 177–202.

Edelbrock, C., & Achenbach, T. M. (1984). The teacher version of the child behavior profile: I. Boys aged 6–11. *Journal of Consulting and Clinical Child Psychology, 52*, 207–217.

Ekman, P. (1984). Expression and the nature of emotion. In K. R. Scherer & P. Ekman (Eds.), *Approaches to emotion* (pp. 319–344). Hillsdale, NJ: Erlbaum.

Fischer, K. W., Shaver, P. R., & Carnochan, P. (1990). How emotions develop and how they organize development. *Cognition and Emotion, 4*(2), 81–127.

Gauvin, M., & Rogoff, B. (1989). Collaborative problem solving and children's planning skills. *Developmental Psychology, 25*, 139–151.

Hogan, A. E., Quay, H. C., Vaughn, S., & Shapiro, S. K. (1989). Revised Behavior Problem Checklist: Stability, prevalence, and incidence of behavior problems in kindergarten and first-grade children. *Psychological Assessment, 1*, 103–111.

Izard, C. E. (1977). *Human emotions*. New York: Plenum Press.

Kohn, M., & Rossman, B. L. (1972). A social competence scale and symptom checklist for the preschool child: Factor dimensions, their cross-instrument generality, and longitudinal persistence. *Developmental Psychology, 6*, 430–444.

Kohlberg, L., LaCrosse, J., & Ricks, D. (1972). The predictability of adult mental health from childhood behavior. In B. B. Wolman (Ed.), *Manual of Child Psychopathology*. New York: McGraw-Hill.

La Frenière, P. J., Dubeau, D., Janosz, M., & Capuano, F. (1990). Profil socio-affectif de l'enfant d'âge préscolaire [Socio-affective profile of preschool children]. *Revue Canadienne de Psycho-Education, 19*(1), 23–41.

La Frenière, P. J., & Sroufe, L. A. (1985). Profiles of peer competence in the preschool: Interrelations between measures, influence of social ecology, and relation to attachment history. *Developmental Psychology, 21*, 56–69.

McGrew, W. C. (1972). *An ethological study of children's behavior*. New York: Academic Press.

Peterson, D. R. (1961). Behavior problems of middle childhood. *Journal of Consulting Psychology, 25*, 205–209.

Plutchik, R. (1980). *Emotion: A psychoevolutionary synthesis*. New York: Harper & Row.

Provost, M., & La Frenière, P. J. (1991). Social participation and peer competence in preschool children: Evidence for discriminant and convergent validity. *Child Study Journal, 21*(1), 57–72.

Quay, H. C. (1983). A dimensional approach to behavior disorder: The revised Behavior Problem Checklist. *School Psychology Review, 12*, 244–249.

Roper, R., & Hinde, R. A. (1978). Social behavior in a play group: Consistency and complexity. *Child Development, 49*, 570–579.

Sroufe, L. A. (1979). Socioemotional development. In J. Osofsky (Ed.), *Handbook of infant development* (pp. 462–515). New York: Wiley.

Sroufe, L. A., Schork, E., Motti, F., Lawroski, N., & La Frenière, P. J. (1984). The role of affect in social competence. In C. E. Izard, J. Kagan, & R. Zajonc (Eds.),

Emotions, cognition and behavior. Cambridge, England: Cambridge University Press.

Waters, E., & Sroufe, L. A. (1983). A developmental perspective on competence. *Developmental Review, 3,* 79–97.

APPENDIX
Sample Items of the Preschool Socioaffective Profile

Social Competence

1. Negotiates solutions to conflicts with other children
2. Cooperates with other children in group activities
3. Comforts or assists another child in difficulty
4. Attentive towards younger children
5. Works easily in group

Anxiety-Withdrawal

1. Maintains neutral facial expression (does not smile or laugh)
2. Timid, afraid (e.g., avoids new situations)
3. Inhibited or uneasy in the group
4. Inactive, watches the other children play
5. Goes unnoticed in a group

Anger-Aggression

1. Gets angry when interrupted
2. Irritable, gets mad easily
3. Forces other children to do things they do not want to do
4. Opposes the teacher's suggestions
5. Defiant when reprimanded

7

A "Common-Language" Version of the California Child Q-Set for Personality Assessment

Avshalom Caspi

University of Wisconsin, Madison

Jack Block and Jeanne H. Block

University of California, Berkeley

Brett Klopp, Donald Lynam, and Terrie E. Moffitt

University of Wisconsin, Madison

Magda Stouthamer-Loeber

Western Psychiatric Institute

University of Pittsburgh

J. Block and J. H. Block's (1980) California Child Q-Set (CCQ), a unique instrument used by professional observers to assess children's personalities, has contributed important information about the nature of personality development. The authors of this article introduce language-simplifying modifications to the items in the original CCQ for this assessment procedure to be used with a wide range of nonprofessional observers (e.g., parents with little formal education). Reliability and validity assessments show that the "common-

Reprinted with permission from *Psychological Assessment*, 1992, Vol. 4(4), 512–523. Copyright © 1992 by the American Psychological Association, Inc.

This work was supported by several agencies: the Antisocial and Violent Behavior Branch of the National Institute of Mental Health (NIMH; Grant MH44548 to Terrie Moffitt); the University of Wisconsin Graduate School; the McArthur Foundation—National Institute of Justice Program on Human Development and Criminal Behavior; and the Office of Juvenile Justice and Delinquency Prevention, Office of Justice Programs, U.S. Department of Justice (Grant 86—JN-CX-0009 to Rolf Loeber and Magda Stouthamer-Loeber). Avshalom Caspi was supported by a Spencer Fellowship from the National Academy of Education. Jack Block was supported by NIMH Grant MH16080.

Points of view or opinions in this document are those of the authors and do not necessarily represent the official position or policies of the U.S. Department of Justice.

language" version of the CCQ can be used with lay persons to yield reliable, valid, and valuable information about the links between personality functioning and problems in adaptive functioning in diverse populations.

Responding to a need for a flexible but clinically rich assessment tool that can be used in diverse populations and with multiple informants and observers, we developed a "common-language" Q-sort, a modification and adaptation of J. Block and J. H. Block's (1969, 1980) observer-based instrument for describing the personality styles of children. The purpose of this article is to introduce the modified version of the California Q-set (CCQ) to researchers and clinicians who may then choose to use it in their own research programs when lay persons must provide the observations desired.

Although there are a number of instruments for the assessment of children's social and emotional adjustment (e.g., Achenbach & Edelbrock, 1983; Quay & Peterson, 1983), these are primarily concerned with behavior problems and dimensions of psychopathology (Martin, 1988). Many other instruments are devoted to assessing temperamental variations (Goldsmith & Rothbart, 1991), but there are few clinically rich instruments that capture and reflect the wide variations of children's personalities, their characteristic ways of approaching and responding to the social world, their distinctive styles of coping with uncertainty and ambiguity, their strengths and weaknesses, resources and vulnerabilities, and competencies and inadequacies (Earls & McGuire, 1991).

A major exception is the CCQ. This age-appropriate counterpart of the adult California Q-set (CAQ; Block, 1961/1978) contains a set of 100 statements describing a wide range of personality, cognitive, and social attributes. The CCQ-set does not represent any one theoretical viewpoint; it reflects a general language for describing variations in children's personalities and has proven valuable in different research settings (J. Block & J. H. Block, 1980).

But the CCQ, as currently constituted, although useful when professional observers are available, is limited in its applications because the psychological vocabulary of the Q-sort may be too complex when lay observers must be used. We set out to construct a modified set of items that can be used with a wide range of nonprofessional observers (e.g., parents with little formal education). In this article, we describe the development of the modified instrument and present evidence relating to its validity using data collected on over 400 children in the Pittsburgh Youth Study.

Q-METHODOLOGY

Q-sorting involves a set of rules for assigning scores to a set of items from a descriptive item pool, or Q-set. The observer or judge's task is to sort the items into a forced, nine-category distribution that ranges from *extremely uncharacteristic or negatively salient* (1) to *extremely characteristic or salient* (9) of the child judged. The remaining cards are distributed in intermediate piles, with those items that seem *neither characteristic nor uncharacteristic* of the person going into the middle pile (5). The Q-sort method offers several advantages in psychological and psychiatric research (Block, 1961/1978; Ozer, in press).

1. The Q-Sort Method Is an Ipsative Approach That Represents the Configuration of Personality Variables Within the Individual.

The Q-sort produces an ipsative or person-centered description, because the sorter explicitly compares each attribute with other attributes within the same individual. For example, placing the item "is cheerful" in the most descriptive pile of cards implies that, compared with other traits, cheerfulness stands out as uniquely salient within this individual's personality. In contrast, standard rating scales produce variable-centered descriptions because the rater implicitly compares the individual with other individuals on each attribute; a rating of "very cheerful" implies that the individual is very cheerful compared with other individuals. The ipsative approach is thus consistent with Allport's (1937) claim that personality should be described intra- rather than inter-individually. It provides an approach in which the person, not the variable, is the focus of analysis (see Bem, 1983).

Among the advantages enjoyed by the ipsative Q-sort method are these four: (a) the significance of the particular behavior (item) being described is generally distinguished from the frequency of that behavior (item); (b) sorters generally remain unaware of the particular constructs that will be scored from the information they provide; (c) response biases are reduced by the fixed distribution because this procedural step brings the judgments of different sorters into metrical equivalence; and (d) sorters make comparisons of characterological qualities within a person rather than comparisons between persons with regard to various qualities (Block, 1957; Moskowitz, 1986; Waters, Noyes, Vaughn, & Ricks, 1985). These features may be helpful in developmental research on psychopathology as well as in research with minority populations. When we use conventional rating procedures, we assume that raters are knowledgeable about the norms for each item they are rating—not so in Q-methodology. Because sample norms are not involved in making Q-ratings, it is easier to compare different samples and also to merge samples.

2. The Q-Sort Can Be Used With Different Raters as Well as in Different Research Contexts.

Q-sorting has been done by clinicians on the basis of archival records (e.g., Block, 1971), by teachers (e.g., Funder, Block, & Block, 1983), parents (e.g., Mischel, Shoda, & Peake, 1988; Waters & Deane, 1985), examiners (e.g., Block, Block, & Keyes, 1988), observers (e.g., Renken et al., 1989), and subjects themselves and their acquaintances (e.g., Funder & Colvin, 1988). However, in these various research contexts, the sorters have been well educated. Hence the need for a simpler, common-language version of this flexible instrument when lay populations of less intelligence and education must be used.

3. The Q-Sort Provides a Descriptive Personality Profile That Can Be Used to Assess a Variety of Personality Constructs.

A perennial difficulty in longitudinal research is that, with hindsight, investigators realize they have overlooked some critical individual difference variable. The Q-sort is valuable because it provides a descriptive personality profile that can be used to assess a variety of personality variables that were not assessed directly during data collection.

As initially proposed by Block (1957), this can be accomplished by first preparing a hypothetical Q-sort that describes a desired personality type and then correlating each individual's Q-sort with the hypothetical template. The resulting correlations are descriptive indexes of similarity between two Q-sort characterizations, with possible values ranging from -1 (complete dissimilarity) to $+1$ (complete similarity). Conceptually, these correlations reflect the degree to which the salience and organization of attributes within each individual resemble the criterion definition of a particular personality type.

Using this method of criterion sorting, it is possible to derive scores for personality variables that were not conceived when the initial data were collected. Although for some variables the standard language of the Q-set may prove inadequate, this general method lends itself to valid applications in costly longitudinal research.

4. The Q-Sort Method Yields Information That Is Amenable to Different Types of Data-Analytic Strategies.

As we have just seen, each individual's Q-sort can be "scored" by correlating it with a criterion profile. Other data-analytic strategies include the following:
1. Cluster analysis of persons. We can correlate the Q-sort profiles of individuals in the sample and subject these to cluster analysis to produce an empirically

derived typology of personality (e.g., Block, 1971; York & John, 1992; Ozer & Gjerde, 1989).

2. Factor analysis of items. Although the Q-sort is an ipsative assessment procedure, ipsative ratings can be factor analyzed to yield meaningful psychological portraits of children and adults (e.g., Shedler & Block, 1990).

3. A priori scale construction. Items that are thought to tap a particular construct can be averaged to create scales for use in later analyses (Renken et al., 1989).

4. Item analysis. It is often desirable to wend one's way through the clinical thicket of the 100 Q-items and to draw detailed portraits of particular persons or groups. For example, careful item analysis of the CCQ may help to reveal subtle distinctions between correlated variables (e.g., Block & Gjerde, 1986).

PHASE 1: CONSTRUCTION OF THE "COMMON-LANGUAGE" Q-SORT

To construct a simpler version of the CCQ, we translated the psychological vernacular of this instrument to ordinary, everyday language. We accomplished this by (a) rewriting difficult Q-items, (b) establishing the readability level of the modified Q-items, and (c) safeguarding against possible distortion of the original item pool.

Rewriting Difficult Q-Items

Members of our research team independently identified difficult CCQ items and rewrote them using simpler language. The rewritten items were compiled alongside the original items and distributed to (a) psychologists with experience using the CCQ, (b) psychologists with experience working with disadvantaged and minority populations, and (c) field workers from the Pittsburgh Youth Study.[1] The judges read the items and (a) assessed whether the modifications distorted the original items, (b) determined which items were too difficult for lay observers, and (c) contributed refinements to a penultimate version of the modified item set.

To further refine the modified Q-set, we recruited through state social service agencies a group of 27 women that was composed of Blacks and Whites. None of the women had attended college, and a majority had not completed high school. Each woman Q-sorted one of her children who was between 9 and 15 years of age and served as an informant, alerting us to problems with the items. Notes were taken, and the sessions were followed by a review period in which the participants offered criticisms and suggestions. Members of our research team reexamined the revisions and convened to make final decisions. A total of 89 items were modified

[1] For their suggestions, comments, and refinements, we thank Daryl Bem, Patsy Byers, Betty Black, Inge Bretherton, Rosemary Costanzo, David Funder, Deb Johnson, Fred Meyers, Mary Neid, Dan Ozer, Dave Riley, and Michael Thornton.

into language that was easier to understand. Table 1 provides examples of some original CCQ descriptive statements alongside their modified counterparts.

Readability of the Q-Sort

To assess the readability level of the CCQ, we relied on the Harris and Jacobson (1982) Wide Range Readability Formula, which uses two variables to calculate the readability level of a written text: the percentage of difficult words and sentence length. For this analysis we treated each Q-item as a passage.

As shown in Column 1 of Table 2, our analysis yielded an overall reading level of greater than (Grade) 11.3 for the CCQ. In contrast, the modified common-language version yielded an overall reading level of (Grade) 4.8. In fact, the modified version's reading level resembles the reading level of many self-report measures designed for use with child and adolescent populations (e.g., Prout & Chizik, 1988).

Table 2 also shows the number of items that contained at least one word above specified grade levels (Harris & Jacobson, 1982). Only 7% of the items in the original version were below the 4th grade reading level. In contrast, 43% of the items in the modified version were below this grade of reading level. Similarly, 36% of the items in the original version were above the 8th grade reading level. In contrast, only 6% of the items in the modified version contained a word above the 8th grade reading level (Items 12, 17, 56, 57, 63, and 91).

TABLE 1
Illustrations of Original and Modified California Child Q-Set

Original	Modified
Has transient interpersonal relationships; is fickle.	His friendships don't last long; he changes friends a lot.
Shows a recognition of the feelings of others; is empathic.	He is able to see how others feel; he can put himself in their place.
Tends to become rigidly repetitive or immobilized when under stress.	He freezes up when things are stressful, or else he keeps doing the same thing over and over.
Becomes anxious when the environment is unpredictable or poorly structured.	He gets nervous if he's not sure what's going to happen or when it's not clear what he's supposed to do.
Tries to manipulate others by ingratiation (e.g., by charm, coyness, or seductiveness).	He tries to get others to do what he wants by playing up to them. He acts charming in order to get his way.

TABLE 2
Readability and Grade Levels for Items and Words in the Original
and Modified California Child Q-Set (CCQ)

CCQ version	Overall readability level	Number of items	Number of items with words at or above grade					
			4	5	6	7	8	>8
California Child Q-Set	>11.3[a]	100	93	86	72	65	53	36
Common-Language Child Q-Set	4.8	100	57	46	29	20	11	6

[a] The Harris-Jacobson (1982) table for converting raw scores to readability scores extends to a raw score of 8.0, which corresponds to a readability score of 11.3. The raw score of the CCQ was 9.70. It is thus fair to suggest that the CCQ readability score reported in this table greatly underestimates the reading level required for using the CCQ.

Assessing the Reliability and Structural Equivalence of the Common-Language Q-Set

We carried out a series of small alternate-form reliability studies to examine the structural equivalence of the two CCQ versions. The research question was whether the similarity between raters using different versions of the CCQ resembled the similarity between raters using the same, original version of the CCQ. If we did not distort the original item pool, we should find that agreement between raters when each uses the original and modified version of the CCQ to describe a child is similar to agreement between raters when each uses the original CCQ item set to describe that child.

Parent study. We recruited eight intact families, each with 2 children between 5 and 15 years of age. The first child in each family was sorted independently by each parent using the original item set. The second child in each family was sorted independently by one parent using the original item set and by the second parent using the modified item set. (The reliability evaluation was thus based on 32 Q-sorts.)

We averaged the two Q-sort formulations available for each child to form a composite Q-sort description. The estimated item reliability for the mother-father composite, based on interrater correlations for each of the 100 original CCQ items, was .51. (This is similar to interrater correlations reported in other research using Q-sorts by parents; e.g., Shoda et al., 1990, reported average reliabilities of .59.) The estimated item reliability for the mother-father composite, based on interrater correlations for each of the 100 original and modified items, was .56. It is apparent that agreement between parents when using the original and modified versions of the CCQ is similar to their agreement when using the original version only.

Teacher study. We recruited three teachers and six student-teachers from a university preschool. Each teacher Q-sorted three children, each between 4 and 6 years old, using different versions of the CCQ. (This reliability evaluation was thus based on 27 Q-sorts.) This design enabled us to calculate agreement between teachers when using the original CCQ as well as when using the common-language Q-set. In addition, we could calculate agreement between teachers when using the original and modified Q-sets.

We averaged the multiple Q-sort formulations available for each child to form a composite Q-sort description. The estimated item reliability of the composite of three teachers, based on interrater correlations for each of the 100 original CCQ items, was .71. (This is similar to interrater correlations reported in other research using Q-sorts by research examiners; e.g., Funder & Block, 1989, reported average reliabilities of .72.) The estimated item reliability of the composite description of three teachers, based on interrater correlations for each of the 100 modified items, was .72. Likewise, the estimated item reliability of the composite description of three teachers, based on interrater correlations of each of the 100 original and modified items, was .72. It appears that teacher agreement when using the modified and original version of the CCQ is similar to teacher agreement when using only the modified or original versions of the CCQ.

Expert study. We obtained criterion definitions of the construct of antisocial behavior from seven clinical psychology Ph.D. students and doctoral-level professionals. Each expert constructed two Q-sort profiles of an antisocial adolescent male between 12 and 14 years old using the original and modified CCQ, respectively. The order in which the profiles were constructed was randomly determined, and they were completed several months apart.

This design, based on 14 Q-sorts, enabled us to calculate agreement within raters as they used the two Q-sets to make clinical judgments. The estimated item reliability of these Q-sorts, based on correlations between each of the 100 original and 100 modified CCQ items, was .82, which suggests that experts treat the items from the two versions of the CCQ similarly when making clinical judgments.

In summary, the reliability of the common-language version of the CCQ is similar to the reliability of the original version and appears adequate for research. In addition, evidence from three studies of parents, teachers, and experts favors the hypothesis that the two CCQ versions are structurally equivalent.

PHASE 2: VALIDATION OF THE COMMON-LANGUAGE Q-SORT

In this phase, we sought to determine the validity of the modified CCQ when used with a wide range of lay observers. We conducted this evaluation as part of the Pittsburgh Youth Study, which offers a large sample of children from varied social and ethnic backgrounds with considerable diversity in behavioral functioning. This study is limited to boys.

Method

Subjects. The sample was randomly selected from 4th grade boys enrolled in public schools in Pittsburgh, Pennsylvania. An initial screening assessment of the sample took place in the spring of 1987 ($N = 149$) and the spring of 1988 ($N = 619$). The boys and one of their principal caregivers (usually the mother) were separately interviewed in the home in such a way that they could not overhear each other. The interview in the home usually lasted less than an hour. The overall cooperation rate of the children and their caregivers was 84.7% (Loeber, Stouthamer-Loeber, Van Kammen, & Farrington, 1989).

The interview for the boys was the Self-Reported Antisocial Behavior Scale (SRA; Loeber et al., 1989). The main caregiver was given the Child Behavior Checklist (Achenbach & Edelbrock, 1983). In addition, the boys' teachers completed the Child Behavior Checklist (Edelbrock & Achenbach, 1986).

The information provided by the three informants was used to rank the boys on antisocial and delinquent acts. Boys ranking in the top 30% were retained in the study, together with an additional 30% randomly selected from the remainder. This led to a sample of 508 boys to be continued in the study. Since the study's inception, the sample has been reduced to 484 subjects (4.7% attrition).

The mean age for the 4th graders was 10.2 at the time of the first interview. After screening, the percentage of Black boys was 53.5. This compares to 53.9% for the population of 4th grade classrooms from which the children had been selected. Slightly less than half of the sample (44.2%) lived in households where the main caregiver had been separated, divorced, widowed, or never married. High school had not been completed by 21.2% of the mothers or acting mothers, whereas at the other extreme 5.5% had earned a college degree. For fathers or acting fathers living with the child, the corresponding figures were 9.4% and 6.5%.

During the summer months of 1990, the subjects and a main caregiver were invited to the University to participate in a series of experimental studies. The child and accompanying caregiver were paid $30 each for their participation.

Q-sorting procedure. A Q-sort was completed by the caregiver with the assistance of a trained examiner, using a large table with special markings to designate the various categories of a completed Q-sort. Throughout the session, the examiner offered explanations, reading assistance, and numerous standardized probes to facilitate completion of the Q-sort. The Q-sorts took between 40 and 80 min to complete.

We secured Q-sorts for 425 boys (87.8% of the targeted study members, $N = 484$; 83.6% of the original study members, $N = 508$). Eighty-five percent of the Q-sorts were completed by mothers; 7% were completed by fathers; 4%, by grandmothers; 2%, by older siblings; and the remainder, by other relatives or acquaintances. Eleven Q-sorts were discarded because of invalidity (e.g., caregiver was intoxicated; did not speak English well).

We performed analyses to determine whether there were differences between sample members for whom we had Q-sort data and sample members for whom we were unable to secure these data. There were no significant differences between the two groups on risk status (low, high), $x^2(1, N = 508)<1$, race (non-White, White), $x^2(1, N = 508)<1$, or social background (Hollingshead socioeconomic status [SES]), $t(506)<1$.

Measures used to evaluate the validity of common-language Q-sorts.

Self-reports of delinquency. Different self-report measures were given to the boys at screening and at the 5th grade assessment. At screening the boys completed the Self-Report Antisocial Behavior Scale, an age-adjusted version of the Self-Reported Delinquency (SRD) questionnaire (Elliott, Huizinga, & Ageton, 1985) consisting of 33 items covering delinquent acts and substance use. At follow-up the boys completed a 40-item version of the SRD and a 16-item substance use questionnaire (Elliot et al., 1985).

For the present study, we used a classification scheme that places a boy in the category of the most serious behavior ever committed. The severity ratings developed by Wolfgang, Figlio, Tracy, and Singer (1985) were used to classify delinquent behaviors according to seriousness: *Level 1 Delinquency* refers to damage to property, firesetting, theft at home, shoplifting, theft outside the home, theft at school, or fraud. Subjects were required to have committed two of the Level 1 behaviors to qualify for this category. *Level 2 Delinquency* refers to theft of a bicycle, theft from a car, picking pockets, joy riding, carrying a weapon, or gang fighting. *Level 3 Delinquency* refers to breaking and entering, strongarming, or selling drugs. A value of zero was given to those subjects who did not qualify for any level.

Caregiver reports of psychiatric symptoms. The *Diagnostic Interview Schedule for Children* (DISC; Costello, Edelbrock, Kalas, Kessler, & Klaric, 1982) was administered to the subjects' caregivers when the boys were in the 5th grade. For the present study, we examined the prevalence of disruptive disorders; included here are boys meeting the *Diagnostic and Statistical Manual of Mental Disorders (DSM-III-R*; American Psychiatric Association, 1987) criteria for a diagnosis of any type of disruptive behavior disorder. Qualifying boys have a possible or probable diagnosis of at least one of the following: attention-deficit hyperactivity disorder, oppositional defiant disorder, or conduct disorder.

Teacher ratings of behavior problems. The boys' teachers completed the

Teacher Report Form (TRF) when the boys were in the 5th grade. The TRF is the teacher version of the Child Behavior Checklist, a questionnaire designed to index externalizing and internalizing behavior problems (Edelbrock & Achenbach, 1986).

Results

Personality correlates of self-reported delinquency. Table 3 shows the mean item placements for each Q-item that differed significantly by the boys' delinquency classification. The four groups differed significantly across 41 of the 100 items ($p < .05$)—more than 8 times the number that would be expected by chance. Of these items, 33 were significant beyond the .01 level; of these, 26 were significant beyond the .001 level.

The correlates of self-reported delinquency were also psychologically meaningful. The definitive Q-item *Is aggressive* discriminated between the four groups of boys ($p < .001$). Other large positive correlates of juvenile delinquency included *Tries to blame other people for things he has done, Usually pushes limits and tries to stretch rules, Tries to be the center of attention, Tries to get others to do what he wants, Exaggerates about things that happen to him,* and *Likes to dominate other people.* The larger negative correlates included *Gets along well with other people, Is considerate and thoughtful of other people, Shows concern about what is right and what is wrong, Is obedient, Can be trusted, Pays attention well and can concentrate on things, Plans things ahead,* and *Thinks about his actions and behavior.* These and the remaining significant items in Table 3 collectively suggest that the early-adolescent offender lacks empathy, cannot be trusted, is impulsive, and is a bully.

Personality correlates of childhood disruptive disorders. Table 4 shows the mean item placements for each Q-item that significantly discriminated between boys with and without *DSM-III-R* disruptive disorders. The two groups differed significantly across 70 of the 100 items ($p < .05$), 14 times the number that would be expected by chance. Of these items, 56 were significant beyond the .01 level; of these, 44 were significant beyond the .001 level.

Once again the correlates were psychologically meaningful. Among the positive correlates of disruptive disorders were these Q-items: *Tries to blame other people for things he has done, Tries to see what and how much he can get away with, Tries to get others to do what he wants, Is aggressive,* and *Likes to dominate other people.* The negative correlates of disruptive disorders included *Is obedient, Is calm and relaxed, Is easygoing, Makes good and close friendships, Is warm and responsive, Pays attention well and can concentrate on things,* and *Plans things ahead.* The many other significant items (shown in Table 4) elaborate the links between personality functioning and disruptive disorders in early

TABLE 3

Mean Scores and Analysis of Variance Results for Q-Items by Delinquency Classification

Item no.	Q-Item	Delinquency classification level				F ratio
		Level 0 (n = 104)	Level 1 (n = 112)	Level 2 (n = 92)	Level 3 (n = 106)	
2	He is considerate and thoughtful of other people.	6.45	6.08	5.84	5.57	6.79***
3	He is a warm person and responds with kindness to other people.	6.88	6.53	6.36	6.21	3.46*
4	He gets along well with other people.	6.95	6.76	6.34	5.92	11.04***
6	He is helpful and cooperates with other people.	6.48	6.08	5.78	5.74	6.06***
10	His friendships don't last long; he changes friends a lot.	2.46	2.67	2.80	3.21	3.66**
11	He tries to blame other people for things he has done.	3.58	4.13	4.2	5.04	10.12***
13	He tries to see what and how much he can get away with. He usually pushes limits and tries to stretch the rules.	4.62	5.55	5.51	6.45	14.35***
15	He shows concern about what's right and what's wrong.	6.30	6.03	5.74	5.09	10.11***
18	He lets other kids know it when he's upset or angry. He doesn't hold back his feelings when he feels upset or angry with them.	5.35	5.84	5.61	6.24	5.43***
19	He is open and straightforward.	5.82	5.23	5.50	5.26	2.74*
20	He tries to take advantage of other people.	2.73	2.77	3.23	3.61	6.84***
21	He tries to be the center of attention.	4.05	4.58	4.85	5.59	10.34***
22	He tries to get others to do what he wants by playing up to them. He acts charming in order to get his way.	3.34	3.84	4.14	4.70	10.33***
27	He looks different from other kids his own age.	5.54	5.29	5.75	5.70	2.66*
31	He is able to see how others feel; he can put himself in their place.	5.19	4.93	4.67	4.18	7.54***
32	He gives, lends, and shares things.	6.53	6.04	6.13	5.82	3.54*

#	Description					
34	He is restless and fidgety; he has a hard time sitting still.	4.12	4.50	4.87	4.91	2.99*
47	He has high standards for himself. He needs to do very well in the things he does.	5.91	5.41	5.33	4.98	4.63**
54	His moods are unpredictable—they change often and quickly.	3.53	4.03	4.47	4.54	5.24***
55	He worries about not getting his share of toys, food, or love. He seems afraid he won't get enough.	2.97	3.61	3.74	4.00	4.57***
56	He is jealous and envious: he wants what other people have.	2.77	3.30	3.42	3.97	8.55***
57	He exaggerates about things that happen to him; he blows things out of proportion.	3.45	3.96	4.44	4.79	9.84***
62	He is obedient and does what he is told.	5.99	5.21	5.27	4.56	13.48***
64	He is calm and relaxed, easy-going	5.86	5.27	4.96	4.66	8.25***
65	When he wants something, he wants it right away. He has a hard time waiting for things he wants and likes.	4.62	5.13	4.89	5.81	5.12**
66	He pays attention well and can concentrate on things.	5.60	4.93	4.67	4.15	12.31***
67	He plans things ahead; he thinks before he does something. He "looks before he leaps."	5.02	4.59	4.17	3.69	12.47***
76	He can be trusted; he's reliable and dependable.	7.11	6.29	6.13	5.60	13.17***
80	He teases and picks on other kids.	4.36	5.03	5.17	5.69	8.74***
85	He is aggressive.	2.99	3.71	3.63	4.65	13.91***
86	He likes to be by himself: he enjoys doing things alone.	4.96	4.12	4.02	3.92	5.90***
88	He is self-confident and sure of himself; he makes up his own mind on his own.	5.96	5.94	5.46	5.24	5.69***
90	He is stubborn.	4.93	5.83	5.77	6.44	9.34***
91	His emotions don't seem to fit the situation. (For example, he either overreacts, doesn't seem to care, or sometimes his reactions just don't make sense.)	3.60	3.91	4.55	4.53	7.40***
93	He's bossy and likes to dominate other people.	3.43	3.94	3.86	4.83	9.84***
94	He whines or pouts often.	3.24	3.37	3.91	3.99	3.44**

Continued

TABLE 3 (*cont.*)

Mean Scores and Analysis of Variance Results for Q-Items by Delinquency Classification

Item no.	Q-Item	Delinquency classification level				F ratio
		Level 0 ($n = 104$)	Level 1 ($n = 112$)	Level 2 ($n = 92$)	Level 3 ($n = 106$)	
95	He lets little problems get to him and he is easily upset. It doesn't take much to get him irritated or mad.	4.41	4.60	4.96	5.19	3.35*
96	He is creative in the way he looks at things; the way he thinks. works or plays is very creative.	6.17	5.95	5.74	5.36	4.51**
98	He is shy; he has a hard time getting to know people.	3.89	3.36	3.24	3.18	2.75*
99	He thinks about his actions and behavior; he uses his head before doing or saying something.	4.95	4.57	3.96	3.43	19.19***
100	Other kids often pick on him; he's also often blamed for things he didn't do.	3.39	3.41	4.03	4.07	4.18**

* $p < .05$. ** $p < .01$. *** $p < .001$.

TABLE 4
Mean Scores and t Test Results for Q-Items by Diagnosis of Disruptive Disorder

Item no.	Q-Item	Diagnosis of disruptive disorder		t test
		No (n = 337)	Yes (n = 77)	
2	He is considerate and thoughtful of other people.	6.15	5.29	4.71***
3	He is a warm person and responds with kindness to other people.	6.66	5.84	4.14***
4	He gets along well with other people.	6.74	5.48	7.19***
6	He is helpful and cooperates with other people.	6.18	5.38	4.02***
7	He likes physical affection. (For example, he likes to hug; he likes to be held.)	5.82	5.23	2.04*
9	He makes good and close friendships with other people.	6.64	5.64	4.48***
10	His friendships don't last long; he changes friends a lot.	2.61	3.57	3.69***
11	He tries to blame other people for things he has done.	3.99	5.31	5.38***
12	He starts to act immature when he faces difficult problems or when he is under stress. (For example, he whines or has tantrums.)	3.74	4.74	4.02***
13	He tries to see what and how much he can get away with. He usually pushes limits and tries to stretch the rules.	5.24	6.84	6.26***
14	He is eager to please.	5.17	4.77	1.96*
15	He shows concern about what's right and what's wrong. (For example, he tries to be fair.)	6.05	4.66	5.79***
16	He is proud of the things he's done and made.	7.22	6.71	2.74**
17	He acts very masculine.	5.16	5.56	2.53*
19	He is open and straightforward.	5.58	4.87	3.36**
20	He tries to take advantage of other people.	2.89	3.88	4.07***
21	He tries to be the center of attention. (For example, by showing off, or by offering to do things.)	4.54	5.75	4.64***
22	He tries to get others to do what he wants by playing up to them.	3.73	5.14	6.19***
23	He acts charming in order to get his way. He is nervous and fearful.	2.86	3.30	2.40*

Continued

TABLE 4 (*cont.*)

Mean Scores and t Test Results for Q-Items by Diagnosis of Disruptive Disorder

25	He thinks things out and you can explain things to him like you can to a grown up.	5.91	5.00	4.22***
30	Most adults seem to like him.	6.97	6.57	2.32*
31	He is able to see how others feel; he can put himself in their place.	4.96	3.79	5.83***
32	He gives, lends, and shares things.	6.31	5.31	4.41***
34	He is restless and fidgety; he has a hard time sitting still.	4.34	5.69	5.04***
35	He holds things in. He has a hard time expressing himself; he's a little bit uptight.	4.15	4.68	2.21*
36	He finds ways to make things happen and get things done.	5.11	4.48	3.60***
37	He likes to compete; he's always testing and comparing himself to other people.	4.79	5.32	2.32*
38	He has an unusual way of thinking about things—for better or for worse, he puts things together in his head in a different way than other people would.	3.82	4.51	2.95**
39	He freezes up when things are stressful, or else he keeps doing the same thing over and over.	3.20	3.88	3.04**
40	He is curious and exploring; he likes to learn and experience new things.	6.39	5.77	3.22**
41	He is determined in what he does; he does not give up easily.	6.03	5.32	3.47**
46	He tends to go to pieces under stress; he gets rattled when things are tough.	3.10	4.04	3.85***
47	He has high standards for himself. He needs to do very well in the things he does.	5.58	4.65	4.08***
49	He has specific habits or patterns of behavior. (For example, he taps his fingers, bites his fingernails, stutters or bites his lips.)	5.53	5.94	2.24*
51	He is well-coordinated. (For example, he does well in sports.)	6.64	6.17	2.11*
52	He is careful not to get hurt (physically).	4.93	3.97	4.47***
53	He has a hard time making up his mind; he changes his mind a lot.	4.02	4.64	2.37*
54	His moods are unpredictable—they change often and quickly.	3.87	5.39	5.98***
55	He worries about not getting his share of toys, food, or love. He seems afraid he won't get enough.	3.37	4.51	3.87***

#	Item			
56	He is jealous and envious; he wants what other people have.	3.12	4.43	5.31***
57	He exaggerates about things that happen to him; he blows things out of proportion.	3.88	5.59	6.43***
59	He is neat and orderly in the way he dresses and acts.	5.56	4.68	3.67***
62	He is obedient and does what he is told.	5.51	4.13	6.74***
64	He is calm and relaxed; easy-going.	5.51	3.81	7.74***
65	When he wants something, he wants it right away. He has a hard time waiting for things he wants and likes.	4.88	6.18	4.49***
66	He pays attention well and can concentrate on things.	5.11	3.65	7.60***
67	He plans things ahead; he thinks before he does something. He "looks before he leaps."	4.65	3.17	7.24***
68	He has a way with words; he can express himself well with words.	5.25	4.32	4.21***
71	He often asks grown-ups for help and advice.	5.20	3.97	5.96***
73	He has a sense of humor—he likes to laugh at funny things.	7.14	6.74	2.27*
74	He usually gets wrapped up in what he's doing.	5.64	5.22	2.25*
75	He is cheerful.	6.21	5.71	3.07**
76	He can be trusted; he's reliable, and dependable.	6.59	4.95	7.54***
77	He feels unworthy; he has a low opinion of himself.	2.78	3.82	4.05***
78	His feelings get hurt easily if he is made fun of or criticized.	5.67	6.36	2.75**
79	He is suspicious—he doesn't really trust other people.	3.04	3.57	2.29*
80	He teases and picks on other kids (including his own brothers and sisters).	4.88	5.88	4.19***
81	He can talk about unpleasant things that have happened to him.	5.41	4.68	3.00**
85	He is aggressive. (For example, he picks fights or starts arguments.)	3.42	5.19	6.60***
86	He likes to be by himself; he enjoys doing things alone.	4.38	3.75	2.45*
88	He is self-confident and sure of himself; he makes up his own mind on his own.	5.82	4.94	4.63***
89	He is able to do many things well; he's skillful.	6.34	5.64	3.78***
90	He is stubborn.	5.54	6.69	4.30***
91	His emotions don't seem to fit the situation. (For example, he either overreacts, doesn't seem to care, or sometimes his reactions just don't make sense.)	3.91	5.10	5.44***
93	He's bossy and likes to dominate other people.	3.76	5.16	5.04***
94	He whines or pouts often.	3.45	4.35	3.03**

Continued

TABLE 4 (*cont.*)
Mean Scores and t Test Results for Q-Items by Diagnosis of Disruptive Disorder

95	He lets little problems get to him and he is easily upset. It doesn't take much to get him irritated or mad.	4.52	5.95	6.00***
96	He is creative in the way he looks at things; the way he thinks, works or plays is very creative.	5.94	5.22	3.41**
99	He thinks about his actions and behavior; he uses his head before doing or saying something.	4.53	2.96	8.01***
100	Other kids often pick on him; he's also often blamed for things he didn't do.	3.55	4.40	3.62**

* $p < .05.$ ** $p < .01.$ *** $p < .001.$

adolescence, suggesting that boys with disruptive disorders are emotionally volatile and lacking in fundamental interpersonal skills.

Personality correlates of externalizing and internalizing disorders. Table 5 shows the significant Q-sort personality correlates of teacher ratings of externalizing behavior problems. Fifty items yielded significant correlations at the .05 level, about 10 times the number that would be expected by chance. Of these 50 items, 37 were significant beyond the .01 level; of these, 29 were significant beyond the .001 level.

Many of the Q-items that correlated with caregiver and self-reports of disruptive behavior were also correlated with teacher reports of externalizing behavior problems. Once again, the definitive item *Is aggressive* correlated significantly with behavior problems. The other correlates show that boys with externalizing problems try to be the center of attention, try to take advantage of others, are restless and fidgety, and have unpredictable moods. In addition, these boys show little concern for what is right and what is wrong, do not pay attention, are not obedient, fail to plan things ahead, and cannot be trusted.

Table 5 also shows the significant Q-sort personality correlates of teacher ratings of internalizing problems. Twenty items yielded significant correlations at the .05 level, about four times the number that would be expected by chance. Of these items, 9 were significant beyond the .01 level; of these, 5 were significant beyond the .001 level. Although fewer in number, the items collectively portray an emotionally constricted and socially inhibited boy who is insecure and easily intimidated. The positive Q-item correlates of internalizing problems include *Worries about things for a long time, Needs to have people tell him that he is doing OK,* and *Gets nervous if he is not sure what is going to happen or when it is not clear what he is supposed to do.* The negative correlates include *Determined in what he does, Openly shows the way he feels,* and *Self-confident and sure of himself.* This coherent pattern of statistically significant findings is especially compelling because few of the boys in this sample experienced internalizing difficulties.

The Q-sort can also be used to reveal similarities and differences in the functioning of children with different presenting problems. For example, when the information in the two columns of Table 5 is combined, it can be seen that children with internalizing problems and those with externalizing problems both experienced some difficulty in forming good and close friendships and tended to "freeze up" under stress. They diverged, however, on other important dimensions (e.g., feeling unworthy, shyness).

TABLE 5

Q-Items Correlates of Externalizing Behavior Problems

Item no.	Q-Item	Correlations	
		Externalizing problems	Internalizing problems
2	He is considerate and thoughtful of other people.	-.19***	
3	He is a warm person and responds with kindness to other people.	-.10*	
4	He gets along well with other people.	-.28***	
6	He is helpful and cooperates with other people.	-.17***	
9	He makes good and close friendships with other people.	-.17***	-.13*
10	His friendships don't last long; he changes friends a lot.	.15**	
11	He tries to blame other people for things he has done.	.24***	
12	He starts to act immature when he faces difficult problems or when he is under stress. (For example, he whines or has tantrums.)	.11*	
13	He tries to see what and how much he can get away with. He usually pushes limits and tries to stretch the rules.	.22***	
15	He shows concern about what's right and what's wrong. (For example, he tries to be fair.)	-.33***	
20	He tries to take advantage of other people.	.22***	
21	He tries to be the center of attention. (For example, by showing off, or by offering to do things.)	.30***	
22	He tries to get others to do what he wants by playing up to them. He acts charming in order to get his way.	.17***	
23	He is nervous and fearful.		.14**
24	He worries about things for a long time.		.18***
25	He thinks things out and you can explain things to him like you can to a grown up.	-.18***	
26	He enjoys playing, running, and exercise.		-.11*
29	He is protective of others. He protects people who are close to him.		-.10*
30	Most adults seem to like him.	-.10*	
31	He is able to see how others feel; he can put himself in their place.	-.15**	
34	He is restless and fidgety; he has a hard time sitting still.	.21***	
35	He holds things in. He has a hard time expressing himself; he's a little bit uptight:		.12*

No.	Item	Col 1	Col 2
37	He likes to compete; he's always testing and comparing himself to other people.	-.10*	
39	He freezes up when things are stressful, or else he keeps doing the same thing over and over.	.12*	.13*
41	He is determined in what he does; he does not easily give up.	-.10*	
46	He tends to go to pieces under stress; he gets rattled when things are tough.	.15***	.11*
48	He needs to have people tell him that he's doing well or ok. He is not very sure of himself.	-.14**	
51	He is well-coordinated.		.12*
53	He has a hard time making up his mind; he changes his mind a lot.		.19***
54	His moods are unpredictable—they change often and quickly.		.10*
56	He is jealous and envious; he wants what other people have.		
57	He exaggerates about things that happen to him; he blows things out of proportion.	-.10*	.22***
58	He openly shows the way he feels, whether it's good or bad.	.18***	
60	He gets nervous if he's not sure what's going to happen or when it's not clear what he's supposed to do.		
62	He is obedient and does what he is told.	-.19***	-.31***
63	He is fast-paced; he moves and reacts to things quickly.		-.23***
64	He is calm and relaxed; easy-going.		
65	When he wants something, he wants it right away. He has a hard time waiting for things he wants and likes.		.17***
66	He pays attention well and can concentrate on things.		-.30***
67	He plans things ahead; he thinks before he does something. He "looks before he leaps."		-.25***
68	He has a way with words; he can express himself well with words.		-.13*
70	He daydreams; he often gets lost in thought or a fantasy world.		-.11*
74	He usually gets wrapped up in what he's doing.		-.13*
76	He can be trusted; he's reliable, and dependable.		-.25***
77	He feels unworthy; he has a low opinion of himself.	.16***	-.16***
78	His feelings get hurt easily if he is made fun of or criticized.	.13*	
79	He is suspicious—he doesn't really trust other people.		.13*
80	He teases and picks on other kids (including his own brothers and sisters).		.14**
81	He can talk about unpleasant things that have happened to him.		-.10*
84	He is a talkative child; he talks a lot.		.11*
85	He is aggressive. (For example, he picks fights or starts arguments.)		.26***
86	He likes to be by himself; he enjoys doing things alone.		-.14**
87	He tries to copy and act like the people he admires and looks up to.	.10*	

Continued

TABLE 5 (cont.)
Q-Items Correlates of Externalizing Behavior Problems

Item no.	Q-Item	Correlations	
		Externalizing problems	Internalizing problems
88	**He is self-confident and sure of himself; he makes up his own mind on his own.**	-.12*	-.14***
89	**He is able to do many things well; he's skillful.**	-.13*	
90	He is stubborn.	.22***	
91	His emotions don't seem to fit the situation. (For example, he either over-reacts, doesn't seem to care, or sometimes his reactions just don't make sense.)	.17***	
93	He's bossy and likes to dominate other people.	.18***	
95	He lets little problems get to him and he is easily upset. It doesn't take much to get him irritated or mad.	.16***	.12*
96	He is creative in the way he looks at things; the way he thinks, works or plays is very creative.	-.20***	
97	He likes to dream up fantasies: he has a good imagination.	-.15**	
98	He is shy; he has a hard time getting to know people.	-.19***	.16***
99	He thinks about his actions and behavior; he uses his head before doing or saying something.	-.27***	
100	Other kids often pick on him: he's also often blamed for things he didn't do.	.21***	

* $p < .05$. ** $p < .01$. *** $p < .001$.

Summary

We have seen considerable overlap in the Q-items that discriminate between self-reported delinquents, boys with disruptive disorders, and students with externalizing problems. The indexes used to define these three groups of boys are generally thought to tap the same construct of antisocial behavior (e.g., Bank & Patterson, in press). How similar, then, are the personality profiles of these three groups? Does the same configuration of personality attributes characterize them?

To evaluate this hypothesis, we converted the various aforementioned statistical tests (e.g., F test, t test) into comparable measures of effect magnitude (Friedman, 1968). First, we converted to a correlation coefficient each of the 100 F tests from our analysis of the Q-item correlates of self-reported delinquency (see Table 3). This yielded a vector of 100 correlations, one correlation between group membership and each Q-item. Second, we converted to a correlation coefficient each of the 100 t tests from our analysis of the Q-item correlates of disruptive disorders (see Table 4). This too yielded a vector of 100 correlations, one correlation between group membership and each Q-item. Third, we created a vector of 100 correlations from our analysis of the Q-item correlates of externalizing problems (see Table 5). We then examined the relations between these three vectors. A high and positive correlation between the three vectors would indicate that the pattern and magnitude of Q-items that discriminate between one of our external criteria (e.g., self-reported delinquency) is similar to the pattern and magnitude of the Q-items that discriminate between another of our external criteria (e.g., teacher reports of externalizing problems).

Indeed, the vector of 100 Q-item correlations from our analysis of self-reported delinquency was strongly related to the vector of 100 Q-item correlations from our analysis of teacher reports of externalizing problems ($r = .76$, $p < .001$). Similarly, the vector correlation between the Q-items describing self-reported delinquents and the Q-items describing boys with disruptive disorders was .78, $p < .001$. Finally, the vector correlation between Q-items describing boys with externalizing problems and boys with disruptive disorders was .72, $p < .001$. Thus, whether antisocial behavior is measured by self-, caregiver-, or teacher-reports, the Q-sort appears to yield a consistent personality description of antisocial boys.

Operationalizing Antisocial Behavior

As we noted in the introduction, the Q-sort is a valuable assessment tool because it provides a descriptive personality profile that can be used in constructing many different personality variables. For example, to bring order to the various empirical relations just described, we wished to derive a Q-sort index of antisocial behavior so that we could assign a single score to each boy. We accomplished this through a criterion sorting procedure in which we first asked 10 experts to describe, using the common-language item set, a prototypical antisocial adolescent male between 12 and 14 years of age.[2] To construct the criterion definition of an antisocial adolescent from the expert descriptions, we averaged the experts' ratings across each item. The reliability of this composite was .97.

Using this criterion Q-sort, we then assessed the antisocial tendency of each subject in our sample by calculating the similarity between his actual Q-description and the criterion description of antisocial behavior: The subject's "score" on antisocial behavior was thus the correlation between his own Q-sort profile and the experts' composite profile of antisocial behavior. A high correlation suggested that the subject closely resembled the criterion definition of antisocial behavior; a low correlation suggested that the subject was different from the criterion definition of antisocial behavior. (In our sample, the scores ranged from −.70 to .66.) This measure of antisocial behavior was then related to each subject's scores on the various external criteria of disruptive behavior.

The results in Table 6 show significant convergence across the different measures of antisocial behavior. The SRD inquires directly about illegal behaviors engaged in by antisocial children; the DISC taps antisocial symptoms associated with disruptive disorders; and the TRF refers to antisocial behaviors directed at other persons in school settings. The correlation of the Q-sort index of antisocial behavior with boys' self-reported delinquency was .37, $p < .001$; with mothers' reports of their boys' disruptive disorders, .47, $p < .001$; with teacher reports of externalizing behavior problems, .36, $p < .001$. Table 6 also presents evidence for divergent validity; the correlation between our antisocial index and teacher reports of internalizing behavior problems was .02, *ns*.

CONCLUSION

The CCQ (J. Block & J. H. Block, 1980) is an observer-based instrument for describing the personality styles of children with a broadband and clinically rich item set. It has been used in previous studies of personality coherence, contributing important information about the nature of social development (e.g., J. H. Block & J. Block, 1980; Shedler & Block, 1990). In this article, we presented language-simplifying modifications to the CCQ so that it may be used now with greater ease by lay observers of diverse backgrounds. The common-language version of the CCQ is not intended to supplant the original version of the CCQ.

---

[2]We thank Robert Cairns, Ken Dodge, David Farrington, Rolf Loeber, Joan McCord, Terrie Moffitt, Gerald Paterson, Herbert Quay, Lee Robins, and Jennifer White for using the Q-sort to formalize their conceptualization of antisocial behavior.

TABLE 6
Correlations Between Validation Study Measures

	Measures from different informants				
	1	2	3	4	5
1 Q-sort derived antisocial index	—	.37**	.47**	.36**	.02
2 Self-reported delinquency		—	.24*	.46**	.10
3 Mothers' reports of disruptive disorders			—	.23*	−.01
4 Teachers' reports of externalizing problems				—	.36**
5 Teachers' reports of internalizing problems					—

*$p < .01$. **$p < .001$.

Rather, it is intended to broaden the application that this assessment procedure may enjoy in diverse clinical and research settings.

The findings reported here suggest that the common-language version of the CCQ items is as reliable as the original item pool. Moreover, the common-language version, like the original form, can yield valuable and valid information about the links between personality functioning and problems in adaptive functioning.

REFERENCES

Achenbach, T. M., & Edelbrock, C. S. (1983). *Manual for the Child Behavior Checklist and Revised Child Behavior Profile.* Burlington: University of Vermont.

Allport, G. W. (1937). *Personality.* New York: Holt.

Bank, L., & Patterson, G. R. (in press). The use of structural equation modeling in combining data from different types of assessment. In J. Rosen & P. McReynolds (Eds.), *Advances in psychological assessment* (Vol. 8). New York: Plenum Press.

Bem, D. J. (1983). Constructing a theory of the triple typology: Some (second) thoughts on nomothetic and idiographic approaches to personality. *Journal of Personality, 51,* 566–577.

Block, J. (1957). A comparison between ipsative and normative ratings of personality. *Journal of Abnormal and Social Psychology, 54,* 50–54.

Block, J. (1971). *Lives through time.* Berkeley, CA: Bancroft.

Block, J. (1961/1978). *The Q-sort in personality assessment and psychiatric research*. Palo Alto, CA: Consulting Psychologists Press.

Block, J., & Block, J. H. (1980). *The California Child Q-Set*. Palo Alto, CA: Consulting Psychologists Press.

Block, J., Block, J. H., & Keyes, S. (1988). Longitudinally foretelling drug use in adolescence: Early childhood personality and environmental precursors. *Child Development, 59*, 336–355.

Block, J., & Gjerde, P. (1986). Distinguishing between antisocial behavior and undercontrol. In J. Block, D. Olweus, & M. Radke-Yarrow (Eds.), *The development of prosocial and antisocial behavior* (pp. 177–206). New York: Academic Press.

Block, J. H., & Block, J. (1969). *The California Child Q-Set*. Unpublished manuscript. Department of Psychology, University of California, Berkeley.

Block, J. H., & Block, J. (1980). The role of ego-control and ego-resiliency in the organization of behavior. In W. A. Collins (Ed.), *Minnesota symposia on child psychology* (Vol. 13, pp. 39–101). Hillsdale, NJ: Erlbaum.

Costello, A., Edelbrock, C., Kalas, R., Kessler, M., & Klaric, S. (1982). *Diagnostic Interview Schedule for Children*. Bethesda, MD: National Institute of Mental Health.

Earls, F., & McGuire, J. (1990). *Assessment of individual differences in children*. Unpublished report. Program on Human Development and Criminal Behavior. School of Public Health, Harvard University.

Edelbrock, C., & Achenbach, T. M. (1986). *Manual for the teacher's report form and teacher version of the child behavior profile*. Burlington: University of Vermont.

Elliott, D. Z., Huizinga, D., & Ageton, S. S. (1985). *Explaining delinquency and drug use*. Beverly Hills, CA: Sage.

Friedman, H. (1968). Magnitude of experimental effect and a table for its rapid estimation. *Psychological Bulletin, 70*, 245–251.

Funder, D. C., & Block, J. (1989). The role of ego-control, ego-resiliency, and IQ in delay of gratification in adolescence. *Journal of Personality and Social Psychology, 57*, 1041–1050.

Funder, D. C., Block, J. H., & Block, J. (1983). Delay of gratification: Some longitudinal personality correlates. *Journal of Personality and Social Psychology, 44*, 1198–1213.

Funder, D. C., & Colvin, C. R. (1988). Friends and strangers: Acquaintanceship, agreement, and the accuracy of personality judgment. *Journal of Personality and Social Psychology, 55*, 149–158.

Goldsmith, H. H., & Rothbart, M. K. (1991). Contemporary instruments for assessing early temperament by questionnaire and in the laboratory. In J. Strelau & A. Angleitner (Eds.), *Explorations in temperament* (pp. 249–272). New York: Plenum Press.

Harris, A. J., & Jacobson, M. D. (1982). *Basic reading vocabularies*. New York: Macmillan.

Loeber, R., Stouthamer-Loeber, M., Van Kammen, W. B., & Farrington, D. P. (1989). Development of a new measure of self-reported antisocial behavior for young children: Prevalence and reliability. In M. W. Klein (Ed.), *Cross-national research in self-*

reported crime and delinquency (pp. 203–225). The Hague: Kluwer Academic Publishers.

Martin, R. P. (1988). *Assessment of personality and behavior problems.* New York: Guilford Press.

Mischel, W., Shoda, Y., & Peake, P. K. (1988). The nature of adolescent competencies predicted by preschool delay of gratification. *Journal of Personality and Social Psychology, 54*, 687–696.

Moskowitz, D. S. (1986). Comparison of self-reports, reports by knowledgeable informants, and behavioral observational data. *Journal of Personality, 54*, 294–317.

Ozer, D. (in press). The Q-sort method in research on personality development. In D. Funder, C. Tomlinson-Keasey, R. D. Parke, & K. Widaman (Eds.), *Studying lives through time: Approaches to personality development.* Washington, DC: American Psychological Association.

Ozer, D., & Gjerde, P. (1989). Patterns of personality consistency and change from childhood through adolescence. *Journal of Personality, 57*, 483–507.

Prout, H. T., & Chizik, R. (1988). Readability of child and adolescent self-report measures. *Journal of Consulting and Clinical Psychology, 56*, 152–154.

Quay, H., & Peterson, D. R. (1983). *Revised Behavior Problem Checklist—Interim manual.* Coral Gables, FL: University of Miami.

Renken, B., Egeland, B., Marvinney, D., Mangelsdorf, S., & Sroufe, L. A. (1989). Early childhood antecedents of aggression and passive-withdrawal in early elementary school. *Journal of Personality, 57*, 257–282.

Shedler, J., & Block, J. (1990). Adolescent drug use and psychological health: A longitudinal inquiry. *American Psychologist, 45*, 612–630.

Shoda, Y., Mischel, W., & Peake, P. K. (1990). Predicting adolescent cognitive and self-regulatory competencies from preschool delay of gratification: Identifying diagnostic conditions. *Developmental Psychology, 26*, 978–986.

Waters, E., & Deane, K. E. (1985). Defining and assessing individual differences in attachment relationships: Q-methodology and the organization of behavior in infancy and early childhood. In I. Bretherton & E. Waters (Eds.), Growing points in attachment research. *Monographs of the Society for Research in Child Development, 50* (Serial No. 209).

Waters, E., Noyes, D. M., Vaughn, B. E., & Ricks, M. (1985). Q-sort definitions of social competence and self-esteem: Discriminant validity of related constructs in theory and data. *Developmental Psychology, 21*, 508–522.

Wolfgang, M., Figlio, R. M., Tracey, P. E., & Singer, F. I. (1985). *The national survey of crime severity.* Washington, DC: U.S. Government Printing Office.

York, K., & John, O. (1992). The four faces of Eve. *Journal of Personality and Social Psychology, 63*, 494–508.

Part III

CHILDREN OF PSYCHIATRICALLY
ILL PARENTS

In the first paper in this section, Fish, Marcus, Hans, Auerbach, and Perdue review the hypothesis that pandysmaturation (PDM) may be an indicator of a genetic propensity to schizophrenia or schizotypal personality disorder. As initially defined by Fish in 1975 and further elaborated in a paper reprinted in the 1977 Annual Progress, criteria for PDM included: (1) a transient retardation of the mean gross motor and/or visual motor developmental quotient, followed by an acceleration of the rate of development and a return to more normal levels; and (2) an abnormal profile of function on a single developmental examination, such that earlier items are failed while later-occurring, more complex items are passed; both of which are (3) accompanied by a parallel retardation in skeletal growth. A modification of these criteria were applied to the data of the Jerusalem Infant Development Study, in which the children of schizophrenic, affectively ill, personality-disordered, and normal parents have been followed for at least 10 years. Bayley Mental and Motor Developmental Quotients at 4, 8, and 12 months, together with information regarding height, head circumference, and weight were examined and related to parental diagnosis and to later cognitive and motor impairments. Children with PDM in infancy were significantly more likely to have had parents who were schizophrenic than were children whose parents had other psychiatric disorders or were normal. Moreover, children with PDM in infancy were significantly more likely to have exhibited an array of cognitive and motor difficulties in middle childhood. These findings, when considered together with the results of 9 other studies of children of schizophrenics, lead the authors to suggest that children with PDM may well be more likely than other offspring of schizophrenic parents to develop schizophrenic spectrum disorders during adolescence and adulthood. The results and thoughtful discussion are of particular interest in light of the growing body of evidence suggesting anatomic and functional CNS deficits in adults with schizophrenia.

In the next paper, Radke-Yarrow, Nottelmann, Martinez, Fox, and Belmont employ a longitudinal design to examine the course of social-emotional development of young children of affectively ill (bipolar disorder and unipolar depression) and well parents. The program of research is directed toward furthering understanding of the mechanisms underlying the well-documented aggregation of problems in the offspring of affectively ill parents. Pairs of siblings were studied: the younger between 1 ½ and 3 ½ years and the older between 5 and 8 years at the time of initial evaluation. All offspring were examined three years later. Psychiatric assessment and mother's report focused on children's disruptive behavior, anxiety, and depressive characteristics. The frequency of problem behavior changed over time in relation to mother's diagnosis. By middle and late childhood, significantly more children of affectively ill than well mothers had depressive, disruptive, and multiple behavior problems. The developmental course of children of unipolar and bipolar mothers differed significantly. Offspring of unipolar mothers developed problems earlier, and both siblings were more likely to have behavior problems. The subjects of this methodologically elegant study and their families are to be followed into adolescence and hopefully beyond, providing the opportunity for systematic exploration of relations between problem behavior during early and middle childhood and psychiatric disorder later in life.

8

Infants at Risk for Schizophrenia: Sequelae of a Genetic Neurointegrative Defect

A Review and Replication Analysis of Pandysmaturation in the Jerusalem Infant Development Study

Barbara Fish
University of California, Los Angeles

Joseph Marcus and Sydney L. Hans
University of Chicago

Judith G. Auerbach
Hebrew University of Jerusalem, Israel

Sondra Perdue
University of Texas Health Science Center, San Antonio

A 1975 report stated that a schizophrenic genotype may be manifested in infants by a neurointegrative defect called **pandysmaturation.** *Recent evidence supports this: (1) 12 studies found delayed development in schizophrenics' infants and in preschizophrenics; (2) "blind" psychometric evaluations favored an adult schizotypal disorder in four to six of seven high-risk subjects with pandysmaturation in the*

Reprinted with permission from *Archives of General Psychiatry*, 1992, Vol. 49, 221–235. Copyright © 1992 by the American Medical Association.

This research was supported in part by the following: the Della Martin Foundation, Los Angeles, Calif; Grant MH-31653 from the National Institute of Mental Health, Bethesda, MD; and by research grants from the Scottish Rite Schizophrenia Research Program, Northern Masonic Jurisdiction USA, Lexington, MA; the William T. Grant Foundation, New York, NY; the Harriett Ames Charitable Trust, New York, NY; the Stephen R. Levy Research Fund to Dr Fish; the US-Israel Binational Science Foundation, Jerusalem; the Israel Chief Scientist Office; the Scottish Rite Schizophrenia Research Program support to the JIDS; the William T. Grant Foundation, New York, NY; the Sturman Center

New York study; and (3) finally, in a partial replication of this method using the Jerusalem data, blind diagnoses of "probable" and "possible" pandysmaturation were significantly related to a parental diagnosis of schizophrenia and to cognitive and motor neurointegrative deficits at 10 years. Obstetrical complications were unrelated to diagnosis, pandysmaturation, or outcome in the overall sample. However, we found a small subgroup of schizophrenic offspring in whom the most severe motor deficits at follow-up were related to obstetrical complications, pandysmaturation, and low birth weight.

The provocative findings emerging from current investigations into the neurology and genetics of schizophrenia make a review of recent data on the development of infants at risk for schizophrenia especially timely. Many of those studying anatomic and functional central nervous system defects in adult schizophrenics believe that their data point to some neurodevelopmental disorders occurring as early as pregnancy[1-3] or the first year of life.[4-6] Some have also suggested a possible effect of obstetrical complications[4,7] or low birth weight.[7-9] However, most of these investigators seem unaware that the ongoing prospective studies of infants genetically at risk for schizophrenia might shed light on these questions.

In 1975 and 1977, Fish[10,11] described "pandysmaturation" (PDM), an index that had been proposed as "a 'marker' in infancy for the inherited neurointegrative defect in schizophrenia" in the first of these prospective infant studies. The aim in 1952 had been to detect infants who were genetically vulnerable to later schizophrenia and to study the evolving neurobiologic manifestations of schizophrenia from the first months of life,[12] since "it is difficult to prove, from the data on adult patients, whether the physiological dysfunctions are the cause of schizophrenia or only the end-result of many years of severe tension or of conditions secondary to hospitalization."[13]

The model of schizophrenia on which the study was based grew out of the delineation of the clinical features of schizophrenic children reported by Bender,[14] the first to emphasize underlying deviations in neurologic maturation. Fish's model postulated that what was inherited in schizophrenia, at least in individuals with the earliest onset and most chronic course, was a neurointegrative defect. In

of Human Development, Jerusalem, Israel; Olivetti Foundation, Boston, MA; and a gift from Sarah Cowan to the JIDS.

Aaron Auerbach, PhD, and Chaim Cohen, MA, assisted in collecting the JIDS follow-up data; Linda Henson, MA, analyzed the data in the JIDS that were provided for this replication analysis; Arthur H. Parmelee, MD, gave advice on analyzing the obstetrical complications of the JIDS; and Robert F. Asarnow, PhD, provided suggestions on two earlier versions of this report.

Sondra Perdue, DrPH, conducted the statistical analyses for this article. Statistical consultation for the derivation of the Cognitive and Motor scores of the JIDS follow-up data was provided by Leland Wilkinson, PhD, Department of Psychology, University of Illinois at Chicago.

a sample of infants who are statistically at higher risk for schizophrenia because they were born to schizophrenic mothers, only a subset would be expected to actually carry the genetic trait. It was hoped to detect such infants by analyzing early neurologic development for specific features of defective neural integration.

Infants who showed signs of neurointegrative defect that were hypothesized to be specific for the schizophrenic phenotype were predicted to be those who would later manifest what is now defined as "schizotypal personality disorder." Kendler[15] has cogently summarized the evidence demonstrating that the genetic predisposition for schizophrenia "not only 'codes' for the classic, psychotic disorder but also increases liability to 'schizophrenia-like' personality disorders." Fish[13] did not expect to predict which schizotypal individuals would actually become psychotic, based on events as remote as infancy.

This model is similar to the one detailed by Meehl[16,17] and the more recent model of Asarnow et al.[18] All three emphasize an underlying neurointegrative defect leading to schizotypal symptoms, but not necessarily to schizophrenia. This is only one of many diathesis/stress models of schizophrenia, such as those developed by Rosenthal[19] and Gottesman and Shields.[20]

Three operational criteria were used to define the index of PDM. These were drawn primarily from the histories of infant development in several childhood schizophrenics whose cases were reported by Bender and Freedman.[21] The first was a **transient retardation** of the mean gross motor and/or visual motor developmental quotient (DQ), followed by an acceleration of the rate of development, and a return to more normal levels. Second, associated with such retardation, there must be an **abnormal profile of function** on a single developmental examination, in which earlier simple items are failed while later-occurring, more complex items are passed. This profile is analogous to the intratest scatter often seen on psychometric testing of adult schizophrenics; it is different from the pattern in ordinary mental retardation or diffuse organic brain disorder.[11] And, finally, the transient lags and the abnormal profile must be accompanied by a parallel **retardation in skeletal growth.**[12,22,23]

It is conceivable that some developmental retardation associated with PDM or other neurointegrative signs might become permanent. Indeed, certain visual motor defects did persist from 2 to 10 years of age.[24] However, during early infancy it would have been impossible to differentiate a permanent retardation from any number of stable neurologic disorders totally unrelated to the schizophrenic genotype. Therefore, the first criterion was arbitrarily limited to **transient** lags that then recovered. It must be emphasized that simple retardation or fluctuations in infant DQs were considered benign, *unless* they were associated with the other two criteria: an abnormal profile and a lag in skeletal growth.[12(p20)]

Although the neurointegrative defect of schizotypal individuals was considered an enduring trait, its phenotypic manifestations would inevitably change as the capacities of the central nervous system matured. Pandysmaturation was only the earliest manifestation, a transitional index that could be identified during the period of rapid growth in the first 2 years of life. It usually began by 9 months of age. Later manifestations of the putative basic neurointegrative defect have been found in older children, adolescents, and adults, and may include the following: the neurointegrative deficits Marcus[25] found using a comprehensive neurologic battery in the first Israeli high-risk children at 7 to 10 years of age; the disturbance in smooth-pursuit eye movements that Holzman et al[26,27] found in schizophrenics with thought disorder and in their relatives; the "soft" or nonlocalizing neurologic signs found in some adolescent[28] and adult schizophrenics, particularly those with thought disorders[29] or with a premorbid history of asociality[30]; and certain attention and information-processing deficits found in studies of children and adolescents at risk for schizophrenia[18,31-34] and in schizophrenic children or adults during the acute or remitted state.[18,32,33]

Current advances in behavioral genetics could be accelerated by biologic markers in infants and young children that reflect a genetic liability to schizophrenia or schizotypal disorders. Recent reviews of potential markers[35,36] have pointed to the well-documented findings in children and adolescents at risk, using the specific tests of attention and information processing noted above.[18,31-34] However, highly regarded investigators who study older children at risk have dismissed PDM as a marker in infancy, having misinterpreted the infant high-risk data as "contradictory." This apparently is because they were unaware of critical differences between the measures used in the various infant studies.[37]

We therefore propose the following: (1) We will review briefly the studies of high-risk infants, highlighting new data relating to PDM that are particularly relevant for issues raised by current research into adult schizophrenia. These data have emerged in the 1980s from the large prospective studies in Jerusalem, Israel,[38-40] and Rochester, NY,[41-43] and the adult follow-up of the original New York subjects whose cases were reported by Fish.[23,44,45] (2) We will clarify the difference between the measures used in these studies and measures in other studies that have no relevance to PDM. (3) We will present a partial replication of Fish's method, using data from the Jerusalem Infant Development Study (JIDS). This replication enlarges the area of agreement across the high-risk infant studies and provides new data regarding the antecedents of neurologic dysfunction in middle childhood.

REVIEW OF NINE PROSPECTIVE STUDIES OF INFANTS AT RISK FOR SCHIZOPHRENIA

1. The New York Infant Study: Schizophrenic Offspring From Birth to Adulthood

This study was begun in 1952 to test the hypothesis that specific neurointegrative disorders in infancy predict vulnerability to later schizophrenia and schizotypal disorder.[12,22] Twelve offspring of chronic schizophrenic mothers and 12 controls from similar low socioeconomic status backgrounds have been studied from their births in 1952–1953 and 1959–1960[23,44,45] up until the present (1991). Nine high-risk infants were reared by supportive grandmothers or adoptive parents. Predictions consisted of ranking the infants according to the severity of PDM, which was defined by the three criteria summarized above. Data to score PDM were derived from an analysis of their Gesell[46] scores and measures of physical growth[47] that were repeated 10 times between birth and 2 years.

Seven high-risk infants (five in warm, stable homes) and one control had PDM.[23,45] Pandysmaturation was related to being the offspring of a schizophrenic mother ($P<.05$) but was not related to obstetrical complications. Pandysmaturation was also related to the severity of later psychiatric and cognitive disorder ($P<.01$) at 10 years of age.

Four high-risk infants (subjects 1, 5, 6, and 7),[45] all with PDM, also had low-normal birth weights (2610 to 2970 g). The birth weights of the remaining three infants with PDM (3690 to 4500 g) were as high as those without PDM (3000 to 5160 g). Three controls, with no PDM, had birth weights similar to the small PDM infants (2640 to 2940 g), so that the mean for the high-risk infants (3540 g) was nonsignificantly different from the controls' (3600 g).

The mean head circumference at birth of the four small PDM infants was also smaller (32.4 cm) than the other infants with PDM (34.9 cm) and those with no PDM (34.7 cm). Similarly, the three small controls also had mean head circumferences that were 2 cm smaller than the other controls. The mothers of two of the three small controls had had moderate to severe obstetrical complications, while none of the mothers of the high-risk infants with PDM did.[45] However, the complications culled from the prenatal and obstetrical charts at the time excluded common "nonoptimal events," such as induction of labor and analgesia, which are included in the summary scores used by later prospective studies that began with pregnancy.[38,41]

Since the 1977 report,[11] 23 subjects (96%) completed 15-, 18-, and 20–22-year follow-up examinations. To date, 11 high-risk subjects and six symptomatic controls have been reinterviewed at 27 to 34 years (one sick high-risk subject is homeless and unreachable). Blind adult diagnoses will be obtained subsequently. One 30-year-old high-risk subject has been chronically schizophrenic since 19 years.[44] Fish,[45] nonblind, provisionally diagnosed six other high-risk subjects as having schizotypal or paranoid personality. Six of these seven have had severe social-affective symptoms since 3 to 6 years of age, requiring 6 to 21+ years of treatment, including three subjects who were hospitalized.[45] Four of these six "sick" adults have "negative" symptoms and remain severely impaired. These include the currently schizophrenic man and three of the four low-birth-weight subjects with PDM. All seven schizophrenic or schizotypal subjects had PDM as infants.[45]

On Gottesman's blind evaluations of these subjects' 1974 to 1975 Minnesota Multiphasic Personality Inventories, five of the six sick subjects were considered to have "schizophrenia," "borderline schizophrenia," or "paranoid personality disorder," and one had "cyclothymic personality disorder" (five subjects were then only 15 years old).[45] Hagin considered four of the six sick subjects to be schizotypal on her blind evaluation of the entire adult psychological battery ($X^2 = 3.03$; $P < .10$). Johnston's blind evaluations of clear Thought Disorder on the adult Wechsler Adult Intelligence Scale and Rorschach test, scored as in Johnston and Holzman,[48] also included four of the six subjects. Of these six high-risk subjects with PDM who were chronically disturbed, three were evaluated as schizotypal or clearly thought disordered by all three judges ($X^2 = 3.28$; $P < .10$), and a fourth was evaluated as schizotypal or clearly thought disordered by two judges. The remaining two were each evaluated as schizotypal by only one judge each. Hagin's ratings of severe to moderately severe disorder were related to PDM ($X^2 = 5.2$; $P < .025$) and included all seven high-risk subjects with PDM.

The later high-risk infant studies used comparable developmental tests, although they did not analyze these data to derive an index of PDM. Their developmental scores do provide data that can be compared with Fish's first criterion of **developmental retardation.** Table 1 summarizes the six major controlled studies as well as three smaller and less systematic ones. It notes which of the three criteria for PDM were measured and whether there was a significant preponderance of lower scores in the schizophrenics' offspring. Three large studies of preschizophrenic children are also summarized.

2. The Jerusalem Infant Development Study (JIDS)

Marcus[25] hypothesized a genetic model similar to that of Fish and looked for neurointegrative disorders to provide an early marker for the schizophrenic genotype.[38-40] There were 19 schizophrenic offspring (10 chronic), 23 offspring of patients with other mental illness (10 affective disorders, 13 personality or neurotic disorders), and 16 offspring from a normal control group with no mental ill-

Table 1.—Elements of Pandysmaturation (PDM) Found in 12 Studies*

Source, Site; Year Begun	Developmental Test	Gross Motor Lag	Visual Motor Lag	Physical Growth Lag	Abnormal Profile of Development	Total N of Sample (N = Schiz)	Schiz Significantly Worse at Age, mo	Outcome (at Age, y)
9 Prospective Studies of Infants at Risk for Schizophrenia								
Fish,[11,12,45] New York; 1952	Gesell	+	+	+	+	24 (12)	PDM 2-18	Schizotypal + 1 schiz (23-38)
Marcus et al,[38-40]* Jerusalem, Israel; 1973	Bayley	+	+	...	...	58 (19)	4, 8, 12	Neurol, cognitive (8-13)
Sameroff et al,[41-43]* Rochester, NY; 1970	Bayley	+	+	...	...	167 (29)	4, 12	Cognitive, social (4, 13)
Mednick et al,[50]* Denmark; 1971	Pediatric	+	...	...	...	249 (83)	5 d, 4, 12	Neurol (11-13)
Hanson et al,[52] Minnesota CPP; 1976	Bayley	0	+	...	...	135 (33)	8	Motor, cognitive, behavior (4, 7)
Marcuse and Cornblatt,[53]* New York State CPP; 1986	Bayley	0	0	...	...	110 (17)	NS	Neurol (7)
Ragins et al,[54]* Pittsburgh, Pa; 1975	Bayley	+	+	+	...	32 (14)	Prehension walking <12, 13	...
Sobel,[55] New York, NY: schiz parents 2; 1961	Pediatric	+	...	...	...	4 (4) 0 control	2 of 4 were retarded	...
Grunebaum et al,[56,57]* Boston, Mass; 1974	Piaget object permanence	...	+	...	...	30 (15 = psychotic)	Object permanence 12	...
3 Studies of Records of Children Who Became Schizophrenic as Adults								
O'Neal and Robins,[58]* St Louis, Mo; 1958	Pediatric	+	...	...	...	85 (28)	Difficulty walking	Schiz adults
Watt,[59] Boston, Mass; 1972	Pediatric	+	...	...	...	92 (23)	Neurol disorders	Schiz adults
Ricks et al,[60,61]* Boston, Mass; 1966	Pediatric	+	...	...	...	485 (185)	Slow development neurol impairment	Schiz adults

*Developmental lags: plus sign indicates present; 0, none found; and ..., not examined. CPP indicates Collaborative Perinatal Project; schiz, schizophrenic; NS, not significant; and neurol, neurologic.

ness (based on the rediagnoses done at follow-up). One infant had two schizophrenic parents.

The JIDS administered the Bayley Scales of Infant Development[49] at 4, 8, and 12 months of age. The schizophrenic offspring had Mental scores that were at least 10 points lower than the normal group at all three ages and had lower Psychomotor scores at 8 months.[38] This would be consistent with the presence of more PDM in the schizophrenic offspring, since more infants of schizophrenics met the first criterion of a developmental retardation. Most of the 13 "poorly performing" schizophrenic offspring had delays in postural control, reaching behaviors, and fine coordination, deficits that were similar to the New York infants with PDM.

Four of the 13 subjects also had birth weights of 2300 to 2440 g; one of these had a schizophrenic father and one had two schizophrenic parents, these being two of a total of four schizophrenic fathers in the sample. Four additional infants had low-normal birth weights (2500 to 2950 g). Mild to severe obstetrical complications were summed for a total obstetrical complication score, using the same scale as the Rochester study below.[41] The lower Mental and Psychomotor scores were not related to obstetrical complications, similar to the New York infants with PDM, but these data have not yet been fully analyzed and will be the subject of a separate report.

At about 10 years of age, 45 of the original sample were reexamined, as well as their siblings in the same age range (J.M., S.L.H., and J.G.A. and Aaron G. Auerbach, PhD, unpublished data, May 1991). Approximately half (44%) of the schizophrenic offspring showed signs of neurobehavioral dysfunctioning in cognitive and motor areas, compared with 24% of the other mental illness group and 15% of the normal group.

3. The Rochester Longitudinal Study

This project[41-43] emphasized multiple, general environmental risk factors, leading to general incompetencies in the children, and eschewed a genetic model leading to schizotypal outcomes in the offspring. However, the Bayley Scale was administered at 4 and 12 months to the offspring of 29 mothers with schizophrenia, 98 with other psychiatric disorders (58 neurotic depression, 40 personality disorder), and a normal control group of 57. While the authors concluded that, among the huge number of variables studied, there was "a paucity of differences" attributable to schizophrenia, the schizophrenic offsprings' Bayley scores were significantly lower at 4 and 12 months, similar to the JIDS.[41] These lower scores were not related to obstetrical complications, similar to the New York and JIDS data. However, the schizophrenic offsprings' mean birth weight (3126 g) was significantly lower than the normal group's mean birth weight (3390 g).

4. The Danish Obstetrical Study

Mednick et al[50] analyzed detailed records of neonatal and subsequent motor development of infants of 83 schizophrenic mothers or fathers, 83 with character disorders, and 83 controls with no mental illness. The children of schizophrenics were differentiated from the controls in having "absence or weakness of motor reflexes" at birth that persisted at 5 days of age, although the difficulties in the controls usually had cleared up by that time. Significantly more children of schizophrenics also had retarded motor development compared with the controls, including delays in head control after 4 months and in walking with support, as well as trends toward delayed sitting, standing, and walking, which did not quite reach statistical significance. Significantly more schizophrenic offspring had low-normal birth weights (2550 to 3000 g) and only in the schizophrenics' infants were these related to the delays in motor development. There were no other differences in obstetrical complications between the groups. These findings are similar to what was seen in the New York, JIDS, and Rochester studies. A subgroup of this sample was later identified that had multiple signs of neurologic dysfunction at 11 to 13 years with a pattern that was similar to that in the Israeli childhood study.[51]

5. The Minnesota Collaborative Perinatal Project (CPP) Study

Hanson et al[52] examined prospective developmental data on 33 children of consensus-diagnosed schizophrenic parents, 36 nonschizophrenics, and 66 normal controls, all of whom had been tested on the Bayley Scale at 8 months, and on many other measures from pregnancy to 7 years of age, as participants in the CPP. The authors found that three indicators, which had been selected a priori, characterized five of the 116 children, and these five children constituted 17% of the schizophrenic offspring. The indicators applied to the 4-year and 7-year test data were as follows: "1) poor motor skills, 2) large intraindividual inconsistencies in performance on cognitive tasks, and 3) observations of 'schizoid'-like behaviors," which were specified further. "All 5 children have an enduring pattern of maladjustment, and have exhibited behaviours often reported in the premorbid development of schizophrenia. Most have severely schizophrenic parents."

The authors "found no differences to suggest that children of these schizophrenics, as a group, have a greater risk for pre/perinatal difficulties."

> The results of repeated measures of physical growth, the results of psychological testing, and the results of repeated neurological examinations also show that the children of schizophrenic parents, on the *average* (our emphasis), are in no way consistently different from the comparison samples for the traits measured.

We asked Hanson if this absence of any "consistent" difference for *all* the psychological testing (8 months, 4 years, and 7 years) obscured any differences in the 8-month Bayley scores, and he gave us those data (May 1989): "The mean 8-month Mental scores of the high-risk group (78.3) were significantly lower than those of their matched normal controls (80.2), at the .005 level." The subjects are being followed up at age $25 \pm$ years.

Moreover, from the descriptions of the children's behavior in the case histories, it is evident that three of the five children who were presumed to be at greatest risk for schizophrenia had deviations on the 8-month Bayley test that were consistent with Fish's data. Case C showed "Performance erratic on mental scale of Bayley, but generally in upper end of the normal range in all areas of development except social." Case D showed "Lower half of normal range on Bayley, did not sit well, pull to standing or roll over. Unresponsive, placid, low energy level, poor muscle tone." Case E was "One to two months behind in all areas of development, weak tremulous child, very emotional, easily upset, titubation noted" (staggering gait). At the 4-year and 7-year testing, case D had "occasional lapses into bizarre, irrelevant chatter" and "irrelevant rambling associations [which] were sometimes incongruous and contradicting," which makes one suspect the beginning of disordered thinking.

6. The New York State CPP Study

Marcuse and Cornblatt[53] examined the prospective data on 17 children of consensus-diagnosed schizophrenic parents and 68 matched normal controls from the New York State sample of the CPP, who had been tested on the same measures as the Minnesota CPP sample above. They found nonsignificantly lower birth weights in the high-risk group and no significant differences from the control groups on the measures of obstetrical complications, the 8-month Bayley scores, or the outcome measures at 1, 4, and 7 years, except that the schizophrenic group was markedly deficient in school achievement, especially in reading, even when controlled for IQ.

However, they identified a subgroup of high-risk children who scored poorly on obstetrical complications and neurologic variables: five children scored in the poorest 25% of the high-risk group, showing the highest number of obstetrical complications, and they also scored in the worst 25% of the sample on several neurologic signs. "It is possible that high-risk children having both indicators may be especially vulnerable." Three of these five high-risk children also had the lowest 8-month Bayley Motor scores of the entire sample. Obviously, the absence of group differences on the Bayley scores obscured the deviant performance of a subgroup of high-risk children whom the authors thought might be "especially vulnerable."

7. The Pittsburgh Study

Ragins et al[54] studied the infants of 14 schizophrenic and 18 "non-schizophrenic" mothers, using the Bayley scale; six in each group were examined once between 4 and 8 months, and 10 in each group were examined once between 12 and 19 months. "No baby weighed less than 5 lbs at birth, but 4 offspring of a schizophrenic fell to or below the 3rd percentile during the first year of life." Four of the schizophrenic group "were not walking alone by 13 months." Compared with the controls, the schizophrenic group "were delayed in prehension skills." The authors concluded that "these differences in growth and development are most parsimoniously related to the difference in the quality of nurturance," which was grossly inadequate in the schizophrenics' homes. The authors did not report whether retarded growth was associated in any infants with a delay in walking or prehension. The fragmentary data reported on a few infants examined at different ages make a group analysis difficult, but the observations are consistent with those of the larger, controlled studies.

8. Offspring of Two Schizophrenic Parents

Sobel[55] examined eight infants born to two schizophrenic parents. He observed the infants with their mothers "monthly" and did "a routine pediatric examination." No systematic measures were made, but Sobel reported that "three of the 4 newborns who went to their original schizophrenic parents developed clear-cut signs of emotional disorders in infancy. None of the 4 newborns . . . who went to foster parents developed any such clear-cut signs of emotional disorder in their first 18 months."

Two of the three infants with "chronic depression" also had retarded motor development, according to the brief anecdotal information provided on the four infants reared by their parents. In one, "Head raising was delayed. Baby M. did not sit until 12 months of age. She was generally hypoactive." In the second, "Baby L. gradually became hypoactive and she began to show regression in her motor development as well. At age 7 months [she] lost the ability to sit up after she had been capable of sitting for a month." No developmental data were reported for the four foster home-reared infants.

9. The Boston Study

As part of a larger intervention study of children of psychotic mothers, Grunebaum et al[56] tested the object permanence of 15 1-year-olds and found that they "did significantly less well . . . than their matched [non-psychotic] controls." "However, these findings were accounted for primarily by the very poor

performance of three subjects . . . who had not had birth complications. Two of
their mothers were diagnosed as schizophrenic and the third was diagnosed as
psychotic depressive." However, the total numbers of schizophrenic or depressed
mothers in the 1-year-old group was not reported, making any group analysis
impossible. A later summary by these authors reported some mean Bayley scores
under 1 year for 14 infants of psychotic mothers, but unfortunately these data also
were not analyzed according to the mothers' diagnoses.[57]

Records of the Development of Adult Schizophrenics

In addition to the direct observations made in these nine prospective studies,
evidence of early disorders of motor development in schizophrenics comes from
three large-scale controlled studies that analyzed the records of children who were
later diagnosed as having schizophrenia. Retrospective studies usually cannot
obtain reliable information on visual motor development. Generally, only the most
severe motor retardation is recorded. While this may be fairly reliable, it will tend
to underestimate the incidence of motor delays that would be measurable in prospective studies.

In the 30-year follow-up of O'Neal and Robins,[58] the childhood records of 28
former patients of a child guidance clinic who became schizophrenic as adults
were compared with 57 former patients later diagnosed as having no mental illness. Difficulty in walking was among the early developmental symptoms that
significantly differentiated the preschizophrenic children from the others. Less
than 25% of these schizophrenics were hospitalized long term as adults.

Watt[59] studied the childhood public school records of 23 schizophrenics and 69
matched classroom controls. He found that severe organic handicaps, including
"neurologic disorders," significantly differentiated the preschizophrenics from
their controls and constituted one of the five factors that postdicted a schizophrenic outcome.

Ricks and Nameche,[60] like O'Neal and Robins,[58] studied the child guidance
records of clinic patients who were later followed up. Their sample included 185
subjects later diagnosed as having schizophrenia, 200 with character disorders,
alcoholism, or depressive disorders, and 100 matched controls who had achieved
positive social and vocational adjustments as adults. They found slow motor
development and other "symptoms suggesting neurologic impairment" in 20% of
the preschizophrenics compared with 10% of the controls. Furthermore, in the
preschizophrenics there was "less evident external or clearly traceable causation"
in the form of birth and subsequent neurologic trauma. These symptoms were
more frequent in the chronic preschizophrenic group than in the "released"
preschizophrenics.[61]

ALL 'NEUROMOTOR' OR 'SENSORIMOTOR' INFANT TESTS ARE NOT ALIKE

These 12 studies of preschizophrenics and infants at risk for schizophrenia show an impressive consistency in finding more delayed gross motor and visual motor infant development in schizophrenic offspring, which would meet Fish's first criterion for PDM. This occurred despite some differences in their methods and, often, in the philosophies of the authors. Yet two earlier reviews[37,62] considered the high-risk infant data to be inconsistent. This is because the reviewers compared the **psychometric** data obtained on Gesell and Bayley tests at 2 to 12 months of age in the high-risk studies reviewed above with the **primitive** functions elicited on standard infant neurologic tests,[52,53,63] neonatal Brazelton examinations,[38,41] and electroencephalograms.[41] They ignored the vast differences between these two classes of data.

As in the rest of science, findings in infants can only be confirmed or disconfirmed if one compares similar measures at comparable ages, as we have done above. **Psychometric infant tests,** such as the Gesell and Bayley, measure the rate of development in achieving numerous standardized milestones and yield DQs.[64] Unlike these two tests, which measure similar functions from birth to 3 years of age, the **Brazelton** examination is applicable only up to 1 month and does not yield a DQ.[64,65] Furthermore, only six of its visual, auditory, and motor items overlap the Gesell and Bayley in the first month, while 21 items evaluate state and other physiologic responses. Unless the six sensory and motor items from the Brazelton examination are analyzed separately, as was done in the JIDS,[38] Brazelton scores cannot even be compared with neonatal Gesell or Bayley scores.

Most of the **neurologic tests** administered to infants primarily evaluate primitive reflex behaviors and have even fewer items that overlap the Gesell or Bayley. One cannot conclude that electroencephalograms, neonatal Brazelton examinations, or neurologic examinations in study A do not confirm the retarded DQs on the Bayley or Gesell tests (with possible PDM) in study B. This is as illogical as saying that electroencephalograms or the standard adult neurologic examinations in study A do not confirm retarded scores on the Wechsler Adult Intelligence Scale in study B. These are simply not interchangeable measures of central nervous system functioning.

A REPLICATION ANALYSIS OF THE JERUSALEM DATA FOR 'PROBABLE PDM'

One of the three criteria for PDM in Fish's New York study was a transient retardation of gross motor and/or visual motor development in the first year of life. The data from the 11 studies by others, summarized above, add up to convincing documentation that delays of gross motor development occur more often in infants at genetic risk for schizophrenia and in preschizophrenics than in nonschizophrenics and normal controls. In addition, the JIDS, Rochester, and the Minnesota CPP studies all found lower visual motor scores in the schizophrenic offspring, and the Pittsburgh study reported delays in prehension, all using the Bayley scale.

However, while the group data repeatedly show significantly more developmental retardation during the first year in schizophrenics' infants, lower scores alone are too common and nonspecific a finding to delineate the subgroup that is genetically vulnerable. That single criterion alone, apart from the other two criteria for PDM, cannot predict schizotypal outcomes for individual children.

In 1952, Fish[12] assumed that transient, simple delays in one aspect of development were benign. Accordingly, to predict schizotypy, she looked for an abnormal profile of *disorganized* development, as defined in our introduction for the second criterion of PDM. The first analysis of the 1952 cohort[12] revealed that retarded and disorganized development was also accompanied by a **retardation of skeletal growth** in the first two infants who showed PDM. A parallel delay in skeletal growth became the third of the three criteria for PDM; all three were required for predicting outcomes of the 1959 cohort.[23,45]

Of the other prospective studies, only the Pittsburgh study looked at growth data. They found a drop to the third percentile in four schizophrenic offspring, but they did not state whether these delays in physical growth accompanied any of the delays in walking or prehension that they observed. Thus, only Fish's New York study had used the third criterion for PDM, consisting of an associated lag in skeletal growth, to differentiate probable PDM from benign lags.

We therefore proposed to analyze the data on growth and Bayley scores that had been collected by the JIDS, in a partial replication analysis, using Fish's method. Infants with "probable PDM" were defined as those who had lags in their Bayley scores at the same time as lags in skeletal growth. Confirming a diagnosis of PDM, by analyzing these test scores for an abnormal profile, as defined for the second of the three criteria for PDM, will not be feasible until Fish's cumbersome hand tabulation is replaced by the computer program now being developed by Fish and others at UCLA.

We hypothesized (1) that probable PDM should occur more often among the schizophrenic offspring than in the offspring in the comparison nonschizophrenic and normal control groups and (2) that probable PDM should be associated with more severe motor and cognitive impairments at the 10-year follow-up examination. We anticipated that the Bayley Motor scale would be less sensitive to neurointegrative disorder than the Gesell. In addition, the JIDS growth data were incomplete, and the JIDS used only three examinations between 1 and 12 months compared with seven in the New York study. All these factors were expected to limit the results.

METHOD

The JIDS sample has been summarized earlier and the details of infant behavior are given in earlier articles.[38-40] For this analysis, the Bayley Mental and Motor DQs of infants in the JIDS at 4, 8, and 12 months and their growth data at the same ages (when available) were evaluated by Fish, who was blind to parental diagnosis. Growth data in the JIDS files were supplemented by additional data retrieved from the well-baby clinic records. Fish considered that infants did not have PDM if all their Bayley DQs were above 90. Since there were only three age points and no ability to analyze the profile of development, Fish set Bayley DQs of less than 80 as the threshold for probable PDM, rather than using 90, as in her New York data.

Height, head circumference, and weight had been converted to six categories of percentile scores, since they were to be tabulated by hand. Fish also set stringent criteria for growth lags, ie, height or head circumference in the 25th percentile or below, since missing data might make it impossible to evaluate an actual decline. Thus, only a drop across categories could be detected (26th to 50th percentile to the 25th or less; 11th to 25th percentile to the 10th or less). This might yield either false-negative results (by obscuring declines within a percentile category) or false-positive results (if a single measurement resulted from static retarded growth, not a decline). If the two measures disagreed, height was considered more important, because it is usually the more reliable measure. Fish then examined these growth lags in relation to the Bayley DQs of individual infants. To differentiate probable PDM from benign variations required a determination that a Mental or Motor score below 80 was accompanied by a decline in height and/or head circumference percentile.

RESULTS

Distribution of PDM Categories

Of the 58 infants in the JIDS, 25 had no DQs below 90 and were considered not to have PDM (**E**, Table 2). All growth data and DQs for the 33 infants with one or more DQs below 90 were tabulated. Only 14 infants had height or head circumference data available at ages when Bayley DQs fell below 90. Two of the 14 had clear declines, at 8 months, of Motor and/or Mental DQs (of 27 to 52 points) to retarded levels (50 to 69 points), which were associated with height, head circumference, and weight in the 10th percentile, with a documented decline in head circumference or weight. These two were diagnosed as having probable PDM (**A**, Table 2) (ie, they would have PDM if the profile of

Table 2.—Blind Diagnoses of 'Probable Pandysmaturation' (PDM) and 'Possible Pandysmaturation' in Four Parent Diagnostic Groups of Jerusalem Infant Development Study (JIDS)*

Blind Diagnosis of PDM	JIDS: Diagnostic Groups			
		Other Mental Illness		
	Schizophrenia	Affective	Personality	Normal
A. *Probable PDM: development plus growth retarded*	2	...	...	...
B. Development resembles PDM; no growth data, PDM unknown	5	1	...	...
Total Candidates for PDM	7	1	...	...
C. Development unlike PDM: no growth data, PDM unknown	3	4	5	1
D. *Not PDM: no growth lag*	1	4	3	4
E. *Not PDM: no Bayley score <90*	8	7	5	11
Total Probably Not Candidates for PDM	12	9	13	16
Total Subjects	19	10	13	16

*PDM categories by parent diagnosis: schizophrenic vs nonschizophrenic ($\chi^2 = 12.8$; $df = 3$; $P = .005$) (see Table 3, paragraph a). Diagnoses and numbers in italics represent definite evaluations based on both skeletal growth and DQ.

development was also abnormal). In 12 of the 14 infants, the growth data ruled out PDM (**D**, Table 2).

Fish also ranked the 19 infants with Bayley DQs below 90 whose PDM was "possible" but unknown because they had no growth data. Only six had developmental curves resembling PDM, with drops in their Mental DQs to 50 to 76 (**B**, Table 2). The curves of the remaining 13 did not resemble PDM (**C**, Table 2): five had drops only of the Motor score at 8 months, which Fish considered an artifact of the insensitive 4-month Bayley Motor score (only one of the 58 infants scored <90 at 4 months); a sixth infant dropped precipitously from high 4- and 8-month DQs to 53 and 55 at 12 months, suggesting some neurologic or other physical cause rather than PDM (in all of Fish's high-risk infants with PDM, PDM had begun by 9 months). The lowest DQs of the final seven were too minimally retarded (80 to 86 DQs).

Fish's blind diagnoses of probable PDM (**A**), possible PDM (**B** or **C**), and "not PDM" (**D + E**) were analyzed in relation to parental diagnosis, antecedent factors (birth weight and obstetrical complications), and follow-up status by one of us (S.P.). Obstetrical complications had been recorded prospectively, and yielded a total score, as in the Rochester study.[41] At approximately 10 years of age, 45 of the original 58 subjects were reexamined (J.M., S.L.H., and J.G.A. and Aaron G. Auerbach, PhD, unpublished data, May 1991). Our replication analysis used only the summary scores for cognitive and motor impairment that had been derived from 14 separate tests (Marcus et al, unpublished data, May 1991). Tests loading mainly on the cognitive factor included Porteus mazes, Raven matrices, mirror drawing, auditory-visual integration, digit cancellation, and matching familiar figures. Those loading on the motor factor included postures, associated movements, fine motor coordination, involuntary movements, mirror movements, reflexes, and eye movements. The Bender test loaded on both factors.

A Significant Relation Between PDM and Parental Schizophrenia

As predicted, the relation between the likelihood of PDM (four categories, **A**, **B**, **C**, and **D + E**) and a parental diagnosis of schizophrenia was significant ($P = .005$, paragraph a). Details of statistical comparisons and tests are shown in Table 3 and are referenced by paragraph letters (paragraphs a through u) in the text. Because PDM categories had been ranked, more powerful statistical tests used for ordinal data often could be used, rather than strictly categorical (nominal) data tests. Ranking of PDM was in the direction of increasing likelihood of PDM, called "increasing PDM," where probable PDM (**A**) > (possible PDM [**B**] > possible PDM [**C**]) > not PDM (**D + E**). For all the analyses, other than the relation between PDM and schizophrenia, PDM categories **B** and **C** were combined as possible PDM. This was done because the differentiation between these

Table 3.—Analyses of Pandysmaturation (PDM), Birth Weight, Obstetrical Complications, and Motor and Cognitive Impairment Scores at 10 Years in Jerusalem Infant Development Study

Comparison			Statistic	No. of Subjects	Significance P
a. PDM categories vs diagnosis, % (n)			$\chi^2 = 12.8$	58	.005
	Schizophrenia	Nonschiz	$df = 3$		
Prob PDM = A	100.0 (2)	0 (0)			
Poss PDM = B	83.3 (5)	16.7 (1)			
Poss PDM = C	23.1 (3)	76.9 (10)			
Not PDM = D + E	24.3 (9)	75.7 (28)			
b. Birth weight vs PDM ranks			$r = -.28$	55	.04
Prob PDM	Mean	2880		2	Means for reference only
Poss PDM	Mean	3035		17	
Not PDM	Mean	3266		36	
c. Birth weight vs diagnosis			ANOVA $F\,(3,51) = 2.35$	55	.07
Schizophrenia	Mean	2995		19	
Affective disorder	Mean	3246		9	
Personality disorder	Mean	3388		12	
Normal group	Mear	3210		15	
Birth weight to schiz vs nonschiz			$F\,(1,53) = 5.85$		.02
d. Obstetrical complication scores vs PDM ranks			$r = .06$	52	NS
e. Obstetrical complication scores vs diagnosis			ANOVA $F\,(3,48) = 0.16$	52	.92 NS

				n	Significance	
Schizophrenia	Mean	3.23		17		
Affective disorder	Mean	3.0		8		
Personality disorder	Mean	2.92		13		
Normal	Mean	2.71		14		
f. PDM ranks vs cognitive score			$r = .33$	45	.03	
Prob PDM	Mean	1.256		2		Means for reference only
Poss PDM	Mean	0.191		11		
Not PDM	Mean	-0.089		32		
g. PDM ranks vs motor score			$r = .32$	45	.03	
Prob PDM	Mean	1.237		2		Means for reference only
Poss PDM	Mean	0.288		11		
Not PDM	Mean	-0.139		32		

h. Diagnosis vs cognitive, motor and normal clusters, % (n)

	Cognitive	Motor	Normal		n	Significance
Schiz	26.7 (4)	33.3 (5)	40.0 (6)	$\chi^2 = 10.60\ (df = 4)$	45	.03
Other diagnoses	11.1 (2)	0.0 (0)	88.9 (16)			
Normal	8.3 (1)	16.7 (2)	75.0 (9)			

i. PDM categories vs clusters % (n)

	Cognitive and/or Motor	Normal		n	Significance
Prob PDM	100.0 (2)	0.0 (0)	$\chi^2 = 5.12\ (df = 2)$	45	.08
Poss PDM	36.4 (4)	63.6 (7)			
Not PDM	25.0 (8)	75.0 (24)			

j. PDM ranks vs follow-up scores, schiz group

		n	Significance
Cognitive	$r = .55$	15	.03
Motor	$r = .24$	15	NS

Table 3.—Analyses of Pandysmaturation (PDM), Birth Weight, Obstetrical Complications, and Motor and Cognitive Impairment Scores at 10 Years in Jerusalem Infant Development Study (cont)

Comparison		Statistic	No. of Subjects	Significance P
k. Obstetrical complications vs motor scores schiz group		$r = .66$	14	.01
Outside motor cluster	Mean	2.67	9	Means for reference only
Within motor cluster	Mean	4.8	5	
l. Obstetrical complications vs motor scores, all subjects		$r = .19$	41	NS
m. Birth weight vs motor scores, schiz group		$r = -.46$	15	.08
Outside motor cluster	Mean	3158	10	Means for reference only
Within motor cluster	Mean	2910	5	
n. Birth weight vs motor scores, all subjects		$r = -.21$	44	NS
q. PDM rank vs motor score, schiz in motor cluster		$r = .87$	5	.05
r. Birth weight vs motor score, schiz in motor cluster		$r = -.81$	5	.09
s. Obstetrical complications vs motor score, schiz in motor cluster		$r = .79$	5	.11
t. Birth weight vs PDM rank, schiz in motor cluster		$r = -.82$	5	.09
u. Obstetrical complications vs motor score, schiz in motor cluster, controlling for birth weight		Partial correlation coefficient $r = .94$	5	.05

*Schiz indicates schizophrenia; NS, not significant; prob, probable; poss, possible; and ANOVA, analysis of variance.

two groups was made (blindly) on clinical grounds. Such judgments could not be replicated by others or on different samples.

Lower birth weight was correlated with increasing PDM ($P = .04$, paragraph b). It was also weakly related to diagnosis ($P = .07$, paragraph c), but it significantly differentiated the schizophrenic from the nonschizophrenic offspring ($P = .02$, paragraph c). In contrast to this, there was no significant relation between PDM and obstetrical complications (paragraph d) for the sample as a whole. This was in keeping with the lack of correlation between obstetrical complications and diagnosis (paragraph e).

A Significant Relation Between PDM, Schizophrenia, and Impairment at 10 Years

As predicted, increasing PDM was significantly related to higher impairment scores at the 10-year follow-up on both the cognitive ($P = .03$, paragraph f) and the motor tests ($P = .03$, paragraph g) for the sample as a whole. Multivariate analysis examining the relationships between increasing PDM and increasing cognitive and motor scores when controlling for any effects of obstetrical complications found that obstetrical complications actually had no effect on these relationships.

The Figure presents high-resolution graphs that show the exact location of each of the 45 children on a plot of their cognitive and motor scores, with subjects having probable PDM and possible PDM identified. A three-group cluster analysis identified both "arms" of the follow-up data, a **"cognitive problem" cluster** (at left in the Figure) and a **"motor problem" cluster**, as different from the "normal" cluster. There are seven children in each of the problem groups. These are balanced across the three PDM categories, with the cognitive cluster and the motor cluster each containing 50% of the probable PDM, 18% of the possible PDM, and 12% of the "not PDM" groups.

The separate plots of the subjects, when divided by parental diagnosis (Figure), depict the clear relationship that exists between parental diagnosis and problem clusters ($P = .03$, paragraph h). This is due to the schizophrenic group, with 60% (9/15) in the problem clusters compared with 11% (2/18) for "other" diagnoses, and 25% (3/12) for the "normal" group. Overall, 64% (9/14) of those in the problem clusters have schizophrenic parents, even though those children represent only 33% (15/45) of the sample.

Even though only two infants had probable PDM, and the separate cells of PDM within each cluster are too small to yield any statistically significant relationships, there is a significant relationship between PDM and "*any* follow-up problem" in the motor and/or cognitive clusters combined ($P = .08$, paragraph i). Collapsing the two abnormal clusters is appropriate, since the PDM categories are distributed equally in both. We note further that, of the two subjects with probable PDM, one lies at the extreme tip of the motor cluster and the other is the second worst in the cognitive cluster (Figure, Schiz).

A scan of subjects with probable plus possible PDM across the three diagnostic groups suggests that PDM predicts later abnormality only in the schizophrenic group. This would be predicted by our hypothesis that PDM reflects a schizophrenic genotype. The significant relationship between PDM category and follow-up status *within the schizophrenic group* of 15 subjects proves to hold only for the cognitive scores ($P = .03$, paragraph j).

PDM, Obstetrical Complications, Birth Weight, and Motor Impairment at 10 Years in the Schizophrenic Offspring

Subject 55, with the worst PDM and the worst motor score, also had one of the highest obstetrical complication scores in the entire sample. We therefore examined the relationship between obstetrical complications and motor scores within the schizophrenic group and found it highly significant ($P = .01$, paragraph k). This contrasts with the nonsignificant relationship between obstetrical complications and motor scores for the entire sample (paragraph l). Similarly, subject 55 also was one of four schizophrenic offspring with a birth weight less than 2500 g; birth weight, as well, bears a significant relationship to motor scores for the schizophrenic group ($P = .08$, paragraph m), but not for the sample as a whole (paragraph n).

Because these relationships apparently led to the worst neurologic status at 10 years, we ranked the five schizophrenic offspring in the motor cluster by their decreasing motor impairment scores. We found that this also ranked them by decreasing PDM category, decreasing obstetrical scores, and except for the fourth subject, also ranked them by increasing birth weight (Table 4). Several of the correlation magnitudes within the schizophrenic offspring in the motor cluster are very high, but the significance levels are low because of the very small numbers: for PDM vs motor, $r = .87$ ($P = .05$, paragraph q); for birth weight vs motor, $r = .81$ ($P-.09$, paragraph r); and for obstetrical complications vs motor, $r = .79$ ($P = .11$, paragraph s). There is also an interesting relation between birth weight and PDM ($r = -.82$, $P = .09$, paragraph t). The partial correlation coefficient for obstetrical complications vs motor scores within the schizophrenic offspring in the motor cluster, when controlling for birth weight, is $r = .94$ ($P = .05$, paragraph u). That is, the effect of obstetrical complications in this small subgroup is not merely a "low birth weight" effect.

The clinical summary of subject 55, the worst of the two children with probable PDM, noted that, in addition to her poor neurologic and cognitive scores at 9 years (despite an average IQ), she had a "psychotic-like" Bender-Gestalt test

Table 4.—Pandysmaturation (PDM) Category, Birth Weight, Obstetrical Complication (OC) Score, and Motor Impairment Score for All Infants in the Jerusalem Infant Development Study in the Motor Cluster at 10-Year Follow-up*

Subject No.	Motor Score	PDM Category	Birth Weight, g	OC Score	Specific OC: *Possible Anoxia*
			Schizophrenic Offspring in the Motor Cluster		
55	2.429	Probable	2440	7	*Pregnancy:* Medication, asthma, previous miscarriages, **premature labor—stopped and cervix sutured.** *Birth:* analgesia 50 to 100 mg, induced labor. *Neonate:* physiologic jaundice
61	2.204	Possible	2790	6	*Pregnancy:* Medication. *Birth:* analgesia >100 mg. *Neonate:* **resuscitation, cyanosis, physiologic jaundice**
58	1.670	Possible	2820	5	*Pregnancy:* Medication, mother >35 y, multipara >6. *Birth:* analgesia >100 mg
45	0.836	None	3550	5	*Pregnancy:* Mother hospitalized at 6 mo with flu and dehydration. *Birth:* analgesia 50 to 100 mg, induced labor, vacuum. *Neonate:* **resuscitation**
62	0.808	None	2950		*Pregnancy:* **Premature labor stopped**
			Offspring of Normal Parents in the Motor Cluster		
23	1.930	None	3600	1	*Birth:* Induced labor
6	1.613	None	3560	2	*Birth:* Induced labor. *Neonate:* **cyanotic, placed in incubator**

result; she daydreamed in class, was fearful, shy, and tormented by peers. At 11.5 years she also showed signs of "cognitive slippage" (J.M., S.L.H., and J.G.A. and Aaron G. Auerbach, PhD, unpublished data, May 1991, for a full vignette).

COMMENT

Replication Analysis of PDM in the JIDS

Despite its anticipated shortcomings, this partial replication of Fish's method confirmed our initial predictions. It did so even though we were limited to applying only two of her three criteria to data from the JIDS; Fish's blind evaluations of PDM were based only on delayed development and a parallel delay in skeletal growth. Yet these evaluations were highly correlated with a parental diagnosis of schizophrenia. This supports our hypothesis that PDM is a marker for a schizophrenic genotype. Herein, as in Fish's original New York study, obstetrical complications did not contribute to the developmental delays involved in PDM.

The evidence for genetic specificity is, in fact, even stronger than in the original New York study. Thus, the JIDS included a mentally ill comparison group, yet probable PDM did not occur with any parental diagnosis other than schizophrenia. Ragins et al[54] attributed retarded growth and development to the "inadequate nurturance" given by psychotic mothers (only schizophrenics, in the Pittsburgh study). However, the offspring of neurotic *depressed* mothers appeared to be "most at risk" when compared with children of schizophrenics and controls in the Rochester study.[41(p58)] The depressed mothers "showed less involvement with their infants"; their infants "had poorer responsivity to people"; followed by "a variety of less adaptive behaviors." In the JIDS, probable PDM due to inadequate nurturance, therefore, should have occurred more often in the infants of severely depressed mothers than in the infants of schizophrenics. However, none occurred in the depressed group.

As we predicted, PDM also proved to be significantly related to both poorer cognitive and motor neurointegrative functioning at the 10-year follow-up within the overall sample. The two children with probable PDM had poor cognitive scores, and one also had the worst motor score. Those with possible PDM in the schizophrenic group were distributed across the abnormal and normal clusters at follow-up. One would expect this if some had PDM and others did not. (We could not confirm whether they had probable PDM, since their growth data were unavailable.)

In contrast to this distribution, all of those with possible PDM in the nonschizophrenic mentally ill group were in the normal cluster at 10 years. This suggests that none of them had PDM. In other words, they probably had the type of nonspecific developmental lags that may occur in infants born to well or mentally ill parents, lags that do not indicate a schizophrenic genotype and are usually not followed by serious sequelae in childhood.

Within the schizophrenic group, PDM was only significantly related to cognitive dysfunction at 10 years. When the JIDS subjects are retested in adolescence, the cognitive deficits at 10 years will, we think, be most highly correlated with the measures of thought disorder[66,67] and with abnormal functioning on the Span of Apprehension and other tests of attention and cognitive processing.[32,33] These are all proven markers for a schizotypal trait.

The validity of PDM as a presumptive genetic marker in infancy can ultimately be proved only by an adult diagnosis of schizophrenia or schizotypal personality disorder. These impaired JIDS subjects are just now entering the risk period for schizophrenia. Their resemblance to Fish's[45] subjects during infancy and late prepuberty suggests that some may follow a similar schizotypal course in adulthood. This replication analysis provides only indirect evidence from the intermediate 10-year follow-up. In the National Institute of Mental Health Israeli Kibbutz-City Study, begun in 1965, eight of the nine subjects who were later diagnosed as having adult schizophrenia had shown cognitive and motor deficits in childhood that were similar to those observed in this study, using similar procedures.[40]

Evidence Since 1975 That PDM Is an Inherited Congenital Neurointegrative Defect

The evidence that PDM manifests an inherited congenital neurointegrative defect appears even stronger in 1991 than it did in 1975.[1,10] The results of our replication analysis add weight to our hypothesis that PDM is a marker in infancy of a schizophrenic genotype. Blind diagnoses of probable and possible PDM were made from JIDS data that included offspring of nonschizophrenic mentally ill parents. We differentiated benign developmental lags from probable PDM by using retarded skeletal growth, the second criterion for PDM. It was not possible to apply the third criterion of an abnormal profile; however, adding the second criterion of PDM identified only schizophrenic offspring.

To the extent that relevant data are available in the large high-risk studies, the JIDS, Rochester, Danish Obstetrical, and Minnesota CPP studies all found consistently lower motor and/or mental development in schizophrenics' offspring in the first year of life. This meets Fish's[45] first criterion for PDM. Only the New York State CPP study did not. In Fish's[45] study, extrinsic factors such as obstetrical complications, socioeconomic status, and race were not related to PDM. Similarly, the lower scores in the JIDS, Rochester, Danish Obstetrical, and Minnesota CPP studies were not related to obstetrical complications. Instead, the JIDS, Rochester, and Danish Obstetrical studies found that low-normal birth weights were associated with a parental diagnosis of schizophrenia, as in half of the New York infants with PDM.

Finally, there is accumulating evidence from the expert blind psychological evaluations of Fish's original subjects. So far, these favor an adult schizotypal disorder or schizophrenia in at least four of the six high-risk infants with PDM who have been chronically disturbed since childhood (including one chronic schizophrenic). Final validation of the predictive value of PDM will depend on the blind consensus diagnoses that will be obtained subsequently on the New York and on the JIDS subjects as adults.

Do Mild Obstetrical Complications Trigger PDM In Utero, With Immaturity, Lower Birth Weight, and Later Neurologic Deficits?

Some intriguing questions are raised by our unexpected findings of a small subgroup of schizophrenic offspring in the motor cluster. These infants had the most severe neurologic deficits at follow-up in addition to their abnormal cognitive functioning. How can one best explain the relationships between the severity of motor symptoms, PDM, obstetrical complications, and lower birth weight in this subgroup? For the sample as a whole, obstetrical complications behaved like a random factor, as in the other high-risk studies. Obstetrical complications were not related to a parental diagnosis of schizophrenia; they were not related to DQs below 90 or to PDM in infancy; and they were not related to cognitive or motor dysfunctions in childhood, even as an additive risk factor.

Nevertheless, we were able to demonstrate that within the schizophrenic group, obstetrical complications were followed by significantly higher motor impairment scores at 10 years. It appears that these infants were more vulnerable to neurologic impairment following obstetrical complications because they carried a schizophrenic genotype. If PDM reflects a schizophrenic genotype, as we think, then it is not surprising that PDM is related to the motor impairment found in this subgroup.

But why should low birth weight, as well, be related to the motor deficits and PDM found in these infants? In 1971, Mednick et al[50] considered the low-normal birth weights in the Danish Obstetrical Study to be obstetrical complications, reflecting deleterious factors in utero related to the mothers' schizophrenia. However, in discussing this article in 1971, Fish[68] posed an alternative explanation, observing that the low-birth-weight infants with motor delays of Mednick et al resembled her infants with PDM immediately postpartum, as well as subsequently. She suggested that the most parsimonious explanation of the low birth weights was that PDM, with its delays in growth and development, had simply begun in utero. In addition, Heston[69] pointed out that "the schizophrenic fathers contributed immature infants in a proportion compatible with their total contribu-

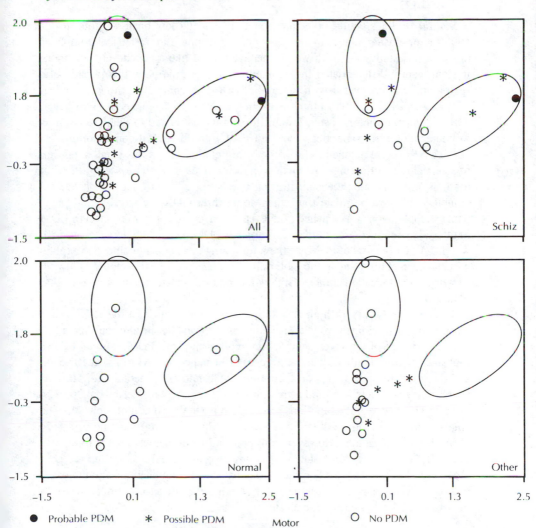

Exact location of subjects from the Jerusalem Infant Development Study on plots of their cognitive and motor impairment scores at 10 years, showing their blind pandysmaturation (PDM) diagnosis and the "cognitive" and "motor" clusters, for "All" subjects and for each parent-diagnosis group. Schiz indicates schizophrenia.

tion of offspring . . . which supports the hypothesis that immaturity at birth is associated with schizophrenic genotypes in a direct relationship." Marcus et al[8] later raised this possibility for the low-birth-weight schizophrenic offspring in the JIDS, where schizophrenic fathers also contributed their share of small infants.

Several findings counter the interpretation that the low birth weights in our JIDS motor cluster occurred simply as a direct response to obstetrical complications. In this study, low birth weight behaved more like a genetic phenomenon. It significantly differentiated the schizophrenic from the nonschizophrenic offspring and was correlated with increasing PDM. In contrast to this, obstetrical complications behaved like a random event, unrelated to diagnosis or PDM. Even within the small motor cluster, low birth weight was related to PDM, as well as to poorer motor outcome, but it was not related to obstetrical complications.

We are therefore inclined to favor the interpretation that in this small subgroup of schizophrenic offspring, low birth weight reflected an earlier onset of PDM in utero as an intervening mechanism; that it was not a direct effect of obstetrical complications. We postulate that when some threshold of relatively mild pregnancy complications was reached (Table 4), this triggered an earlier onset of PDM in utero. The retarded growth that accompanies PDM then resulted in a lower birth weight. An early onset of PDM, as the intervening mechanism, could also explain why the normal offspring in the motor cluster had normal birth weights following obstetrical complications (Table 4); they lacked both schizophrenic genotype and PDM.

Three of the New York high-risk subjects resembled those in the JIDS motor cluster: low-normal birth weights, accompanied by smaller head circumferences, occurred in four of the seven schizophrenic offspring with PDM. Three of these four small high-risk infants had the lowest Performance IQs (61 to 78) at 10 years, and the worst Koppitz scores on their Bender-Gestalt tests (mental age, 5.5 to 7 years). They (subjects 1, 5, and 6) retained these visual motor deficits at 20 to 24 years.[45] Their 10-year dysfunctions resemble those in the JIDS motor cluster. The small high-risk infants in the New York study did not have moderate or severe obstetrical complications. However, common, milder events were not summed, as in the JIDS. The New York State CPP study also identified a subgroup (25% of the high-risk offspring) that had the worst obstetrical complications and the worst neurologic symptoms in childhood. This subgroup appears to resemble the JIDS high-risk children in the motor cluster.

Possible Implications for Adult Schizophrenia of the Low Birth Weights and Obstetrical Complications in the JIDS Motor Subgroup

McNeil[70] reviewed the many studies, including his own, which reveal an increased incidence of obstetrical complications in schizophrenics. He made a convincing case that "obstetrical complications are in some way related to the subsequent development of schizophrenia." If this is so, then the JIDS subgroup at the highest risk for adult schizophrenia should be those with PDM, lower birth weights, and more severe neurologic deficits, following obstetrical complications.

It is tempting to speculate that such a course might explain the findings of Suddath et al,[71] in which the schizophrenic twins of discordant monozygotic pairs had larger ventricles and smaller hippocampi than their normal cotwins. The reanalysis of the earlier discordant monozygotic twin data by McNeil[70] would support this; he demonstrated increased obstetrical complications in the more severely ill schizophrenic twin of the pair.

On the other hand, DeLisi et al[72] found no significant difference between the limbic structures of schizophrenic siblings with and without a history of obstetrical complications, although the limbic structures were smaller in schizophrenics than their normal siblings. Silverton et al[9] also found that ventricular enlargement was unrelated to a composite obstetrical complication score in a subsample of the Danish high-risk study. Instead, enlargement was significantly negatively related to birth weight. However, McNeil[70] demonstrated that there is much false-negative information regarding obstetrical complications in the retrospective histories in psychiatric charts, when he compared these with the original prenatal and obstetrical records. He also pointed out that the midwives' reports used in the Danish studies include mainly *birth* complications, and only *major* pregnancy events. Such factors may explain some of these discrepancies. Certainly many of the "nonoptimal events" in our JIDS subjects with high motor scores would not be provided by pregnancy histories obtained in adulthood (Table 4).

Data on the Genain quadruplets[73] suggest both the relevance and the limitations of predictions from isolated birth weight and growth data when the genetic contribution is identical. Their birth weights were as follows: Nora, 2041 g; Myra, 1928 g; Iris, 1503 g; and Hester, 1361 g; their heights at birth were in the same rank order (43, 42, 40.6, and 35 cm),[73(p542)] as was the retardation of their carpal bone age (as a percent of age) at 22 months (68%, 59%, 54%, and 50%).

In keeping with her growth retardation, Hester also trailed far behind in early development and did not walk until 20 months, while Iris generally lagged only 1 month behind Nora and Myra.[73(p50)] Hester's clinical course was also the worst, with "strange" behavior as a preschooler,[73(p524)] the largest fall in school grades at 14 years[73(p197)] when her IQ dropped from 89 to 77,[73(p195)] and a schizophrenia that ended in long-term hospitalization with a regressed hebephrenic state.[73(p519)] Iris remained second to worst in her drop in grades at 14 years and in her subsequent schizophrenia[73(p528)] with a predominantly hebephrenic course. However, above 1900 g, birth weight did not override other factors: Nora was clearly the best in school through high school[73(p197)] but had the third worst course with repeated hospitalizations and hebephrenic features, while Myra never required hospitalization and her "illness was arrested early."[73(pp518-528)]

Schizophrenia in New York Subjects With PDM Did Not Follow Low Birth Weight

We have two other caveats from Fish's New York study regarding the prognostic significance of low birth weight (and inferred obstetrical complication). First, none of the three schizotypal subjects who had low-normal birth weights, small head circumferences, and persistent fine motor and perceptual symptoms at 10 to 20+ years has had a psychotic break as an adult of 30 to 38 years (subject 5, a homeless woman, could not be reexamined after 22 years).[45]

Second, the 30-year-old man who has been chronically schizophrenic since 19 years[44] had a birth weight of 3840 g, no fine motor symptoms at 10 years, and an average Koppitz score on his Bender test (which was only diagnosed blindly as schizophrenic by Bender herself). Yet he showed declining scores in reading and on intelligence testing from 10 years on, despite private schooling and remedial help. Finally, at 19 years, an extensive neuropsychological study in hospital was interpreted as showing "some form of long-standing, diffuse central nervous system deficit," including "left hemisphere and frontal lobe problems with concentration and symbolic reasoning." To us, his progressive cognitive and psychiatric decline appeared to be a genetically programmed insidious course from birth on, up until the final weeks leading to his first hospitalization. At that point the withdrawal of family and therapist support, and a substitution of lithium carbonate for thioridazine, tipped his fragile balance into what was diagnosed in hospital as an "acute" breakdown. His flat affect had been observed from 1 month of age, and other negative symptoms became evident by 6 to 10 years, long before his first psychotic episode.

Alternative Paths of 'Schizotypal Infants': Following Normal Pregnancies or Those Marked by Several Nonoptimal Events

As viewed from the combined observations of the New York and JIDS studies, the **primary developmental course** for infants with a schizophrenic genotype appears to be as follows: PDM from birth to 2 years; moderate to severe social-affective symptoms beginning between 3 and 6 years; followed by cognitive deficits and moderate to severe psychopathologic features at 10 years; and schizotypal disorders in adolescence and adulthood. At this stage of our analyses, we do not believe that the infant data predict which schizotypal subjects will develop a schizophrenic psychosis. However, the discontinuity between schizophrenia and schizotypal personality disorder is an artifact of *DSM-III* categories.[74] Genetic data demonstrate that these two disorders share the same genetic predisposition.[15]

A **potential alternative pathway** for infants with a schizophrenic genotype, especially if their mothers' pregnancies had been complicated by a series of even *mild* nonoptimal events, is the following: an earlier onset of PDM in utero; lower weight (and probably smaller head circumference) at birth; and more severe neurologic deficits at 10 years, in addition to the cognitive and psychiatric problems of the other subjects with PDM. The adult course of this JIDS subgroup has yet to be determined.

The Significance of PDM for the Neurologic Findings in Adult Schizophrenia, in the Absence of Obstetrical Complications

The life course of the schizophrenic man in the New York study emphasizes an essential finding of the New York and JIDS studies for scientists who are interested in the early origins of the neurologic abnormalities they have discovered in adult schizophrenics. One does not need to invoke the extrinsic insult of obstetrical complications to explain neurologic signs in schizophrenia.

Pandysmaturation itself includes many neurologic manifestations between birth and 2 years. Pandysmaturation was highly correlated with a parental diagnosis of schizophrenia and was not related to obstetrical complications in both the New York and JIDS studies. Furthermore, PDM led to cognitive neurointegrative deficits at 10 years in the JIDS, and subsequent schizotypal symptoms in the New York study, in the absence of obstetrical complications or low birth weight. The fundamental, necessary, and specific etiology of schizotypy and schizophrenia is the genetic one, which we, like Meehl,[16,17] believe is manifested in part by PDM, cognitive, and other specific neurointegrative deficits.

Obstetrical complications could only play a nonspecific, precipitating, or facilitating role in the manifestation of the genetic predisposition. When discordant twin data are examined carefully,[20,75] obstetrical complications appear to function like many other biologic and psychosocial life events that seem to tip some genetically vulnerable individuals into psychosis. But which of these nonspecific factors will serve this function seems to vary from one schizophrenic to another.[20,75]

The finding of Andreasen et al[4,76] of decreased cerebral and cranial size in some schizophrenics may be related to the retardation of skeletal growth during PDM. Pandysmaturation includes a lag in head circumference, which was more marked in the subgroup with low-normal birth weights. In the subjects of Andreasen et al, decreased cranial size was associated with prominent negative symptoms and impaired frontal function. Three (subjects 1, 5, and 7) of the four New York high-risk subjects with PDM and small head circumferences at birth had persistent negative signs that began in early childhood.[45]

We suggest that scientists who are interested in the early origins of the neurologic lesions they are discovering in adult schizophrenics might find records of the gross motor milestones, head circumference, height, and weight of their subjects in obstetrical and pediatric charts. If such data from birth to 1 year of age were analyzed for probable PDM, much as we did herein, they might yield some interesting leads, beyond that provided by low birth weight alone.

The observations of Fish[11-13,22,77] of PDM during the first 2 years of life may reveal something of the locus of the neurointegrative disorder during infancy. The manifestations of PDM reveal a profound, innate dysregulation of the normal timing, sequences, and spatial organization of neurologic development: development even went into reverse, with periods when previously acquired abilities were lost; and periods when the cephalocaudal gradient was temporarily reversed, so that control of the legs was more advanced than that of the head.

In the New York study's 1959 cohort analyzed by Fish and Dixon,[77] when arousal, vestibular, and sensory responses were measured, the periods of PDM were accompanied by decreased arousal, reflected in brief or absent nystagmus after vestibular stimulation and by severe apathy and underresponsiveness in the three infants whose PDM was most severe. The association of disorders of skeletal growth, arousal, tonus, motility, proprioceptive, vestibular, and vasovegetative functions suggested a dysregulation that involved hypothalamic and reticular activating systems in schizotypal infants.[13,78]

These systems might well be affected by a dysfunction resulting from the excess disorientation of hippocampal pyramidal cells found by Kovelman and Scheibel[1] in schizophrenics' brains, structural changes that most probably occurred during fetal development when neuroblasts migrate into the hippocampal primordium. These authors hypothesized that the anatomic disorganization "may conceivably affect patterns of synaptic linkage upon the hippocampal cell, leading to altered information processing in the areas involved." Furthermore, they emphasized that while schizophrenia does not emerge for years thereafter, such delays occur in many other hereditary central nervous system diseases.

Others have also found reduced volume and cellular density in limbic structures.[2,71,72,79-81] These findings, in the absence of "histologic evidence of anoxia"[81] or gliosis, "support the assumption of a *developmental hypoplasia* [our emphasis] of medial temporal lobe structures in schizophrenics rather than an ongoing pathological process."[2] A 1986 workshop of neuroscientists[5] agreed that "there is evidence for changes in limbic structures," and they concluded that "the case that the changes are in some sense developmental is growing." Additional evidence supporting "neurodevelopmentally determined abnormalities" was presented at a 1990 workshop,[82] which cites a report given there by Bogerts and Falkai of reduced hippocampal volumes and histologic abnormalities in the entorhinal region that "were interpreted as indicating **developmental arrest in midgestation**" [our emphasis]. Weinberger[83] even formulated a neurodevelopmental theory, based on "a subtle, static structural brain lesion that involves a diffuse system of periventricular limbic and diencephalic nuclei and their connections to the dorsolateral prefrontal cortex . . . which is presumed to have occurred early in development." In the light of all this accumulating evidence, perhaps it is not too farfetched to hope that, in the not too distant future, the newer noninvasive techniques, in conjunction with PDM, may be used to investigate this question directly in a pilot study of high-risk infants.

REFERENCES

1. Kovelman JA, Scheibel AB. A neurohistological correlate of schizophrenia. *Biol Psychiatry.* 1984;19:1601–1621.

2. Falkai P, Bogerts B, Rozumek M. Limbic pathology in schizophrenia: the entorhinal region: a morphometric study. *Biol Psychiatry.* 1988;24:515–521.

3. Crow TJ, Ball J, Bloom SR, Brown R, Bruton CJ, Colter N, Frith CD, Johnstone EC, Owens DGC, Roberts GW. Schizophrenia as an anomaly of development of cerebral asymmetry. *Arch Gen Psychiatry.* 1989;46:1145–1150.

4. Andreasen N, Nasrallah HA, Dunn V, Olson SC, Grove WM, Ehrhardt JC, Coffman JA, Crossett JHW. Structural abnormalities in the frontal system in schizophrenia: a magnetic resonance imaging study. *Arch Gen Psychiatry.* 1986;43:136–144.

5. Crow TJ, Berndl K, Bogerts B, Cohen RJ, Flor-Henry P, Ingvar DH, Johnstone EC, Lehmann D, Patterson TE, Shagass C, Straube ER, Taylor PJ, Weinberger DR. Structural and functional deviations: group report. In: Helmchen H, Henn FA, eds. *Biological Perspectives of Schizophrenia.* New York, NY: John Wiley & Sons Inc; 1987:254–269.

6. Weinberger DR, Berman KF, Zec RF. Physiologic dysfunction of dorsolateral prefrontal cortex in schizophrenia, I: regional cerebral blood flow evidence. *Arch Gen Psychiatry.* 1986;43:114–125.

7. Cannon TD, Mednick SA, Parnas J. Genetic and perinatal determinants of structural brain deficits in schizophrenia. *Arch Gen Psychiatry.* 1989;46:883–889.

8. Schulsinger F, Parnas J, Petersen ET, Schulsinger H, Teasdale TW, Mednick SA, Moller L, Silverton L. Cerebral ventricular size in the offspring of schizophrenic mothers: a preliminary study. *Arch Gen Psychiatry.* 1984;41:602–606.

9. Silverton L, Finello KM, Schulsinger F, Mednick SA. Low birth weight and ventricular enlargement in a high-risk sample. *J Abnorm Psychol.* 1985;94:405–409.

10. Fish B. Biologic antecedents of psychosis in children. In: Freedman DX, ed. *The Biology of the Major Psychoses: A Comparative Analysis, Association for Research in Nervous and Mental Disease.* New York, NY: Raven Press; 1975;54:49–80.

11. Fish B. Neurobiologic antecedents of schizophrenia in children: evidence for an inherited, congenital neurointegrative defect. *Arch Gen Psychiatry.* 1977;34:1297–1313.

12. Fish B. The detection of schizophrenia in infancy. *J Nerv Ment Dis.* 1957;125:1–24.

13. Fish B. Involvement of the central nervous system in infants with schizophrenia. *Arch Neurol.* 1960;2:115–121.

14. Bender L. Childhood schizophrenia: clinical study of 100 schizophrenic children. *Am J Orthopsychiatry.* 1947;17:40–56.

15. Kendler SK. The genetics of schizophrenia: an overview. In: Tsuang MT, Simpson JC, eds. *Handbook of Schizophrenia: Nosology, Epidemiology and Genetics.* New York, NY: Elsevier Science Publishers; 1988;3:437–462.

16. Meehl PE. Schizotaxia revisited. *Arch Gen Psychiatry.* 1989;46:935–944.

17. Meehl PE. Toward an integrated theory of schizotaxia, schizotypy, and schizophrenia. *J Pers Disorders.* 1990;4:1–99.

18. Asarnow RF, Asarnow JR, Strandburg R. Schizophrenia: a developmental perspective. In: Cicchetti D, ed. *The Emergence of a Discipline: Rochester Symposium on Developmental Psychopathology.* Hillsdale, NJ: Lawrence Erlbaum Associates Inc Publishers; 1990;1:189–219.

19. Rosenthal D. *Genetic Theory and Abnormal Behavior.* New York, NY: McGraw-Hill International Book Co; 1970.

20. Gottesman II, Shields J. *Schizophrenia: The Epigenetic Puzzle.* New York, NY: Cambridge University Press; 1982.

21. Bender L, Freedman AM. A study of the first three years in the maturation of schizophrenic children. *Q J Child Behav.* 1952;1:245–272.

22. Fish B. Longitudinal observations of biological deviations in a schizophrenic infant. *Am J Psychiatry.* 1959;116:25–31.

23. Fish B. Characteristics and sequelae of the neurointegrative disorder in infants at risk for schizophrenia (1952–1982). In: Watt NF, Anthony EJ, Wynne LC, Rolf JE, eds. *Children at Risk for Schizophrenia.* New York, NY: Cambridge University Press; 1984:423–439.

24. Fish B, Hagin H. Visual-motor disorders in infants at risk for schizophrenia. *Arch Gen Psychiatry.* 1973;28:900–904.

25. Marcus J. Cerebral functioning in offspring of schizophrenics: a possible genetic factor. *Int J Ment Health.* 1974;3:57–73.

26. Holzman PS, Proctor LR, Levy DL, Yasillo NJ, Meltzer HY, Hart SW. Eye-tracking dysfunctions in schizophrenic patients and their relatives. *Arch Gen Psychiatry.* 1974;31:143–151.

27. Holzman PS, Kringlen E, Matthysse S, Flanagan SD, Lipton RB, Cramer G, Levin S, Lange K, Levy DL. A single dominant gene can account for eye tracking dysfunctions and schizophrenia in offspring of discordant twins. *Arch Gen Psychiatry.* 1988;45:641–647.

28. Hertzig MA, Birch HG. Neurologic organization in psychiatrically disturbed adolescents. *Arch Gen Psychiatry.* 1968;19:528–537.

29. Tucker GJ, Campion EW, Silberfarb PM. Sensorimotor functions and cognitive disturbance in psychiatric patients. *Am J Psychiatry.* 1974;31:143–161.

30. Quitkin F, Rifkin A, Klein DF. Neurologic soft signs in schizophrenia and character disorders: organicity in schizophrenia with premorbid asociality and emotionally unstable character disorders. *Arch Gen Psychiatry.* 1976;33:845–853.

31. Asarnow JR. Children at risk for schizophrenia: converging lines of evidence. *Schizophr Bull.* 1988;14:613–631.

32. Asarnow R, Granholm E, Sherman T. Span of apprehension in schizophrenia. In: Steinhauer S, Gruzelier JH, Zubin J, eds. *Handbook of Schizophrenia, V: Neuropsychology, Psychophysiology and Information Processing.* New York, NY: Elsevier Science Publishers; 1991:335–370.

33. Nuechterlein KH, Dawson ME. Information processing and attentional functioning in the developmental course of schizophrenic disorders. *Schizophr Bull.* 1984;10: 160–203.

34. Rutschmann J, Cornblatt B, Erlenmeyer-Kimling L. Sustained attention in children at risk for schizophrenia: findings with two visual continuous performance tasks in a new sample. *J Abnorm Child Psychol.* 1986;14:365–385.

35. Erlenmeyer-Kimling L. Biological markers for the liability to schizophrenia. In: Helmchen H, Henn FA, eds. *Biological Perspectives of Schizophrenia.* New York, NY: John Wiley & Sons Inc; 1987:254–269.

36. Erlenmeyer-Kimling L. High-risk research in schizophrenia: a summary of what has been learned. *J Psychiatr Res.* 1987;21:401–411.

37. Erlenmeyer-Kimling L, Cornblatt B. Biobehavioral risk factors in children of schizo-phrenic parents. *J Autism Dev Disord.* 1984;14:357–374.

38. Marcus J, Auerbach J, Wilkinson L, Burack CM. Infants at risk for schizophrenia: the Jerusalem Infant Development Study. *Arch Gen Psychiatry.* 1981;34:703–713.

39. Marcus J, Auerbach JG, Wilkinson L, Burack CM. Infants at risk for schizophrenia: the Jerusalem Infant Development Study. In: Watt NF, Anthony EJ, Wynne LC, Rolf JE, eds. *Children at Risk for Schizophrenia.* New York, NY: Cambridge University Press; 1984:444–464.

40. Marcus J, Hans SL, Nagler S, Auerbach JG, Mirsky AF, Aubrey A. Review of the NIMH Israeli Kibbutz-city study and the Jerusalem Infant Development Study. *Schizophr Bull.* 1987;13:425–438.

41. Sameroff AJ, Seifer R, Zax M. Early development of children at risk for emotional dis-order. *Monogr Soc Res Child Dev.* 1982;47(7, serial No. 199):1–82.

42. Sameroff AJ, Barocas R, Seifer R. The early development of children born to mentally ill women. In: Watt NF, Anthony EJ, Wynne LC, Rolf JE, eds. *Children at Risk for Schizophrenia.* New York, NY: Cambridge University Press; 1984:482–514.

43. Sameroff AJ, Seifer R, Zax M, Barocas R. Early indicators of developmental risk: Rochester Longitudinal Study. *Schizophr Bull.* 1987;13:383–394.

44. Fish B. The antecedents of an 'acute' schizophrenic break. *J Am Acad Child Psychiatry.* 1986;25:595–600.

45. Fish B. Infant predictors of the longitudinal course of schizophrenic development. *Schizophr Bull.* 1987;13:395–409.

46. Gesell A. *Developmental Diagnosis.* 2nd ed. New York, NY: Paul B Hoeber Inc; 1947.

47. Wetzel NC. The baby grid. *J Pediatr.* 1946;29:439–454.

48. Johnston MH, Holzman PS. *Assessing Schizophrenic Thinking.* San Francisco, Calif: Jossey-Bass Inc; 1979.

49. Bayley N. *Bayley Scales of Infant Development*. New York, NY: Psychological Corp; 1969.

50. Mednick SA, Mura M, Schulsinger F, Mednick B. Perinatal conditions and infant development in children with schizophrenic parents. *Soc Biology*. 1971;18: S103–S113.

51. Marcus J, Hans SL, Mednick SA, Schulsinger F, Michelsen N. Neurological dysfunctioning in offspring of schizophrenics in Israel and Denmark: a replication analysis. *Arch Gen Psychiatry*. 1985;42:753–761.

52. Hanson DR, Gottesman II, Heston LL. Some possible childhood indicators of adult schizophrenia inferred from children of schizophrenics. *Br J Psychiatry*. 1976;129:142–154.

53. Marcuse Y, Cornblatt B. Children at high risk for schizophrenia: predictions from infancy to childhood functioning. In: Erlenmeyer-Kimling L, Miller NE, eds. *Life-Span Research on the Prediction of Psychopathology*. Hillsdale, NJ: Lawrence Erlbaum Associates Inc Publishers; 1986:81–100.

54. Ragins N, Schacter J, Elmer E, Preisman R, Bowes AE, Harway V. Infants and children at risk for schizophrenia: environmental and developmental observations. *J Am Acad Child Psychiatry*. 1975;14:150–177.

55. Sobel DE. Children of schizophrenic patients: preliminary observations on early development. *Am J Psychiatry*. 1961;118:512–517.

56. Grunebaum H, Weiss JL, Gallant D, Cohler BJ. Attention in young children of psychotic mothers. *Am J Psychiatry*. 1974;131:887–891.

57. Grunebaum H, Weiss JL, Gallant D, Cohler BJ. *Mentally Ill Mothers and Their Children*. Chicago, Ill: University of Chicago Press; 1975.

58. O'Neal P, Robins LN. Childhood patterns predictive of adult schozophrenia: a 30-year follow-up study. *Am J Psychiatry*. 1958;115:385–391.

59. Watt N. Longitudinal changes in the social behavior of children hospitalized for schizophrenia as adults. *J Nerv Ment Dis*. 1972;155:42–54.

60. Ricks DF, Nameche G. Symbiosis, sacrifice and schizophrenia. *Ment Hyg*. 1966;50:541–551.

61. Ricks DF, Berry JC. Family and symptom patterns that precede schizophrenia. In: Roff M, Ricks DF, eds. *Life History Research in Psychopathology*. Minneapolis, Minn: University of Minnesota Press; 1970;1:31–50.

62. Walker E, Emory E. Infants at risk for psychopathology: offspring of schizophrenic parents. *Child Dev*. 1983;54:1269–1285.

63 McNeil TF, Kaij L. Offspring of women with nonorganic psychoses. In: Watt NF, Anthony EJ, Wynne LC, Rolf JE, eds. *Children at Risk for Schizophrenia*. New York, NY: Cambridge University Press; 1984:465–481.

64. Francis PL, Self PA, Horowitz FD. The behavioral assessment of the neonate: an overview. In: Osofsky JD, ed. *Handbook of Infant Development*. 2nd ed. New York, NY: John Wiley & Sons Inc; 1987:723–779.

65. Brazelton TB, Nugent JK, Lester BM. Neonatal behavioral assessment scale. In:

Osofsky JD, ed. *Handbook of Infant Development*. 2nd ed. New York, NY: John Wiley & Sons Inc; 1987:780–817.

66. Caplan R, Guthrie D, Fish B, Tanguay P, David-Lando G. The kiddie formal thought disorder rating scale (K-FTDS): clinical assessment, reliability, and validity. *J Acad Child Adolesc Psychiatry*. 1989; 28: 208–216.

67. Caplan R, Perdue S, Tanguay P, Fish B. Formal thought disorder in childhood onset schizophrenia and schizotypal personality disorder. *J Child Psychol Psychiatry*. 1990;31:1103–1114.

68. Fish B. Discussion: genetic or traumatic developmental deviation? *Soc Biol*. 1971;18:S117–S119.

69. Heston LL. Schizophrenia in infancy? *Soc Biol*. 1971;18:S114–S116.

70. McNeil TF. Obstetric factors and perinatal injuries. In: Tsuang MT, Simpson JC, eds. *Handbook of Schizophrenia: Nosology, Epidemiology and Genetics*. New York, NY: Elsevier Science Publishers; 1988;3:319–344.

71. Suddath RL, Christison GW, Torrey EF, Casanova MF, Weinberger DR. Anatomical abnormalities in the brains of monozygotic twins discordant for schizophrenia. *N Engl J Med*. 1990;322:789–794.

72. DeLisi LE, Dauphinals ID, Gershon ES. Perinatal complications and reduced size of brain limbic structures in familial schizophrenia. *Schizophr Bull*. 1988;14:185–191.

73. Rosenthal D, ed. *The Genain Quadruplets*. New York, NY: Basic Books Inc Publishers; 1963.

74. American Psychiatric Association, Committee on Nomenclature and Statistics. *Diagnostic and Statistical Manual of Mental Disorders, Third Edition*. Washington, DC: American Psychiatric Association; 1980.

75. Gottesman II, Shields J. *Schizophrenia and Genetics: A Twin Study Vantage Point*. Orlando, Fla: Academic Press Inc; 1972.

76. Andreasen NC, Ehrhardt JC, Swayze VW II, Alliger RJ, Yuh WTC, Cohen G, Ziebell S. Magnetic resonance imaging of the brain in schizophrenia: the pathophysiologic significance of structural abnormalities. *Arch Gen Psychiatry*. 1990;47:35–44.

77. Fish B, Dixon W. Vestibular hyporeactivity in infants at risk for schizophrenia: its association with critical developmental disorders. *Arch Gen Psychiatry*. 1978;35:963–971.

78. Fish B. Contributions of developmental research to a theory of schizophrenia. In: Hellmuth J, ed. *Exceptional Infant, II: Studies in Abnormalities*. New York, NY: Brunner/Mazel Inc; 1971:473–482.

79. Bogerts B, Meertz E, Schonfeldt-Bausch R. Basal ganglia and limbic system pathology in schizophrenia. *Arch Gen Psychiatry*. 1985;42:784–791.

80. Brown R, Colter N, Corsellis JAN, Crow TJ, Frith CD, Jagoe R, Johnstone EC, Marsh L. Postmortem evidence of structural brain changes in schizophrenia: differences in brain weight, temporal horn area and parahippocampal gyrus compared with affective disorder. *Arch Gen Psychiatry*. 1986;43:36–42.

81. Jeste DV, Lohr JB. Hippocampal pathologic findings in schizophrenia: a morphometric study. *Arch Gen Psychiatry*. 1989;46:1019–1024.

82. Waddington JL, Torrey EF, Crow TJ, Hirsch SR. Schizophrenia, neurodevelopment, and disease: the fifth biannual winter workshop on schizophrenia, Badgastein, Austria, January 28 to February 3, 1990. *Arch Gen Psychiatry.* 1991;48:271–273.
83. Weinberger DR. The pathogenesis of schizophrenia: a neurodevelopmental theory. In: Nasrallah HA, Weinberger DR, eds. *The Handbook of Schizophrenia, I: The Neurology of Schizophrenia.* New York, NY: Elsevier Science Publishers; 1986:397–406.

9

Young Children of Affectively Ill Parents: A Longitudinal Study of Psychosocial Development

Marian Radke-Yarrow, Editha Nottelmann, Pedro Martinez, Mary Beth Fox, and Barbara Belmont

National Institute of Mental Health, Bethesda, Maryland

The course of social-emotional development of young children of affectively ill and well parents was assessed. The families were classified by mother's diagnosis: bipolar illness (N = 22), unipolar depression (N = 41), and normal (N = 37). Father's diagnosis also was obtained. Pairs of siblings were studied; the younger was between 1½ and 3½ years and the older between 5 and 8 years when the study began. They were seen again 3 years later. Psychiatric assessment and mother's report were used to evaluate children's disruptive behavior, anxiety, and depressive characteristics. The frequency of problem-level behavior changed over time in relation to mother's diagnosis. By middle and late childhood, significantly more children of affectively ill than well mothers had depressive and disruptive problems and multiple behavior problems. Offspring of unipolar mothers developed problems earlier and both siblings were more likely to have behavior problems.

Few aspects of human study are more complex or controversial than issues of intergenerational transmission of individual qualities and capacities. When a long succession of intergenerational studies over several decades reaches a single con-

Reprinted with permission from *Journal of the American Academy of Child and Adolescent Psychiatry*, 1992, Vol. 31(1), 68–77. Copyright © 1992 by the American Academy of Child and Adolescent Psychiatry.

This work was supported by the National Institute of Mental Health, Bethesda, Maryland, and by the John D. and Catherine T. MacArthur Foundation, Research Network Award on the Transition from Infancy to Early Childhood, Chicago, Illinois.

The authors wish to acknowledge earlier participation by Drs. Leon Cytryn and Donald McKnew in the planning and initial administration of psychiatric assessments, the extensive contributions of

clusion, it is to be taken seriously. Studies of offspring of affectively ill parents offer such a single conclusion; namely, that these offspring, as a group, have higher rates of psychiatric and psychological problems than are found among the offspring of parents without psychiatric problems (Beardslee et al., 1983; Orvaschel et al., 1988; Welner et al., 1977). This conclusion leaves much to be explained, however, and does not represent consensus in all respects. Although elevated rates of problems are present in most of the studies, there is little agreement as to the expected frequency of problems. Reported rates of problems range from 8% (Keller et al., 1986) to 74% (Hammen et al., 1987) in offspring of parents with unipolar depression and from 23% (LaRoche et al., 1985) to 92% (Hammen et al., 1987) in offspring of bipolar parents. Such large differences reflect the variable and often unspecified criteria that have been used to define "problems," the various methods by which problem status is determined, and the variable criteria of parents' psychiatric status.

A most important missing element in this research (Beardslee et al., 1987) is evidence concerning the mechanisms underlying the aggregation of problems in the offspring of affectively ill parents. These issues have not had high priority in offspring research, although hypotheses concerning genetic transmission, environmental stressors, and combinations of these factors are implicit in the writings. It is clear that until such evidence is available, interpretations of parent–offspring concordance in psychiatric disorders must remain somewhat speculative. Unfortunately, there is no easy approach to the investigation of underlying mechanisms; these questions seem certain to require many divergent research efforts that begin to dismantle the unknowns.

One approach that offers promise is developmental. Through this approach, it is possible to chart the stages of psychosocial development over the early life course and to identify the kinds of vulnerabilities that appear at given developmental periods. If there are regularities and patterns in developmental course, and if specific early problems bear a relation to psychopathologies that appear later, one can then search, with sharper focus, for specific indicators and conditions, within and outside the organism, that are signals of later disorder. Because offspring studies have been cross-sectional in design and have been mainly of older children and young adults, it is not possible from these studies to identify early vulnerabilities, the kinds of problems that appear at different developmental periods, or the continuity or discontinuity of specific problems over time. Moreover, the offspring studies have often based prevalence rates on samples composed of

Judy Stilwell, who conducted parents' diagnostic interviews, and Anne Mayfield, who provided liaison with the families.

The statistical consultants were Kathleen McCann, George Washington University, and Gregory Campbell, Laboratory of Statistical and Mathematical Methodology, Division of Computer Research and Technology, National Institute of Health.

wide bands of ages (e.g., 6 to 15 years, McKnew et al., 1979; 6 to 23 years, Weissman et al., 1987; 8 to 16 years, Hammen et al., 1987) without breakdown into developmentally relevant age groupings. There is need, therefore, to inquire prospectively into children's psychosocial functioning over the childhood years to identify successive patterns of behavior and to determine their links to later disorder. The present study has these objectives.

An inherent difficulty in such research lies in problems of assessment of young children. A first question involves the focus of assessment: In which of children's developing capabilities, at specific developmental periods, are vulnerabilities or signs of impairment likely to occur? Which behaviors might be antecedents of later depression? Because the entire range of children's behavior (cognitive, affective, vegetative, social) presents possible links to subsequent disorder, a broad evaluation is indicated.

A second issue concerns the conceptualization of children's problems. *DSM-III* categories are of adult origin; their applicability to the functioning of 2-, 5-, 10-, and 20-year-olds is not likely to be the same. Closely related is the issue of disentangling normative developmental characteristics and developmental problems. For example, lapses in impulse control, emotional control, and anxiety about being separated from mother are normative in the early years. There are few clear guidelines for deciding the significance of these patterns at different ages or determining the point at which these behaviors shift from "normal for age" to "problematic." Moreover, the same underlying process can be expressed in different behavior at different ages.

Just as the concepts used in assessment must be geared to the developmentally changing organism, so too must the instruments of assessment and the sources of information. Multiple methods and sources are a necessity; they are also almost certainly likely to present many disagreements (LaPousse and Monk, 1958; Reich and Earls, 1987). In developmental studies that span the childhood years, multiple informants are not only important, their contributions also vary with the ages of the children studied. Interviews with young children are difficult; however, children's verbal behavior and their behavior in response to the challenge of an interview are highly informative at any age. Parental reports, though invaluable, depend for their validity on parental sensitivity. Parents are good sources of data on some aspects of child functioning and less good on others. Observed behavior is a further source of information. Because each source of data is partial and furnishes specialized information, the combined evidence is probably the best estimate of the child.

In summary, assessment of psychopathology in early childhood is not a well mapped field, conceptually or methodologically. But knowledge about the childhood years is of major importance in gaining an understanding of the causes of psychiatric disorders and for preventive intervention.

THE PRESENT STUDY

The present study had two major research goals: (1) to assess and compare the psychosocial functioning of children of unipolar, bipolar, and normal control parents at specific periods of childhood and (2) to follow the course of psychosocial functioning of individual children through the years of childhood, to gain an understanding of continuities and discontinuities in problem behavior patterns.

The focus was on three domains of child behavior: disruptive-oppositional behavior, depressive qualities of affect and behavior, and anxious-fearful behavior.

Assessments were made at three periods of development that are significant transitional stages in childhood, during which many new capabilities emerge and new socialization demands must be met if development is to proceed successfully: the period from infancy to childhood (1½ to 3½ years), the period of broadening relationships beyond the family to the social world of school and peers (5 to 6 years), and later childhood (8 to 11 years), when significant cognitive changes occur and also when more, and more varied, demands for mastery and social relationships skills come into play. (A further assessment, now in progress, is made between 12 to 16 years. The present report takes the children through the first three developmental periods.)

This report emphasizes the psychiatric assessment of children. It is part of a broader longitudinal family study (Radke-Yarrow, 1989) that includes detailed investigation of parental and family functioning and child behavior from toddlerhood to adolescence. An ultimate goal is to bring together these multiple sources of data to describe the developmental course of child behavior in relation to parental illness and family variables. In the present report, family contextual conditions, examined at a macrolevel, are the psychiatric status of both parents, the socioeconomic level of the family, and family stress, indexed by marital discord.

METHOD

Sample

The sample was a community sample of 100 families, 63 families with parental affective illness and 37 normal control families. There were two children in each family in the following age ranges at the time the family entered the study: 1½ to 3½ years for the younger child ($\overline{X}$ age = 2.6 years, SD = 0.60) and 5 to 8 years for the older child ($\overline{X}$ age = 6.4 years, SD = 1.1). The number of boys and girls was approximately equal in each group except for the bipolar families, in which there were more girls than boys. Mothers ranged in age from 22 to 45 years ($\overline{X}$ age = 32.5 years, SD = 4.4); fathers ranged from 25 to 50 years ($\overline{X}$ age = 35.4,

SD = 4.7). The families were predominantly middle to upper-middle class; there were nine lower socioeconomic families. Most parents were high school or college educated. At the beginning of the study, 92% of the families were intact. The sample was 85% Caucasian, 1% Hispanic, 12% black, and 2% Oriental.

A basic consideration in choosing the sample was to select affectively ill parents who were performing the critical role of primary caregivers of their children. Forty-nine percent, 73%, and 49% of the offspring of the control, bipolar, and unipolar mothers, respectively, had had some day care. However, mother's responsibility for primary care of the child was essential. By this criterion, parents who had been separated from their children because of long or frequent hospitalizations were not eligible. A mother was eligible if she met the Schedule for Affective Disorders and Schizophrenia: Lifetime Version (SADS-L) (Spitzer and Endicott, 1977) Research Diagnostic Criteria for unipolar depression, bipolar illness, or no past or current psychiatric diagnosis. Affective illness was the primary diagnosis; anxiety could be present as part of the clinical picture of depression but not as the primary diagnosis. There was *no* other Axis I diagnoses, past or present. Serious or chronic physical illness in the immediate family, bereavement, or postpartum reactions were exclusionary criteria. If the mother met criteria for eligibility, the father was given a SADS-L interview. For the well families, *both* parents had to be without current or past psychiatric disorder. For the affectively ill families, fathers either were without current or past psychiatric disorder or they met the illness criteria used for the mothers. This provided two subgroups within the affectively ill families: only mother ill, both parents ill.

Participants were recruited through day-care centers, parent groups, local newspapers, and clinicians. The research was described as a study of child development and child rearing in families in which the mother was depressed and in families in which the mother was well. The required ages of children were also indicated. Notices, repeated at intervals over a 2½-year period, provided a telephone number for volunteers. Approximately 500 calls were received.

Telephone interviews were the first level of detailed screening. Two hundred sixty-one families passed this screening. Mothers were then interviewed. The SADS-L interviews were conducted by a psychiatric nurse, trained by a staff member of the New York Psychiatric Institute. Ten interviews were coded independently by a member of the trainer's staff and the nurse, with 100% agreement on the diagnoses.

The sample consisted of 41 mothers with major depression; 19 of the husbands were without a diagnosis, one was bipolar, and 21 had a diagnosis of depression or anxiety symptoms. There were 22 bipolar mothers (five bipolar I, 17 bipolar II); 14 of the husbands were unipolar, and eight were without diagnosis. There were 37 families in which neither parent had a past or current diagnosis. Sixty-five percent of the diagnosed mothers had sought some form of professional help; 28% had been, or were currently, receiving some form of medication; 13% reported suicidal ideation or plans; and 14% had been hospitalized for depression. The range in mother's lifetime GAS scores, an index of severity based on the SADS, ranged from 1 to 70. The median for unipolar mothers was 50 (indicative of serious symptomatology or impairment in functioning). The median for bipolar mothers was 30 (indicative of an inability to function in almost all areas). Mothers' episode status at the time of the children's assessments varied. It was assumed, however, that characteristic patterns of parental behavior, although varying in intensity, have some continuity within and between episodes. This assumption is supported by the research literature (Billings and Moos, 1985; Harder et al., 1980; Weissman and Paykel, 1974). Eighty-two percent of the bipolar mothers and 59% of the unipolar mothers were in episode at the time of the SADS interview, conducted within several months of entrance into the study; 87% of the mothers had one or more episodes during the lifetime of the children.

Because most of the families at the start of the study were still married, the sample differs from the population of affectively ill families, in which rates of separation or divorce are high (Fendrich et al., 1990). However, by Time 2 assessment, 11%, 23%, and 10%, respectively, of control, bipolar, and unipolar families had separated. It was assumed that selective volunteer factors that might be operating (e.g., parents' concern about their children) were operating similarly in the three groups. The research focus was not on prevalence rates in an epidemiological sense, but on comparisons of the characteristics of child development across diagnostic groups. For mothers who had a diagnosis and who became part of the study, it was required that they have available a mental health professional.

Design

An accelerated longitudinal design was used, covering three age periods that will be referred to as early childhood (1½ to 3½ years), middle childhood (5 to 8 years), and late childhood (8 to 12 years). At the first assessment, the younger siblings were in early childhood and the older siblings in middle childhood. At the second assessment, the younger siblings were in middle childhood and the older siblings were in late childhood. Since data on middle childhood were obtained on both siblings (older siblings at Time 1, $\overline{X} = 6.4$ years; and younger siblings at Time 2, $\overline{X} = 5.6$ years), a partial replication was built into the study.

Procedure

Two sources of data were used for the primary analyses: psychiatric assessment and mother's report of child problems. Each source represents a different sample of experience with the child and a different perspective on behavior. Together they were expected to provide a broader evaluation of the child's functioning than each source alone (Zahner et al., 1989). Therefore, the two data sources were expected to provide complementary data, conflicting as well as supportive evidence (Reich and Earls, 1987). For each data source and for each behavioral domain, criteria were established for classifying the child's behavior as problematic (see below). The two sources were combined additively and interfaced as the best estimate of problems.

Assessments of children under 4 years of age. For children under 4 years of age, the psychiatric evaluation of the child was based on a videotaped play session consisting of a standard sequence of situations designed to challenge the child in various ways; namely, the child's ability to separate from mother, relate to an unfamiliar adult, explore the environment, and express and manage affect appropriately. The psychiatrist talked briefly with mother and child before inviting the child to come in to play. The child's separating from mother was observed and evaluated. If the child could not tolerate separation from the mother, the door was left open, and/or the child was given the opportunity to make contact with the mother.

The session had three 10- to 12-minute segments. In the first segment, the child was invited to play with a standard set of relatively neutral toys (blocks, crayons and paper, ball, doll, teddy bear). After 10 minutes, the psychiatrist asked the child to help put away the toys and bring out new toys. In the second segment, a doll house and dolls matched to the child's family provided possibilities for play relevant to the child's family. The psychiatrist helped to involve the child by identifying "mother," "sister," etc., but was generally nondirective. After 10 minutes, a change was made to toys that had high potential for aggressive play (guns, soldiers, punching bag, boxing gloves, pounding blocks).

The psychiatrist evaluated the child on specific behavioral dimensions: (1) separation anxiety, (2) generalized anxiety, (3) disruptive or oppositional behavior, and (4) depressive affect, taking into consideration the age of the child. He made a judgment as to whether the child was exhibiting behavior judged to be of clinical concern. The clinicians' decisions for labeling behavior as problematic were based on the following considerations: (1) whether the behavior was so deviant as to suggest the need for treatment and/or close monitoring and (2) whether the behavior posed a serious risk to, or interference with, the normal course of development. Ten cases were blind-scored by a second psychiatrist; agreement on assigned problem areas was 85%.

The mother reported on the child's problems (Child Behavior Check List [CBCL], Achenbach and Edelbrock, 1979). At the time the study began, there was no scale for anxiety and no scale for preschool-age children. Therefore, the mother's report was used for the children under 4 years only with regard to disruptive or oppositional behavior, which, it was assumed, might be underestimated by the psychiatrist, based on a single evaluation. The norms for the 6- to 11-year-olds were used. The criterion used was *T*-scores at or above the 90th percentile. *Assessment of children from 5 to 11 years of age.* For children 5 years of age and older, the psychiatrist's evaluation was based on a structured psychiatric interview, the Child Assessment Scale (CAS) (Hodges et al., 1981). The interview was designed to access children's fears, moods, somatic concerns, expression of anger, self-image, thought disorders, and also their relationships at home, at school, and with peers. For this study, evaluations were made of anxiety, depression, and disruptive behavior disorders based on the items specified in the instrument manual as indicative of disorder according to *DSM-III* classifications (Hodges et al., 1981). Because of the ages of the children, these designations of disorders are regarded as problems of clinical concern (not diagnoses).

Interviewers (either a psychiatrist or psychologist) were blind to the diagnostic status of parents and sibling and previous assessments of the child. The interviews were analyzed from video and/or audio record by two other child psychiatrists (M.B.F. and P.M.) who had no knowledge of the psychiatric status of parents or sibling. For reliability of scoring, both psychiatrists coded 25 cases. Agreement on assignment of problem status on disruptive, anxious, and depressive dimensions was a κ of 0.83.

Assessments of children's problems from mothers' reports on the CBCL were normed *T*-scores at or above the 90th percentile (above normal range) (Achenbach and Edelbrock, 1979) on narrow-band scales of depressive behavior, delinquent behavior, and aggressive behavior.

It is recognized, as noted earlier, in assessing preschool and early school-age children, the nosological as well as measurement problems present difficulties. The definitions and boundaries of behavior that constitute a problem are not clearly drawn for children, especially for very young children. The best cut points for predictions are not easily determined; quite likely, different cut points are relevant at different ages. For these reasons, assigning "diagnoses" was avoided.

The instruments used in this study (play interview, structured interview, mother's report) are from the armamentarium of child measurement in developmental psychology and child psychiatry. The cut-off points in each of the three instruments, theoretically, pick up the children whose problems are at a "warning" level of deviance, which may be subclinical or clearly clinical. Unfortunately, there are no outside criteria to turn to for validation. Each instrument has assets and limitations. The play interview assessment rests on real behavior, which, however, cannot be evaluated on a finely calibrated scale. The structured interview faces language limitations of the child; very careful interpretation of children's responses is required to ascertain the child's understanding of questions. The child's behavior in the interview can furnish further information on the child.

Mothers' reports are relied upon extensively in the research literature but have limitations of possible insensitivity or bias.

Feedback was given to the parents about their children. Entirely independent of the *blind* assessments, each child was reviewed by two staff members who were responsible for data collection and two child psychiatrists who were not involved in the assessments just described. This group planned the advice to be given to the parents.

Family data. Data on the family context included father's diagnosis, socioeconomic status (Hollingshead, 1975, using data on both parents), marital discord, and family history. Data on marital discord, rated 0 to 4, were obtained in an interview adapted from Brown and Harris (1978). For data on the psychiatric status of first- and second-degree relatives, parents were interviewed (Family History-Research Diagnostic Criteria, Endicott et al., 1975), screening for symptoms of affective illness, schizophrenia, schizo-affective disorders, and alcoholism and drug abuse, including information on the course and treatment of the disorder and the extent of disruption of the person's life. The information was reviewed by a psychiatrist and the "best estimate" of a diagnosis was made. Although the source of the data did not permit making firm diagnoses, it was possible to identify families in which descriptions of relatives indicated disorder-fitting symptom pictures of affective illness.

Overview of data analysis. To summarize, assessments of the dependent variables of disruptive behavior and depression were based on scores combining psychiatric evaluation and mother's CBCL report. Anxiety was based on the psychiatrist's evaluation. Dichotomous variables, designating presence or absence of problem behavior at a "clinical concern" level, were obtained for the younger sibling in early and middle childhood; for the older sibling, in middle and late childhood. The independent variables included maternal diagnosis and variables of family context. The primary analyses are based on maternal diagnosis.

Analysis of the relations among the variables proceeded through two stages: *Stage I*, the association of the various independent variables with each of the child variables was examined separately, based on each source of information. *Stage II*, child variables were combined to form a measure of overall problem status across sources and dimensions.

Two approaches to analysis were implemented. A cross-sectional approach examined the influence of independent variables (main effects) on various outcome measures at each age period, and the influence of the interaction of selected variables on child outcome at each age period. For example, one cross-sectional analysis addressed the influence of maternal diagnosis, child gender, and the interaction of maternal diagnosis and gender on the child's anxiety in middle childhood. If the interaction was significant, then the contribution of maternal diagnosis to child's anxiety was explored separately by child gender.

   The second approach was longitudinal and examined the influence of the child's development over time on the outcome measures of anxiety, disruptive behavior, and depression. In addition to treating time or development as a source of possible variance in its own right, the contribution of the interaction of time and mother's diagnosis was explored. The longitudinal analyses examined the development of the younger sibling from early childhood to middle childhood and the older sibling from middle childhood to late childhood. The analyses yielded the significance of the contribution of maternal diagnosis, time, and their interaction. The contribution of time also was examined *within* each maternal diagnosis to explore, for instance, whether the disruptive behavior of the offspring of unipolar women increases or decreases significantly over time.

Statistical models. Choice of statistical models for cross-sectional and repeated measures analysis of a small sample of categorical data posed a challenge. In particular, to facilitate direct comparison of results, the authors wished to implement comparable statistical models for the cross-sectional and longitudinal approaches. In the cross-sectional approach, the goal was to test the hypothesis of homogeneity; e.g., the probability of a given behavior, such as disruptive behavior, being the same for offspring of all mothers regardless of maternal diagnosis. Similarly, in the longitudinal approach, the goal was to test the hypothesis of marginal homogeneity; e.g., the probability of disruptive behavior being the same at each age period. Marginal probabilities (in this case, the probability of disruptive behavior at specific age periods) were also used to assess the interaction of time and maternal diagnosis.

   In a review of several statistical models of categorical data, weighted least squares methods for fitting linear models to the children's outcome measures emerged as an appropriate technique for meeting the research goals. Another type of model, Cochran-Mantel-Haenszel statistics (Landis et al., 1978), typically computed for randomized experiments, does not provide direct information regarding the interaction of independent variables and time, whereas WLS methods will provide this information (Landis et al., 1988). A third approach to categorical data analysis, maximum likelihood estimation of loglinear models (Bishop et al., 1975), does not make a priori distinction between independent and dependent variables and is not readily applicable to repeated measures analyses and tests of marginal homogeneity (SAS Institute, Inc., 1985). WLS methods for categorical data may be considered an extension of analyses of variance and regression models for continuous data; they readily allow repeated measures analysis and tests of marginal homogeneity, and they make a clear distinction between independent and dependent variables. Weighted least squares estimation techniques for linear modeling of categorical data (Grizzle et al., 1969) and for repeated measurement designs (Koch et al., 1977) first require computing appropriate functions of the data. In the cross-sectional approach, the joint probability is used; e.g., the probability of anxiety in a child of a unipolar mother. The straightforward extension for the longitudinal approach is to use the marginal probability previously noted; e.g., the probability of anxiety in a child of a unipolar mother in early childhood. The next step is to define a linear model of the functions to test each hypothesis of interest. For example, an important hypothesis in the longitudinal approach is the hypothesis of no maternal diagnosis by time interaction. If this hypothesis holds, then the marginal probabilities can be expressed as the sum of a mean, a parameter for maternal diagnosis, and a parameter for time. In the third step, weighted estimation methods fit this model to the data by providing estimates for the parameters, taking into account the correlations of each child's outcome measure over time. A Wald statistic for testing the hypothesis of no interaction is also generated. (This statistic reflects the residual variance in the data left over after model fitting.) Wald statistics have an approximate χ^2 distribution. For every hypothesis of interest, WLS methods generate an χ^2 value and corresponding significance level, thus allowing for straightforward interpretations.

Because of the relatively small sample, cross-sectional analyses were limited to two independent variables (diagnosis and gender, diagnosis and socioeconomic status [SES], diagnosis and marital stress), and longitudinal analyses were limited to maternal diagnosis and time (development).

CROSS-SECTIONAL FINDINGS

The term *problem status* is used to indicate that a child's behavior was of "clinical concern" on a given instrument or combination of instruments. The percentage of children who met this criterion is reported in the tables, separately for each sibling group. Table 1 is a reference table that presents the data at the most detailed level—by source of information. The findings, however, are discussed in terms of best estimates of child functioning, based on the combined data sources (Table 2).

The tables present children's problem status in relation to mother's diagnosis (Tables 1 and 2) and to family diagnosis and family history (Table 3). Any influences of gender, SES, and marital stress are described in the text.

Children's Disruptive, Depressed, and Anxious Behavior, by Mother's Diagnosis

There were systematic diagnosis-related associations that differed by type of problem, source of information, and developmental level.

Disruptive behavior. The prevalence of disruptive behavior differed by mother's diagnosis—at a trend level in early childhood and significantly thereafter

TABLE 1

Percentage of Children with Problems of Clinical Concern by Mother's Diagnosis by Developmental Stage and by Data Source

	Younger Sibling				Older Sibling			
	1½–3½ (yrs)		5–6 (yrs)		5–8 (yrs)		8–11 (yrs)	
Child's Problem—Mother's Diagnosis	Psy[a]	CBCL[b]	Psy	CBCL	Psy	CBCL	Psy	CBCL
Disruptive behavior								
Control	11	3	3	3	3	5	0	3
Bipolar	9	5	0	24	6	22	6	28
Unipolar	17	20	3	22	2	27	10	32
χ^2	NS	6.23**	NS	10.76****	NS	8.79***	5.50*	17.48****
Depression								
Control	0		3	0	11	3	11	3
Bipolar	0		5	19	11	17	33	17
Unipolar	5		15	20	20	15	25	29
χ^2	NS		NS	5.86**	NS	5.44*	NS	13.18****
Anxiety								
Control	35		17		14		34	
Bipolar	9		9		11		44	
Unipolar	34		32		25		25	
χ^2	9.79***		5.69*		NS		NS	
Any of these problems								
Control	43	3	17	3	24	8	37	6
Bipolar	23	5	18	29	17	33	56	33
Unipolar	54	20	49	32	39	32	48	44
χ^2	6.90***	6.23**	11.32****	18.33****	NS	10.17***	NS	22.22****
Comorbidity								
Control	5	0	3	0	3	0	9	0
Bipolar	0	0	0	14	11	6	28	11
Unipolar	7	2	7	10	10	10	17	17
χ^2	5.35*	NS	NS	7.93**	5.49*	NS	NS	10.69**

Note: NS at Time 1 = 37 control, 22 bipolar, 41 unipolar; NS at Time 2 = 35 control, 22 bipolar, 41 unipolar.
* $p < 0.08$, ** $p < 0.05$, *** $p < 0.01$, **** $p < 0.001$.
[a] Psy = Psychiatrist's evaluation.
[b] CBCL = Mother's report.

TABLE 2

Percentage of Children with Problems of Clinical Concern (Combined Data Sources) by Mother's Diagnosis and by Developmental Stage

Child's Problem—Mother's Diagnosis	Younger Sibling		Older Sibling	
	1½–3½ (yrs)	5–6 (yrs)	5–8 (yrs)	8–11 (yrs)
Disruptive behavior				
Control	14	6	8	3
Bipolar	15	24	28	28
Unipolar	34	22	30	42
χ^2	5.36*	6.54**	8.07**	26.27****
Depression				
Control	0	3	14	14
Bipolar	0	24	17	44
Unipolar	5	34	32	42
χ^2	NS	18.69****	NS	10.77****
Anxiety				
Control	35	17	14	34
Bipolar	9	9	11	44
Unipolar	34	32	25	25
χ^2	9.79***	5.69*	NS	NS
Any of these problems				
Control	43	20	32	40
Bipolar	25	38	39	61
Unipolar	56	58	62	68
χ^2	6.29**	14.17****	8.14**	6.34**
Comorbidity				
Control	5	3	3	11
Bipolar	0	14	17	50
Unipolar	15	22	22	32
χ^2	9.14***	8.33**	9.23***	11.51****

Note: NS at Time 1 = 37 control, 22 bipolar, 41 unipolar; NS at Time 2 = 35 control, 22 bipolar, 41 unipolar.
* $p < 0.08$, ** $p < 0.05$, *** $p < 0.01$, **** $p < 0.0001$.

TABLE 3

Percentage of Children with a Problem of Clinical Concern by
Family Diagnosis and Family History and by Developmental Stage

Child's Problem—Family Diagnosis/Family History	N		Younger Sibling		Older Sibling	
			1½–3½ (yrs)	5–6 (yrs)	5–8 (yrs)	8–11 (yrs)
Family diagnosis	T_1 T_2					
No parent ill	36 34		42	20	33	42
One parent ill	22 24		50	54	77	64
Two parents ill	31 36		42	48	39	68
		χ^2	NS	9.64***	15.35****	8.75***
Family diagnosis and family history—no parent ill						
No history	27		44	15	26	30
History	9		33	38	56	78
		χ^2	NS	NS	NS	6.61***
One parent ill						
No history	12		33	42	64	64
History	13		67	67	91	64
		χ^2	3.00*	NS	NS	NS
Two parents ill						
No history	19		53	58	44	67
History	14		29	36	31	69
		χ^2	NS	NS	NS	NS

* $p < 0.08$, ** $p < 0.05$, *** $p < 0.01$, **** $p < 0.0001$.

(Table 2). In middle and late childhood, problem disruptive behavior was present in significantly more children of unipolar and bipolar mothers (between 22% to 42%) than of normal control mothers. The presence of disruptive behavior in these age groups was very low (3% to 8%) in the control group. In the cohort of 5-to 6-year-olds, boys (22%) more often than girls (10%) were problem disruptive ($\chi^2 = 3.99$, $p < 0.05$).

In early childhood, disruptive behavior (assessed by a psychiatrist) was significantly more frequent in families with higher stress than among children in families with lower stress ($\chi^2 = 7.05$, $p < 0.01$). In late childhood, disruptive behavior was significantly more frequent among children in the lower SES families ($\chi^2 = 7.46$, $p < 0.02$)—in particular, in the bipolar group (80%) (based on mother's report) ($\chi^2 = 20.44$, $p < 0.0004$)—than among children in the higher SES families.

Depression. In early childhood, only two girls of unipolar mothers were judged by the psychiatrist to be depressed. In middle and late childhood, when depression was more frequent (Table 2), children of affectively ill mothers were more likely than children of control mothers to have such problems. The difference was significant in middle childhood in the 5- to 6-year-old group ($\chi^2 = 18.69$, $p < 0.0001$) and in the same direction, but not significant, in the 5- to 8-year-old group. In late childhood, the difference between the offspring of affectively ill and control mothers was highly significant ($\chi^2 = 10.77$, $p < 0.0001$).

A gender difference in depression appeared only in middle childhood in mothers' reports on the cohort of younger siblings. Boys (18%) more often than girls (6%) were reported to have problems of depression ($\chi^2 = 3.87$, $p < 0.05$).

Anxiety. Children's anxiety had a unique pattern in relation to mother's diagnosis (Table 2). In early childhood, anxiety (mainly separation anxiety) was rated by the psychiatrist as problematic in a third of the children in the control and unipolar groups; it was remarkably absent in the children of bipolar mothers. (In all groups, separation anxiety was found equally in children currently in day-care and those not in day-care.) The bipolar children manifested almost no anxiety in separating from their mothers or in entering into the play session with the psychiatrist. They quickly formed a relationship and freely explored the environment. Because the bipolar group was slightly older than the other groups, separation anxiety was compared in bipolar, unipolar, and control offspring matched on age. The results were the same. Although the group differences were not statistically significant in middle childhood, again, relatively few offspring of bipolar mothers exhibited high levels of anxiety (9% and 11%). Only in late childhood was anxiety frequent in the bipolar group. The relatively high frequency of anxiety in all of the groups in the preadolescent to adolescent years is in line with findings in the literature (Kashani and Orvaschel, 1990).

Gender differences in anxiety appeared only at the preschool level ($\chi^2 = 5.36$,

p <0.02); preschool girls were anxious more often (37%) than preschool boys (20%). In middle childhood, anxiety was associated with high family SES in the older sibling cohort ($\chi^2 = 7.72$, p <0.02).

Children's Overall Problem Status

Data from all sources and across specific dimensions of disorder were combined (Table 2). Based on this assessment, offspring of affectively ill mothers ages 5 years and older were significantly more likely to exhibit a problem or multiple problems of clinical concern than were children of normal control mothers. Offspring of bipolar mothers were very much favored (reflecting the absence of separation anxiety in the psychiatrist's evaluation).

Offspring of unipolar mothers had the highest rate of problems in the preschool period, and they continued to be the group most likely to have problems. In late childhood, the rates of problems in the offspring of both bipolar and unipolar groups were high (61% and 68%, respectively). The relatively high rate of overall problem status in children of normal controls reflects the age-normative presence of anxiety referred to earlier.

Because the severity of mothers' affective illness varied (indexed by GAS scores), the prevalence of childhood problems was investigated in relation to mothers' severity scores. Using the median GAS score, children of mothers higher and lower in level of functioning were compared on overall problem status. Although poorer maternal functioning was associated with higher frequencies of problems in the offspring in each age group, none of the differences was significant. Likewise, when children of affectively ill mothers receiving medication ($N = 11$), and those not on medication ($N = 52$) were compared, the prevalence of problems did not differ significantly. Problems appeared in 45% and 44% of the younger children of mothers receiving medication and those not receiving medication, respectively, and in 64% and 49% of the older children of mothers receiving medication and those not receiving medication, respectively.

Comorbidity

Throughout childhood, significantly fewer children of normal control mothers than children of unipolar mothers presented problems in more than one domain. In middle and late childhood, fewer control children than children of bipolar mothers presented multiple problems.

Cohort Comparison in Middle Childhood

In middle childhood, data were available on both siblings (the younger at Time 2 and the older at Time 1: columns 2 and 3, Table 2) to provide an overall picture of replication. Similar in the two groups was the percentage of children whose behavior was seen as problematic on disruption. On depression, anxiety, combined problems, and comorbidity, the three offspring groups were ranked similarly on problem status.

Problems of Siblings

Offspring of affectively ill and normal mothers were compared, taking into account the problem status of the two siblings. At Time 1, both siblings presented problems in 35% of unipolar, 18% in bipolar, and 8% in control families. At Time 2, the parallel percentages were 45% unipolar, 28% in bipolar, and 14% in control families. In contrast, both children were without problems in 53% of bipolar, 32% of control, and 18% of unipolar families at Time 1; and, at Time 2, in 33% of bipolar, 53% of control, and 20% of unipolar families.

Children's Problems and Family Diagnosis

Families were classified in terms of (1) diagnoses of both parents (both parents well, mother only ill, both parents ill), and (2) presence of affective disorders in first- and second-degree relatives (Table 3). Contrary to expectation, having two affectively ill parents did not represent a systematically greater risk to the children compared with having only an ill mother. In an effort to explain the unexpected finding, one-parent ill and two-parent ill families were examined for possible differences in unipolar-bipolar composition and SES. No significant differences were found.

Family history of affective illness (as reported by the parents), too, failed to relate to frequencies of children's problems, with one exception (Table 3). In normal control families, more children had problems in those families with affective illness present in first- or second-degree relatives.

LONGITUDINAL FINDINGS

Developmental continuities and discontinuities in children's behavioral patterns and the history, or precursors, of children's problems were investigated in longitudinal analyses.

Group Analyses

From the longitudinal analyses, it is apparent that mother's diagnosis had the greatest impact on children's disruptive problems throughout childhood ($\chi^2 = 7.57$, $p < 0.05$ for the younger cohort and $\chi^2 = 22.79$, $p < 0.001$ for the older cohort). Time or development made no significant contribution. In contrast, the course of children's depressive problems was significantly influenced by both mother's diagnosis (for the younger cohort $\chi^2 = 23.11$, $p < 0.001$ and for the older cohort $\chi^2 = 10.56$, $p < 0.01$) *and* time or development (for the younger cohort $\chi^2 = 12.81$, $p < 0.001$ and for the older cohort $\chi^2 = 5.28$, $p < 0.05$) as well as by time in interaction with diagnosis for the younger cohort ($\chi^2 = 7.81$, $p < 0.05$). From early to middle childhood, time had a significant impact on the unipolar group ($\chi^2 = 8.61$, $p < 0.01$) and a marginally significant impact on the bipolar group ($\chi^2 = 3.56$, $p < 0.06$), with an increase in depressive problems. From middle to late childhood, there was a significant increase in depressive problems with time only on the bipolar group ($\chi^2 = 6.92$, $p < 0.01$).

The longitudinal analyses added little to the understanding of anxiety, which increased significantly in the control and bipolar offspring in the older cohort from middle to late childhood and was relatively high in the unipolar group at all ages (Table 2).

When overall problem status was considered, mother's diagnosis was a significant contributor to the prevalence of problems and comorbidity of problems. Time had significant impact on the problem course of normal control children, whose problems decreased from early to middle childhood ($\chi^2 = 3.96$, $p < 0.05$). From middle to late childhood, time also was a significant factor in the comorbidity of children's problems ($\chi^2 = 9.21$, $p < 0.001$). Comorbidity increased significantly in the bipolar group ($\chi^2 = 6.00$, $p < 0.01$).

Individual Pathways

Preschool-age children from control families who were problem-free remained so 3 years later in 75% of the cases. Preschool-age children from affectively ill families who were problem-free remained problem-free in 50% of the cases. When preschool-age children who *had* problems were reassessed at 5 to 6 years, 20% of the children from the control families and 64% of the children from affectively ill families continued to have problems.

In the older cohort, 40% of the control children who had problems in middle childhood continued to have problems in late childhood. However, 78% of the children from affectively ill families who presented problems initially in middle childhood continued to have problems 3 years later.

In summary, the developmental trajectories were significantly different for children of normal control, bipolar, and unipolar mothers.

DISCUSSION

The data from this study provide a developmental perspective on the problems of young offspring of affectively ill mothers and well mothers. The problems presented by children in early, middle, and late childhood differed in frequency by maternal diagnosis. Children of affectively ill mothers, compared with children of normal control mothers, exhibited more disruptive and depressive problems; their problems increased over time; and they more often presented multiple problems. The longitudinal analyses indicated a different developmental course for children of control, unipolar, and bipolar mothers. The continuity of problems across 3 years also was greater in offspring of affectively ill mothers than in offspring of normal mothers. Gender differences were not strong but in the expected direction. Boys were more disruptive, and girls were more anxious.

The findings identify a number of issues that extend an understanding of the development of at-risk children and pose questions for further study. First, the differences in the developmental course of children of unipolar and bipolar mothers lead to interesting questions. Children of bipolar mothers appeared competent and without problems in the preschool period, mainly because they were able to separate from the mother without anxiety and related easily to the psychiatrist. But, in earlier research (Radke-Yarrow et al., 1985), many of these children were found to have insecure attachment relationships with their mother. Their early "maturity" as evidenced in the psychiatric session may, therefore, represent a precarious method of coping with disorganized mothering. Their early well-being, followed by a rise in depressive and disruptive problems in the latter part of childhood, alerts one to the possible significance of specific developmental timing in the expression of this affective illness. Speculatively, one might raise the question of timing in relation to genetic factors. At the same time, environmental risks (maternal impairments) are likely to have different kinds of impact on children at different developmental periods. Near the end of childhood, children may be most vulnerable to the interpersonal stresses created by parental bipolar illness.

The developmental path of the offspring of unipolar mothers, in contrast, is an early and steady high level of problem behavior. This finding raises questions about the qualities of mothering or the factors inherent in the child that account for this early and severe faltering in normal development.

The lack of differences in problems in children with one ill parent versus children with two ill parents, although unexpected, suggests questions and hypotheses that should be explored: For example, does the illness of both parents so disorganize family functioning that other processes are set in motion that are protective? Are other family members or other social support systems mobilized to provide for the child? Are such experiences the differentiating factors in how well or badly the child is functioning? Does illness of the mother and its consequences in dysfunctional parenting have the predominant impact in the childhood period?

In this study, a restricted but central set of behavior problems was investigated. The early and developmentally distinct patterns in these behaviors suggest the importance of studying a broader sampling of psychosocial functioning beyond the *DSM-III* framework of problems. Little is known regarding children's representations or understanding of their experiences with affectively ill parents. There is little systematic research concerning the styles or strategies that individual children develop to deal with parental illness and the consequences of these styles for children's adaptation.

Evaluation of young children's psychosocial functioning continues to pose difficulties, both conceptual and methodological, and calls for research to improve assessment. Children can inform only to a certain extent about themselves through interview procedures. Their behavior, as an informant, can undoubtedly be used more effectively in research than has been done. Although structured and standard maternal and teacher report forms have made parents and teachers more systematic data sources, individual variations in the sensitivity and commitment of the informant remain a limitation. The question can be raised as to whether depressed and nondepressed mothers are equally good observers and reporters. There is a belief that depressed mothers have distorted perceptions of their children. Richters and Pellegrini (1989) have reviewed this literature and offer some data of their own, indicating that there is not compelling research evidence on this issue. It remains an area for additional study. The present study differs in a number of ways from many of the studies in the offspring literature. It provides systematic longitudinal assessments of young children. The prospective design eliminates the problems inherent in retrospective data. The children are identified by parental diagnostic classifications that distinguish unipolar and bipolar illness, family constellations and conditions, and family history. Ages of children are controlled and specific to important transitional periods of childhood. Sibling data provide the possibility of intrafamily comparisons.

The children in this study are being followed into adolescence. In these later periods, broader assessments of children's psychosocial functioning and behavioral observations of the children and their families are included. These continued evaluations will allow us to investigate further the longitudinal course of problems, to predict outcomes from early childhood to adolescence, and to follow back from adolescence to early childhood.

REFERENCES

Achenbach, T. M. & Edelbrock, C. S. (1979), The child behavior profile: II. Boys aged 12–16 and girls aged 6–11 and 12–16. *J. Consult. Clin. Psychol.,* 47:223–233.

Beardslee, W. R., Bemporad, J., Keller, M. B. and Klerman, G. L. (1983), Children of parents with major affective disorder: a review. *Am. J. Psychiatry,* 140:825–832.

———Schultz, H. S. & Selman, R. L. (1987), Level of social-cognitive development, adaptive functioning, and DSM-III diagnoses in adolescent offspring of parents with affective disorders: implications of the development of the capacity for mutuality. *Developmental Psychology,* 23:807–815.

Billings, A. G. & Moos, R. H. (1985), Children of parents with unipolar depression: a controlled 1-year follow-up. *J. Abnorm. Child Psychol.,* 11:149–166.

Bishop, Y. M., Feinberg, S. E. & Holland, P. W. (1975), *Discrete Multivariate Analysis: Theory and Practice.* Cambridge, MA: The MIT Press.

Brown, G. W. & Harris, T. O. (1978), *Social Origins of Depression: A Study of Psychiatric Disorder in Women.* London: Tavistock.

Endicott, J., Andreasen, N. & Spitzer, R. L. (1975), *Family History*-Research Diagnostic Criteria. New York: New York State Psychiatric Institute, Biometrics Research.

Fendrich, M., Warner, V. & Weissman, M. M. (1990), Family risk factors, parental depression, and psychopathology in offspring. *Developmental Psychology,* 26:40–50.

Grizzle, J. E., Starmer, C. F. & Koch, G. G. (1969), Analysis of categorical data by linear models. *Biometrics,* 25:489–504.

Hammen, C., Gordon, D., Burge, D., Adrian, C., Jaenicke, C. & Hiroto, D. (1987), Maternal affective disorders, illness, and stress: risk for children's psychopathology. *Am. J. Psychiatry,* 144:736–741.

Harder, D. W., Kokes, R. F., Fisher, L. & Strauss, J. S. (1980), Child competence and psychiatric risk. IV. Relationships of parent diagnostic classifications and parent psychopathology severity to child functioning. *J. Nerv. Ment. Dis.,* 168:343–347.

Hollingshead, A. B. (1975), *Four-Factor Index of Social Status.* New Haven, CT: Yale University Sociology Department.

Hodges, K., Kline, J., Fitch, P., McKnew, D. & Cytryn, L. (1981), The child assessment schedule: a diagnostic interview for research and clinical use. *Catalog of Selected Documents in Psychology,* 11:56.

Kashani, J. H. & Orvaschel, H. (1990), A community study of anxiety in children and adolescents. *Am. J. Psychiatry,* 147:313–318.

Keller, M. B., Beardslee, W. R., Dorer, D. J., Lavori, P. W., Samuelson, H. & Klerman, G. R. (1986), Impact of severity and chronicity of parental affective illness on adaptive functioning and psychopathology in children. *Arch. Gen. Psychiatry,* 43:930–937.

Koch, G. G., Landis, J. R., Freeman, J. L., Freeman, Jr., D. H. & Lehnen, R. G. (1977), A general methodology for the analysis of experiments with repeated measurement of categorical data. *Biometrics,* 33:133–158.

Landis, J. R., Heyman, E. R. & Koch, G. G. (1978), Average partial association in three-way tables: a review and discussion of alternate tests. *International Statistical Review,* 46:237–254.

———Miller, M. E., Davis, C. S. & Koch, G. G. (1988), Some general methods for the analysis of categorical data in longitudinal studies. *Statistics in Medicine,* 1:109–137.

LaPousse, R. & Monk, M. A. (1958), An epidemiologic study of behavior characteristics of children. *Am. J. Public Health,* 48:1134–1144.

LaRoche, C., Cheifetz, P., Lester, E. P., Schibuk, L., DiTommaso, E. & Engelsmann, F. (1985), Psychopathology in the offspring of parents with bipolar affective disorders. *Can. J. Psychiatry,* 30:337–343.

McKnew, D. H., Cytryn, L., Efron, A. M., Gershon, E. S. & Bunney, W. E. (1979), Offspring of patients with affective disorders. *Br. J. Psychiatry,* 134:148–152.

Orvaschel, H., Walsh-Allis, G. & Ye, W. (1988), Psychopathology in children of parents with recurrent depression. *J. Abnorm. Child Psychol.,* 16:17–28.

Radke-Yarrow, M. (1989), Family environments of depressed and well parents and their children: issues of research methods. In: *Aggression and Depression in Family Interactions,* ed. G. R. Patterson. Hillsdale, NJ: Lawrence Erlbaum Associates, pp. 48–67.

———Cummings, M. E., Kuczynski, L. & Chapman, M. (1985), Patterns of attachment in two- and three-year-olds in normal families and families with parental depression. *Child Dev.,* 56:884–893.

Reich, W. & Earls, F. (1987), Rules for making psychiatric diagnosis in children on the basis of multiple sources of information: preliminary strategies. *J. Abnorm. Child Psychol.,* 15:601–616.

Richters, J. & Pellegrini, D. (1989), Depressed mothers' judgments about their children: an examination of the depression-distortion hypothesis. *Child Dev.,* 60:1068–1075.

SAS Institute, Inc. (1985), *SAS User's Guide: Statistics, Version 5 Edition.* North Carolina: SAS Institute, Inc.

Spitzer, R. L. & Endicott, J. (1977), *The Schedule for Affective Disorders and Schizophrenia: Lifetime Version.* New York: New York State Psychiatric Institute, Biometrics Research.

Weissman, M. M. & Paykel, E. S. (1974), *The Depressed Woman: A Study of Social Relationships.* Chicago: University of Chicago Press.

———Gammon, G. D., John, K., Merikangas, K. R., Warner, V., Prusoff, B. A. & Sholomskas, D. (1987), Children of depressed parents: increased psychopathology and early onset of major depression. *Arch. Gen. Psychiatry,* 44:847-853.

Welner, Z., Welner, A., McCrary, M. D. & Leonard, M. A. (1977), Psychopathology in children of inpatients with depression: a controlled study. *J. Nerv. Ment. Dis.,* 164:408–413.

Zahner, G. E. P., Leckman, J. F., Benedict, T. L. & Leo-Summers, L. S. (1989), The clinical process of assembling psychodiagnostic information from parents, children, and teachers: recommendations for multiple informant algorithms for the diagnostic interview schedule for children. Prepared for the Epidemiology and Psychopathology Research Branch, Division of Clinical Research of the National Institute of Mental Health.

Part IV

DISRUPTIVE BEHAVIOR DISORDERS

The disruptive behavior disorders, encompassing the often co-occurring DSM-III-R diagnoses of Attention Deficit Hyperactivity Disorder, Oppositional Defiant Disorder, and Conduct Disorder are frequently refractory to treatment and carry considerable long-term morbidity. The four papers in this section address various facets of this major social and psychiatric problem. In the first paper, Quiggle, Garber, Panak, and Dodge examine the role that cognitions play in childhood problem behavior. The subjects were 220 third- through sixth-graders identified as being depressed ($N = 81$), aggressive ($N = 26$), comorbid ($N = 24$), or normal ($N = 89$). Peer nomination and teacher ratings were used to assess level of aggression, and the Children's Depression Inventory provided a self-report measure of depression. Responses to questions about six stories depicting children in situations in which they were rejected, ridiculed, provoked, or experienced failure provided data on social information processing style. Aggressive children demonstrated a hostile attributional bias, were more likely to report that they would engage in aggressive behavior, and indicated that aggression would be easy for them. Children characterized as depressed also showed a hostile attributional bias, although they were more likely to attribute negative situations to internal, stable, and global causes. Children who were comorbid generally showed patterns similar to both aggressive and depressed children. The findings are limited by the hypothetical nature of the experimental situation, as well as by the fact that subjects were a community sample identified on the basis of self-report, teacher report, or peer nomination. Nevertheless, the results raise the possibility that cognitive therapeutic techniques may be of value in the treatment of aggression as well as depression.

As the use of psychopharmacologic agents in the treatment of childhood psychiatric disorder expands, exploration of children's understanding of medication effects assumes increasing importance. In the second paper in this section, Pelham and colleagues explore how children with ADHD account for methylphenidate-induced behavioral change. In two separate experiments, boys between the ages of 7 and 12 underwent a double blind, placebo-controlled medication assessment while attending a summer day-treatment program. Each day the boys were asked to evaluate their behavior, and to indicate whether their performance was attributable to medication, the action of counselors, or their own effort. Objective measures showed improved behavior with methylphenidate, and the boys reported improved behavior when they had received active medication.

A similar attributional pattern was found across drug conditions; the boys attributed success to ability or effort, and failure to the pill or to the actions of counselors. The authors consider this response pattern as self-enhancing and interpret the data as providing little support of the often-expressed concern that that pharmacological treatment of children with ADHD discourages self-regulation of behavior.

The third paper in this section focuses on yet another aspect of the treatment of ADHD with methylphenidate: its effect on covert antisocial behavior. Hinshaw, Heller, and McHale argue persuasively that covert antisocial behavior (stealing, destruction of property, cheating, etc.) carries a high risk for negative outcome and warrants investigation as a construct separate from that of aggression. To study covert behaviors an individual laboratory setting was devised in which ADHD and comparison boys between the ages of 6 and 12 years had the opportunity to take desired items and use an answer key while working on a problem set. The session was surreptitiously videotaped; stealing was measured by counts of objects remaining in the room; property destruction and cheating were coded from the videotapes. The subjects with ADHD were observed while on active medication and on placebo. Observed instances of property destruction and stealing were correlated with parental and staff ratings of similar behaviors. Unmedicated children with ADHD tended to display greater rates of stealing and property destruction than did children in the comparison group. Methylphenidate resulted in a significant reduction in the occurrence of these acts. However, cheating behavior increased while on stimulant medication. A thought-provoking discussion of the findings focuses on questions of the generalizability of results obtained in the laboratory, as well as on the ethical issues raised by the experiment design.

In the final paper in this section, Kruesi and colleagues report the results of a prospective follow-up study of a sample of 29 children and adolescents with disruptive behavior disorders. The subjects, who ranged in age at the time of initial assessment from 6 to 17 years, had all participated in an inpatient evaluation during which lumbar cerebral spinal fluid (CSF) was obtained and psychophysiological studies were performed. All subjects and their parents were located after an interval of two years. Outcome variables included a general measure of overall functioning as well as more specific assessment of aggression, suicide attempts and arrests. A 5-hydroxyindoleacetic acid (5-HIAA) concentration significantly predicted severity of physical aggression during follow-up, while the skin conductance level significantly predicted institutionalization. These biological laboratory measures contributed significantly in multivariate analyses even after clinical measures including aggressivity/previous antisocial behavior, IQ, parental mental health, and socioeconomic status were accounted for. Although interpretation is limited by the wide age-range of the subjects and the relatively brief follow-up interval, the findings are consistent with earlier reports of the predictive import of CSF 5-HIAA concentration and autonomic nervous system activity in children with disruptive behavior disorders. Further clarification of the independent and interactive contributions of both biologic and social factors to the outcome of children with ADHD, Oppositional Defiant Disorder, and Conduct Disorder could provide a basis for the development of more individualized and more effective treatments.

10

Social Information Processing in Aggressive and Depressed Children

Nancy L. Quiggle, Judy Garber,
William F. Panak, and Kenneth A. Dodge
Vanderbilt University, Nashville, Tennessee

Social information processing patterns of children who were identi-fied as being aggressive or depressed, both, or neither were compared in order to address the issue of specificity and to explore whether chil-dren who are comorbid show a unique processing style. Subjects were 220 children in the third through sixth grade. Peer nomination and teacher ratings were used to assess level of aggression, and the Children's Depression Inventory was used to measure level of depres-sion. Aggressive children showed a hostile attributional bias, were more likely to report that they would engage in aggressive behavior, and indicated that aggression would be easy for them. Depressed chil-dren similarly showed a hostile attributional bias, although they were more likely to attribute negative situations to internal, stable, and global causes. Depressed children also reported that they would be less likely to use assertive responses and that they expected that asser-tive behavior would lead to more negative and fewer positive out-comes. Children who were comorbid generally showed patterns similar to both aggressive and depressed children.

During the past few decades, there has been an increased interest in the role that cognitions play in childhood psychopathology and problem behavior (Kendall &

Reprinted with permission from *Child Development*, 1992, Vol. 63, 1305–1320. Copyright © 1992 by the Society for Research in Child Development, Inc.

This research was supported in part by a grant to Garber from the Vanderbilt University Research Council, and a grant to Dodge from the National Institute of Mental Health No. MH42498. Garber was also supported as a Faculty Scholar from the W. T. Grant Foundation (#88121488), and Dodge was supported by a Research Career Development Award from the National Institute of Child Health and Human Development. This paper was written while Dodge was a Fellow at the Center for

Urbain, 1982). This interest stems in part from the hypothesis that humans respond primarily to cognitive representations of their environment and experiences rather than to those experiences themselves (Beck, 1967, 1976; Lazarus, 1968; Lazarus, Kanner, & Polkman, 1980). Thus atypical or problematic responses to a situation are hypothesized to result from biased or inaccurate interpretations of the situation.

In an effort to understand how biases in cognitive processing relate to problem behaviors, attempts have been made to identify the steps involved in competent responding (Dodge, 1986; D'Zurilla & Goldfried, 1971; Flavell, 1974; McFall, 1982; Meichenbaum, Butler, & Gruson, 1981; Newell & Simon, 1972; Rubin & Krasnor, 1986; Schank & Abelson, 1977; Spivack, Platt, & Shure, 1976). In children, deviations from competent responding have been found to be characteristic of such diverse problems as aggression (e.g., Dodge, 1980, 1986), depression (e.g., Hammen & Zupan, 1984; Kaslow, Rehm, Pollack, & Siegel, 1988; Seligman et al., 1984), and impulsivity (e.g., Kendall & Braswell, 1985; Meichenbaum, 1977; Meichenbaum & Goodman, 1971).

Transgressions from normative information processing can take place at any step in a sequential process and can take the form of either distortions or deficits (Dodge, 1986; Kendall, 1985). Either of these types of cognitive patterns might lead to problematic behavior, but the particulars of the transgressions and the points in processing at which they occur are hypothesized to distinguish one form of psychopathology from another. For example, impulsive children show deficits in cognitive processing, whereas depressed children show distortions in their self-evaluations, and depressed and anxious individuals both show cognitive distortions, but differ with regard to the type and content of distortion (Beck, Brown, Steer, Eidelson, & Riskind, 1987; Kendall & Ingram, 1989; Kendall, Stark, & Adam, 1990). Whereas some studies have examined cognitive processing versus cognitive deficits within the same population (e.g., Fuhrman & Kendall, 1986; Kendall et al., 1990; Schwartz, Friedman, Lindsay, & Narrol, 1982), few studies have yet contrasted social information processing across different childhood disorders. Thus, it is unclear whether particular social cognitive patterns are specific to particular disorders or are characteristic of problem behavior in general.

The primary purpose of this study was to examine the social information processing patterns associated with two different childhood problems: aggression and depression. Although these problems appear to differ markedly along a passive-active continuum, they also have been found to co-occur in the same children (e.g., Blumberg & Izard, 1985; Cole & Carpentieri, 1990; Jacobsen, Lahey, &

Advanced Study in the Behavioral Sciences, Stanford, CA, with support by the John D. and Catherine T. MacArthur Foundation. For all support, we are grateful. We also would like to thank Dr. Edward Binkley and the children, parents, teachers, and staff of the Metropolitan Nashville School District who cooperated in this research.

Strauss, 1983; Kazdin, Esveldt-Dawson, Unis, & Rancurello, 1983). Of interest here is the extent to which cognitive patterns associated with each syndrome are specific to that syndrome and to what extent they are shared by both.

Aggression

Some of the research on cognitive factors in childhood aggression has been based on a social information processing model outlined by Dodge (1986). According to this model, individuals' behavioral responses to a social situation follow from a set of sequential information processing steps that are generally outside their conscious awareness except in highly novel or complex situations. These steps are: (*a*) encoding social cues in the environment, (*b*) forming a mental representation and interpretation of those cues, (*c*) searching for possible behavioral responses, (*d*) deciding on a response from those generated, and (*e*) enacting the selected response. Dodge (1986) has argued that biases or deficits at any of these steps can lead to aggressive behavioral responses, and there is now considerable empirical evidence to support this claim.

Regarding cue encoding, aggressive children have been found to search for fewer social cues before making attributions about another's intent than do nonaggressive children (Dodge, 1986; Dodge & Newman, 1981; Finch & Montgomery, 1973; Milich & Dodge, 1984), even when the number of cues available is experimentally controlled (Dodge & Tomlin, 1987). Aggressive children are also more likely to focus on aggressive cues in the environment than are their less aggressive peers, and they have more trouble shifting their attention away from such aggressive cues (Gouze, 1981, 1987).

At the cue interpretation step of processing, aggressive children display a bias toward making attributions of hostile intent regarding the behavior of others (Aydin & Markova, 1979; Dodge, 1980, 1986; Dodge, Murphy, & Buchsbaum, 1984; Dodge & Newman, 1981; Dodge, Pettit, McClaskey, & Brown, 1986; Dodge & Tomlin, 1987; Nasby, Hayden, & dePaulo, 1979). This bias is particularly evident when information is ambiguous or benign (Dodge, 1980; Dodge & Frame, 1981; Dodge et al., 1984), but it also occurs when cues suggest that the peer's action was accidental or made with prosocial intent (Dodge, 1986; Dodge et al., 1984).

In studies of response generation, aggressive children have been found to generate more aggressive responses and fewer assertive responses than nonaggressive children (Asarnow & Callan, 1985; Deluty, 1981, 1983, 1985; Dodge, 1986; Feldman & Dodge, 1987; Forman, 1980; Gouze, 1987). Studies of response decision have found that aggressive children value aggressive responses more and assertive responses less than do their peers (Asarnow & Callan, 1985; Deluty, 1985; Dodge, 1986; Feldman & Dodge, 1987). Moreover, Perry, Perry, and

Rasmussen (1986) found that aggressive children were more confident in their ability to use aggressive responses, and less confident in their ability to inhibit aggression, than were nonaggressive children. The groups were equally confident, however, in their ability to use verbal persuasion and prosocial behaviors. Aggressive children also expected aggression to be more effective in obtaining rewards, in decreasing aversive treatment from others, and in bringing about more positive self-evaluations.

Finally, Dodge et al. (1986) have found that aggressive children are deficient in skills required for the enactment of competent responses to negative situations. There have been no studies, however, investigating the competence of children to carry out the responses that they themselves have selected. Taken together, this literature suggests a pattern of cognitive biases and deficits that may influence children to behave aggressively, although it is not known whether these biases are the cause or the consequence of aggressive behavior.

There have been only a few studies that have addressed the specificity of these cognitive-behavioral patterns. In general, these studies (e.g., Dodge, Price, Bachorowski, & Newman, 1990; McClaskey, 1988; Milich & Dodge, 1984) have found that these social problem-solving deficits are more characteristic of aggressive children than children with other types of externalizing problems (e.g., Attention Deficit Disorder, socialized conduct disorder). No studies thus far have compared social information processing of aggressive versus depressed children.

Depression

One of the most widely studied cognitive theories of depression is that of Beck (1967, 1976; Beck, Rush, Shaw, & Emery, 1979), who has argued that cognitive structures or schemata affect the encoding, storage, and retrieval of information. He postulated that depressed individuals have negatively biased schemata that lead them to filter out positive information selectively and to exaggerate negative information. They then make specific dysphoria-provoking cognitive errors that result in a negative view of the self, current circumstances, and the future.

Although Beck (1967, 1976) did not explicitly break down his theory into the information processing components described above, he clearly addressed some of the same steps. Selective filtering of negative events reflects a bias in cue encoding. Negative views of current circumstances reflect biased attributions at the cue interpretation stage. Similarly, negative views of the future reflect biased expectations that may influence response decisions.

Ingram (1984) offered an information processing analysis of depression that concerns *how* cognitive processes result in depression. According to Ingram, when individuals appraise life events as resulting in meaningful loss, a primitive emotion node for depression is activated in memory. The associative nature of cognitive networks results in increased memory for other depressive events that reactivate the depressive node and create a cognitive recycling process that maintains the depressed effect. Because incoming information summates with activation already in the cognitive network, the depressed individual is primed to perceive and process depressogenic information over other types of information available. Moreover, there will be less cognitive capacity available for efficient enactment of behaviors since the system is engaged in self-focused depressive cognitions.

Ingram's (1984) model focuses on biased processing at various steps of Dodge's (1986) social information processing model. Associative networks in memory are offered as an explanation for biases in cue encoding and response generation. Cue interpretations that include appraisals of meaningful loss are expected to result in depressed affect. Finally, limited cognitive capacity is offered as an explanation for inaccurate or distorted processing of information and decreases in behavioral enactment.

Another important theory of depression is the reformulated learned helplessness model (Abramson, Seligman, & Teasdale, 1978), which asserts that depression follows the experience of a negative event when the individual explains the event in internal, stable, and global terms. This explanatory style results in the expectation that no action will control the outcome of similar events in the future, resulting in helplessness, hopelessness, passivity, and depression (Abramson, Metalsky, & Alloy, 1989).

The learned helplessness model also describes cognitive biases that correspond to several steps in a social information processing model. The depressogenic explanatory style reflects a particular pattern of biases in cue interpretation. In addition, because depressives tend to view most response choices as ineffective, they may be more likely to select passive responses over those that might be more effective.

Much of the empirical evidence regarding social cognitions in depressed individuals can be reviewed from a social information processing perspective. Although considerable research has addressed the stages of cue encoding, cue interpretation, and response decision, the stages of response generation and response enactment have not been investigated as extensively in depressed as compared to aggressive children.

With regard to cue encoding, Hammen and Zupan (1984) found that depressed children both endorse and recall more negative and fewer positive self-referent words than do their nondepressed peers. Depressed children also recall more negative words that they did not endorse as self-referent. These findings suggest that depressed children display a bias toward attending to negative cues, at least when they are viewed as self-referent.

Research examining cue interpretation biases in depressed children has supported the reformulated learned helplessness model (Abramson et al., 1978). Studies have found that relative to nondepressed children, depressed children make internal, stable, and global attributions for negative events (Bodiford, Eisenstadt, Johnson, & Bradlyn, 1988; Kaslow et al., 1988; Kaslow, Rehm, & Siegel, 1984; Seligman & Peterson, 1986; Seligman et al., 1984) and external, specific, and unstable attributions for positive events (Curry & Craighead, 1990; Kaslow et al., 1984, 1988; Nolen-Hoeksema, Girgus, & Seligman, 1986; Peterson & Seligman, 1984; Seligman & Peterson, 1986; Seligman et al., 1984).

The one study to examine response generation in depressed children (Mullins, Siegel, & Hodges, 1985) found that, when presented with hypothetical problems involving social interactions, depressed children generate as many relevant means to a given end as do nondepressed children. Depressed children, however, offer more irrelevant means as well.

Whereas researchers interested in childhood aggression have studied response decision by asking children to select from a list of responses that they or the children themselves have generated, researchers of childhood depression have used less direct procedures. They have assessed children's expectations regarding action, an important piece of information when making a response choice. When asked how well they will do on an experimental task, depressed children expect to do more poorly (Kaslow et al., 1984; McGee, Anderson, Williams, & Silva, 1986), to receive fewer rewards (Layne & Berry, 1983), and to view situations as out of their control (Kaslow et al., 1988) more often than do nondepressed children. Depressed children also display a bias toward viewing the future as hopeless and their own abilities as lacking (Kazdin et al., 1983; Kazdin, Rodgers, & Colbus, 1986). No studies to date have examined how effectively depressed children enact a response once they have chosen one.

Taken together, these findings depict a depressive cognitive pattern of attending to negative cues in the environment, interpreting the negative events as being due to global and stable factors either of the world or of the self, generating irrelevant means of solving problems, expecting to be ineffective in changing the situation to a more desirable one, and ultimately interacting less with others.

Aggression and Depression

How does the social cognitive pattern of depressed children compare to that found for aggressive children? Both groups of children seem to display a bias toward attending to negative cues in the environment. Whereas aggressive children identify others as the source of negative events, depressed children are more likely to identify the source of negative outcomes within themselves. Aggressive children are more likely than nonaggressive children to believe that aggressive responses can alter negative situations in their favor, whereas depressed children tend to believe that no action is likely to have much effect. Finally, aggressive children report that they are more likely to be aggressive in response to negative social situations, whereas depressed children report a greater likelihood of being passive or detached. These statements are hypotheses rather than conclusions, however, because no single study has contrasted the cognitive patterns of aggressive children with those of depressed children. A central issue is the extent to which cognitive patterns associated with each syndrome are specific to that syndrome, and the extent to which they are shared by both. This specificity issue is important because it may have implications for understanding the etiology of both aggression and depression (Garber & Hollon, 1991).

The second important issue addressed in this study was what are the social information processing patterns of children who are *both* aggressive and depressed. There is increasing evidence that depression and aggression, or depression and conduct disorder, co-occur (Asarnow, 1988; Bodiford et al., 1988; Chiles, Miller, & Cox, 1980; Cole & Carpentieri, 1990; Geller, Chestnut, Miller, Price, & Yates, 1985; Jacobsen et al., 1983; Kazdin et al., 1983; Marriage, Fine, Moretti, & Haley, 1986; Mendelson, Reid, & Frommer, 1972; Puig-Antich, 1982). This study examined the social information processing of children with comorbid aggression and depression in contrast to the processing of those children who manifest only one of these problems. Comorbid children could have one of the following cognitive processing patterns: (*a*) they could be similar to either aggressive *or* depressed children; (*b*) they could be the composite of *both* aggressive and depressed children, and thus show features of both groups; (*c*) comorbid children could be quantitatively different from the single groups, and show more severe processing errors, but of essentially the same kind; or (*d*) they could be a qualitatively distinct group that has its own unique pattern of processing social information.

Finally, cognitive factors do not alone affect behavior. Emotion is also an important component of psychopathology (e.g., Beck, 1967; Dodge, 1991; Izard, 1972), whether emotion is seen as a cognitive interpretation of an individual's physiological state (Ekman, Levenson, & Friesen, 1983; Schachter & Singer, 1962) or as a separate system that then influences cognition (Zajonc, 1980). Thus, a final goal of this study was to examine the degree and types of emotions reported by aggressive and depressed children in response to standard problematic stimuli.

METHOD

Subjects

Subjects were 220 children (104 boys, 116 girls) in grades 3–6 (ages 9 to 12 years old) of three public schools in a moderate size metropolitan area. Subjects were taken from a pool of 588 children who had parental permission to participate in the study and had gone through a screening procedure described below. All three schools serviced primarily lower- to middle-income families.

Procedure

Self-report and peer data were collected during school hours in group sessions. All questions were read aloud and children marked their responses on their own answer sheets. Identification numbers, rather than names, were used for recording the peer nominations. Teachers' reports were filled out by the teachers at a time they found convenient.

Aggression. Teacher report of aggression was based on the teacher version of the Child Behavior Checklist (CBCL; Achenbach & Edelbrock, 1986; Edelbrock & Achenbach, 1984) aggression scale. The CBCL aggression scale has been found to have acceptable reliability and construct validity (Achenbach & Edelbrock, 1986). Internal consistency of the scale was .97 (Cronbach's alpha) for this sample.

Peer nominations for aggression were made using Dodge's (1980) peer nomination technique. For each question, children nominated three peers in their own grade whom: (*a*) they liked the most, (*b*) they liked the least, (*c*) starts fights, and (*d*) gets mad. The number of nominations for each item was tallied for each child. These scores were converted to standard scores within a grade level and within a school. Two summary scores were then computed: (*a*) a social preference score, and (*b*) an aggression score. The social preference score was calculated by subtracting the "liked least" standard score from the "liked most" standard score, and then standardizing these difference scores. The aggression score was calculated as the mean of the standard "starts fights" score and the standard "gets mad" score. Scales using similar items have been shown to have good short- and long-term temporal stability for social preference scores as well as for individual items (Carlson, Lahey, & Neeper, 1984; Coie & Dodge, 1983), and to correlate with aggressive behavior as observed by teachers and trained observers (Dodge, Coie, & Brakke, 1982).

Consistent with other studies in the literature (e.g., Asarnow & Callan, 1985; Dodge, 1980), a combination of teacher report and peer nominations of aggression was used to identify aggressive children. Children were considered aggressive if they scored above the median on teacher rated aggression *and* they obtained a score below the median on social preference *and* above the eightieth percentile on peer nominated aggression (*n* = 52).

Depression. Self-reported depression was measured using the Childhood Depression Inventory (CDI; Kovacs & Beck, 1977), a modification of the Beck Depression Inventory (Beck, Ward, Mendelson, Mock, & Erbaugh, 1961) for use with children. Each of 27 items lists three levels (scored as 0, 1, or 2) of some thought, feeling, or behavior associated with depression. For each item, children marked the sentence that best described them during the past 2 weeks. Consistent with other studies of childhood depression (e.g., Kaslow et al., 1984; Nelson, Politano, Finch, Wendel, & Mayhall, 1987), children were categorized as depressed if they had a CDI score of 13 or greater.

The CDI has been found to have acceptable reliability and construct validity (Kovacs), 1981; Saylor, Finch, Spirito, & Bennett, 1984; Seligman & Peterson, 1986; Smucker, Craighead, Craighead, & Green, 1986). It correlates highly with clinicians' ratings of depression and discriminates among depressed children, non-depressed clinic patients, and normal schoolchildren (Kovacs, 1983).

Assessment of Information Processing Patterns

Subjects were interviewed individually by graduate student experimenters who were blind to the status of the children with respect to aggression and depression. Children were read six stories (in random order) and answered a series of questions after each story. Children responded verbally and the experimenter transcribed responses on a form. Open-ended responses were coded later by one of the authors (a female graduate student). Two female reliability raters (one an advanced undergraduate student, the other a graduate student) were trained in the scoring system and coded the responses of a random 10% of the sample. As there were, on average, five open-ended responses (two response generation, three response evaluation) for each of six stories for each of the 22 subjects who were checked for reliability, a total of about 660 responses were analyzed for reliability. Scores were considered in agreement if both raters assigned the response to the same category.

The six information processing stories depicted children in situations in which (a) they tried to enter a group but were rejected (2 Entry stories), (b) a peer ridiculed or bumped them (2 Provocation stories), and (c) they found out that they had failed at an academic task (2 Failure stories). All stories were worded so that the gender of the characters was left ambiguous. An example of an Entry story is: "Let's imagine that several kids are sitting at a lunch table eating lunch. You can see that they are laughing and having a good time and you'd like to join them. You walk up to the table and ask them if they'd make room for you too. One of them tells you 'No.'"

Entry and provocation situations were selected because they have been shown to elicit biased cognitive interpretations in aggressive children (Corsaro, 1981; Dodge, 1983, 1986; Dodge, McClaskey, & Feldman, 1985), and failure situations have been shown to elicit biased cognitive interpretations in depressed individuals

(Kaslow, Tannenbaum, Abramson, Peterson, & Seligman, 1983). After each story, subjects were asked a series of questions designed to assess aspects of social information processing.

Familiarity. The first question asked subjects how often they had been in a situation like the one in the story. Subjects responded using a four-point scale ranging from 1 "almost never" to 4 "very often."

Attribution of intent. Next, subjects were asked how much they thought what happened in the story was due to the deliberate malevolent intent of another (e.g., "How much do you think the kid who said 'No' was trying to be mean?"). They responded on a four-point rating scale ranging from 1 "not at all" to 4 "very much."

Attributional style. A series of 12 paired attributions was read to subjects, who then decided which of the two choices was the more likely reason for what had happened. The format of this section followed that of the Children's Attributional Style Questionnaire (Seligman et al., 1984), but items reflected possible attributions for the specific events in the stories. For each pair, two of the factors along the Internal-External, Global-Specific, and Stable-Unstable dimensions were held constant while the other factor was varied. The number of times that a child chose an internal over an external, a global over a specific, and a stable over an unstable attribution was summed. Each dimension was varied four times across the 12 pairings; a score range of 0 to 4 was possible for each dimension. A composite attribution score (range 0 to 12) was calculated by summing the number of Internal, Global, and Stable attributions. Higher scores indicated a more depressogenic explanatory style.

Affect. Subjects next were asked how they would feel in the situation described to them. Subjects rated how angry, sad, and happy (presented in random order) they would feel in this situation on separate rating scales ranging from 1 "not at all" to 4 "extremely."

Response generation. Children than reported what they thought they would do if this situation happened to them. They were probed for multiple responses (up to six per story). Each response was later coded into one of five mutually exclusive categories: (*a*) aggressive, (*b*) assertive, (*c*) withdrawn, (*d*) pure affect, and (*e*) other. Responses were coded as aggressive if they involved an act of physical or verbal aggression, or retaliation. Assertive responses were those in which the child requested information, bargained, tried again, or worked harder. Passive or withdrawn responses were those that involved doing nothing, taking the blame, begging, giving in, quitting, withdrawing from the situation, or waiting to see what would happen. Pure affect responses were those in which children reported how they thought they would feel even though they had been asked what they would do in the situation (responses such as: "I would feel bad," or "I'd be angry"). Responses that did not fit in any of the first four categories were coded as "other." Intercoder reliability calculated on a random 10% of the responses yielded 92% agreement and a Cohen's kappa of .88.

Response evaluation. Subjects were next read each of three types of responses, supposedly given by other children: aggressive, withdrawal, and assertive (presented in random order). Examples of each type of response for the Entry story given above are (1) aggressive: "One kid just pushed between the kids and sat down anyway"; (2) withdrawal: "One kid put his head down and went and ate by himself"; and (3) assertive: "One kid said 'I think there would be room if you moved over. I'd really like to sit with you.'"

Subjects rated the quality of the response from 1 "very bad" to 4 "very good." Next, they reported what they thought would happen if they engaged in that behavior. This open-ended response was recorded verbatim and later was scored according to whether it expressed a positive or negative outcome for the child. Intercoder reliability yielded 84% agreement and a Cohen's kappa of .66. Next, they rated how likely it was that they would respond as had been described, from 1 "definitely would not" to 4 "definitely would." Finally, they rated how easy or hard it would be for them to react as described, from 1 "very easy" to 4 "very hard."

RESULTS

Gender and Story Effects

Prior to the main analyses, each variable was correlated with gender. Sex of subject was related significantly to only two dependent variables: sad affect ratings were higher for girls than for boys ($r = .22$, $p < .001$), and the proportion of aggressive responses generated was higher for boys than for girls ($r = -.26$, $p < .001$). Gender was covaried in the analyses of these two variables. For all other analyses, boys and girls were combined.

There were significant differences on almost all variables as a function of story type (Entry, Provocation, or Failure), with story type accounting for as little as 1% (e.g., "How happy would you feel in this situation?") to as much as 60% (e.g., attribution of intent) of the variance on a specific variable. However, univariate analyses showed that story type interacted significantly with level of aggression or depression for only one dependent variable (proportion of pure affect responses generated). Therefore, story effects were partitioned out, and the group effects presented below are based on the sum of responses across all six stories.

Status Group Effects

The familiarity variable was analyzed using analysis of variance (ANOVA), whereas the latter six groups of variables were analyzed using multivariate analysis of variance (MANOVA) followed by univariate ANOVAs.[1] Level of aggression and level of depression were treated as fully crossed independent variables (see Table 1 for the means for all variables). Significant main effects for one independent variable and not the other suggest specificity. Significant main effects for both independent variables suggest that the dependent variable reflects a pattern common to both disorders. A significant interaction between the two independent factors suggests that the comorbid group had a unique cognitive pattern of responding. The nonaggressive group included those children who were normal (high in neither aggression nor depression) and the pure depressed group (high in depression but low in aggression), whereas the aggressive group consisted of children high in aggression who were either high or low in depression. The nondepressed group similarly consisted of normal (low in both aggression and depression) and pure aggressive children (high in aggression but low in depression); the depressed group consisted of children high in depression who were either high or low in aggression.

Familiarity

There was a significant main effect for depression, $F(1, 216) = 18.24$, $p < .001$, and a marginally significant effect for aggression, $F(1, 216) = 4.24$, $p < .05$, with regard to children's self-reported familiarity with the situations. This indicates that depressed children, and to some extent aggressive children, were more familiar with the presented problem situations than were their peers. The interaction was nonsignificant.

Attributions

The MANOVA of the attribution of intent and depressogenic attributional style variables revealed a significant multivariate main effect for both aggression, $F(2, 215) = 5.92$, $p < .01$, and depression, $F(2, 215) = 11.64$, $p < .001$. Univariate analyses indicated that aggressive children were significantly more likely than nonaggressive children to attribute hostile intent to another, $F(1, 216) = 7.10$, $p < .01$. This attributional tendency was not specific to aggression, however. Depressed children also made attributions of hostile intent significantly more than did nondepressed children, $F(1, 216) = 7.20$, $p < .01$. Depressed children were also significantly more likely than nondepressed children to attribute negative events to the combination of internal, global, and stable causes (composite score),

---

[1]In order to control experiment-wise Type I error, Holms's modified Bonferroni procedure was used (Holland & Copenhaven, 1988) across the seven MANOVAs within effects. In practice, this led to the rejection of multivariate null hypotheses when $p < .01$. Univariate effects calculated subsequent to significant multivariate effects also were considered significant at $p < .01$, and marginally significant if $.01 < p < .05$.

TABLE 1
Social Cognition as a Function of Depression and Aggression

VARIABLE	NORMAL (n = 89) M	SD	DEPRESSED (n = 81) M	SD	AGGRESSIVE (n = 26) M	SD	COMORBID (n = 24) M	SD	DEP F	AGG F	DEP x AGG F
Familiarity	9.22	(2.81)	11.54	(3.42)	10.38	(3.19)	12.54	(4.20)	18.24***	4.24*	.02
Attributions:											
Hostile intent	11.90	(2.68)	13.12	(2.49)	13.12	(3.42)	14.29	(3.30)	7.20**	7.10**	.00
Composite*	26.07	(6.02)	29.05	(6.65)	27.27	(5.14)	31.38	(5.31)	13.03***	3.23	.33
Affect:[b]											
Sad	14.46	(3.82)	16.02	(4.19)	13.92	(3.82)	15.96	(4.08)	6.54**	.06	.06
Mad	14.84	(3.66)	17.17	(3.75)	16.00	(4.16)	16.83	(3.44)	6.99**	.43	1.51
Happy	7.47	(1.74)	7.22	(1.55)	8.04	(1.91)	7.00	(1.59)	5.09*	.29	1.99
Response generation:[b]											
Aggress	.53	(.61)	.63	(.66)	.66	(.86)	.82	(.82)	2.50	1.46	.24
Withdraw	1.16	(.72)	1.21	(.62)	1.03	(.87)	1.10	(.72)	.26	1.13	.01
Assert	1.92	(.84)	1.74	(.74)	2.04	(1.00)	1.49	(.98)	8.48**	.10	2.17
Pure affect	.28	(.47)	.27	(.47)	.16	(.26)	.48	(.61)	4.58*	.27	4.81*
Response evaluation:											
Aggression:											
Quality	7.81	(1.82)	8.31	(2.41)	8.77	(2.92)	8.62	(3.45)	.21	2.73*	.69
How likely	8.79	(2.45)	9.75	(3.16)	11.35	(3.59)	10.42	(4.22)	.00	10.52**	3.64
How easy	19.15	(4.19)	18.30	(4.34)	16.00	(6.04)	15.75	(5.80)	.53	14.24***	.16
Pos.[c] outcome	.12	(.36)	.11	(.47)	.12	(.59)	.21	(.42)	.32	.39	.55
Neg.[d] outcome	7.39	(1.72)	7.52	(1.97)	7.27	(1.48)	6.71	(1.55)	.58	2.67	1.44
Withdrawal:											
Quality	11.71	(2.38)	12.52	(2.56)	11.23	(2.25)	12.50	(3.05)	6.63*	.38	.32
How likely	11.40	(2.46)	12.05	(2.92)	11.00	(2.67)	11.58	(2.86)	1.99	1.00	.00
How easy	17.38	(3.40)	16.25	(3.68)	16.42	(4.94)	15.50	(4.23)	2.83	1.94	.30
Pos. outcome	1.18	(1.50)	.82	(1.00)	1.08	(1.38)	.42	(1.06)	6.20*	1.48	.51
Neg. outcome	7.11	(2.55)	6.82	(1.98)	7.00	(1.52)	7.62	(1.74)	.22	1.00	1.75
Assert:											
Quality	20.20	(1.96)	19.76	(2.46)	19.92	(2.50)	19.67	(3.63)	.78	.23	.05
How likely	17.76	(2.56)	17.05	(2.64)	17.12	(2.45)	15.67	(4.12)	5.81*	5.12*	.67
How easy	12.19	(3.39)	13.21	(2.90)	11.46	(3.70)	13.00	(4.71)	5.36*	.72	.22
Pos. outcome	4.51	(1.71)	3.80	(1.59)	4.42	(1.75)	2.92	(1.91)	16.37***	3.14	2.16
Neg. outcome	2.08	(1.72)	2.85	(1.96)	2.04	(1.68)	3.79	(1.82)	18.63***	2.36	2.80

[a] The composite score is the combination of the Internal, Stable, and Global scores.
[b] For these variables, the group means were adjusted for the covariate gender.
[c] Pos. = positive.
[d] Neg. = negative.
* p < .05.
** p < .01.
*** p < .001.

$F(1, 216) = 13.03$, $p < .001$. Aggressive children, however, did not differ from their less aggressive peers with respect to explanatory style. There were no significant interactions.

Affect

Because there was a significant effect for gender on affect, multivariate analysis of covariance was conducted with gender as the covariate. The MANCOVA of the three affect questions revealed a significant main effect for depression, $F(3,$

213) = 3.77, $p < .05$. Univariate analyses indicated that depressed children reported that they would feel significantly more anger, $F(1, 215) = 6.99, p <.01$, and showed a marginally significant trend toward reporting more sadness, $F(1, 215) = 6.54, p <.05$, and less happiness, $F(1, 215) = 5.09, p <.05$, than non-depressed children. There were no significant main effects for aggression or significant interactions.

Response Generation

Again, because there was a significant effect for gender on the proportion of responses generated, multivariate analysis of covariance was conducted with gender as the covariate. A MANCOVA was conducted on the proportion of responses generated that were coded in each of the response categories as a function of group status. The main effect for depression was marginally significant, $F(4, 212) = 2.49, p <.05$. Several univariate effects were found, and these are reported in Table 1. There was a marginally significant interaction with regard to pure affect responses, $F(1, 215) = 4.81, p <.05$; post hoc cell contrasts indicated that the comorbid children were more likely to generate purely affective responses than were other children.

Response Evaluation

Aggressive responses. The MANOVA of the response evaluation items concerning aggression revealed a significant main effect for aggressive children, $F(5, 212) = 3.89, p <.01$. Univariate analyses indicated that, in comparison to their less aggressive peers, aggressive children reported that they would be more likely to use aggressive responses, $F(1, 216) = 10.52, p <.01$, and that aggression would be easier for them, $F(1, 216) = 14.24, p <.001$. Children high on depression did not differ significantly from children low on depression for any of these variables; there were no significant interactions.

Withdrawal responses. The MANOVA of the response evaluation items concerning withdrawal revealed a significant main effect for depression, $F(5, 212) = 3.72, p <.01$. Univariate analyses indicated that depressed children showed a trend toward rating withdrawal responses more favorably, $F(1, 216) = 6.63, p <.05$, and toward reporting that withdrawal would lead to more positive outcomes, $F(1, 216) = 6.20, p <.05$, than did their nondepressed peers. Children high on aggression did not differ significantly from children low on aggression for any of these variables, and there were no significant interactions.

Assertive responses. The MANOVA of the response evaluation items with regard to assertiveness revealed a significant main effect for depression, $F(5, 212) = 4.43, p <.01$. Univariate analyses indicated that depressed children were more likely to report that assertion would lead to fewer positive outcomes, $F(1, 216) = 16.37$, $p < .01$, and more negative outcomes, $F(1, 216) = 18.63$, $p < .01$, than did their nondepressed peers. Depressed children also showed a marginally significant trend toward saying that they would use assertive responses less, $F(1, 216) = 5.81$, $p < .05$, and would find assertive responses less easy than would nondepressed children, $F(1, 216) = 5.36$, $p < .05$. There were no significant main effects for aggression, nor any significant interactions.

DISCUSSION

Overall, results of this study are consistent with social information processing models of social competence (e.g., Dodge, 1986) and cognitive theories of depression (e.g., Abramson et al., 1978; Beck, 1967; Ingram, 1984). Aggressive children demonstrated a hostile attributional bias, were relatively more likely to report that they would engage in aggressive behavior and would find it easy to aggress, and showed a tendency toward evaluating aggressive behavior more favorably than did their nonaggressive peers. These results are consistent with earlier findings that aggressive children value aggressive responses more (Asarnow & Callan, 1985; Deluty, 1985; Dodge, 1986; Feldman & Dodge, 1987) and are more confident in their ability to use aggressive responses (Perry et al., 1986).

As hypothesized, children with high levels of self-reported depressive symptoms showed the depressogenic attributional style outlined by Abramson et al. (1978). Interestingly, they also showed a hostile attributional bias. In addition, compared to nondepressed children, depressed children were more likely to report that engaging in assertive behavior would result in fewer positive and more negative outcomes, and showed a trend toward generating fewer assertive responses, reporting that they would be less likely to use assertive responses, and would find assertion less easy. Although depressed children were no more likely to generate passive or withdrawn responses, they did tend to evaluate withdrawal more favorably and to expect that withdrawal would lead to more positive outcomes. They also reported that they would feel greater anger as well as somewhat more sadness in these situations than did their nondepressed peers. Thus, the results of this study are consistent with the existing empirical literature that has found social cognitive deficits and biases in both aggressive and depressed children.

Specificity. The specificity issue is concerned with the extent to which different types of social information processing patterns are uniquely characteristic of one group. Depressed children, and to some extent aggressive children, tended to report that the negative situations described in the stories happened to them more often than did children who were neither depressed nor aggressive. It is possible that both depressed and aggressive children actually experience more negative situations than do normal children. On the other hand, it is also possible that these children are biased toward noticing, remembering, or reporting negative events. Observational studies are needed in order to assess objectively the extent to which depressed and aggressive children actually experience such negative circumstances.

Similarly, both aggressive and depressed children were more likely than their peers to attribute hostile intent to another in negative situations. A more in-depth evaluation of the thoughts that led children to their hostile attributions is necessary to determine whether or not the same cognitive processes are associated with the hostile attributions of both groups. It might be that depressed children explain others' negative intentions in terms of their own faults and failures (e.g., in stable and global internal terms). In contrast, aggressive children might be more likely to see others' hostile intentions as unrelated to their own behaviors (external), and therefore deserving of aggressive, retaliatory action. This is consistent with the finding in the present study that depressed children tended to make internal, stable, and global attributions for the negative situations, whereas aggressive children did not. Thus, although both depressed and aggressive children shared a common tendency to attribute hostile intent to others, they differed with regard to their explanatory style.

Aggressive and depressed children also differed in their reported affective responses to the negative situations, with depressed children reporting more anger and somewhat more sadness. An association between anger and depression is consistent with other studies in the literature (e.g., Blumberg & Izard, 1985; Izard, 1972; Toolan, 1974). Somewhat surprising, however, was the lack of association between reported anger and aggression. This could have been due to several factors.

It is possible that aggressive children do not actually experience anger more than do other children. Rather, they might experience comparable levels of anger, but might not have learned appropriate ways of managing it behaviorally. It could also be that aggressive children have difficulty accurately labeling their feelings. Although they might experience the heightened levels of arousal that normally would be called anger, aggressive children might not have learned the appropriate affect label. Finally, it is possible that aggressive children actually experience relatively more anger, but they are less willing to report negative feelings. Future studies should replicate these affect results and test among these alternative explanations for the lack of reported anger by aggressive children.

Whereas aggressive children reported that they would be more likely to be aggressive and would find aggression relatively easy, depressed children tended to generate relatively fewer assertive responses, expected fewer positive and more negative consequences for assertive behavior, and tended to expect more positive outcomes for withdrawal. These findings indicate that depressed children report that they become affectively aroused but behaviorally passive and ineffective in response to negative situations. They are more likely to anticipate that action will lead to negative outcomes, whereas inaction might lead to improvement. In such a world it might, indeed, be better not to act, but to leave action to others. Such passivity could result from a belief that these negative circumstances are uncontrollable (Seligman, 1975; Weisz, Weiss, Wasserman, & Rintoul, 1987), or an expectation that they cannot produce the kinds of responses (e.g., assertive) that will effectively alter these situations (Bandura, 1977, 1982).

Thus, both aggressive and depressed children showed information processing patterns that were different from normals, and were consistent with their respective ways of typically responding to difficult negative situations. That is, aggressive children favored aggression, whereas depressed children viewed assertiveness less favorably and showed a tendency toward favoring withdrawal. Overall, these findings are interesting in that different types of deviations in information processing are associated with particular forms of psychopathology. Depressed and aggressive children have different, albeit comparably less competent ways of responding to negative interpersonal and achievement situations. Thus, these results provide further evidence that Dodge's (1986) social information processing model of social competence is a more general perspective that can be used as a guide for understanding depressive withdrawal as well as aggression. *Comorbidity.* Comorbid children showed the cognitive patterns of both the aggressive and depressed groups in an additive manner, suggesting that they simply express the cognitive characteristics of both groups from which they are composed. That is, for those variables associated with aggression, comorbid children responded more like aggressive children, and for those variables associated with depression, they responded like depressed children. Thus, comorbid children showed essentially the same patterns that would be expected for the single groups. There was only a suggestion of a unique cognitive pattern with regard to one variable—response generation. Comorbid children showed a tendency toward generating more purely affective responses to the negative situations.

It may be that comorbid children are as aggressive as their aggressive peers, but become more frustrated when they do not obtain their desired goals through their behaviors. This may result in their feeling more angry and helpless, similar to depressed children. In contrast to depressed children, however, comorbid children may focus more on the frustration and anger they feel rather than the helplessness. Whereas depressed children eventually give up and withdraw, comorbid children might continue to try aggression, and continue to be frustrated and upset when they fail to achieve their goals.

It is also possible that the comorbid group consisted of two subgroups of children, some of whom are more like depressed children with respect to the underlying causal processes, but who develop secondary aggressive cognitions and behaviors, and a second subgroup who are more like aggressive children, but who develop secondary depression. Since the distinction between primary and secondary disorders (Robins & Guze, 1972) is defined in terms of the chronology of onset, however, it is impossible to conclude from the current cross-sectional study whether in fact this notion of two subgroups of either primary depressed or primary aggressive children is correct. Longitudinal studies are needed that more precisely assess the onset of depression and aggression, and that evaluate the social information processing of children prior to their development of either depressive or aggressive symptomatology. Such prospective studies will also allow us to explore the extent to which the hypothesized cognitive processing deficits are a cause, concomitant, or consequence of aggression and depression.

Several limitations of this research are noteworthy since they provide directions for future investigations. First, all findings from this study were based on children's verbal responses to hypothetical situations. Whether or not children exhibit the kinds of cognitive patterns found here while they actually are in the situations needs to be tested. Experimental studies are needed in which children are exposed to situations like those described in the hypothetical stories and their cognitions are recorded and their behaviors observed. Observational studies of children in real-life situations will help to determine whether the attributions and expectations of these children reflect different experiences, or are biased interpretations of a reality that is fairly common to all.

An important issue for future studies concerns the question of the origins of the various cognitive processing patterns of depressed and aggressive children. When and how did these children begin to view their worlds differently? What socialization experiences may have contributed to the development of the observed cognitive patterns? A recent study by Dodge and colleagues (Dodge, Bates, & Pettit, 1990) suggests that the experience of physical violence as a child may be an important predictor of social information processing deficits and subsequent aggression. Others (e.g., Garber, Braafladt, & Zeman, 1991; Hammen, 1988; Hammen, Burge, & Stansbury, 1990; Seligman & Peterson, 1986) are beginning to examine the contribution of maternal psychopathology, maternal cognitive style, and patterns of mother-child interactions to the development of depressogenic cognitive styles in children.

Another important question is to what extent these various cognitive patterns are caused and/or maintained by the social interactions that these children encounter. Conversely, to what extent do these children's less competent ways of interacting with others contribute to the negative situations in which they often find themselves? Clearly, there are multidirectional influences of environmental circumstances, cognitions, and behaviors. Longitudinal research examining the developmental course of cognitive processing variables is needed to facilitate the early identification of children who are at risk for depression and aggression before their cognitive patterns are set.

It is also important to emphasize that the present study was conducted with a community sample of children identified on the basis of self-report, teacher report, and peer nominations. The extent to which these findings are generalizable to a clinically referred sample of children who have diagnoses of a mood disorder and/or conduct disorder—aggressive type needs to be investigated further. In addition, future studies will also need to address the problem of sample selection based on different procedures and informants.

In sum, this study found differences in the ways in which aggressive versus nonaggressive and depressed versus nondepressed children process social information. Processing deficits common to both aggressive and depressed children as well as cognitive patterns that were specific to each group were identified. Comorbid children were found to most often exhibit the biases of both the aggressive and depressed children in an additive manner. The findings were consistent with information processing models (e.g., Abramson et al., 1978; Beck, 1967; Dodge, 1986; Ingram, 1984) that assert that cognitive processes play an important role in psychopathology.

REFERENCES

Abramson, L. Y., Metalsky, G. I., & Alloy, L. B. (1989). Hopelessness depression: A theory-based subtype of depression. *Psychological Bulletin*, 96, 358–372.

Abramson, L. Y., Seligman, M. E. P., & Teasdale, J. (1978). Learned helplessness in humans: Critique and reformulation. *Journal of Abnormal Psychology*, 87, 49–74.

Achenbach, T. M., & Edelbrock, C. (1986). *Manual for the Teacher's Report Form and Teacher Version of the Child Behavior Profile*. Burlington: University of Vermont, Department of Psychiatry.

Asarnow, J. R. (1988). Peer status and social competence in child psychiatric inpatients: A comparison of children with depressive, externalizing, and concurrent depressive and externalizing disorders. *Journal of Abnormal Child Psychology*, 16, 151–162.

Asarnow, J. R., & Callan, J. W. (1985). Boys with peer adjustment problems: Social cognitive processes. *Journal of Consulting and Clinical Psychology*, 53, 80–87.

Aydin, O., & Markova, I. (1979). Attribution tendencies of popular and unpopular children. *British Journal of Social and Clinical Psychology*, 18, 291–298.

Bandura, A. (1977). Self-efficacy: Toward a unifying theory of behavioral change. *Psychological Review*, 84, 191–215.

Bandura, A. (1982). Self-efficacy mechanism in human agency. *American Psychologist*, 37, 122–147.

Beck, A. T. (1967). *Depression: Clinical, experimental, and theoretical aspects*. New York: Hoeber.

Beck, A. T. (1976). *Cognitive therapy and the emotional disorders*. New York: International Universities Press.

Beck, A. T., Brown, G., Steer, R., Eidelson, J. I., & Riskind, J. (1987). Differentiating anxiety and depression: A test of the cognitive content specificity hypothesis. *Journal of Abnormal Psychology*, 96, 179–183.

Beck, A. T., Rush, A. J., Shaw, B. F., & Emery, G. (1979). *Cognitive therapy of depression.* New York: Guilford.

Beck, A. T., Ward, C. H., Mendelson, M., Mock, J., & Erbaugh, J. (1961). An inventory for measuring depression. *Archives of General Psychiatry*, 4, 561–571.

Blumberg, S. H., & Izard, C. E. (1985). Affective and cognitive characteristics of depression in 10- and 11-year-old children. *Journal of Personality and Social Psychology*, 49, 194–202.

Bodiford, C. A., Eisenstadt, T. H., Johnson, J. H., & Bradlyn, A. S. (1988). Comparison of learned helplessness cognitions and behavior in children with high and low scores on the Children's Depression Inventory. *Journal of Clinical Child Psychology*, 17, 152–158.

Carlson, C. L., Lahey, B. B., & Neeper, R. (1984). Peer assessment of the social behavior of accepted, rejected, and neglected children. *Journal of Abnormal Child Psychology*, 12, 187–198.

Chiles, J., Miller, M., & Cox, G. (1980) Depression in an adolescent delinquent population. *Archives of General Psychiatry*, 37, 1179–1184.

Coie, J. D., & Dodge, K. A. (1983). Continuities and changes in children's social status: A five-year longitudinal study. *Merrill-Palmer Quarterly*, 29, 261–282.

Cole, D. A., & Carpentieri, S. (1990). Social status and the comorbidity of child depression and conduct disorder. *Journal of Consulting and Clinical Psychology*, 58, 748–757.

Corsaro, W. A. (1981). Friendship in the nursery school: Social organization in a peer environment. In S. Asher & J. M. Gottman (Eds.), *The development of children's friendships* (pp. 207–241). New York: Cambridge University Press.

Curry, J. F., & Craighead, W. E. (1990). Attributional style in clinically depressed and conduct disordered adolescents. *Journal of Consulting and Clinical Psychology*, 58, 109–115.

Deluty, R. H. (1981). Alternative-thinking ability of aggressive, assertive, and submissive children. *Cognitive Therapy and Research*, 5, 309–312.

Deluty, R. H. (1983). Children's evaluations of aggressive, assertive, and submissive responses. *Journal of Clinical Child Psychology*, 12, 124–129.

Deluty, R. H. (1985). Cognitive mediation of aggressive, assertive, and submissive behavior in children. *International Journal of Behavioral Development*, 8, 355–369.

Dodge, K. A. (1980). Social cognition and children's aggressive behavior. *Child Development*, 51, 162–170.

Dodge, K. A. (1983). Behavioral antecedents of peer social status. *Child Development*, 54, 1386–1399.

Dodge, K. A. (1986). A social information processing model of social competence in children. In M. Perlmutter (Ed.), *Eighteenth Annual Minnesota Symposium on Child Psychology* (pp. 77–125). Hillsdale, NJ: Erlbaum.

Dodge, K. A. (1991). Emotion and social information processing. In J. Garber & K. A. Dodge (Eds.), *The development of emotion regulation and dysregulation* (pp. 159–181). New York: Cambridge University Press.

Dodge, K. A., Bates, J. E., & Pettit, G. S. (1990). Mechanisms in the cycle of violence. *Science*, 250, 1678–1683.

Dodge, K. A., Coie, J. D., & Brakke, N. P. (1982). Behavior patterns of socially rejected and neglected preadolescents: The roles of social approach and aggression. *Journal of Abnormal Child Psychology*, 10, 389–409.

Dodge, K. A., & Frame, C. L. (1982). Social cognitive biases and deficits in aggressive boys. *Child Development*, 53, 620–635.

Dodge, K. A., McClaskey, C. L., & Feldman, E. (1985). A situational approach to the assessment of social competence in children. *Journal of Consulting and Clinical Psychology*, 53, 344–353.

Dodge, K. A., Murphy, R. M., & Buchsbaum, K. (1984). The assessment of intention-cue detection skills in children: Implications for developmental psychopathology. *Child Development*, 55, 163–173.

Dodge, K. A., & Newman, J. P. (1981). Biased decision making processes in aggressive boys. *Journal of Abnormal Psychology*, 90, 375–379.

Dodge, K. A., Pettit, G. S., McClaskey, C. I., & Brown, M. (1986). Social competence in children. *Monographs of the Society for Research in Child Development*, 51 (2, Serial No. 213).

Dodge, K. A., Price, J. M., Bachorowski, J. A., & Newman, J. R. (1990). Hostile attributional tendencies in severely aggressive adolescents. *Journal of Abnormal Psychology*, 99, 385–392.

Dodge, K. A., & Tomlin, A. M. (1987). Utilization of self-schemas as a mechanism of interpretational bias in aggressive children. *Social Cognition*, 5, 280–300.

D'Zurilla, T. J., & Goldfried, M. R. (1971). Problem-solving and behavior modification. *Journal of Abnormal Psychology*, 78, 107–126.

Edelbrock, C. S., & Achenbach, T. M. (1984). The teacher version of the Child Behavior Profile: I. Boys aged 6–11. *Journal of Consulting and Clinical Psychology*, 52, 207–217.

Ekman, P., Levenson, R. W., & Friesen, W. V. (1983). Automatic nervous system activity distinguishes among emotions. *Science*, 221, 1208–1210.

Feldman, E., & Dodge, K. A. (1987). Social information processing and sociometric status: Sex, age, and situational effects. *Journal of Abnormal Child Psychology*, 15, 211–227.

Finch, A. J., Jr., & Montgomery, L. E. (1973). Reflection-impulsivity and information seeking in emotionally disturbed children. *Journal of Abnormal Child Psychology*, 1, 358–362.

Flavell, J. H. (1974). The development of inferences about others. In T. Mischel

(Ed.), *Understanding other persons* (pp. 66–116). Totowa, NJ: Rowman & Littlefield.

Forman, S. G. (1980). Self-statements of aggressive and nonaggressive children. *Child Behavior Therapy*, 2, 49–60.

Fuhrman, M. J., & Kendall, P. C. (1986). Cognitive tempo and behavioral adjustment in children. *Cognitive Therapy and Research*, 10, 45–50.

Garber, J., Braafladt, N., & Zeman, J. (1991). The regulation of sad affect: An information processing perspective. In J. Garber & K. A. Dodge (Eds.), *The development of emotion regulation and dysregulation* (pp. 208–240). New York: Cambridge University Press.

Garber, J., & Hollon, S. (1991). What can specificity designs say about causality in psychopathology research? *Psychological Bulletin*, 110, 129–136.

Geller, B., Chestnut, E. C., Miller, M. D., Price, D. T., & Yates, E. (1985). Preliminary data on DSM-III: Associated features of major depressive disorder in children and adolescents. *American Journal of Psychiatry*, 142, 643–644.

Gouze, K. R. (1981, April). *Children's initial aggression level and the effectiveness of intervention strategies in moderating TV effects on aggression.* Paper presented at the biennial meeting of the Society for Research in Child Development, Boston.

Gouze, K. R. (1987). Attention and social problem solving as correlates of aggression in preschool males. *Journal of Abnormal Child Psychology*, 15, 181–197.

Hammen, C. (1988). Self-cognitions, stressful events, and the prediction of depression in children of depressed mothers. *Journal of Abnormal Child Psychology*, 16, 347–360.

Hammen, C., Burge, D., & Stansbury, K. (1990). Relationship of mother and child variables to child outcomes in a high-risk sample: A causal modeling analysis. *Developmental Psychology*, 26, 24–30.

Hammen, C., & Zupan, B. A. (1984). Self-schemas, depression, social problem solving and social competence in preadolescents: Is inconsistency the hobgoblin of little minds? *Cognitive Therapy and Research*, 9, 685–702.

Holland, B. S., & Copenhaven, M. D. (1988). Improved Bonferroni-type multiple testing procedures. *Psychological Bulletin*, 104, 145–149.

Ingram, R. E. (1984). Toward an information-processing analysis of depression. *Cognitive Therapy and Research*, 8, 443–478.

Izard, C. (1972). *Patterns of emotions: A new analysis of anxiety and depression.* New York: Academic Press.

Jacobsen, R. H., Lahey, B. B., & Strauss, C. C. (1983). Correlates of depressed mood in normal children. *Journal of Abnormal Child Psychology*, 11, 29–40.

Kaslow, N. J., Rehm, L. P., Pollack, S. L., & Siegel, A. W. (1988). Attributional style and self-control behavior in depressed and nondepressed children and their parents. *Journal of Abnormal Child Psychology*, 16, 163–175.

Kaslow, N. J., Rehm, L. P., & Siegel, A. W. (1984). Social-cognitive and cognitive correlates of depression in children. *Journal of Abnormal Child Psychology*, 12, 605–620.

Kaslow, N. J., Tanenbaum, R. L., Abramson, L. Y., Peterson, C., & Seligman, M. E. P. (1983). Problem solving deficits and depressive symptoms among children. *Journal of Abnormal Child Psychology*, 11, 497–502.

Kazdin, A. E., Esveldt-Dawson, K., Unis, A. S., & Rancurello, M. D. (1983). Child and parent evaluations of depression and aggression in psychiatric inpatient children. *Journal of Abnormal Child Psychology*, 11, 401–413.

Kazdin, A. E., Rodgers, A., & Colbus, D. (1986). The hopelessness scale for children: Psychometric characteristics and concurrent validity. *Journal of Consulting and Clinical Psychology*, 54, 241–245.

Kendall, P. C. (1985). Toward a cognitive-behavioral model of child psychopathology and a critique of related interventions. *Journal of Abnormal Child Psychology*, 13, 357–372.

Kendall, P. C., & Braswell, L. (1985). *Cognitive-behavioral therapy for impulsive children*. New York: Guilford.

Kendall, P. C., & Ingram, R. E. (1989). Cognitive-behavioral perspectives: Theory and research on depression and anxiety. In P. C. Kendall & D. Watson (Eds.), *Anxiety and depression: Distinctive and overlapping features* (pp. 27–53). New York: Academic Press.

Kendall, P. C., Stark, K. D., & Adam, T. (1990). Cognitive deficit or cognitive distortion in childhood depression. *Journal of Abnormal Child Psychology*, 18, 225–270.

Kendall, P. C., & Urbain, E. (1982). Social-cognitive approaches to therapy with children. In J. R. Lachenmeyer & M. S. Gibbs (Eds.), *Psychopathology in childhood* (pp. 298–326). New York: Gardner.

Kovacs, M. (1981). Rating scales to assess depression in school-aged children. *Acta Paedopsychiatra*, 46, 305–315.

Kovacs, M. (1983). *Interview Schedule for Children: Form C and Follow-up Form*. Unpublished report, Pittsburgh, PA.

Kovacs, M., & Beck, A. T. (1977). An empirical-clinical approach toward a definition of childhood depression. In J. G. Schulterbrandt & A. Raskin (Eds.), *Depression in childhood: Diagnosis, treatment, and conceptual models* (pp. 1–25). New York: Raven.

Layne, C., & Berry, E. (1983). Motivational deficit in childhood depression and hyperactivity. *Journal of Clinical Psychology*, 39, 523–531.

Lazarus, R. S. (1968). Emotions and adaptation: Conceptual and empirical relations. In W. J. Arnold (Ed.), *Nebraska Symposium on Motivation* (pp. 175–266). Lincoln: University of Nebraska Press.

Lazarus, R. S., Kanner, A. D., & Folkman, S. (1980). Emotions: A cognitive-phenomenological analysis. In R. Plutchik & H. Kellerman (Eds.), *Emotion: Theory, research, and experience: Vol. I. Theories of emotion* (pp. 189–217). New York: Academic Press.

Marriage, K., Fine, S., Moretti, M., & Haley, G. (1986). Relationship between depression and conduct disorder in children and adolescents. *Journal of the American Academy of Child Psychiatry*, 25, 687–691.

McClaskey, C. L. (1988). *Symptoms of ADHD, ADD, and aggression in children: Teacher ratings, peer sociometrics, and judgments of hypothetical behavior.* Unpublished doctoral dissertation, Indiana University.

McFall, R. M. (1982). A review and reformulation of the concept of social skills. *Behavioral Assessment*, 4, 1–35.

McGee, R., Anderson, J., Williams, S., & Silva, P. A. (1986). Cognitive correlates of depressive symptoms in 11-year-old children. *Journal of Abnormal Child Psychology*, 14, 517–524.

Meichenbaum, D. (1977). *Cognitive-behavior modification: An integrative approach.* New York: Plenum.

Meichenbaum, D., Butler, L., & Gruson, L. (1981). Toward a conceptual model of social competence. In J. D. Wine & M. D. Smye (Eds.), *Social competence* (pp. 36–60). New York: Guilford.

Meichenbaum, D., & Goodman, J. (1971). Training impulsive children to talk to themselves: A means of developing self-control. *Journal of Abnormal Psychology*, 77, 115–126.

Mendelson, W. B., Reid, M. A., & Frommer, E. A. (1972). Some characteristic features accompanying depression, anxiety, and aggressive behavior in disturbed children under five. In A. L. Annell (Ed.), *Depressive states in childhood and adolescence* (pp. 151–158). New York: Halsted.

Milich, R., & Dodge, K. A. (1984). Social information processing in child psychiatric populations. *Journal of Abnormal Child Psychology*, 12, 471–490.

Mullins, L. L., Siegel, L. J., & Hodges, K. (1985). Cognitive problem-solving and life event correlates of depressive symptoms in children. *Journal of Abnormal Child Psychology*, 13, 305–314.

Nasby, W., Hayden, B., & dePaulo, B. M. (1979). Attributional bias among aggressive boys to interpret unambiguous social stimuli as displays of hostility. *Journal of Abnormal Psychology*, 89, 459–468.

Nelson, W. M., Politano, P. M., Finch, A. J., Wendel, N., & Mayhall, C. (1987). Children's Depression Inventory: Normative data and utility with emotionally disturbed children. *Journal of the American Academy of Child and Adolescent Psychiatry*, 26, 43–48.

Newell, H., & Simon, H. (1972). *Human problem solving.* Englewood Cliffs, NJ: Prentice-Hall.

Nolen-Hoeksema, S., Girgus, J. S., & Seligman, M. E. P. (1986). Learned helplessness in children: A longitudinal study of depression, achievement and explanatory style. *Journal of Personality and Social Psychology*, 51, 435–442.

Perry, D. G., Perry, L. C., & Rasmussen, P. (1986). Cognitive social learning mediators of aggression. *Child Development*, 57, 700–711.

Peterson, C., & Seligman, M. E. P. (1984). Causal explanations as a risk factor for depression: Theory and evidence. *Psychological Review*, 91, 347–374.

Puig-Antich, J. (1982). Major depression and conduct disorder in prepuberty. *Journal of the American Academy of Child Psychology*, 21, 118–128.

Robins, E., & Guze, S. (1972). Classification of affective disorders: The primary-secondary, the endogenous-reactive, and the neurotic-psychotic concepts. In T. A. Williams, M. A. Katz, & J. A. Shield (Eds.), *Recent advances in the psychobiology of the depressive illnesses* (pp. 283–293). Washington, DC: NIMH, Government Printing Office.

Rubin, K. H., & Krasnor, L. R. (1986). Social-cognitive and social-behavioral perspectives on problem solving. In M. Perlmutter (Ed.), *Eighteenth Annual Minnesota Symposium on Child Psychology* (Vol. 18, pp. 1–65). Hillsdale, NJ: Erlbaum.

Saylor, C. A., Finch, A. J., Spirito, A., & Bennett, B. (1984). The Child Depression Inventory: A systematic evaluation of psychometric properties. *Journal of Consulting and Clinical Psychology*, 52, 955–967.

Schachter, S., & Singer, J. (1962). Cognitive, social, and physiological determinants of emotional state. *Psychological Review*, 69, 379–399.

Schank, R., & Abelson, S. (1977). *Scripts, plans, goals, and understanding*. Hillsdale, NJ: Erlbaum.

Schwartz, M., Friedman, R. J., Lindsay, P., & Narrol, H. (1982). The relationship between conceptual tempo and depression in children. *Journal of Consulting and Clinical Psychology*, 58, 488–490.

Seligman, M. E. P. (1975). *Helplessness: On depression, development and death*. San Francisco: Freeman.

Seligman, M. E. P., & Peterson, C. (1986). A learned helplessness perspective on childhood depression: Theory and research. In M. Rutter, C. E. Izard, & P. B. Read (Eds.), *Depression in young people: Developmental and clinical perspectives* (pp. 223–249). New York: Guilford.

Seligman, M. E. P., Peterson, C., Kaslow, N. J., Tanenbaum, R. L., Alloy, L. B., & Abramson, L. Y. (1984). Attributional style and depressive symptoms among children. *Journal of Abnormal Psychology*, 93, 235–238.

Smucker, M. R., Craighead, W. E., Craighead, L. W., & Green, B. J. (1986). Normative and reliability data for the children's depression inventory. *Journal of Abnormal Child Psychology*, 14, 25–39.

Spivack, G., Platt, J., & Shure, M. B. (1976). *The problem-solving approach to adjustment*. San Francisco: Jossey-Bass.

Toolan, J. M. (1974). Masked depression in children and adolescents. In S. Lesse (Ed.), *Masked depression* (pp. 142–154). New York: Jason Aronson.

Weisz, J. R., Weiss, B., Wasserman, A. A., & Rintoul, B. (1987). Control-related beliefs and depression among clinic-referred children and adolescents. *Journal of Abnormal Psychology*, 96, 58–63.

Zajonc, R. B. (1980). Feeling and thinking: Preferences need no inferences. *American Psychologist*, 35, 151–175.

11

Methylphenidate and Attributions in Boys with Attention-Deficit Hyperactivity Disorder

William E. Pelham
Western Psychiatric Institute and Clinic
University of, Pittsburgh, Pennsylvania

Debra A. Murphy
Medical College of Wisconsin, Milwaukee

Kathryn Vannatta
University of Oregon, Eugene

Richard Milich
University of Kentucky, Lexington

Barbara G. Licht
Florida State University, Tallahassee

**Elizabeth M. Gnagy, Karen E. Greenslade,
Andrew R. Greiner, and Mary Vodde-Hamilton**
Western Psychiatric Institute and Clinic
University of Pittsburgh, Pennsylvania

In Experiment 1, 28 attention-deficit hyperactivity disorder (ADHD) boys underwent a double-blind, placebo-controlled medication assessment in a summer day-treatment program. Daily, boys were

Reprinted with permission from *Journal of Consulting and Clinical Psychology*, 1992, Vol. 60(2), 282–292. Copyright © 1992 by the American Psychological Association, Inc.

This research was conducted while William E. Pelham was supported in part by grant AA06267 from the National Institute on Alcohol Abuse and Alcoholism.

The study was conducted during the 1987 and 1988 Summer Treatment Programs (STP) conducted by the Attention Deficit Disorder (ADD) Program at the Western Psychiatric Institute and Clinic (WPIC). We would like to thank WPIC for its support and to express our appreciation to the ADD and STP program staffs, particularly Lynn Martin, for their helpful cooperation.

asked questions to assess their attributions for and evaluations of their behavior. Objective measures showed improved behavior with methylphenidate; however, boys tended to attribute their performance to effort rather than to medication, particularly when medicated. Experiment 2 involved 38 ADHD boys the following summer and replicated the procedures in Experiment 1, with the addition of a no-pill condition and a comparison of attributions for success and failure outcomes. Simply taking a pill (no-pill vs. placebo comparison) did not show significant effects, whereas the results of Experiment 1 were replicated with placebo-methylphenidate comparisons. Across drug conditions a self-enhancing attributional pattern was obtained; the majority of attributions for success were to ability or effort, whereas attributions for failure were to the pill or to counselors.

Psychostimulant medications (e.g., methylphenidate [MPH; Ritalin] are a routine component of treatment regimens for children with an attention-deficit hyperactivity disorder (ADHD). More than 6% of elementary-school children receive the medications (Safer & Krager, 1988). Beneficial, acute, stimulant effects have been documented in the areas of classroom behavior (e.g., Pelham, Bender, Caddell, Booth, & Moorer, 1985), peer relations (Cunningham, Siegel, & Offord, 1985), and mother-child interactions (Barkley, Karlsson, Strzelecki, & Murphy, 1984). Despite the evidence supporting the short-term efficacy of psychostimulants, there is concern that despite a positive acute effect on *behavior*, medication may have concurrent adverse effects on *cognitive-motivational* factors.

Few studies have examined the relationship between medication and cognitive-motivational factors. Some have argued that pharmacological treatment gives ADHD children a cognitive schema that discourages self-regulation and instead encourages the belief that performance outcomes are relatively independent of self-effort (e.g., Henker & Whalen, 1980; O'Leary, 1980). The mechanisms underlying this relationship are thought to be the children's causal attributions for their behavior and motivational states that may result from their beliefs about medication. Along with other cognitive-motivational constructs, children's causal attributions are reliable predictors of their responses in a variety of situations. For example, compared with mastery-oriented children, helpless children make fewer adaptive, internal attributions in success situations and in failure situations make more maladaptive ability attributions, exhibit more negative affect, and show declines in persistence and performance (e.g., Dweck & Leggett, 1988; Elliott & Dweck, 1988). Concerns regarding putative, detrimental medication effects have derived in part from such results. ADHD children are thought to exhibit a helpless cognitive style that medication may exacerbate.

In the first study of this area, Henker and Whalen (1980) interviewed medicated ADHD children regarding their attributions concerning causes of and solutions for their problems. The children were considerably more likely to list medication than personal factors such as effort and ability as the solution for their problems. In addition, children's medication solution attributions were positively correlated with their beliefs about the biological basis of their hyperactivity. Although this was an important seminal study, it has limitations, including procedural issues and sample characteristics, that limit its generalizability and validity. Brown and Borden (1989) used a similar format to assess solution attributions following cognitive therapy and MPH and reported no significant differences among treatment groups in children's solution attributions. Furthermore, in contrast to Whalen and Henker's results, the majority of the children made more effort than medication attributions.

These studies provide somewhat contradictory results regarding attributions and medication. One possible source of these differences is that none of the investigations assessed medication-related attributions for specific situations or tasks. For example, Henker and Whalen (1980) specifically structured their interview to use hypothetical situations to learn about children's broad, general beliefs regarding their medication. In addition to assessment of such *general* beliefs, attributional studies with other populations of children have also involved asking about causal attributions for *specific* outcomes that the children have recently experienced—most often success or failure in a learning or problem-solving task in a laboratory manipulation (e.g., Diener & Dweck, 1978; Licht & Dweck, 1984). This is an important distinction because a child may believe on a very general level that medication is helpful; yet, he may not attribute the specific successes and failures experienced throughout a typical day to his medication.

Several recent studies of ADHD and pharmacology have assessed medication-related attributions for specific tasks. For example, Milich, Licht, Murphy, and Pelham (1989) found that ADHD boys chose medication significantly less often than either effort or ability as an explanation for their successes. Milich, Carlson, Pelham, and Licht (1991) and Carlson, Pelham, Milich, and Hoza (1991) reported similar findings about children's attributions using solvable and insolvable word puzzles, particularly following successful outcomes, which were made more likely with medication. Thus, the results of the few empirical studies that have been conducted on the relationship between pharmacotherapy and ADHD children's attributions for specific outcomes are not consistent with anecdotal clinical folklore.

The present studies were designed to examine ADHD boys' causal attributions in a double-blind, within-subject, placebo-controlled medication trial. We extended the contexts in which these attributions have been studied and examined a number of within-subject variables that might be related to attributional results.

Several secondary questions were also addressed: (a) the relationship between ADHD boys' perceptions of their behavior and their actual behavior and (b) MPH effects on ADHD children's self-ratings of their happiness and self-esteem.

EXPERIMENT 1

Method

Subjects. Subjects were 28 ADHD boys[1] ranging in age from 7 years 2 months to 11 years 8 months ($M = 8$ years 10 months) and attending the 1987 Western Psychiatric Institute and Clinic (WPIC) Summer Treatment Program (STP), an 8-week, day-treatment program. All subjects met the criteria for a *Diagnostic and Statistical Manual of Mental Disorders*, 3rd ed., rev. (*DSM-III-R;* American Psychiatric Association, 1987) diagnosis of ADHD, based on a structured parent interview and a number of standardized parent and teacher rating scales. Of the 28 subjects, 11 also met *DSM-III-R* criteria for diagnosis of oppositional/defiant disorder, and another 10 subjects met criteria for a *DSM-III-R* diagnosis of conduct disorder (see Table 1 for subject characteristics). Twelve of the boys had received medication for ADHD before participating in the summer program.

Procedure

Setting. A day in the STP lasted from 8:00 a.m. until 5:00 p.m. on weekdays and was divided into the following activities: two academic classroom periods, each staffed by a special education teacher and an aide; an art class; swimming; three supervised, group, outdoor recreational activities (e.g., soccer); and lunch. For all activities except the academic classrooms, five counselors supervised 12 children grouped by sex and age. The 28 boys in this study were distributed across five groups. In all settings throughout the day a point and feedback system was constantly in effect in which boys earned points for appropriate behavior (Pelham, 1991).

Medication procedure. During the last 6 weeks of the program, the boys underwent a randomized, double-blind, placebo-controlled, within-subject, clinical medication assessment that has been described in detail elsewhere (e.g., Pelham & Hoza, 1987; Pelham et al., 1990). Children in the current study received a low dose of MPH (.15 mg/kg or .3 mg/kg, depending on the child's weight) and a high dose of MPH (.3 mg/kg or .6 mg/kg, depending on the child's weight). Five chil-

---

[1]Subjects for the Milich, Licht, Murphy, and Pelham (1989) study were participants in the summer program in which Experiment 1 of the current study was conducted. Twenty-two of the 26 subjects in that study were also subjects in Experiment 1 of the present study. Milich et al. assessed children's evaluations of and attributions for their performance on a single task (a continuous performance task) on one placebo day and one .3 mg/kg methylphenidate day, and these assessments occurred immediately following the task. In contrast, Experiment 1 assessed children's evaluations of and attributions for an entire day's performance on multiple days and doses for a wide range of behaviors.

TABLE 1

Means and Standard Deviations for Subject Characteristics in Experiment 1 and 2

| | Experiment 1[a] | | Experiment 2 | | | |
| | | | Entire sample[b] | | Forced-choice sample[c] | |
Item	M	SD	M	SD	M	SD
Age (in months)	106.4	15.1	119.4	21.3	120.9	1.5
Full-scale IQ[d]	102.7	12.47	106.2	13.1	103.2	12.0
Woodcock-Johnson Achievement[e]						
Reading	95.9	13.2	96.8	14.1	91.7	14.8
Arithmetic	97.1	18.1	99.6	15.6	94.9	13.2
Written language	96.7	18.5	99.0	13.3	93.8	13.8
DSM–III–R items endorsed in a parent structured interview[f]						
ADHD	11.3	1.8	11.1	2.1	11.7	1.5
ODD	6.1	2.5	4.9	2.3	4.9	2.1
CD	2.0	1.9	1.5	1.6	1.9	1.4
Abbreviated Conners Rating Scale[g]						
Parent	20.5	5.1	18.9	5.4	18.2	5.2
Teacher	16.9	6.7	15.0	5.9	14.9	5.5
IOWA Conners Teacher Rating Scale[h]						
Inattention/Overactivity	10.7	3.4	9.7	3.5	9.7	3.7
Aggression	6.9	5.2	4.6	4.1	5.1	4.6
Disruptive behavior disorders Teacher rating scale[i]						
Inattention	16.9	6.5	15.0	6.6	15.2	5.7
Impulsivity	15.6	7.3	13.3	6.8	14.1	6.7
Oppositional/defiant	11.5	9.3	8.5	7.1	9.0	6.9

Note. DSM–III–R = *Diagnostic and Statistical Manual of Mental Disorders*, 3rd ed., rev. ADHD = attention-deficit hyperactive disorder. ODD = oppositional/defiant disorder. CD = conduct disorder.
[a] n = 28. [b] n = 38. [c] n = 17. [d] Wechsler Intelligence Scale for Children—Revised. [e] Achievement cluster standard scores for the Woodcock-Johnson Psycho-educational Battery. [f] Mean number of symptoms endorsed in the interview. [g] Goyette, Conners, and Ulrich, 1978. [h] Pelham, Milich, Murphy, and Murphy, 1989. [i] Pelham, Gnagy, Greenslade, and Milich, in press.

dren received a protocol that included .15 mg/kg and .3 mg/kg, and 23 received a protocol that included .3 mg/kg and .6 mg/kg. Children were assigned to the .3/.6 protocol unless they were overweight and would have received a weight-adjusted dose that the program physician decided was too high, in which case they received the .15/.3 protocol. Each subject received an identical capsule of either a low dose, a high dose, or placebo before 8:00 a.m. and at midday, with the medication condition randomized daily. Children knew that they would be receiving different types of medication, but they were not told that some capsules would be inactive.

Frequency counts of positive (e.g., rule-following) and negative (e.g., noncompliant) behaviors were made throughout the day, and children's behavior and academic performance were tracked daily in the classroom settings. The number of time-outs that children received and whether their daily report cards were positive or negative were recorded daily. The three-to-five target symptoms on these daily reports were individualized, depending on a child's presenting symptoms, and positive reports were awarded by parents. All of these measures were used to evaluate response to medication. Their reliabilities are adequate (Pelham & Hoza, 1987).

Questionnaire administration procedure. At the end of each day, research assistants who did not work clinically with the children administered questionnaires. The children were read the following instructions: "I am just going to ask you some questions about your day. This is not a test. I just want to know how you felt about your day." They were promised confidentiality regarding their responses and were asked to be careful and honest. First, a set of questions presented in a 10-point Likert format were asked. As shown in Table 2, some of these questions inquired about attributions (effort, ability, pill, counselors), some dealt with the boys' perceptions of their performance in several domains (e.g., rule-following, time out), and one each asked about mood and self-esteem. The anchor points for the Likert questions were phrased similarly, with the high scores indicating a positive endorsement for all but the time-out question. For example, the two anchor points for the question "How hard did you try to do well today?" were "*I did not try at all* (1)" and "*I tried very hard* (10)."

Following the Likert-scale questions, the boys were asked whether they had had an overall good day or a bad day, and they were then presented with a series of forced-choice questions regarding their attributions. They were offered pairs of explanations for their good (or bad) day (defined according to their response to the previous question), and they were asked to choose the better explanation. The forced-choice questions (see last three questions, Table 2) reflected the attributional domains of effort (e.g., you tried hard), medication (e.g., the pill helped you), or their counselors (e.g., the way the counselors treated you). Each attribution was paired against the others in a random order, with all possible pairs

TABLE 2

Means and Standard Deviations, and Analysis of Variance Results for each Dependent Variable in Experiment 1

Variable	Placebo		Low dose		High dose		F^a
	M	SD	M	SD	M	SD	
Attribution							
How hard did you try to do well today?	9.22	1.11	9.73	0.50	9.66	0.56	4.24[b]
How good are you at earning points?	9.48	0.89	9.74	0.32	9.80	0.39	2.41[c]
How much did the pill help you today?	7.23	3.00	7.31	3.03	7.49	3.20	0.56
How much did the counselors' giving and taking points help you today?	8.60	2.25	9.00	1.54	9.13	1.57	4.34[b]
Behavior							
Did you have a good day or a bad day?	8.60	2.04	9.55	0.88	9.53	0.93	6.10[d]
How well did you follow the rules today?	8.89	1.58	9.65	0.48	9.69	0.53	5.84[d]
How did you do with time out today?	2.37	2.17	1.67	1.32	1.22	0.55	7.37[e]
How well did you mind the counselors today?	9.26	1.10	9.8	0.47	9.80	0.37	6.36[d]
Mood-self-esteem							
How well did you get along with other kids today?	9.19	1.16	9.57	0.63	9.64	0.83	4.69[b]
How happy or sad were you today?	8.43	2.09	9.42	1.03	9.55	0.75	7.70[e]
How much did you like yourself today?	8.79	1.80	9.51	0.97	9.59	0.89	5.40[f]
Forced choice							
Effort	1.52	0.40	1.68	0.41	1.69	0.34	4.64[f]
Pill	0.85	0.51	0.67	0.59	0.66	0.57	5.00[b]
Counselors	0.63	0.49	0.64	0.48	0.64	0.47	0.04

Note. Attribution, behavior, and mood-self-esteem questions are rated on 10-point scales, and the means represent averages first over days within children, then over children within drug condition. On the forced-choice questions, each question could be endorsed twice daily. The means presented are the number of endorsements per day, averaged as noted above.
[a] $N = 28$, $df = (2, 54)$.   [b] $p < .025$.   [c] $p < .10$.   [d] $p < .005$.   [e] $p < .0025$.   [f] $p < .01$.

presented (example: "You said you had a good day. Was that because you tried hard or because the pill you took today helped you?"). Therefore, each day a child could choose each of the three attributions (effort, pill, counselors) from zero to two times. Both the rating scale and the forced-choice format have been used successfully to investigate attributions in children by other investigators (e.g., Diener & Dweck, 1980; Licht, Kistner, Ozkaragoz, Shapiro, & Clausen, 1985). The questionnaire was administered approximately 16 times per child, distributed across medication conditions. The dependent measures were boys' scores, averaged over days, for each question for each medication condition.

Results

Manipulation check. In order to ensure that the children's behavior was actually affected by the medication, analyses were performed on several dependent measures from the clinical medication assessment. Thus, one-way analyses of variance (ANOVAs) with three levels of drug (placebo, low dose, high dose) were conducted on the daily frequencies of six observational and product categories that overlapped with the questions asked on the attribution questionnaires. The boys (a) received more points for following rules on medication than on placebo days, $F(2, 54) = 24.11$, $p < .0001$ ($M = 75.8\%$ for placebo compared with $M = 84\%$ for low dose and $M = 88.4$ for high dose); (b) were less noncompliant with counselor requests on medication compared with placebo days, $F(2, 54) = 11.02$, $p < .001$ ($M = 4.3$ for placebo compared with $M = 2.1$ for low dose and $M = 1.4$ for high dose); (c) received fewer time-outs on medication than on placebo days; $F(2, 54) = 8.35$, $p < .001$ ($M = 1.2$; $M = 0.5$; and $M = 0.3$, respectively); (d) were more likely to receive a positive daily report card on medication than on placebo days, $F(2, 54) = 14.05$, $p < .0001$ ($M = 52.9\%$; $M = 70.0\%$; and $M = 79.8\%$, respectively); (e) had higher frequencies of positive peer interactions with MPH, $F(2, 54) = 21.87$; $p < .0001$ ($M = 172.9$; $M = 196.4$; $M = 216.0$, respectively); and (f) had lower frequencies of negative verbal interactions with other children, $F(2, 54) = 15.23$, $p < .0001$ ($M = 5.2$; $M = 3.3$; $M = 2.0$, respectively). Furthermore, 22 of the 28 boys were determined by the program staff at termination to be positive responders to MPH.

Questionnaire responses. Questionnaire responses were analyzed in a series of one-way (drug: placebo, high dose, low dose) ANOVAs, and the results along with condition means and standard deviations are shown in Table 2. Preliminary analyses of the effect of protocol: (.15 vs. .3, or .3 vs. .6) revealed no significant effect of protocol nor any interactions between protocol and drug on any dependent measure (all $Fs < 1.5$). All analyses shown in Table 2 are therefore collapsed over protocol, combining .15 mg/kg (in a .15/.3 protocol) and .3 mg/kg (in a .3/.6

protocol) into a low dose condition and .3 mg/kg (in a .15/.3 protocol) and .6 mg/kg (in a .3/.6 protocol) into a high-dose condition.

As Table 2 reveals, both the Likert and forced-choice questions showed that the boys increased their effort attributions on MPH compared with placebo days. Their attributions to the pill actually decreased with medication on the forced-choice question, trading off with effort, and were unchanged on the Likert rating. Ability attributions (How good are you at earning points?) did not vary with medication condition. Attributions to counselors' assistance improved on the Likert rating and were unchanged on the forced-choice questions. The questions regarding behavior (e.g., rule-following, compliance), mood, and self-liking all revealed positive effects of medication.

Subgroup analyses. In order to assess whether response to medication influenced attributions, the ANOVAs were also repeated using response (positive or negative/non) as a grouping variable. Results on the Likert ratings revealed no main effects or interactions ($p > .05$) of response. On the forced-choice questions, there was an interaction ($p < .005$) between response and drug on the effort question, such that positive responders to medication were more likely than nonresponders to exhibit the medication-related effects shown in Table 2.

In order to determine whether previous experience with medication influenced attributions, the ANOVAs were repeated with previous medication as a grouping variable. On the forced-choice questions, there were no main effects or interactions ($p > .05$) of previous medication. However, on the Likert scale questions, there were significant ($p < .05$) interactions between previous medication and drug on all questions except the ones involving the pill and the counselors, with previously medicated boys making more negative (i.e., lower) ratings than medication-naive boys on placebo days.

Discussion

This study demonstrated that: (a) MPH improved the boys' behavior (manipulation check); (b) the boys *reported* improved behavior with MPH (self-ratings of behavior); and (c) most important, the boys were more likely to make *adaptive* attributions (i.e., effort) and *no* more likely to make possibly maladaptive attributions (i.e., the pill) when medicated compared with placebo days. Thus, concerns that MPH induces dysfunctional attributions in medicated ADHD boys were not supported by this study. In contrast, the medication-related increase in effort attributions suggests that medicated boys adopt attributional styles that would generally be considered positive. Indeed, on the forced-choice questions, for both MPH conditions, subjects chose effort as a causal explanation for their success or failure 56% of the time, compared with medication (22%) and counselor attributions (21%). Indeed, such a self-enhancing attributional pattern is characteristic of normal children and adults (Miller & Porter, 1988; Taylor & Brown, 1988). In addition to these major findings, the results also showed that the boys reported themselves to be happier and reported that they liked themselves better on days when they were medicated compared with days when they received placebo.

The study had several limitations. First, boys said they had bad days so infrequently that the data could not be analyzed separately for success (good days) and failure (bad days). Normal children typically make *internal* (effort or ability) attributions for success and *external* attributions for failure (Elliott & Dweck, 1988). It is possible that our attributional results—increased effort and decreased pill attributions when medicated—depended in part on whether the boy had a successful outcome—a good day (e.g., high percentage of following rules, positive daily report card)—or an unsuccessful outcome—a bad day (e.g., many time-outs, negative daily report card). Because the boys were more likely to have good days *when medicated* in our setting, the increase in internal attributions on medication days might be a function of medication-induced success rather than medication per se. To address this issue, children's days must be separated into successful and unsuccessful outcomes and medication effects and attributions examined as a function of outcome.

A second limitation of the study is that children received a pill every day. Therefore, it could be argued that children were less likely to choose medication than counselors or effort as a causal explanation for their performance, given that on some (i.e., MPH) days their pill may have improved their behavior, whereas on other (i.e., placebo) days it may not. As such, children may have had difficulty perceiving a systematic relationship between taking a pill and their behavior. To clarify this issue, it would be necessary to include a no-pill condition to separate pharmacological effects of MPH from placebo expectancy effects.

EXPERIMENT 2

Method

Subjects. Subjects were 38 ADHD boys ranging in age from 7 years 3 months to 13 years 9 months (M = 9 years 11 months) and attending the 1988 WPIC Summer Treatment Program. All subjects again met criteria for ADHD. Eighteen also met criteria for oppositional/defiant disorder, and another 8 met criteria for conduct disorder (see Table 1 for subject characteristics). Twenty-five of the 38 boys had received medication for ADHD before they participated in the summer program.

Procedure

Setting and medication. This investigation was conducted one year after

Experiment 1. The counselors were different, but the activities, treatment, dependent measures, and clinical medication assessment procedures were the same. However, in the current study, boys received either a .3 mg/kg dose of MPH, a placebo, or no pill, with condition randomized daily.[2]

Questionnaire administration procedure. These were modified slightly from Experiment 1. At the end of each day, research assistants asked the boys the Likert questions (except that on no-pill days, the wording was modified such that boys were asked how much the pill would have helped them had they received it). Following these questions, clinical staff gave the boys their daily report cards on which their treatment goals were individualized and tracked. Each boy had a criterion for a positive daily report card that was subsequently rewarded by his parents. After receipt of the daily report, the children were administered a set of forced-choice questions reflecting the attributional domains of effort, medication, counselors, and ability (e.g., you're good/not good at doing the things on your daily report card). In order to determine the stem to be used in asking each question, instead of asking the boy what kind of day he had (as in Experiment 1), his daily report card was used to define whether he had a good or a bad day. Across conditions, the average number of days each boy was administered the questionnaire totaled 13.3. The forced-choice questions were analyzed separately for days on which the boys received positive and negative report cards.

Results

Manipulation check. One-way ANOVAs with 2 levels of drug (placebo, MPH) were conducted on the medication assessment measures. The boys (a) received more points for following rules on medication ($M = 80.0\%$) than on placebo days ($M = 74.2\%$), $F(1, 37) = 27.18$, $p < .0001$; (b) were less noncompliant with counselor requests on medication ($M = 2.3$) compared with placebo days ($M = 5.3$), $F(1, 37) = 22.48$, $p < .001$; (c) received fewer time-outs on medication ($M = 0.4$) than on placebo days ($M = 0.8$), $F(1, 37) = 11.04$, $p = .005$; (d) were more likely to receive a positive daily report card on medication ($M = 66.6\%$) than on placebo days ($M = 52.6\%$), $F(1, 37) = 8.87$, $p < .01$; (e) had higher frequencies of positive peer interactions with MPH ($M = 94.2$) than on placebo ($M = 81.7$), $F(1, 37) = 12.12$, $p < .005$; and (f) had lower frequencies of negative verbal interactions with other children, $F(1, 37) = 6.71$, $p < .025$ (MPH: $M =$

---

[2]Twenty-two of the 38 subjects in this study were also participating in a protocol in which they received other types of stimulant medication (pemoline, Dexedrine Spansule, and Slow-Release Ritalin) on days not included in this experiment (Pelham et al., 1990). However, as we have documented previously, there is no carryover from one day to the next in stimulant effects in this setting, so the inclusion of subjects who received different stimulants on days not included in Experiment 2 did not influence our results.

1.6; placebo: $M = 4.2$). Finally, 22 boys were determined to be positive responders to medication and 16 were not.

Questionnaire Responses Analyses involved two sets of planned ANOVAs. The first ANOVA contrasted no-pill and placebo days and assessed the effect of taking a pill; the second contrasted placebo with active drug and evaluated the effect of MPH.

As Table 3 shows for the Likert questions, the first set of comparisons shows no difference between no-pill and placebo days. The second set reveals that the boys were significantly more likely to report on MPH than on placebo days that they tried hard, had a good day, followed the rules better, had fewer time-outs, and were more compliant with the counselors. In addition, there were trends ($p < .10$) for the boys to say more often on medication days than on placebo days that they were happy and that they liked themselves.

A second set of planned comparisons was conducted for the forced-choice items. A positive or negative daily report card was used to evaluate attributions for naturally occurring success and failure outcomes.[3] Results are summarized in Table 4.

The 2 (pill: placebo, no-pill) $\times$ 2 (day type: success, failure) ANOVAs revealed significant effects of day type for the effort, $F(1, 16) = 22.88$, $p < .001$; pill, $F(1, 16) = 23.12$, $p < .001$; and ability, $F(1, 16) = 7.22$, $p < .05$, attributions. The boys made significantly more effort and ability attributions on positive daily report days ($M = 2.53$ [$SD = 0.58$] for effort; $M = 1.83$ [0.63] for ability) than on negative days ($M = 1.71$ [0.83] for effort and $M = 1.20$ [0.93] for ability) and significantly more pill attributions on negative ($M = 1.64$ [0.87]) than on positive days ($M = 0.61$ [0.56]). Across day type, boys tended to make more pill attributions ($M = 1.27$ [0.87]) and fewer counselor attributions ($M = 1.14$ [0.98]) on placebo days than on no-pill days ($M = 0.98$ [0.90] for pill and $M = 1.34$ [0.98] for counselors).

Regarding MPH effects, 2 (drug: placebo, .3 mg/kg MPH) $\times$ 2 (day type) ANOVAs revealed significant effects of day type for the effort, $F(1, 16) = 12.89$, $p < .01$; pill, $F(1, 16) = 21.82$, $p < .001$; and ability, $F(1, 16) = 6.81$, $p < .05$ attributions. The boys made significantly more effort, $M = 2.46$ (0.59), and ability, $M = 1.79$ (0.64), attributions on positive daily report days than on negative daily report days, $M = 1.63$ (0.97) for effort; $M = 1.28$ (0.85) for ability, and significantly more pill attributions on negative, $M = 1.79$ (0.75), than on positive, $M = 0.82$ (0.64), days. No effects were revealed for drug or the interaction ($Fs < 1.0$).

As Table 4 illustrates, regardless of medication or pill conditions, boys were

---

[3]The sample size for these comparisons ($n = 17$) is smaller than the overall sample because 21 children did not receive both positive and negative reports in all drug conditions and therefore did not have data for all possible combinations of drug and success/failure conditions.

TABLE 3

Means, Standard Deviations, and Analysis of Variance Results for Each Rating Scale Item as a Function of Drug Condition in Experiment 2

Variable	No pill		Placebo		Methylphenidate		N vs. P[a]	P vs. M[b]
	M	SD	M	SD	M	SD	F[c]	F[c]
Attribution								
How hard did you try to do well today?	9.21	1.10	9.11	1.53	9.41	0.90	0.21	2.91[d]
How good are you at earning points?	9.14	1.09	9.11	1.03	9.20	1.29	0.06	0.27
How much did the pill help you/how much would it have helped you today?	6.01	3.05	6.22	2.95	6.55	2.89	0.27	1.30
How much did the counselors' giving and taking points help you today?	8.04	2.06	8.19	1.97	8.33	1.79	0.30	0.34
Behavior								
Did you have a good day or a bad day?	8.51	1.61	8.72	1.73	9.12	1.18	0.74	4.56[e]
How well did you follow the rules today?	8.56	1.43	8.71	1.67	9.13	1.06	0.37	4.40[e]
How did you do with time out today?	1.56	0.71	1.76	0.90	1.42	0.82	1.41	4.18[e]
How well did you mind the counselors today?	9.17	1.08	8.95	1.44	9.29	0.92	1.60	4.49[e]
How well did you get along with other kids today?	9.25	0.97	9.31	1.05	9.50	0.90	0.10	2.01
Mood–self-esteem								
How happy or sad were you?	8.60	1.58	8.65	1.80	8.98	1.14	0.05	3.18[d]
How much did you like yourself?	8.82	1.52	8.67	1.87	9.12	1.31	0.35	3.21[d]

Note. Items are rated on 10-point scales and averaged over children and over days within a drug condition. [a] N vs. P = no pill versus placebo. [b] P vs. M = placebo versus methylphenidate. [c] $N = 38$, $df = (1, 37)$. [d] $p < .10$. [e] $p < .05$.

TABLE 4

Means and Standard Deviations for First-Choice Questions as a Function of Success (Positive Daily Report Card) and Failure (Negative Daily Report Card) in Experiment 2

| | No drug | | | | Placebo | | | | Methylphenidate | | | |
| | Success | | Failure | | Success | | Failure | | Success | | Failure | |
Variable	M	SD	M	SD	M	SD	M	SD	M	SD	M	SD
Effort	2.60	0.55	1.85	0.81	2.47	0.64	1.56	0.86	2.44	0.55	1.69	1.10
Pill	0.52	0.66	1.44	0.88	0.71	0.45	1.83	0.83	0.95	0.78	1.75	0.69
Counselors	1.13	0.86	1.56	1.07	0.92	0.91	1.36	1.02	0.91	0.88	1.24	1.13
Ability	1.76	0.65	1.15	1.03	1.90	0.62	1.25	0.84	1.68	0.65	1.32	0.87

Note. $N = 17$. Each attribution could be chosen from 0 to 3 times on any day, and the means presented are the number of endorsements averaged over children and days within drug and success/failure conditions.

three times more likely to make effort attributions and two times more likely to make ability attributions than pill attributions on positive daily report days. Relative to positive days, however, on negative daily report days they reduced their effort and ability attributions by 34% and 28%, respectively, and increased their pill attributions by more than 100%. On negative report days, they made more pill attributions than either effort or ability attributions.

Subgroup analyses

Response to medication. Separate Drug (no pill vs. placebo and placebo vs. .3 mg/kg MPH) × Response (positive or negative/non) ANOVAs (with day type—success or failure—added for the forced-choice analyses) were conducted for the Likert scale and forced-choice questions. No main effects of or interactions with response ($p < .05$) were found in the no pill versus placebo comparisons for either Likert or forced-choice questions. In the placebo versus MPH comparisons, a significant interaction, $F(1, 36) = 6.03, p < .025$, was obtained between response and drug for the Likert question, "How much did the pill help you today?" Nonresponders said that the pill helped them less than did the responders, but the difference between the groups was greater in the MPH condition ($Ms = 7.5$ and 5.2, for responders and nonresponders, respectively) than in the placebo condition ($Ms = 6.6$ and 5.7). In addition, a significant interaction was revealed between response and day type for the forced-choice ability item, $F(1, 15) = 4.99, p < .05$. On failure days, nonresponders were much less likely to make ability attributions ($M = 0.7$) than were responders ($M = 1.6$), whereas the two groups did not differ on success days (both $Ms = 1.8$).

Previous medication. Comparable analyses revealed that the only significant main effect of previous medication was on the pill forced-choice item in the no pill versus placebo comparison, $F(1, 15) = 6.47, p < .05$. Boys without a history of medication were less likely to make attributions to the pill ($M = 0.85$) than were previously medicated boys ($M = 1.27$). On the forced-choice counselor item in the no pill versus placebo comparison, there was a significant interaction between previous medication and day type, $F(1, 15) = 5.02, p < .05$. On failure days, boys without a previous history of medication made more counselor attributions ($M = 1.91$) than did boys with a previous history ($M = 1.22$), while the difference between the groups was considerably less on success days ($Ms = 1.16$, .95). These two patterns suggest that there was a trade-off between the two external attributions, pill and counselor, such that boys with a previous history of medication used the pill as their external attribution of choice, while those without a history blamed counselors for their failures. There were no ($p < .05$) main effects of or interactions with previous medication on the no pill versus placebo Likert questions or on any variable in the placebo versus MPH comparisons.

Pill attributions. Finally, to determine whether there was a subset of boys within the group who were showing dysfunctional attributions, several additional analyses were conducted. Each child's choices on the forced-choice questions were tallied for days when the children received a pill (including both placebo and active drug days). The relative proportions with which they made pill, effort, ability, and counselor attributions were computed separately for success (positive daily report) and failure (negative daily report) days, and resulting distributions were examined. Given our original hypotheses, of special interest was the distribution of pill attributions, which showed considerable variability. A median split was performed for pill attributions made on success and failure days, and analyses were conducted using the proportion of pill attributions as a grouping variable. Boys above the median of 33% for attributions to the pill on positive daily report days were defined as the high pill attribution for success (HPA/success) group; they made pill attributions an average of 53% ($SD = 11$) of the possible times that such an attribution could be made. Boys below the median were defined as the low pill attribution for success (LPA/success) group; they made pill attributions an average of 13% ($SD = 12$) of the possible occasions. A second median split was performed for pill attributions on negative daily report card days, and analyses were repeated using these attributions as a grouping variable. Boys above and below the median of 60% for attributions to the pill on negative report days were defined, respectively, as the high pill attribution for failure (HPA/failure) group (blamed the pill an average of 77% [$SD = 11$] of the possible times) and the low pill attribution for failure (LPA/failure) group, 35% ($SD = 15$) of attributions were to the pill.

Three sets of analyses were performed to investigate differences between the HPA and LPA groups. First, attributions to the other forced-choice domains were assessed as a function of boys' attributions to the pill. Second, behavioral measures from the day treatment program were studied to examine the relationship between pill attributions and behavior patterns. Finally, groups were compared on diagnostic and descriptive measures to examine possible sources of covariation that might explain obtained differences between the HPA and LPA groups.

In the analysis of the forced-choice responses, only attributions on negative daily report days were examined using the success grouping, and only attributions on positive daily report days were examined for the failure subgrouping, thus preventing confounding of the grouping and dependent variables. The proportion of attributions made to ability, effort, and counselors were compared for (a) pill attributions for success (HPA/success vs. LPA/success) and (b) pill attributions for failure (HPA/failure vs. LPA/failure). HPA/success boys tended to be more likely to attribute their failures to ability ($M = 43\%$, $SD = 26$) than did the LPA/success boys, $M = 28\%$ (23), $t(36) = -1.79$, $p < .10$. Conversely, HPA/failure boys were more likely to attribute their successes to effort, $M = 93\%$ (10), than were the LPA/failure boys, $M = 79\%$ (18), $t(34) = -2.85$, $p < .01$. No effects were found for counselor attributions.

In order to assess behavioral differences between the HPA/success and LPA/ success groups, a set of one-way (pill attribution for success: low, high) ANOVAs was performed on the dependent measures from the clinical medication assessment, collapsed over placebo and no-pill days.[4] As Table 5 indicates, unmedicated boys who attributed success to the pill (HPA/success boys) behaved significantly *worse* than unmedicated boys who did not attribute success to the pill (LPA/ success boys) on many dependent measures across both academic and social settings.

To examine behavior as a function of failure attributions, corresponding ANOVAs compared HPA/failure and LPA/failure groups (see also Table 5). Unmedicated boys who attributed failure to the pill (HPA/failure boys) behaved significantly *better* than unmedicated boys who did not attribute failure to the pill (LPA/failure boys) on many dependent measures across settings.

In order to explore other areas in which HPA and LPA groups might covary, a 2 (success attribution to pill: HPA/success, LPA/success) × 2 (failure attribution to pill: HPA/failure, LPA/failure) multivariate analyses of variance (MANOVA) was performed on numerous baseline variables, including age, IQ, academic achievement, parent and teacher rating scales, and family history of affective/ anxiety disorders. Differences were found on only one of the 17 variables (arithmetic achievement). In addition, chi-square analyses of the association between the HPA and LPA dichotomies and previous medication history and response to medication revealed no significant relationships. Thus, the HPA and LPA group differences cannot be explained on the basis of baseline differences on demographic, diagnostic, medication history, medication response, or familial variables. Finally, in order to determine whether the boys who attributed success to the pill were the same boys who blamed the pill for failure, a 2 (HPA/success, LPA/success) × 2 (HPA/failure, LPA/failure) chi-square was conducted. There was no relationship between pill attributions for success and failure, with all four cells having similar numbers of subjects.

Discussion

Experiment 2 was designed both to replicate and to clarify the results of Experiment 1 and yielded three main findings. First, the manipulation check again revealed improved functioning with medication, and the boys' ratings reflected this improvement. Second, there were minimal or no differences in attributions between no-pill and placebo conditions, demonstrating that the results of

---

[4]Days on which the subjects received medication were not included in the analyses because our interest was in how attributions might mediate children's *unmedicated* behavior. When the HPA/ success and LPA/success groups were compared on behavioral indices on medication days, the group differences found on unmedicated days were eliminated.

TABLE 5

Analysis of Variance Results for Behavioral Measures as a Function of Proportion of Attributions Made to the Pill in Experiment 2

Dependent measure	Pill attributions for success					Pill attributions for failure				
	Low		High			Low		High		
	M	SD	M	SD	F^a	M	SD	M	SD	F^b
Following rules[c]	76.8	7.6	70.8	10.5	4.02^d	70.0	11.2	77.4	5.5	6.18^e
Noncompliance[f]	3.5	3.0	7.0	6.3	4.73^g	7.4	6.5	3.1	2.3	6.82^e
Positive peer interactions[f]	90.4	39.1	78.6	36.5	0.93	77.6	41.6	94.1	34.0	1.71
Conduct problems[f]	0.3	0.2	0.7	1.1	2.85^d	0.8	1.1	0.2	0.2	4.33^g
Negative verbalizations[f]	3.0	5.4	4.4	6.6	0.57	5.6	8.2	2.1	1.9	3.20^d
Following rules in classroom[c]	94.9	10.4	79.5	25.4	5.99^e	78.7	26.9	94.4	7.6	5.71^e
Seatwork completed[c]	79.9	14.4	70.9	22.6	2.17	69.4	22.1	79.6	15.1	2.59
Seatwork correct[c]	89.7	6.2	83.6	7.8	7.28^e	84.1	7.8	88.9	7.1	3.56^d
Positive daily report received[c]	63.1	24.1	48.5	21.6	3.85^d	55.0	21.1	53.1	25.2	0.06
Time-outs assigned[f]	0.5	0.4	1.2	1.3	4.64^g	1.3	1.3	0.4	0.3	6.90^e

Note. n for success attributions = 38. n for failure attributions = 36.
[a] F value for between-groups main effect, df = (1, 36).   [b] df = (1, 34).   [c] Percentages.   [d] p < .10.   [e] p < .025.   [f] Daily frequency counts.   [g] p < .05.

Experiment 1 were not confounded by the fact that the boys always ingested a pill. Pill-taking did not affect the boys' attributions. Third, success and failure played a large role in the boys' attributions. They made significantly more effort and ability attributions on daily report (success) days and significantly more pill attributions on negative daily report (failure) days, and this pattern did not interact with drug condition. These results thus clarified one of the findings from Experiment 1—the increased number of effort attributions made on medication days. Given that MPH in Experiment 1 resulted from a confounding of success and medication. When success and failure outcomes were examined separately, effort attributions were equally likely across medication conditions.

The most important findings of the two studies are these relationships among attributions, medication, and success and failure. We found no evidence for the samples as a whole that psychostimulant medication produced debilitating attributions in ADHD children. In fact, by increasing the likelihood that the boys had successful days, medication actually had a *positive* emanative effect by increasing their rates of internal (effort) attributions. As a group the boys in both studies showed across pill and medication conditions a "healthy" attributional pattern that has been labeled as self-enhancing, self-serving, or positive illusory (Alloy & Abramson, 1988; Taylor & Brown, 1988; Weary, Stanley, & Harvey, 1989). That is, they blamed their failures on an external factor, their pill, and they took credit for their successes by making internal (effort or ability) attributions.

We have also found this attributional pattern in two laboratory studies in which success and failure and MPH have been experimentally manipulated (Carlson et al., 1991; Milich et al., 1991). Thus, in four independent studies we have failed to find adverse psychostimulant effects on ADHD boys' attributions. The only other empirical investigation of this issue merely noted that medication may enter ADHD children's attributional matrices, but it was unable to draw any conclusions about whether the effects were beneficial or unsalutary (Whalen, Henker, Hinshaw, Heller, & Huber-Dressler, 1991). The bulk of the empirical evidence suggests that ADHD boys have a positive illusory attributional style that is not disrupted by their medication. To the contrary, to the extent that their attributional style is mediated by medication-induced success, medication may actually enhance their positive illusions. Such positive illusions may play an important role in preventing and ameliorating untoward reactions, such as depression, to stressful life events (Taylor & Brown, 1988; Weary et al., 1989). Thus, it may be adaptive for ADHD children to have this attributional style because their pervasive functional impairment might otherwise have severe repercussions on their affect and self-esteem.

At the same time, we found considerable variability in children's attributions to the pill, and these individual differences were meaningfully related to the boys' behavior when unmedicated. Boys above the median in pill attributions for success were significantly more likely than the LPA/success boys to make ability attributions on failure days. Thus, boys who gave external credit for positive events gave internal blame for negative events. This attributional style has been labeled *depressive realism*, as it is viewed as a relatively realistic appraisal of reality by relatively incompetent (depressed) individuals (Alloy & Abramson, 1988). In contrast, the LPA/success boys showed the positive illusory style that characterizes healthy individuals—relatively fewer success attributions to the pill and fewer ability attributions to failure. Furthermore, without MPH the HPA/success boys behaved significantly worse across situations than the LPA/success boys. This pattern would be expected if depressogenic attributions are associated with decreased effort in the face of difficult situations (that is, behavior *without* medication).

The subgrouping based on pill attributions for failure (from a different set of days) revealed similar results—HPA/failure boys (above the median in pill attributions for failure) tended to be more likely to attribute their successes to effort than did LPA/failure boys, thus exhibiting a self-enhancing attributional style. Compared with the LPA/failure boys, they showed better unmedicated behavior and performance—the pattern that would be expected if positive illusions give rise to enhanced self-efficacy in the face of difficulty (Alloy & Abramson, 1988; Taylor & Brown, 1988).

These findings suggest that our interpretation of the group results should be qualified. Perhaps a subgroup of ADHD boys have a depressogenic attributional style. If they are taking medication, the external attribution they make for success may be to their pill, and to that extent perhaps this style may be facilitated by psychostimulant medication. Given possible overlap between ADHD and affective disorders (Biederman, Newcorn, & Sprich, 1991), and given reports that such depressogenic styles predict subsequent depressive symptomatology in children (Seligman et al., 1984), further study is needed. Indeed, studies of individual differences have recently been noted as an important direction for attributional research (Weary et al., 1989). Replication is particularly needed given the post hoc nature of our subgroup analyses.

Previous medication history and response to medication revealed minimal effects that were not replicated across studies and that can be easily summarized. Medication responders or previously medicated children were more likely to show the self-rating and attributional effects that characterized the sample as a whole. Previously medicated or responder children were apparently more aware of the effects of the medication on their behavior (responders by definition had larger effects), and they made self-ratings and attributions consistent with that awareness and effects.

The manipulation checks revealed large, beneficial stimulant effects on all dependent measures. The boys' self-ratings paralleled these beneficial effects in each of the domains queried—noncompliance, time out, rule-following, getting along with other children (in Experiment 1), and overall evaluation of their day (i.e., their daily report card). Both experiments also showed that ADHD children reported themselves to be happier and to like themselves more on days when they received MPH compared with placebo days. Self-liking and happiness were assessed only with single questions rather than standard instruments, and the results need to be considered in that light. This apparent salutary impact of medication on children's happiness and self-esteem runs counter to concern regarding putative dysphoric stimulant effects (Whalen, Henker, Collins, McAuliffe, & Vaux, 1979). Our results may reflect in part the constant monitoring and frequent feedback given in our setting. The boys' increased sense of well-being may have resulted from the medication-improved behavior and the resulting increase in positive staff feedback. In the same way it induces internal attributions by increasing the boys' successes, MPH may enhance their happiness and self-liking by initiating a chain of behaviors in which the child behaves appropriately and significant others respond positively to that behavior.

Several limitations and qualifications of our studies warrant mention. First, our results were obtained in a day-treatment setting with a highly structured behavioral point system, and the effects of medication on attributions and perceptions must be interpreted in that light. Some studies have shown that stimulant and behavioral interventions interact (Pelham, 1989), and the boys' attributions may have been influenced by the behavioral context. Because our results contradict prevailing beliefs about putative, medication-induced, dysfunctional cognitions, it would be important to demonstrate generalization to contexts without concurrent behavioral interventions.

A second limitation concerns the fact that we assessed only children of elementary-school age. Because response to MPH is inversely correlated with age (Taylor et al., 1987), older ADHD children may have fewer opportunities to make effort attributions for medication-induced successes. Furthermore, as children grow older, they begin to view ability as limiting the usefulness of effort in performance, therefore becoming increasingly vulnerable to the debilitating effects of failure (Licht & Kistner, 1986). Thus, attributions to medication may become more dysfunctional with increasing age.

Finally, although larger and more comprehensive than previous investigations, our studies assessed attributions in an acute medication trial. Because ADHD children typically receive stimulants for years rather than days, it would be critical to study attributions after extended pharmacotherapy. Perhaps consistent and long-term association between medication and success/failure outcomes may induce or magnify the dysfunctional style shown by some of our HPA/LPA subgroups. Furthermore, whether the positive illusions shown by many of our children will have functional *long-term* value needs to be evaluated.

REFERENCES

Alloy, L. B., & Abramson, L. Y. (1988). Depressive realism: Four theoretical perspectives. In L. A. Alloy (Ed.), *Cognitive processes in depression* (pp. 223–265). New York: Guilford Press.

American Psychiatric Association. (1987.) *Diagnostic and statistical manual of mental disorders* (3rd ed., rev.). Washington, DC: Author.

Barkley, R. A., Karlsson, J. Strzelecki, E., & Murphy, J. V. (1984). Effects of age and Ritalin dosage on the mother-child interactions of hyperactive children. *Journal of Consulting and Clinical Psychology, 52,* 739–749.

Biederman, J., Newcorn, J., & Sprich, S. (1991). Comorbidity of attention deficit hyperactivity disorder with conduct, depressive, anxiety, and other disorders. *American Journal of Psychiatry, 148,* 564–577.

Brown, R., & Borden, K. (1989). Attributional outcomes: The subtle messages of treatments for attention deficit disorder. *Cognitive Therapy and Research, 13,* 147–160.

Carlson, C., Pelham, W. E., Milich, R., & Hoza, B. (1991). *ADHD boys' performance and attributions following success and failure: Drug effects and individual differences.* Manuscript submitted for publication.

Cunningham, C. E., Siegel, L. S., & Offord, D. R. (1985). A developmental dose-response analysis of the effects of methylphenidate on the peer interactions of attention deficit disordered boys. *Journal of Child Psychology and Psychiatry, 26,* 955–972.

Diener, C. I., & Dweck, C. S. (1978). An analysis of learned helplessness: Continuous changes in performance, strategy, and achievement cognitions following failure. *Journal of Personality and Social Psychology, 36,* 451–462.

Diener, C. I., & Dweck, C. S. (1980). An analysis of learned helplessness: 2. The processing of success. *Journal of Personality and Social Psychology, 39,* 940–952.

Dweck, C. S., & Leggett, E. L. (1988). A social-cognitive approach to motivation and personality. *Psychological Review, 95,* 256–273.

Elliott, E. S., & Dweck, C. S. (1988). Goals: An approach to motivation and achievement. *Journal of Personality and Social Psychology, 54,* 5–12.

Goyette, C. H., Conners, C. K., & Ulrich, R. F. (1978). Normative data on revised Conners parent and teacher rating scales. *Journal of Abnormal Child Psychology, 6,* 221–236.

Henker, B., & Whalen, C. K. (1980). The many messages of medication: Hyperactive children's perceptions and attributions. In S. Salzinger, J. Antrobus, & J. Glick (Eds.), *The ecosystem of the "sick" kid* (pp. 141–166). San Diego, CA: Academic Press.

Licht, B. G., & Dweck, C. S. (1984). Determinants of academic achievement: The interaction of children's achievement orientations and skill area. *Developmental Psychology, 20,* 628–636.

Licht, B. G., & Kistner, J. A. (1986). Motivational problems of learning-disabled children: Individual differences and their implications for treatment. In J. K. Torgesen & B. Y. L. Wong (Eds.), *Psychological and educational perspectives on learning disabilities* (pp. 225–255). San Diego, CA: Academic Press.

butions of learning disabled children: Individual differences and their implications for persistence. *Journal of Educational Psychology*, 77, 208–216.

Milich, R., Carlson, C. L., Pelham, W. E., & Licht, B. (1991). Effects of methylphenidate on the persistence of ADHD boys following failure experiences. *Journal of Abnormal Child Psychology*, 19, 519–536.

Milich, R., Licht, B. G., Murphy, D. A., & Pelham, W. E. (1989). ADHD boys' evaluations of and attributions for task performance on medication versus placebo. *Journal of Abnormal Psychology*, 98, 280–284.

Miller, D. T., & Porter, C. A. (1988). Errors and biases in the attribution process. In L. Y. Abramson (Ed.), *Social cognition and clinical psychology: A synthesis* (pp. 3–30). New York: Guilford Press.

O'Leary, K. D. (1980). Pills or skills for hyperactive children. *Journal of Applied Behavior Analysis*, 13, 191–204.

Pelham, W. E. (1989). Behavior therapy, behavioral assessment, and psychostimulant medication in treatment of attention deficit disorders: An interactive approach. In J. Swanson & L. Bloomingdale (Eds.), *Attention deficit disorders: 4. Current concepts and emerging trends in attentional and behavioral disorders of childhood* (pp. 169–195). London: Pergamon Press.

Pelham, W. E. (1991). *Children's summer day treatment program 1991 program manual.* Unpublished manuscript, University of Pittsburgh School of Medicine, Western Psychiatric Institute and Clinic, Pittsburgh.

Pelham, W. E., Bender, M. E., Caddell, J., Booth, S. & Moorer, S. (1985). The dose-response effects of methylphenidate on classroom academic and social behavior in children with attention deficit disorder. *Archives of General Psychiatry*, 42, 948–952.

Pelham, W. E., Gnagy, E. M., Greenslade, K. E., & Milich, R. (in press). Teacher-rated *DSM-III-R* symptoms of the disruptive behavior disorders: Prevalence, age effects, factor analyses, and conditional probabilities in a normative sample. *Journal of the American Academy of Child Psychiatry.*

Pelham, W. E., Greenslade, K. E., Vodde-Hamilton, M. A., Murphy, D. A., Greenstein, J. J., Gnagy, E. M., & Dahl, R. E. (1990). Relative efficacy of long-acting CNS stimulants on children with attention deficit-hyperactivity disorder: A comparison of standard methylphenidate, sustained-release methylphenidate, sustained-release dextroamphetamine, and pemoline. *Pediatrics*, 86, 226–237.

Pelham, W. E., & Hoza, J. (1987). Behavioral assessment of psychostimulant effects on ADHD children in a summer day treatment program. In R. Prinz (Ed.), *Advances in behavioral assessment of children and families* (Vol. 3, pp. 3–33). Greenwich, CT: JAI Press.

Pelham, W. E., Milich, R., Murphy, D. A., & Murphy, H. A. (1989). Normative data on the IOWA Conners teacher rating scale. *Journal of Clinical Child Psychology*, 18, 259–262.

Safer, D. J., & Krager, J. M. (1988). A survey of medication treatment for hyperactive/inattentive students. *Journal of the American Medical Association*, 260, 2256–2258.

Seligman, M. E. P., Kaslow, N. J., Alloy, L. B., Peterson, C. P., Tanenbaum, R. L., &

Abramson, L. Y. (1984). Attributional style and depressive symptoms among children. *Journal of Abnormal Psychology, 93*, 235–238.

Taylor, S. E., & Brown, J. D. (1988). Illusion and well-being: A social psychological perspective on mental health. *Psychological Bulletin, 103*, 193–210.

Taylor, E., Schachar, R., Thorley, G., Wieselberg, H. M., Everitt, B., & Rutter, M. (1987). Which boys respond to stimulant medication? A controlled trial of methylphenidate in boys with disruptive behavior. *Psychological Medicine, 17*, 121–143.

Weary, G., Stanley, M. A., & Harvey, J. H. (1989). *Attribution*. New York: Springer-Verlag.

Whalen, C., Henker, B., Collins, B., McAuliffe, S., & Vaux, A. (1979). Peer interaction in a structured communication task: Comparisons of normal and hyperactive boys and of methylphenidate (Ritalin) and placebo effects. *Child Development, 50*, 388–401.

Whalen, C., Henker, B., Hinshaw, S., Heller, T., & Huber-Dressler, A. (1991). Messages of medication: Effects of actual versus informed medication status on hyperactive boys' expectancies and self-evaluations. *Journal of Consulting and Clinical Psychology, 59*, 602–606.

12

Covert Antisocial Behavior in Boys with Attention-Deficit Hyperactivity Disorder: External Validation and Effects of Methylphenidate

Stephen P. Hinshaw
University of California, Berkeley

Tracy Heller
University of California, Los Angeles

James P. McHale
University of California, Berkeley

Covert antisocial behaviors such as stealing, destroying property, and cheating carry high risk for delinquency. An individual laboratory setting was devised in which youngsters could take desired objects and use answer keys to assist with worksheets. Twenty-two boys with attention-deficit hyperactivity disorder (ADHD) and 22 comparison boys were observed on two occasions, with the ADHDs receiving a methylphenidate-placebo crossover. Laboratory stealing and property destruction were positively correlated with maternal and staff ratings of parallel behaviors. Methylphenidate resulted in significant reductions of these acts, but it also effected an increase in cheating, presumably because of its enhancement of task involvement. The generalizability of the laboratory findings, actions of stimulants in

Reprinted with permission from *Journal of Consulting and Clinical Psychology*, 1992, Vol. 60(2), 274–281. Copyright © 1992 by the American Psychological Association, Inc.

This research received primary support from National Institute of Mental Health Grant 45064, awarded to Stephen P. Hinshaw. The Fernald Child Study Center of University of California, Los Angeles, housed the research project and provided partial support.

We gratefully acknowledge the diligent work of research assistants Payam Ajang, Lisa Capps, Colleen Cantwell, Sara DeVault, Karen Garland, and Katherine Leddick and the videotape coding of Katrina Foley, Pamela Hurley, and Melissa Simpson.

this domain, and the ethics of experimental investigations of covert antisocial behavior are discussed.

Antisocial behavior is stable (Huesmann, Eron, Lefkowitz, & Walder, 1984; Olweus, 1979) and highly predictive of academic and social problems and of long-term maladjustment (e.g., Robins, 1966; Stattin & Magnusson, 1989; West & Farrington, 1977). Within this domain, the distinction between overt aggression and covert antisocial behavior (e.g., stealing, lying, truancy) has a long psycho-metric history (see Quay, 1986). This division was again documented by Loeber and Schmaling (1985a), who subjected the most prevalent antisocial behaviors of childhood to multidimensional scaling. A bipolar dimension emerged, with one end consisting of such confrontive acts as arguing, attacking/hitting others, fight-ing, threatening, and throwing tantrums (overt antisocial behaviors) and the other pole comprising such clandestine activities as destructiveness, fire-setting, lying/cheating, stealing, and truancy (covert behaviors).

These two categories display trajectories, predictive validities, and family interactions that are partially distinct. First, aggression declines between child-hood and adolescence, but covert activities increase over this span (Loeber, 1982). Second, covert versus overt behaviors in childhood show differential predictive power: Adolescents who self-report theft are prone to later burglary convictions, whereas those with self-reported aggression are likely to commit subsequent aggressive offenses (Wadsworth, 1979; see also Moore, Chamberlain, & Mukai, 1979).[1] Third, families of overtly aggressive children often exhibit coercive interchanges, whereas parents of covertly antisocial youngsters tend to display poor child monitoring (Patterson & Stouthamer-Loeber, 1984). In short, the domain of covert antisocial actions warrants inves-tigation as a separable construct.

Children with attentional deficits are at high risk for the development of anti-social behavior. (The terms *hyperactivity, attentional deficits*, and *ADHD* [attention-deficit hyperactivity disorder] are used interchangeably herein.) Indeed, prospective studies have documented that elevated rates of delinquency and substance abuse plague hyperactive children in adolescence and young adult-hood (Barkley, Fisher, Edelbrock, & Smallish, 1990; Gittelman, Mannuzza, Shenker, & Bonagura, 1985; Satterfield, Hoppe, & Schell, 1982). Although the overtly aggressive characteristics of ADHD children have been increasingly investigated through direct observations (e.g., Hinshaw, Henker, Whalen, Erhardt,

---

[1]It is conceivable that early stealing predicts delinquency primarily because the latter is often defined in terms of property crime (Loeber & Stouthamer-Loeber, 1987). Yet Mitchell and Rosa (1981) found that early stealing predicted a wide range of adult criminality; furthermore, lying and truancy are not simply youthful versions of later criminal activities. Also, we note that cheating is often paired with lying in the assessment of dishonest behavior (e.g., Achenbach & Edelbrock, 1983).

& Dunnington, 1989; Murphy, Pelham, & Lang, in press), extremely few data are available regarding the display of covert antisocial acts in this group. One explanation for this dearth of evidence involves the concealed nature and low base rates of these behaviors. Indeed, covert acts (stealing, lying, property destruction) displayed by ADHD boys attending a summer treatment program occurred less than once per day, with the mean rates of stealing near zero (Hoza, 1989). Such low base rates warrant development of alternative methods for documentation of covert behaviors in ADHD youngsters.

Evidence is converging that the most widely used treatment for ADHD, stimulant medication, reduces overtly aggressive acts in naturalistic settings (e.g., Gadow, Nolan, Sverd, Sprafkin, & Paolicelli, 1990; Hinshaw et al., 1989; Murphy et al., in press; see review of Hinshaw, 1991) and yields benefit for both aggressive and nonaggressive subgroups (Barkley, McMurray, Edelbrock, & Robbins, 1989; Klorman et al., 1988). The effects of stimulants on covert antisocial acts are, however, indeterminate. Murphy et al. (in press) and Pelham et al. (1990) found that methylphenidate decreased a *conduct problems* category that combined physical aggression with covert acts of stealing, property destruction, and lying. Yet separate analyses of these behaviors yielded extremely low base rates; in the covert realm, medication reduced only property destruction (Hoza, 1989).

Clarification of medication effects on covert behaviors would be important both clinically and theoretically. Despite producing significant short-term benefits for a majority of children with ADHD, stimulant intervention has not yet been shown to alter the course of the disorder (e.g., Weiss & Hechtman, 1986). One plausible explanation is that these medications do not affect such crucial variables as covert antisocial behaviors, which display considerable predictive validity for negative outcomes (e.g., Loeber & Stouthamer-Loeber, 1987). More theoretically, if stimulants *were* shown to reduce risk for covert activities, elucidation of underlying mechanisms for such actions would be critical. In short, a central aim for the present investigation was to clarify the effects of methylphenidate on the display of covert antisocial behaviors.

To summarize, covert actions are at least partially distinct from overtly aggressive acts, and they carry high risk for negative outcomes. Their display may be particularly problematic for youngsters with ADHD, who are, by definition, impulsive and poorly self-regulated. In order to observe such behaviors directly, we surreptitiously videotaped an individual laboratory setting, in which ADHD as well as comparison boys had the opportunity to take desired items and to use an answer key while working on a problem set. Stealing was measured by counts of objects remaining in the room; property destruction and cheating were coded from the videotapes. For validation purposes, we correlated these measures with relevant maternal rating scales and with staff ratings. In order to achieve the goal of ascertaining stimulant effects on the covert acts, we performed a methylphenidate-placebo crossover with the ADHD participants.

METHOD

Overview of Procedures

This investigation took place during a summer research program for ADHD and comparison boys, aged 6–12 years. Before the 5-week program, parents completed rating scales about their sons, and we performed extensive assessments of each child and family. During the program, participants were divided into equal-sized younger (6- to 9-year) and older (9.5- to 12-year) cohorts for all activities. The boys could earn points for participating in the daily class and play events; these were redeemable for backup reinforcers at a weekly "store." ADHD boys received stimulant medication trials during the summer, and all participants received global staff ratings of risk for covert antisocial behavior during the final week. The entire program was conducted in accordance with American Psychological Association ethical principles and with full approval from the University of California, Los Angeles (UCLA) Medical Human Subjects Protection Committee.

The experimental study of covert actions took place during the final week of the program. Each boy participated in a laboratory session on two consecutive days, Wednesday and Thursday of Week 5, with the ADHD boys participating once on placebo and once on 0.3 mg/kg of methylphenidate. Debriefing was performed at the end of the second experimental day. Following the program, a controlled trial of systematic parent and child treatment was initiated for the ADHD participants.

Subjects

The 22 boys with ADHD were recruited through physicians, medical clinics, and parent self-help groups. All had received primary diagnoses of ADHD from physicians; all were receiving ongoing treatment with stimulant medication; and none had mental retardation, neurologic dysfunction, psychosis, or significant emotional disturbances (e.g., major depression).[2] For parent ratings and interviews, we asked families to appraise their sons' unmedicated behavior. (Because

---

[2]Twenty-seven ADHD and 23 comparison boys were enrolled in the program, but 3 ADHD youngsters and 1 comparison child were absent during the final week. In addition, 2 ADHD participants had Verbal IQ scores below 70, and they were therefore excluded from data analysis. Of the 22 participating ADHD youngsters, 2 had previously displayed tics and were receiving clonidine in the community; they remained on clonidine during the methylphenidate trials.

of the medicated nature of the sample, teacher ratings were considered less valid, and we did not consider these.)

Regarding parent scales, each boy exceeded the traditional cutoff of 15 from either mother or father on the Conners Abbreviated Symptom Questionnaire (Goyette, Conners, & Ulrich, 1978). Furthermore, parents rated their sons on a randomized list of the *Diagnostic and Statistical Manual of Mental Disorders*, 3d ed., rev. (*DSM-III-R*; American Psychiatric Association, 1987) criteria for disruptive behavior disorders, with scores of 2 (*pretty much*) or 3 (*very much*) on the 4-point scale signifying symptom presence. All subjects but 3 met or surpassed the *DSM-III-R* criterion of eight symptoms for ADHD, with the remainder missing this cutoff by one item. Also, from structured interviews with parents, all 22 boys met or surpassed the cutoff of five symptoms for attention problem disorder on Loney's (1987) Divergent and Convergent Items (DACI). Finally, parents noted that each boy had an onset of ADHD at or before the age of 6 years. As for the important issue of additional externalizing diagnoses (see Hinshaw, 1987), parent ratings on the *DSM-III-R* checklists revealed that 10 of the 22 participants qualified for a diagnosis of oppositional-defiant disorder, and 4 other youngsters met criteria for conduct disorder. Two ADHD boys had severe (1.5 *SD*) discrepancies between IQ and reading that would qualify as learning disabilities.

As for medication, the ADHD boys had been receiving stimulant treatment (17 were on methylphenidate, 3 on dextroamphetamine, and 2 on pemoline) for periods ranging from 4 months to 7 years (*Mdn* = 2 years) before participating in the program. In all cases families and physicians agreed to methylphenidate trials for the summer.

The comparison boys were recruited through school flyers and newspaper advertisements for a summer enrichment program. None of the 22 youngsters met criteria for any behavior disorder on any of the parent rating scales; one comparison boy met criteria for a learning disability. Table 1 summarizes pertinent behavioral, demographic, and cognitive data for the ADHD and comparison samples. The ADHD boys scored lower on Verbal IQ than did the comparison boys; the mathematics difference approached significance.

Experimental Procedures

Boys were oriented to the laboratory sessions in groups of four on each day of the study, with each tetrad comprising 2 ADHD and 2 comparison youngsters. An experimenter explained to each group that the purpose of the activity was to see how well boys could work without an adult present. The experimenter then modeled work on a sample worksheet (hidden word searches for the older cohort; hidden picture searches for the younger cohort). Boys were told that they would

TABLE 1

Scores of Attention-Deficit Hyperactivity Disorder (ADHD) and Comparison Boys on
Rating Scale, Demographic, and Cognitive Variables

Variable	ADHD (n = 22)	Comparison (n = 22)	p^a
CASQ (maternal rating)	20.9	3.4	<.001
CBCL Hyperactivity scale (maternal rating)	73.4	56.3	<.001
Age (years)	9.3	9.7	ns
Ethnicity (% White)	77.3	77.3	ns
Family status (% from two-parent, biological family)	59.0	77.3	ns
Wechsler Intelligence Scale for Children—Revised, Verbal IQ	106.3	117.0	<.05
Woodcock-Johnson Psycho-educational Battery (percentile scores)			
Reading cluster	53.0	62.6	ns
Mathematics cluster	63.0	79.0	(.06)

Note. CASQ = Conners Abbreviated Symptom Questionnaire; CBCL = Child Behavior Checklist.
^{a} Based on two-tailed, independent-sample t tests for continuous variables or single-df chi-square tests for categorical variables.

have 8 min (Day 1) and 6 min (Day 2) to work. Problems on the worksheets progressed from relatively easy to quite difficult.

In order to determine whether different contingencies for task performance would affect rates of covert antisocial behaviors, we assigned boys randomly to either high- or regular-incentive conditions across both days of the investigation. In the former, the tetrad members were informed that boys who got all problems correct, as detected at the end of the work session when worksheets were scored, would receive 15 bonus points, equivalent to approximately a morning's worth of reinforcers; others would receive their usual allotment of 2 points for participation in a special activity. Regular-incentive participants were told that they could earn 2 points if they got at least half of the problems correct.

At the close of the tetrad's orientation, a research assistant individually escorted each boy to a separate room, reiterated the ground rules, emphasized the contingency in effect, and explained that she would reenter to grade the boy's work when time was up. In discussing the grading, she pointed out the answer key that she would use, which was clipped in the front position on her clipboard. (Answer keys were prepared such that the last answer was partially obscured for the older cohort and one figure was not circled for the younger cohort.) After handing the boy his worksheet, she then left the room, "accidentally" (and silently) leaving her clipboard on the table near the boy. If a boy left the room, he was directed back inside by the assistant, who stayed in the hallway near the door. If he brought the clipboard out to her, she accepted it.

At the time limit, each assistant reentered the room, picked up the clipboard, collected the boy's worksheet, and left for a minute, allegedly to score the sheet. The research assistants explained to each boy in the high-incentive condition that no one had scored 100%; they then awarded 2 points to the boy. All boys in the regular condition were given 2 points.

The individual work rooms were each approximately 3 m² in size. Each contained a chair and large work table, with little additional furniture. A "letter organizer" was placed on the right side of each table, which contained the following, in peripheral view of the boy: a $1 bill, 3 quarters (4 quarters on Day 2, in order to vary the stimulus conditions slightly), a pack of baseball cards, and a 23 × 31 cm manila envelope. This unclasped envelope contained an additional $1 bill, 2 small matchbox cars, and an additional answer key for the worksheet. All rooms also contained one-way mirrors, behind which video cameras recorded the session.

In order not to bias the experiment for the second day, we provided no debriefing on Day 1. (Brief, open-ended, postsession interviews with each boy following the work session yielded little scorable data regarding his truthfulness in reporting on his work.) After all children had finished the study on Day 2, the director of the program debriefed the boys in groups. He explained the purpose of the study—to see how boys would respond when working on their own—and stated explicitly that taking things and cheating were not right. He also stated that boys could return any items that were taken.

Medication Procedures

The ADHD boys were assigned randomly to one of two medication orders: methylphenidate on Day 1 and placebo on Day 2 (order MP) or the reverse (order PM). Medications were dispensed on site, privately and in double-blind fashion, at 8:30 a.m. and 11:45 a.m. All experimental procedures took place between 45 and 150 min after receipt of medication. We constrained randomization so that each medication order contained approximately equal numbers of boys from each age cohort and each incentive condition.

Because of the short half-life of methylphenidate, dosage changes across 2-day periods of a day are quite sensitive to medication effects (e.g., Murphy et al., in press). We selected dosages of methylphenidate considered low (0.3 mg/kg). Medication and placebo tablets, packaged by the UCLA pharmacy, were prepared in 2.5 mg increments and placed in opaque capsules to disguise the taste differential. To ensure that medication was never below 0.3 mg/kg, the 2.5 mg-incremented dosages were always rounded up, so that the actual weight-adjusted dosage range was 0.30–0.38 mg/kg. Absolute dosages ranged from 7.5 to 15 mg.

Experimental Measures

Stealing. Experimenters (different from the individual assistants) made counts of objects in the rooms immediately following each individual work session, noting (a) the amount of money that had been taken (out of $2.75 on Day 1 and $3 on Day 2), (b) the number of toy cars stolen, and (c) whether the pack of baseball cards had been taken. Floor areas were checked, in order to ensure that money or objects had not been thrown as opposed to taken. Because of the objectivity of these unobtrusive measurements, reliability was not formally assessed, although on the occasions that two experimenters were present, the agreement was always perfect. Given the utility of continuous, as opposed to dichotomous, measures of covert behavior (see Hartshorne & May, 1928), we created a composite stealing variable (0–5) by reducing the amount of money taken to a 3-point scale (0 = *none*; 1 = *$1 or less*; 2 = *more than $1*) and adding this score to the number of cars stolen (0–2) and to the dichotomous variable of whether the baseball card pack was taken (0 = *no*; 1 = *yes*).

Property destruction. We assessed this variable by having trained undergraduate observers watch each videotaped experimental session, write down the sequence of events, and make a 4-point rating (0 = *none*; 1 = *scribbling on worksheet*; 2 = *crumpling papers*; 3 = *writing on furniture or wall, ripping papers, breaking pencils, throwing objects*). The observers were unaware of group (ADHD vs. comparison) status, medication status, or incentive condition of the participants. The three observers' scores were correlated across the 88 taped sessions, with a mean pairwise correlation of $r = .67$. When rater is considered a fixed effect, the alpha coefficient across raters is equivalent to an intraclass correlation coefficient (Shrout & Fleiss, 1979), appropriate for use as a reliability estimate when averaged scores are analyzed. The alpha reliability for property destruction was .86.

Mean scores across the three raters were entered for each session, except for those 10 instances in which disagreements were greater than 1 point. Written narratives supplied by each observer revealed that such discrepancies resulted from the occasional scoring of 3 for minor doodling or scribbling on the table. In order not to overestimate property destruction, we resolved such disagreements by entering the average of the lower scores given.[3]

Cheating. The same observers made a 3-point appraisal of the boy's use of the

---

[3] The "room-check" experimenters noted six clear instances of property destruction (e.g., destroyed materials), four of which were confirmed by the videotape analyses. The other two instances involved boys' ripping and throwing of objects outside of camera range. For these cases, we assigned scores of 3.

answer key, with $0 = $ *no cheating* (never looking at the answer key or attempting to return it), $1 = $ *occasional looking between the key and the worksheet*, and $2 = $ *repeated use*. The average pairwise correlation between raters was $r = .89$, yielding an alpha of .96. Mean scores across the three raters were entered as the child's score in all instances.

Rating Measures

Parents. Parents completed separate Child Behavior Checklists (CBCL; Achenbach & Edelbrock, 1983) before the start of the program, with regard to their son's behavior while unmedicated. We used maternal ratings, for which the response rate was 100%. The narrow-band externalizing scale that taps covert antisocial behavior for boys aged 6–11 is the 12-item Delinquency scale, which contains such items as lying/cheating, stealing, destroying property, fire-setting, truancy, and the like. (The item composition for Delinquency changed only slightly for our 3 subjects aged 12 years.) The 1-week test-retest reliability for this scale is .95; the 6-month stability coefficient is .71 (Achenbach & Edelbrock, 1983).

We also created narrower a priori scales from the CBCL, in order to match more specifically our laboratory indices of covert antisocial activity (see Loeber & Schmaling, 1985b). We defined *stealing* with Item 81 (steals at home) and Item 82 (steals outside the home); coefficient alpha in our sample $= .55$ (no test-retest data were available). We composed *property destruction* from Item 20 (destroys own property), Item 21 (destroys others' property), and Item 106 (vandalism); alpha $= .71$. Finally, we indexed *cheating* with Item 43 (lies/cheats) and Item 69 (secretive); alpha $= .52$.

Program staff. During the final week of the program, eight senior staff members made 4-point, global ratings, based on the entire program, of each child's overall risk for commission of covert antisocial behaviors ($0 = $ *none*; $3 = $ *severe risk*; see Hinshaw et al., 1989, for justification of similar procedures for appraising overall aggression). The alpha reliability of these ratings was .96; mean scores across the raters were used for each boy.

RESULTS

Base Rates of Laboratory Measures

We first present several rates of laboratory actions that reflect the extent of engagement in covert behavior. Across both days of the study, 38% of the sessions involving comparison boys and 64% of those with ADHD participants included the taking of at least one object; regarding stealing of money, the respective rates were 18% and 43%. As for property destruction, 14% of the comparison sessions and 36% of the ADHD sessions showed scores averaging over 0.5 on our 0–3 scale across the days. For cheating, the respective rates (for scores above 0.5 on our 0–2 scale) were 25% and 52%. For the ADHD boys, rates were elevated in placebo sessions as compared with medication sessions (see parametric analyses below).

Relationships Among Measures

Table 2 presents intercorrelations among the maternal CBCL scales, global staff ratings, and laboratory indices of covert behavior. Regarding the laboratory measures, we used placebo data for the ADHD boys, in order to increase variability of the scores. For the comparison youngsters, we used Day 1 data for a random half and Day 2 scores for the other half, parallel to the ADHD boys, for whom placebo scores were evenly divided across the 2 days.

As would be expected from subscales that largely originated from an established empirical factor (i.e., the CBCL Delinquency scale), the maternal CBCL scales were significantly intercorrelated with one another, and each was associated with the staff rating of risk for covert antisocial behavior. Indeed, the association between the 12-item Delinquency scale and the mean staff rating was substantial ($r = .64$). The laboratory indices were mildly to moderately correlated with the Delinquency scale. Stealing was consistently associated with its respective a priori scale and with the staff appraisal of risk for covert tendencies; for property destruction, these associations were also significant. For cheating, however, the correlations were not significant. The three covert laboratory measures were nonsignificantly intercorrelated.[4]

Not included in the table were the background variables of income and Verbal IQ, each of which has been shown to correlate negatively with covert antisocial behavior in large-scale investigations (e.g., West & Farrington, 1977). These background variables did not correlate significantly with any rating scale or laboratory measure in the present data (all $ps > .05$).

Effects of Group Status and Methylphenidate on Laboratory Indices

We began our parametric analyses with 2 (incentive condition: high, regular) × 3 (subject order: comparison, medication-placebo [MP], placebo–medication [PM]) × 2 (Day 1, Day 2) analyses of variance (ANOVAs), in which incentive

---

[4]To ascertain whether the laboratory indices showed any discrimination from overt aggression, we considered correlating them with the 23-item, narrow-band Aggression scale from the CBCL in addition to the Delinquency scale. In our sample, however, these two CBCL narrow-band externalizing scales were highly intercorrelated ($r = .82$), precluding a meaningful distinction between the criterion variables.

TABLE 2

Intercorrelations Among Ratings and Laboratory Covert Behaviors

Variable	1	2	3	4	5	6	7	8
1. CBCL Delinquency	—	.69***	.83***	.53***	.64***	.41**	.39**	.34*
2. CBCL Stealing		—	.59***	.51***	.50***	.45**	.24	.36*
3. CBCL Property Destruction			—	.41**	.55***	.28	.30*	.40**
4. CBCL Cheating				—	.35*	.13	.25	.29
5. Staff rating					—	.39**	.48**	.23
6. Laboratory stealing						—	.22	.20
7. Laboratory property destruction							—	.07
8. Laboratory cheating								—

Note. CBCL = Child Behavior Checklist.
* $p < .05$. ** $p < .01$. *** $p < .001$.

condition and subject order were between-subjects factors and day was a within-subject factor. Another set of ANOVAs substituted the between-subjects factor of age cohort (older, younger) for incentive condition, as our small sample size precluded four-way factorials. Because they did not correlate with the outcome measures, Verbal IQ and income were not included as covariates. Also, because of our interest in examining effects on the distinct covert behaviors, we did not perform multivariate analyses of variance (see Huberty & Morris, 1989); more appropriately, we selected an alpha level of .01 for experimentwise protection.

The ANOVAs yielded information regarding overall effects of day, incentive condition, and age cohort, but interactions involving subject order were decomposed through a priori, planned contrasts of specific cell means, with appropriate error terms from the omnibus analyses (Winer, 1971; see also Whalen, Henker, Collins, McAuliffe, & Vaux, 1979). Medication effects for the ADHD boys were tested by contrasting the sum of the two medication cells (Day 1 for the MP order plus Day 2 for the PM order) with the placebo sum (Day 1 for PM plus Day 2 for MP). To appraise effects of ADHD versus comparison status, we contrasted the medication score as well as the placebo score with the comparison boys' average score across the 2 days. Finally, in order to detect differential medication effects within the MP versus PM orders for the ADHD youngsters, we also performed post hoc medication–placebo comparisons separately for each other.

The ANOVAs yielded no main effects or interactions of incentive condition or cohort for any outcome, and these factors were not considered further. A main effect of day emerged for stealing, $F(1, 40) = 13.63$, $p < .001$, with higher overall scores on Day 2 ($M = 1.48$) than Day 1 ($M = 09.75$). The day effect was also significant for cheating, $F(1, 40) = 29.46$, $p < .001$, with higher scores on Day 1 ($M = 1.00$) than Day 2 ($M = 0.39$). There was no day effect for property destruction.

An effect of medication status emerged for stealing, $F(1, 40) = 9.67$, $p < .01$;

see Figure 1a. The ADHD boys had higher scores when receiving placebo (M = 1.95) than when taking methylphenidate (M = 1.09). Although placebo stealing tended to be elevated above that of the comparison boys (M = 0.70), $F(1, 40)$ = 5.90, p <.05, the mean level on medication was not significantly different from the comparison youngsters' mean, $F(1, 40)$ = 0.22. Regarding the different medication orders, there was a clear increase in stealing from Day 1 to Day 2 for the MP order, $F(1, 40)$ = 22.7, p <.001, but the PM group showed no change across days, $F(1, 40)$ = 0.13, *ns* (see Figure 1a).

For property destruction, the medication effect was significant, $F(1, 40)$ = 9.01, p <.01, with methylphenidate producing lower scores (M = .36) than placebo (M = 1.08). There was a marginal tendency for the placebo rate to be elevated above that of the comparison boys (M = 0.29), $F(1, 40)$ = 3.61, p <.10, but the medication level was nearly identical to that of the comparison boys, $F(1, 40)$ = 0.03, *ns*. The MP order did not show a significant increase in property destruction across days, $F(1, 40)$ = 2.33, *ns*, but the PM order significantly reduced property destruction from Day 1 to Day 2, $F(1, 40)$ = 7.40, p <.01.

Regarding cheating, there was a medication effect in the opposite direction to those for stealing and property destruction: Active medication (M = 1.24) effected an increase over placebo (M = 0.65), $F(1, 40)$ = 15.36, p <.001 (see Figure 1b). The medication mean was elevated above that of the comparison boys (M = .44), $F(1, 40)$ = 6.58, p <.05, but the placebo average was not significantly different from the comparison boys' level, $F(1, 40)$ = 0.31, *ns*. For the MP

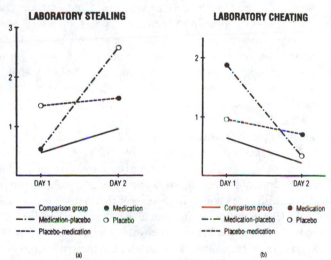

Figure 1. (a) Mean laboratory stealing scores by subject order and by day; (b) mean laboratory cheating scores by subject order and by day.

order, there was a significant reduction of cheating from Day 1 to Day 2, $F(1, 40)$ = $41.15, p < .001$, but no medication-related change was found for the PM order, $F(1, 40) = 0.69$, *ns.*

DISCUSSION

The ADHD children's performance of covert antisocial behaviors was examined in an individual laboratory setting. Rates of the covert antisocial behaviors of stealing and destroying property in this setting were elevated above those found in naturalistic investigations (see Hartshorne & May, 1928), and these laboratory behaviors were associated with parent and staff ratings of similar activities, yielding initial evidence for their validity. Furthermore, whereas unmedicated ADHD children tended to display greater rates of stealing and property destruction than did comparison youngsters, the stimulant methylphenidate significantly reduced these covert actions, with medicated levels not different from those of the comparison boys. An opposite pattern occurred for cheating, in that methylphenidate increased this behavior.

Regarding our attempts to validate the laboratory measures against adult ratings, we should note immediately that such ratings are not infalliable criterion measures. Indeed, developmental psychopathologists continue to grapple with the lack of definitive criteria against which to validate most of their constructs (e.g., Achenbach, McConaughy, & Howell, 1987). Nonetheless, stealing and property destruction were associated with CBCL ratings of general covert actions (Delinquency scale) and of modality-specific behaviors (a priori stealing and property destruction scales, respectively); they were also correlated with global staff ratings of risk for commission of covert antisocial actions. On the other hand, cheating was correlated less consistently with the ratings. It would be helpful, in future investigations, to include self-report measures of covert behavior as additional criterion variables, given their stability and predictive validity (Farrington, 1973).

Methylphenidate led to decreases in stealing and property destruction, replicating Hoza's (1989) finding for the latter variable. In each case, placebo levels tended to be elevated above those of the comparison boys, but medication scores did not differ from those of the comparison youngsters, suggesting the normalization of covert acts with medication. To the extent that our laboratory indices are valid, these results lead to the important conclusion that even low dosages of stimulants effect reductions in these important covert antisocial behaviors. The medication effects, however, were qualified by differential patterns of response across the two medication orders. For stealing, children in the MP order greatly increased this behavior across days, but boys in the PM order showed no difference across Days 1 and 2. Although it is conceivable that this differential effect reflects sampling differences, the results are opposite for property destruction, for which the responsive boys were those in the PM order. Without repetitions of the same condition (i.e., MM and PP as well as MP and PM orders), full disentangling of treatment condition from time of administration is problematic.

Informal observations suggested that some laboratory stealing (as well as most property destruction) was quite impulsive in nature, with coins or toys literally falling out of the boys' pockets or hands as they left the experimental room. Other stealing acts, however, seemed to involve careful strategizing (e.g., scrutinizing the desk and envelope before planfully taking and concealing objects). Although we did not attempt systematic classification of such subtypes (chiefly because some children did not stay in camera range for the entire session and because of the levels of inference involved in making such judgments), methylphenidate may have been particularly effective in reducing stealing and property destruction linked to impulsivity (e.g., Whalen, 1989).

Methylphenidate effects on cheating were also significant but in the opposite direction: The medication increased cheating behavior. Differential medication effects were also found for the two orders here, in that only the MP order showed increased cheating (on Day 1) with methylphenidate. One possible explanation for the overall medication effect is that cheating was associated with greater task involvement in our laboratory work sessions (see Hartshorne & May, 1928). In support of this contention, informal observations suggested that task interest was quite high on the first day of the study, with considerable enthusiasm expressed for doing well on the worksheets. Given the known actions of stimulants on task involvement and motivation (e.g., Milich, Carlson, Pelham, & Licht, 1991), and given the inconsistent correlation of laboratory cheating with parent or staff ratings, our laboratory cheating measure may index, in part, motivation to perform optimally on academic-like tasks.

The research that we performed is in the experimental tradition of such investigators as Buckle and Farrington (1984), Diener, Fraser, Beaman, and Kelem (1976), and Switzer, Deal, and Bailey (1977), who observed—or inferred from permanent products—covert antisocial acts in natural or laboratory settings. Our decision to pursue this investigation was not made lightly, particularly given the need to repeat the procedures across two days (for purposes of the medication crossover) and to videorecord the laboratory sessions surreptitiously (in order to ensure that the behaviors exhibited were truly covert). First, given the rise in violence and theft in our society (Loeber, 1990), there is an urgent need to obtain valid observational data on the key domain of covert behaviors in childhood (Farrington, 1979), particularly in high-risk groups like ADHD youngsters. Second, the children in our study were participants in a highly structured program, which attempted to facilitate rule-governed behavior; the overall message to them and their families was one of the development of self-control. Third, full debriefing took place at the conclusion of the investigation, and it emphasized that taking objects and cheating were not right. Fourth, shortly after the program, we (a) initiated intensive behavioral parent management and cognitive-behavioral child groups for half of the ADHD participants, (b) coordinated the obtaining of community services for the remaining half, and (c) issued feedback and reports to each family. Thus, we did not expose the children to our procedures in the absence of treatment and advocacy.

Still, providing the opportunity to take objects and to use answer keys facilitated the display of covert behaviors in the lab. Furthermore, we recorded behaviors from behind one-way mirrors, after having informed the child that he would be working without observation. We feel that the ethical risks entailed by these procedures were outweighed by the overall program format, the explicit debriefing, and the valuable information obtained about the validity and medication-responsiveness of covert behaviors. Farrington (1979) has contended that experimental investigations of covert behavior carry the promise of facilitating development of pertinent interventions; we concur with his conclusion that risks posed by such research are outweighed by the promise of better prediction and prevention of delinquency-related behaviors.

Despite the medication effects that we found, stimulant medication is quite unlikely to be a panacea for preventing delinquency risk in youngsters with ADHD. For one thing, the generalizability of our indices is still unknown, despite some evidence for concurrent validity; for another, children are usually unmedicated during after-school or weekend hours, those often-unsupervised times that are critical for commission of covert actions. Furthermore, covert behaviors and delinquency are typically embedded in cultural and familial networks that are not amenable to intervention directed solely toward the child. Indeed, linkages between the impulse control and cognitive deficits displayed by ADHD children and their propensity for antisocial behavior are complex, spanning biological, familial, social, and cultural pathways (Loeber, 1990; Moffitt, 1990). Effective intervention strategies will need to be multifaceted, and they will require implementation early in developmental trajectories.

REFERENCES

Achenbach, T. M., & Edelbrock, C. (1983). *Manual for the Child Behavior Checklist and Revised Child Behavior Profile*. Burlington, VT: Author.

Achenbach, T. M., McConaughy, S. H., & Howell, C. T. (1987). Child/adolescent behavioral and emotional problems: Implications of cross-informant correlations for situational specificity. *Psychological Bulletin*, 101, 213–232.

American Psychiatric Association. (1987.) *Diagnostic and statistical manual of mental disorders* (3rd. ed., rev.). Washington, DC: Author.

Barkley, R. A., Fischer, M., Edelbrock, C. S., & Smallish, L. (1990). The adolescent outcome of hyperactive children diagnosed by research criteria: 1. An 8-year prospective follow-up study. *Journal of the American Academy of Child and Adolescent Psychiatry*, 29, 546–557.

Barkley, R. A., McMurray, M. B., Edelbrock, C. S., & Robbins, K. (1989). The response of aggressive and nonaggressive ADHD children to two doses of methylphenidate. *Journal of the American Academy of Child and Adolescent Psychiatry*, 28, 873–881.

Buckle, A., & Farrington, D. P. (1984). An observational study of shoplifting. *British Journal of Criminology*, 24, 63–73.

Diener, E., Fraser, S. C., Beaman, A. L., & Kelem, R. T. (1976). Effects of deindividuation variables on stealing among Halloween trick-or-treaters. *Journal of Personality and Social Psychology*, 33, 178–183.

Farrington, D. P. (1973). Self-reports of deviant behavior: Predictive and stable? *Journal of Criminal Law and Criminology*, 64, 99–110.

Farrington, D. P. (1979). Experiments on deviance with special reference to dishonesty. In L. Berkowitz (Ed.), *Advances in experimental social psychology* (Vol. 12, pp. 207–252). San Diego, CA: Academic Press.

Gadow, K. D., Nolan, E. E., Sverd, J., Sprafkin, J., & Paolicelli, L. (1990). Methylphenidate in aggressive-hyperactive boys: 1. Effects on peer aggression in public school settings. *Journal of the American Academy of Child and Adolescent Psychiatry*, 29, 710–718.

Gittelman, R., Mannuzza, S., Shenker, R., & Bonagura, N. (1985). Hyperactive boys almost grown up: 1. Psychiatric status. *Archives of General Psychiatry*, 42, 937–947.

Goyette, C. H., Conners, C. K., & Ulrich, R. F. (1978). Normative data on revised Conners Parent and Teacher Rating Scales. *Journal of Abnormal Child Psychology*, 6, 221–236.

Hartshorne, H., & May, M. (1928). *Studies in deceit* (Book one of *Studies in the nature of character*). New York: MacMillan.

Hinshaw, S. P. (1987). On the distinction between attentional deficits/hyperactivity and conduct problems/aggression in child psychopathology. *Psychological Bulletin*, 101, 443–463.

Hinshaw, S. P. (1991). Stimulant medication and the treatment of aggression in children with attentional deficits. *Journal of Clinical Child Psychology*, 20, 301–312.

Hinshaw, S. P., Henker, B., Whalen, C. K., Erhardt, D., & Dunnington, R. E. (1989). Aggressive, prosocial, and nonsocial behavior in hyperactive boys: Dose effects of methylphenidate in naturalistic settings. *Journal of Consulting and Clinical Psychology*, 57, 636–643.

Hoza, J. (1989). *Response to stimulant medication among children with attention deficit hyperactivity disorder*. Unpublished doctoral dissertation, Florida State University.

Huberty, C. J., & Morris, J. D. (1989). Multivariate analysis versus multiple univariate analyses. *Psychological Bulletin*, 105, 302–308.

Huesmann, L. R., Eron, L. D., Lefkowitz, M. M., & Walder, L. O. (1984). Stability of aggression over time and generations. *Developmental Psychology*, 20, 1120–1134.

Klorman, R., Brumaghim, J. T., Salzman, L. F., Strauss, J., Borgstedt, A. D., McBride, M. C., & Loeb, S. (1988). Effects of methylphenidate on attention-deficit hyperactivity disorder with and without aggressive/noncompliant features. *Journal of Abnormal Psychology*, 97, 413–422.

Loeber, R. (1982). The stability of antisocial and delinquent child behavior: A review. *Child Development*, 53, 1431–1446.

Loeber, R. (1990). Development and risk factors of juvenile antisocial behavior and delinquency. *Clinical Psychology Review*, 10, 1–41.

Loeber, R., & Schmaling, K. B. (1985a). Empirical evidence for overt and covert patterns of antisocial conduct problems: A meta-analysis. *Journal of Abnormal Child Psychology*, 13, 337–352.

Loeber, R., & Schmaling, K. B. (1985b). The utility of differentiating between pure and mixed forms of antisocial child behavior. *Journal of Abnormal Child Psychology*, 13, 315–336.

Loeber, R., & Stouthamer-Loeber, M. (1987). Prediction. In H. C. Quay (Ed.). *Handbook of juvenile delinquency* (pp. 325–382). New York: Wiley.

Loney, J. (1987). Hyperactivity and aggression in the diagnosis of attention deficit disorder. In B. B. Lahey & A. E. Kazdin (Eds.), *Advances in clinical child psychology* (Vol. 10, pp. 99–135). New York: Plenum Press.

Milich, R., Carlson, C. L., Pelham, W. E., & Licht, B. G. (1991). Effects of methylphenidate on the persistence of ADHD boys following failure experiences. *Journal of Abnormal Child Psychology*, 19, 519–536.

Mitchell, S., & Rosa, P. (1981). Boyhood behaviour problems as predictors of criminality: A fifteen-year follow-up study. *Journal of Child Psychology and Psychiatry*, 22, 19–33.

Moffitt, T. E. (1990). Juvenile delinquency and attention deficit disorder: Boys' developmental trajectories from age 3 to age 15. *Child Development*, 61, 893–910.

Moore, D. R., Chamberlain, P., & Mukai, L. H. (1979). Children at risk for delinquency: A follow-up comparison of aggressive children and children who steal. *Journal of Abnormal Child Psychology*, 7, 345–355.

Murphy, D. A., Pelham, W. E., & Lang, A. R. (in press). Aggression in boys with attention deficit-hyperactivity disorder: Methylphenidate effects on naturalistically observed aggression, response to provocation, and social information processing. *Journal of Abnormal Child Psychology*.

Olweus, D. (1979). Stability of aggressive reaction patterns in males: A review. *Psychological Bulletin*, 86, 852–875.

Patterson, G. R., & Stouthamer-Loeber, M. (1984). The correlation of family management practices and delinquency. *Child Development*, 55, 1299–1307.

Pelham, W. E., Greenslade, K. E., Vodde-Hamilton, M., Murphy, D. A., Greenstein, J. J., Gnagy, E. M., & Dahl, R. E. (1990). Relative efficacy of long-acting stimulants on ADHD children: A comparison of standard methylphenidate, Ritalin SR-20, Dexedrine spansule, and pemoline. *Pediatrics*, 86, 226–237.

Quay, H. C. (1986). Classification. In H. C. Quay & J. S. Werry (Eds.), *Psychopathological disorders of childhood* (3rd ed., pp. 1–34). New York: Wiley.

Robins, L. N. (1966). *Deviant children grown up: A sociological and psychiatric study of sociopathic personality.* Baltimore: Williams & Wilkins.

Satterfield, J. H., Hoppe, C. M., & Schell, A. M. (1982). A prospective study of delinquency in 110 adolescent boys with attention deficit disorder and 88 normal adolescent boys. *American Journal of Psychiatry, 139,* 795–798.

Shrout, P. E., & Fleiss, J. L. (1979). Intraclass correlations: Uses in assessing interrater reliability. *Psychological Bulletin, 86,* 420–428.

Stattin, H., & Magnusson, D. (1989). The role of early aggressive behavior in the frequency, seriousness, and types of later crime. *Journal of Consulting and Clinical Psychology, 57,* 710–718.

Switzer, E. B., Deal, T. E., & Bailey, J. S. (1977). The reduction of stealing in second graders using a group contingency. *Journal of Applied Behavior Analysis, 10,* 267–272.

Wadsworth, M. E. J. (1979). *Roots of delinquency.* Oxford, England: Robertson.

Weiss, G., & Hechtman, L. (1986). *Hyperactive children grown up.* New York: Guilford Press.

West, D. J., & Farrington, D. P. (1977). *The delinquent way of life: Third report of the Cambridge study in delinquent development.* London: Heinemann.

Whalen, C. K. (1989). Attention deficit-hyperactivity disorder. In T. H. Ollendick & M. Hersen (Eds.), *Handbook of child psychopathology* (2nd ed., pp. 131–169). New York: Plenum Press.

Whalen, C. K., Henker, B., Collins, B. E., McAuliffe, S., & Vaux, A. (1979). Peer interaction in a structured communication task: Comparisons of normal and hyperactive boys and of methylphenidate (Ritalin) and placebo effects. *Child Development, 50,* 388–401.

Winer, B. J. (1971). *Statistical principles in experimental design* (2nd ed.). New York: McGraw-Hill.

13

A 2-Year Prospective Follow-up Study of Children and Adolescents with Disruptive Behavior Disorders

Prediction by Cerebrospinal Fluid 5-Hydroxyindoleacetic Acid, Homovanillic Acid, and Autonomic Measures

Markus J. P. Kruesi, Euthymia D. Hibbs, Theodore P. Zahn,
Cynthia S. Keysor, Susan D. Hamburger,
John J. Bartko, and Judith L. Rapoport
National Institute of Mental Health, Bethesda, Maryland

A 2-year prospective follow-up study of 100% (N = 29) of a sample of children and adolescents with disruptive behavior disorders found that the baseline lumbar cerebrospinal fluid monoamine metabolite concentration and autonomic nervous system activity predicted some subsequent outcomes. The 5-hydroxyindoleacetic acid concentration significantly predicted severity of physical aggression during follow-up. The skin conductance level significantly predicted institutionalization. Correlations were in predicted directions with lower cerebrospinal fluid 5-hydroxyindoleacetic acid concentrations and autonomic activity correlated with poor outcome. Moreover, in multivariate analyses, which included nonlaboratory measures as predictors, cerebrospinal fluid and autonomic measures still contributed significantly to the prediction. However, hypothesized predictions of cerebrospinal fluid 5-hydroxyindoleacetic acid concentrations for suicide attempts and of low autonomic nervous system activity for arrests

Reprinted with permission from *Archives of General Psychiatry*, 1992, Vol. 49, 429–435. Copyright © 1992 by American Medical Association.

Presented in part at the New Research Program of the 144th Annual Meeting of the American Psychiatric Association, New Orleans, La, May 13, 1991.

were not supported thus far. Patients are still at risk; consequently, these results must be considered preliminary. Nonetheless, the results suggest that further investigation of relationships between biological factors and outcome of children with disruptive behavior disorders is warranted.

Disruptive behavior disorders (DBDs) constitute a heterogeneous group, encompassing diagnoses (*DSM-III-R*) of attention-deficit hyperactivity disorder, oppositional defiant disorder, and conduct disorder. These overlapping groups are characterized by age-inappropriate behaviors, including hyperactivity, impulsivity, and aggression, with substantial overlap among the three disorders.[1] "Pure" conduct disorder or "pure" oppositional disorder are relatively rare in clinical samples, with most cases also qualifying for an attention-deficit disorder diagnosis.[1] Follow-up studies of hyperactive children have found a wide range of outcomes, with about half being undiscernible from that of normal controls and a substantial minority (about 25%) having antisocial outcomes.[2-4]

Conduct disorder predicts criminal[5] and substance abuse outcomes[6] of hyperactive children. However, childhood conduct disturbance is common, while only about a third have it persist into adulthood[7]; in contrast, adult antisocial personality disorder is almost always preceded by conduct disorder in childhood.[8,9] Thus, as with hyperactivity, conduct disturbance alone does not predict which disruptive individuals go on to chronicity. Aggression is an important behavioral dimension within conduct disorder, as well as for a broad range of (overlapping) poor outcomes, including subsequent aggression,[10-12] illegal drug involvement,[10] delinquency,[13] and criminal activities.[12,14-18] Aggression is an acknowledged behavioral precursor in about 75% of male chronic offenders.[19]

Follow-up studies of delinquents have concentrated primarily on psychosocial measures for prediction of outcome.[20] However, as Rutter et al[21] have argued, biological factors may well be more important than environmental factors in the subgroup of conduct disorders that persist into adult life. With the exception of a few adoption studies,[22-24] data on the predictive value of biological measures are limited, and few such variables have differentiated aggressive and antisocial subjects from controls.

Two biological measures that have most consistently differentiated adult antisocial and/or aggressive populations in independent studies, ie, cerebrospinal fluid (CSF) 5-hydroxyindoleacetic acid (5-HIAA) concentration and autonomic nervous system (ANS) activity, were selected as possible predictors. Reduced concentrations of the serotonin metabolite, 5-HIAA, in lumbar CSF significantly correlated with aggression in children and adolescents with DBDs, and patients with DBDs had significantly lower CSF 5-HIAA concentrations than pediatric patients with obsessive-compulsive disorder.[25] In adults, follow-up of depressed adults has found low CSF 5-HIAA concentrations to predict suicide attempts,[26-27] while for adult offenders,[28] reduced CSF 5-HIAA concentrations are a risk factor for subsequent aggressive behavior. Similarly, Brown et al[29] reported that a reduced CSF 5-HIAA concentration predicted future discharge as unsuitable for military service.

Low autonomic activity has been related to criminal and aggressive outcomes.[30,31] The following four peripheral indexes of baseline ANS activity were found to predict outcome: (1) rate of spontaneous fluctuations of skin conductance (SFs/min), (2) mean skin conductance level (SCL), (3) mean heart rate (HR), and (4) trials to habituation of skin conductance-orienting responses to a series of brief innocuous tones. A 9-year follow-up of adolescents found that those who were sentenced for a crime during the follow-up interval had significantly lower resting base levels of SFs/min, SCL, and HR.[30] In younger children, low skin conductance activity at the age of 3 years predicted fighting at the age of 9 years.[31] Fast habituation of skin conductance responses characterized inpatients who made violent suicide attempts both retrospectively and on 1-year follow-up.[32] Thorell[33] found lower SFs/min and fewer and smaller skin conductance-orienting responses in suicidal patients compared with that in both nonsuicidal patients and normal controls.

In the present study, the predictive power of CSF 5-HIAA and ANS activity measures is examined in a group of 29 children and adolescents who initially were referred for assessment of DBDs. The patients had lumbar CSF monoamine metabolite concentrations and autonomic measures collected at the first evaluation (time 1). These laboratory measures were part of studies of CSF 5-HIAA concentrations and autonomic reactivity in relation to severity and type of aggression or DBDs (T.P.Z. and M.J.P.K., unpublished data, November 1991).[25]

The main hypothesis that drove this study was that low concentrations of CSF 5-HIAA would predict follow-up among patients with DBDs, specifically severe outcomes in the form of physical aggression and suicide attempts. Other hypothesized relationships that were based on findings from studies, as noted above, were as follows: low CSF homovanillic acid (HVA) concentrations predict suicide attempts; low SFs/min, SCL, and HR each predict arrest; and fast habituation (low trials to habituation) predicts suicide attempts. We also speculated that low 5-HIAA concentrations or ANS activity might predict other adverse outcomes, such as lower global functioning, institutionalization, and substance abuse.

SUBJECTS AND METHODS

Subjects were 29 children and adolescents, with a mean age of 11.3 years (SD, 3.6 years; age range, 6 to 17 years) with DBDs who had had lumbar CSF collected and psychophysiological studies performed during an inpatient evaluation for children and adolescents with DBDs.[25]

During the initial evaluation, we reviewed all available records from previous therapists, hospitals, residential treatment facilities, schools, etc. With the use of the previous data and structured interviews of the child and of at least one parent about the child,[34-36] *DSM-III-R*[37] diagnoses were made. Diagnoses at follow-up were made based on previous information, plus structured and clinical interviews of both patient and at least one parent. Demographic characteristics and diagnoses of the sample are listed in Tables 1 and 2, respectively.

At initial evaluation, parent(s) were interviewed with the Schedule for Affective Disorders and Schizophrenia.[38] The IQ was assessed with the use of the Wechsler Intelligence Scale for Children-Revised[39] or Wechsler Adult Intelligence Scale–Revised,[40] where age appropriate. Additional patient characteristics, details of CSF collection, assay of monoamine metabolites, and age correction have been described elsewhere.[25] All subjects were free of medications for at least 3 weeks before collection of the lumbar puncture and ANS activity measures.

The ANS activity measures that were performed during the baseline evaluation were the determination of the SCL and HR, which were recorded during a 3-minute rest period and a series of 10 tones (80 dB, 1000 Hz) of 1.5 seconds' duration, presented every 20 to 30 seconds to which no response was required. Skin conductance was measured via a constant (0.5-V) voltage system from 0.64

TABLE 1
Demographics of Sample (N = 29) at Time 1 Baseline Evaluation
and at Follow-up*

Demographical Variable	Baseline Evaluation	Follow-up
Age, y	11.3 (3.6)	13.8 (3.9)
Wechsler IQ		
Verbal	103.9 (12.4)	. . .
Performance	103.4 (13.8)	. . .
Full scale	103.3 (12.7)	. . .
Length of follow-up, mo	. . .	26.2 (8.9)
Sex		
M	27 (93)	. . .
F	2 (7)	. . .
Race		
B	5 (17)	. . .
W	22 (76)	. . .
Other	2 (7)	. . .

*For age, Wechsler IQ, and length of follow up, data are given as mean (SD); for sex and race, data are given as number (percentage).

TABLE 2
Diagnoses of Sample at Time 1 Baseline Evaluation and at
Follow-up*

DSM-III-R Diagnoses†	Baseline Evaluation		Follow-up	
	No. (%)	Mean Age (SD), y	No. (%)	Mean Age (SD), y
ADHD	16 (55)	9.8 (3.1)	16 (55)	13.3 (4.1)
Undifferentiated ADD	3 (10)	15.0 (1.7)	4 (14)	13.0 (3.7)
Conduct disorder/ASP	18 (62)	12.8 (3.0)	12 (41)	17.1 (2.2)
Oppositional defiant disorder	4 (14)	9.5 (5.1)	7 (24)	11.1 (2.2)
Affective/anxiety disorder	4 (14)	12.3 (4.3)	4 (14)	11.3 (1.5)
Developmental disorders	7 (24)	9.1 (3.0)	3 (10)	10.7 (1.5)
Substance abuse	2 (7)	16.0 (0)	7 (24)	17.0 (1.4)
Other disorders, including personality disorders other than antisocial	6 (21)	11.7 (4.3)	3 (10)	16.3 (3.1)
No diagnosis	0	. . .	1 (3)	. . .

*ADHD indicates attention-deficit hyperactivity disorder; ADD, attention-deficit disorder; and ASP, antisocial personality disorder.
†Total exceeds 29 as multiple diagnoses were made. Age at follow-up is, in some cases, younger because membership in a diagnostic group was not identical at follow-up.

cm^2 of silver/silver chloride electrodes on the middle and ring fingertips of the left hand with the use of 0.5% potassium chloride in agar electrode paste. The HR was recorded with a tachograph from lead II. The four variables presented here are the SFs/min during the 3-minute rest period, the mean SCL, the HR during the rest period, and the number of trials to habituation of the skin conductance responses to the tones. These had minimum amplitudes of 0.02 microSiemens and onset latencies of 0.8 to 4 seconds. Habituation was defined as two consecutive tones with no elicited response.

Interim Procedure

After initial evaluation, patients were referred to community practitioners for individualized treatment, depending on the results of assessment, family needs and/or preferences, and local treatment opportunities. Follow-up interviews were scheduled after a minimum interval of 14 months.

Follow-up

All 29 patients with DBDs (100%) who had had lumbar punctures were located and interviewed in person. Parent(s) of 24 children were interviewed in person, and parent(s) of another five subjects were interviewed by telephone. The mean ($\pm$SD) follow-up interval between the lumbar puncture and subsequent interview for subjects was 26 ($\pm$8.9) months; the range was 14 to 65 months; and the mode was 24 months. The mean age at follow-up was 13.8 ($\pm$3.9) years, and the age range was 8 to 22 years.

Structured interviews of the patient and parent, including sections of the Diagnostic Interview for Children and Adolescents and the Diagnostic Interview for Children and Adolescents–Parent version[34-36] that covered disruptive behaviors, socialization, affective disorders, and alcohol and other substance abuse, were conducted. Checklist reports about the patient's aggressive actions and their frequencies (N. E. Harnett, PhD, RN, and M.J.P.K., unpublished data, June 1991) were completed by the patient and by a custodial parent. The Child Behavior Checklist[41] was completed by a parent of all subjects who were aged younger than 17 years at follow-up.

Outcome Measures

Outcome measures were selected for aggression, suicide attempts, and arrest(s), as well as for other aspects of overall functioning during the follow-up interval. Based on interview data, as well as review of all other available information, two investigators (E.D.H. and M.J.P.K.) made diagnoses and completed ratings for the following measures to cover the interval from the time of lumbar puncture to the time of follow-up: (1) the Modified Overt Aggression Scale[42] (ie, its Physical Aggression subscale, Autoaggression subscale, and total score); (2) suicide attempt(s) (ie, from self-report of the individual and/or other sources); (3) arrest(s) during follow-up based on parent and/or patient report; (4) the Children's Global Assessment Scale,[43] which evaluates the overall functioning of a patient on a continuum of psychological health and illness; (5) institutionalization, which was defined as the child having been confined during the follow-up interval in psychiatric or substance abuse hospitalization, residential treatment, and/or correctional facilities; and (6) substance abuse diagnosis at follow-up, with the best clinical diagnosis by consensus, utilizing all available information.

Statistical Analysis

The age of the subject was anticipated to be a major confounding factor within the baseline and outcome variables. Some forms of aggression (eg, suicide and homicide) are more frequent in adolescents and young adults than in prepubertal children.[44,45] Age was also significantly (inversely) correlated with 5-HIAA, HVA, HR, and SFs/min measures at baseline. Correlations between age and all baseline measures are shown in Table 3.

The initial analysis used Pearson Product-Moment Correlation Coefficients[46] to establish the bivariate relationships between age and the predictor (baseline laboratory and clinical measures) and outcome variables. Partial correlations, removing the effects of age from both sets of variables, were then calculated to

TABLE 3
Baseline Measures Entered Into Multiple Regression and
Discriminant Function Analyses to Predict Outcome and Their
Correlation with Age (N = 26)*

	r	P
Nonlaboratory measures		
Age of child in months	. . .	. . .
Brown-Goodwin Lifetime History of Aggression	.50	.01
Socioeconomic status of the family	-.26	NS
Presence/absence of antisocial diagnoses in parent(s)	.07	NS
CBCL Aggressive subscale score	-.24	NS
CBCL Social Competence subscale score	-.28	NS
Iowa Conners' Inattention/Overactivity Ward Teacher rating	-.73	.0001
GAS lowest level of functioning— past 6 mo	-.09	NS
Full-scale IQ	.05	NS
Biological laboratory measures		
CSF 5-HIAA concentration	-.59	.002
CSF HVA concentration	-.69	.0001
SFs/min	-.31	NS
SCL	-.20	NS
Trials to habituation of skin conductance–orienting responses to a series of brief tones (trials to habituation)	-.09	NS
Resting HR	-.37	.06

*NS indicates not significant; CBCL, Child Behavior Checklist; GAS, Children's Global Assessment Scale; CSF, cerebrospinal fluid; 5-HIAA, 5-hydroxyindoleacetic acid; HVA, homovanillic acid; SFs/min, rate of spontaneous skin fluctuations per minute; SCL, skin conductance level; and HR, heart rate.

determine whether the hypothesized relationships between predictor and outcome variables existed after the effects of age were partialed out. Although we had one-tailed hypotheses, we conservatively used two-tailed levels of significance.

If a significant relationship was found *after* accounting for the influence of age, we conducted a second tier of analyses. This was performed to explore whether baseline laboratory measures contributed to prediction above and beyond that obtained from the clinical measures. For continuous rating scale outcomes, a non-stepwise multiple regression analysis was performed in which all of the nonlaboratory variables (age, the Children's Global Assessment Scale score, socioeconomic status, IQ, aggression, parental antisocial personality disorder diagnosis, and rating scale scores) were entered as a group. This determined the amount of outcome variance that was accounted for by nonlaboratory measures alone. A second hierarchical regression analysis was then performed; this analysis included the nonlaboratory and the biological laboratory variables (5-HIAA, HVA, and ANS activity measures) as a group to determine the additional variance in the outcome measure that was accounted for by the biological laboratory variables. This was determined by the change in the R^2 from the first regression analysis to the second. A stepwise regression analysis was then performed that included *all* of the predictor variables, to determine which variable had the strongest influence on the outcome variable.

As shown in Table 3, as an exploration, a wide scope of baseline (time 1) measures were introduced into the model for the multivariate analyses.

For dichotomous outcome variables (eg, institutionalization), a BMDP[47] stepwise discriminant analysis with jackknife validation, with the use of the same nonlaboratory and biological predictor variables, was conducted to explore which baseline variables might discriminate between the presence or absence of the outcome. Discriminant function analyses utilized prior probabilities due to differing group sizes.

Patients came from a wide variety of school settings, and nine of the original 29 patients lacked ratings from their usual school—most often because of truancy, expulsion, or other conduct disturbance. So, ratings of inattention/overactivity,[48] derived from the Conners' Teacher Rating Scale,[49] utilized National Institute of Mental Health hospital schoolteacher ratings in preference to the child's usual outside teacher.

Because the repeatedly observed strong correlation of CSF 5-HIAA concentrations with concentrations of HVA, which is a dopamine metabolite, has raised questions about the possible interactions between serotonin and dopamine turnover,[50] as well as questions about the specificity of the CSF 5-HIAA concentration as a marker associated with aggression and suicide, both HVA and 5-HIAA measures were included in the correlation, multiple regression, and discriminant function analyses.

TABLE 4
Correlation and Partial Correlations Correcting for Age of CSF Monoamine Metabolite

			CSF Predictor							
			5-HIAA Concentration				HVA Concentration			
	Age, Correlation		Correlation		Partial Correlation		Correlation		Partial Correlation	
Outcome Measure	r	P	r	P	r	P	r	P	r	P
MOAS										
Physical Aggression subscale score	.70	.0001	-.72	.0001	-.53	.006	-.53	.006	-.08	...
Auto-Aggression subscale score	.35	.08	-.23	...	-.03	...	-.34	.09	-.13	...
Total score	.69	.0001	-.60	.001	-.34	.09	-.57	.002	-.17	...
Suicide attempt	.37	.07	-.38	.06	-.22	...	-.48	.01	-.34	.09
Arrest	.63	.0005	-.42	.03	-.08	...	-.30	.14	.25	...
GAS	-.57	.002	.43	.03	.14	...	.52	.006	.21	...
Institutionalization	.80	.0001	-.47	.02	-.005	...	-.57	.002	-.05	...
Substance abuse	.59	.001	-.23	...	.18	...	-.28	.17	.22	...

RESULTS

Clinical Course and Overall Functioning

The group continued to experience significant difficulties. For example, 12 (41%) of the 29 subjects had been hospitalized, incarcerated, and/or placed in residential treatment, and four (14%) of the 29 subjects had made suicide attempts. The mean (± SD) Children's Global Assessment Scale score at follow-up was 54 (±11.4), which was in the lower half of a 10-point range, indicating that "disturbance would be apparent to those who encounter the child in a dysfunctional setting or time but not to those who see the child in other settings."[43] This range is in between that describing "isolated or sporadic antisocial acts" and that describing "frequent episodes of aggressive or other antisocial behavior with some preservation of meaningful social relationships."

A variety of treatments had been given to the group: 24 (83%) of the 29 subjects had had medication trials or ongoing medication management during follow-up, nine (31%) of the 29 subjects had received inpatient or residential treatment, nine (45%) of 20 subjects who had not had inpatient or residential treatment had individual therapy, and three (15%) of the same 20 subjects had had family therapy. Only one of the 29 subjects could be described as not having had any formal treatment during the follow-up interval. A wide range of other interventions that were aimed at amelioration, such as out-of-home placements, new school placements, tutoring, and juvenile justice system sanctions, also occurred.

Concentrations and ANS Activity Concentrations Measures Collected at Baseline and Outcome Measures*

Age, Correlation		SCL				SFs/min				HR				Trials to Habituation			
		Correlation		Partial Correlation		Correlation		Partial Correlation		Correlation		Partial Correlation		Correlation		Partial Correlation	
r	P	r	P	r	P	r	P	r	P	r	P	r	P	r	P	r	P
.70	.0001	-.005	...	.19	...	-.11	...	.16	...	-.17	...	.14	...	.14	...	.28	.17
.35	.08	.01	...	.09	...	-.17	...	-.07	...	-.35	.08	-.25	...	.05	...	.09	...
.69	.0001	.01	...	.21	...	-.16	...	.09	...	-.31	.12	-.08	...	.07	...	.19	...
.37	.07	-.17	...	-.11	...	-.19	...	-.09	...	-.41	.04	-.32	.12	.03	...	.07	...
.63	.0005	-.18	...	-.07	...	-.04	...	.21	...	-.21	...	.03	...	.05	...	.13	...
.57	.002	.03	...	-.11	...	-.15	...	-.04	...	-.02	...	-.30	.14	-.24	...	-.35	.08
.80	.0001	-.44	.02	-.47	.02	-.40	.04	-.27	.19	-.13	...	.29	.15	-.19	...	-.20	...
.59	.001	-.24	...	-.16	...	-.19	...	-.01	...	-.10	...	.16	...	.04	...	.11	...

Correlational Analysis

No outliers were present. Age correlated significantly with six of eight outcome measures and with two of six baseline laboratory measures as seen in Tables and 3 and 4. Pearson and partial correlations among baseline CSF measures, baseline ANS activity measures, and outcome measures are shown in Table 4. Because of missing baseline data, the sample size was limited to 26.

As shown, 10 of 16 correlations between raw values for CSF measures and outcome were significant ($P<.05$, two tailed). After partialing out the effect of age, one of the hypothesized predictions from the CSF, ie, the inverse correlation between the 5-HIAA concentration and severity of aggression during follow-up, remained highly significant ($P = .006$). However, the hypothesized prediction of the 5-HIAA concentration for suicide attempts was not supported. Statistical trends for inverse correlations between the total score on the Modified Overt Aggression Scale and the 5-HIAA concentration, and between suicide attempts and the HVA concentration were found after partialing out the effect of age. This is a conservative approach, in that if one-tailed P values had been used, as hypothesized, these relationships would reach conventional levels ($P\leqslant.05$) of statistical significance.

Table 4 also shows correlations and partial correlations (accounting for age) between ANS activity measures and outcome variables. Three of 32 possible correlations between raw values were significant. The inverse correlation between SCL and institutionalization remained significant in the predicted direction, after the effect of age was partialed out, with the adverse outcome associated with a lower SCL. Hypothesized prediction of trials to habituation for suicide attempts and of SFs/min, SCL, and HR for arrest were not supported.

Multivariate analyses then explored whether the laboratory measures had any predictive value beyond that offered by more commonly collected clinical measures.

Because physical aggression was related to the 5-HIAA concentration after partialing out the effect of age, multiple regression analyses were carried out to explore whether the laboratory measures had any predictive import for physical aggression beyond that offered by more commonly collected clinical measures. First, a hierarchical multiple regression was carried out with the use of all the baseline nonlaboratory measures as shown in Table 3. As shown in Table 5, the multiple R^2 was .65 for the nonlaboratory measures. A second multiple regression that entered the nonlaboratory measures and the laboratory measures as a set resulted in a multiple R^2 of .91. Thus, laboratory variables significantly explained $(P<.02)$[51] an additional 26% of the variance in the physical aggression outcome variable. Adjusted R^2 values,[51] which corrected for the number of predictor variables that were entered in a multiple regression, showed a greater difference and were also significant. As an additional assessment of the relative import of laboratory and clinical measures, all predictors were competed into a stepwise multiple regression; the 5-HIAA measure was entered into the model first and accounted for 52% of the variance in physical aggression.

Another laboratory measure, ie, SCL, was significantly correlated with the dichotomous outcome of institutionalization. To explore this contribution relative

TABLE 5
Multiple Regression Analyses*

	Cumulative R^2	Adjusted R^2
Multiple regression—hierarchical		
Nonlaboratory measures	.65	.48
Biological laboratory measures and nonlaboratory measures	.91†	.80†
Multiple regression—stepwise		
5-HIAA	.52	.52
Age	.64	.62
Antisocial diagnosis—parent	.70	.67
IQ	.75	.72

*Amount of variance (R^2) in Physical Aggression subscale of the Modified Overt Aggression Scale (outcome) that was predicted by nonlaboratory and laboratory baseline measures. 5-HIAA indicates 5-hydroxyindoleacetic acid.

†Amount of additional variance explained over model that used only nonlaboratory measures was statistically significant ($P<.02$).

TABLE 6
Discriminant Analysis: Prediction of Institutionalization During
2-Year Follow-up of DBDs (N = 26)*

Institutionalization, Total Group (+ = 11, − = 15)	Cumulative R^2	Jackknife Classification, %
Age (+, older)	.64	−100
SCL (+, lower)	.72	+91†
HR (+, lower)	.84	96

*DBDs indicates disruptive behavior disorders; plus sign, the outcome occurred (eg, 11 were institutionalized); minus sign, outcome did not occur; SCL, skin conductance level; and HR, heart rate.
†Before the jackknife procedure, 100% of those who were institutionalized were correctly classified by the three predictor variables.

to clinical measures, a stepwise discriminant function analysis was conducted by utilizing all of the baseline variables. Results are shown in Table 6.

The biological laboratory measures, ie, SCL and HR, added significantly to the prediction.

COMMENT

This 2-year prospective follow-up study found that laboratory-based biological parameters, such as the CSF 5-HIAA concentration and SCL, offered significant predictive information for severity of physical aggression and institutionalization as outcomes for children with DBDs. Hypothesized relationships among 5-HIAA concentrations, trials to habituation, and suicide attempts were not found. Low ANS activity also failed to predict arrest.

The biological laboratory measures that did predict outcome not only had significant correlations with follow-up after partialing out the effect of age, but contributed significantly in the multivariate analyses even after clinical measures, which numerous earlier studies had identified as important predictors, such as aggressivity/previous antisocial behavior[8-10,52,53] and IQ,[10,53] as well as family factors, including parental mental health[10,52-55] and socioeconomic status,[56] were forced into the model first. To our knowledge, this is the first report that has combined CSF and clinical measures in a prospective study of DBDs. The findings from this present report confirm earlier suggestions[57,58] of the predictive validity of the CSF 5-HIAA concentration in children with disruptive disorders, are generally consistent with the findings from other studies with regard to the predictive import of ANS activity,[30,59] and suggest that further study of biological factors in adverse outcomes among patients with DBDs is warranted.

Observed trends in the partial correlations are consistent with those of other studies and would have reached significance if one-tailed statistics had been used. Our results extend the findings from adult studies that lower CSF HVA concentrations can predict future suicide attempts[26,27] in children and adolescents. The trend for fast habituation to predict better global functioning at follow-up is not consistent with the idea that lower ANS activity is associated with worse outcomes. However, that trend is similar to findings in acute schizophrenia,[60,61] relating slow habituation to poor short-term outcome, and to similar findings from a recent 3- to 5-year follow-up study of children and adolescents with obsessive-compulsive disorder.[62]

Just how much laboratory measures add to the prediction by comparison with data from studies that utilized clinical variables only[9,53] is difficult to quantify. Methodological, sample, and definitional differences, and limits of data accessible from other studies, as well as limitations inherent in this study, prevent more precise quantification.

There are several other limitations to this study. Age at intake correlated with all outcome measures at a significance level of $P \leqslant .08$, and our initial wide age spread was thus unfortunate. However, even within more narrow age samples, such as that of Loney et al,[10] age at referral predicted involvement with alcohol, probably reflecting the fact that for many outcomes, there are age-related periods of risk. Thus, one perspective is that it is even more remarkable that the laboratory measures showed any predictive value. Nonetheless, future studies must focus on a more narrow age range to avoid these limitations.

The follow-up interval is relatively brief; patients are still "at risk," and ultimate outcome is still unknown. Loeber et al[63] documented continuities and discontinuities in aggressive behavior and suggested that 4-year follow-up intervals give greater accuracy. However, even briefer follow-up intervals in adult subjects found prediction of CSF 5-HIAA or HVA measures for suicide attempts during (1-year) follow-up intervals,[26,32] while Virkkunen et al[28] found significantly lower CSF 5-HIAA concentrations in those who committed a new offense during the 3 years following release from correctional facilities.

Our relatively short follow-up period may have yielded a low estimate of the predictive power of autonomic measures. Correlations between ANS activity measures and outcome measures were generally in an inverse direction, as expected. However, only one correlation between ANS activity measures and outcomes reached statistical significance after the effect of age was partialed out. The ANS activity measures did not, as hypothesized, predict which eight of 26 subjects had been arrested during the follow-up. The follow-up studies of pediatric samples that found ANS activity measures predicted later aggression or criminality[31,59] had follow-up intervals of 6 to 9 years. Yet, cross-sectional studies of relationships between ANS activity measures and aggressive or conduct disturbance in this and other pediatric samples have not consistently shown significant associations.[64]

Some synergistic risk factors have not yet entered the picture for many of these patients. Alcohol, for example, may significantly increase risk for individuals with low 5-HIAA concentrations.[27]

The consistency of findings in pediatric cases with those in adults makes the further study of relationships of CSF monoamine metabolite concentrations and autonomic activity in pediatric samples with severe intractable aggression of both clinical and research importance.

REFERENCES

1. Reeves JC, Werry JS, Elkind GS, Zametkin A. Attention deficit, conduct, oppositional, and anxiety disorders in children, II: clinical characteristics. *J Am Acad Child Adolesc Psychiatry.* 1987;26:144–155.

2. Gittelman R, Mannuzza S, Shenker R, Bonagura R. Hyperactive boys almost grown up, I: psychiatric status. *Arch Gen Psychiatry,* 1985;42:937–947.

3. Weiss G, Hechtman L, Milroy T, Perlman T. Psychiatric status of hyperactives as adults: a controlled prospective 15-year follow-up of 63 hyperactive children. *J Am Acad Child Adolesc Psychiatry.* 1985;24:211–220.

4. Mannuzza S, Klein RG, Bonagura R, Malloy P, Giampino TL, Addalli KA. Hyperactive boys almost grown up, V: replication of psychiatric status. *Arch Gen Psychiatry.* 1991;48:77–83.

5. Mannuzza S, Gittelman-Klein R, Konig PH, Giampino TL. Hyperactive boys almost grown up, IV: criminality and its relationship to psychiatric status. *Arch Gen Psychiatry.* 1989;46:1073–1079.

6. August GJ, Stewart MA, Holmes CS. A four-year follow-up of hyperactive boys with and without conduct disorder. *Br J Psychiatry.* 1983;143:192–198.

7. Rutter M. Pathways from childhood to adult life. *J Child Psychol Psychiatry.* 1989;30:23–51.

8. Robins LN. *Deviant Children Grown Up.* Baltimore, Md: Williams & Wilkins; 1966.

9. Robins LN. Sturdy childhood predictors of adult antisocial behavior: replications from longitudinal studies. *Psychol Med.* 1978;8:611–622.

10. Loney J, Kramer J, Milich RS. The hyperactive child grows up: predictors of symptoms, delinquency and achievement at follow-up. In: Gadow JD, Loney J, eds. *Psychosocial Aspects of Drug Treatment for Hyperactivity: AAAS Selected Symposium.* Boulder, Colo: Westview Press Inc; 1981;44:381–416.

11. Pfeffer CR, Plutchik R, Mizruchi MS. Predictors of assaultiveness in latency age children. *An J Psychiatry.* 1983;140:31–35.

12. Huesmann LR, Eron LD. Cognitive processes and the persistence of aggressive behavior. *Aggress Behav.* 1984;10:243–251.

13. Roff JD, Wirt RD. Childhood aggression and social adjustment as antecedents of delinquency. *J Abnorm Child Psychol.* 1984;12:111–126.

14. Stattin H, Magnusson D. The role of early aggressive behavior in the frequency, seriousness, and types of later crime. *J Consult Clin Psychol.* 1989;57:710–718.

15. Feldhusen JF, Aversano FM, Thurston JR. Prediction of youth contacts with law enforcement agencies. *Criminal Justice Behav.* 1976;3:235–253.

16. Ensminger ME, Kellam SG, Rubin BR. School and family origins of delinquency: comparison by sex. In: van Dusen K, Mednick S, eds. *Prospective Studies of Crime and Delinquency.* Boston, Mass: Kluwer/Nijhoff; 1983:73–97.

17. Douglas JWB. The school progress of nervous and troublesome children. *Br J Psychiatry.* 1966;112:1115–1116.

18. Morris HH, Escoll PJ, Wexler MSW. Aggressive behavior disorders in children: a follow-up study. *Am J Psychiatry.* 1956;112:991–997.

19. Loeber R, Stouthamer-Loeber M. Prediction. In: Quay HC, ed. *Handbook of Juvenile Delinquency.* New York, NY: John Wiley & Sons Inc; 1987:324–382.

20. Loeber R, Dishion T. Early predictors of male delinquency: a review. *Psychol Bull.* 1983;94:68–99.

21. Rutter M, MacDonald H, Le Couteur A, Harrington R, Bolton P, Bailey A. Genetic factors in child psychiatric disorders, II: empirical findings. *J Child Psychol Psychiatry.* 1990;31:39–83.

22. Mednick SA, Gabrielli WF, Hutchings B. Genetic influences in criminal convictions: evidence from an adoption cohort. *Science.* 1984;224:891–894.

23. Cloninger CR, Sigvardson S, Bowman M, von Knorring AL. Predisposition to petty criminality in Swedish adoptees. *Arch Gen Psychiatry.* 1982;39:1242–1247.

24. Crowe RR. An adoption study of antisocial personality. *Arch Gen Psychiatry.* 1974;31:785–791.

25. Kruesi MJP, Rapoport JL, Hamburger S, Hibbs E, Potter WZ, Lenane M, Brown GL. CSF monoamine metabolites, aggression and impulsivity in disruptive behavior disorders of children and adolescents. *Arch Gen Psychiatry.* 1990;47:419–426.

26. Traskman L, Asberg M, Bertilsson L, Sjostrand L. Monoamine metabolites in CSF and suicidal behavior. *Arch Gen Psychiatry.* 1981;38:631–636.

27. Roy A, Dejong RA, Linnoila M. Cerebrospinal fluid monoamine metabolites and suicidal behavior in depressed patients. *Arch Gen Psychiatry.* 1989;46:609–612.

28. Virkkunen M, De Jong J, Bartko J, Goodwin FK, Linnoila M. Relationship of psychobiological variables to recidivism in violent offenders and impulsive fire setters: a follow-up study. *Arch Gen Psychiatry.* 1989;46:604–606.

29. Brown GL, Ballanger JC, Minichiello MD, Goodwin FK. Human aggression and its relationship to cerebrospinal fluid 5-hydroxyindoleacetic acid, 3-methoxy-4-hydroxyphenylglycol, and homovanillic acid. In: Sandler M, ed. *Psychopharmacology of Aggression.* New York, NY: Raven Press; 1979:131–148.

30. Raine A, Venables PH, Williams M. Relationships between central and autonomic measures of arousal at age 15 and criminality at age 24. *Arch Gen Psychiatry.* 1990;47:1003–1007.

31. Venables PH. Childhood markers for adult disorders. *J Child Psychol Psychiatry.* 1989;30:347–364.

32. Edman G, Asberg M, Levander S, Schalling D. Skin conductance habituation and cerebrospinal fluid 5-hydroxyindoleacetic acid in suicidal patients. *Arch Gen Psychiatry.* 1985;43:586–592.

33. Thorell LH. Electrodermal activity in suicidal and non-suicidal depressive patients and in matched healthy subjects. *Acta Psychiatr Scand.* 1987;76:420–430.

34. Herjanic B, Campbell W. Differentiating psychiatrically disturbed children on the basis of a structured interview. *J Abnorm Child Psychol.* 1977;5:127–134.

35. Welner Z, Reich W, Herjanic B, Jung K, Amado H. Reliability, validity and child agreement studies of the Diagnostic Interview for Children and Adolescents (DICA). *J Am Acad Child Adolesc Psychiatry.* 1987;26:649–653.

36. Herjanic B, Reich W. Development of a structured psychiatric interview for children: agreement between child and parent on individual symptoms. *J Abnorm Child Psychol.* 1982;10:307–324.

37. American Psychiatric Association, Committee on Nomenclature and Statistics. *Diagnostic and Statistical Manual of Mental Disorders, Revised Third Edition.* Washington, DC: American Psychiatric Association; 1987.

38. Endicott J, Spitzer RL. A diagnostic interview: the Schedule for Affective Disorders and Schizophrenia. *Arch Gen Psychiatry.* 1978;35:837–844.

39. Wechsler D. *Wechsler Intelligence Scale for Children–Revised.* New York, NY: Psychological Corp; 1974.

40. Wechsler D. *Wechsler Adult Intelligence Scale–Revised.* New York, NY: Psychological Corp; 1981.

41. Achenbach TM, Edelbrock C. *Manual for the Child Behavior Checklist and Revised Child Behavior Profile.* Burlington, Vt: University of Vermont Department of Psychiatry; 1983.

42. Kay SR, Wolkenfield F, Murrill LM. Profiles of aggression among psychiatric patients, I: nature and prevalence. *J Nerv Ment Dis.* 1988;176:539–546.

43. Shaffer D, Gould MS, Brasic J, Ambrosini P, Fisher P, Bird H, Aluwahlia S. A Children's Global Assessment Scale. *Arch Gen Psychiatry.* 1983;40:1228–1231.

44. Daly M, Wilson M. Killing the competition. *Hum Nature.* 1990;1:81–107.

45. Hoberman HM, Garfinkel BD. Completed suicide in children and adolescents. *J Am Acad Child Adolesc Psychiatry.* 1988;27:689–695.

46. SAS Institute. *User's Guide: Statistics, Version 5.* Cary, NC: SAS Institute; 1985.

47. Dixon WJ, Brown MB, Engelman L, Frane JW, Hill MA, Jennrich RI, Toporek JD. *BMDP Statistical Software: 1983 Printing With Additions.* Berkeley, Calif: University of California Press; 1983.

48. Loney J, Milich R. Hyperactivity, inattention, and aggression in clinical practice. In: Wolraich M, Routh D, eds. *Advances in Developmental and Behavioral Pediatrics.* Greenwich, Conn: JAI Press Inc; 1985:113–147.

49. Conners CK. A teacher rating scale for use in drug studies with children. *Am J Psychiatry.* 1969;126:884–888.
50. Agren H, Mefford IN, Rudorfer MV, Linnoila M, Potter WZ. Interacting neurotransmitter systems: a non-experimental approach to the 5HIAA-HVA correlation in human CSF. *J Psychiatr Res.* 1986;20:175–193.
51. Draper NR, Smith H. *Applied Regression Analysis.* 2nd ed. New York, NY: John Wiley & Sons Inc; 1981:91.
52. Weiss G, Minde K, Werry JS, Douglas VI, Nemeth E. Studies on the hyperactive child, VIII: five-year follow-up. *Arch Gen Psychiatry.* 1971;24:409–414.
53. Weiss G, Hechtman L. *Hyperactive Children Grown Up.* New York, NY: Guilford Press; 1986.
54. Mendelson WB, Johnson NE, Stewart MA. Hyperactive children as teenagers: a follow-up study. *J Nerv Ment Dis.* 1971;153:273–278.
55. Barkley RA, Fischer M, Edelbrock CS, Smallish L. The adolescent outcome of hyperactive children diagnosed by research criteria, I: an 8-year prospective follow-up study. *J Am Acad Child Adolesc Psychiatry.* 1990;29:546–557.
56. Duyme M. Antisocial behavior and postnatal environment: a French adoption study. *J Child Psychol Psychiatry.* 1990;31:699–710.
57. Kruesi MJP, Linnoila M, Rapoport JL, Brown GL, Petersen R. Carbohydrate craving, conduct disorder and low 5-HIAA. *Psychiatry Res.* 1985;16:83–86.
58. Kruesi MJP. Cruelty to animals and CSF 5-HIAA. *Psychiatry Res.* 1989;28:115–116.
59. Raine A, Venables PH, Williams M. Autonomic-orienting responses in 15-year-old male subjects and criminal behavior at age 24. *Am J Psychiatry.* 1990;147:933–937.
60. Zahn TP, Carpenter WTJ, McGlashan TH. Autonomic nervous system activity in acute schizophrenia, II: relationships to short-term prognosis and clinical state. *Arch Gen Psychiatry.* 1981;38(3):260–266.
61. Frith CD, Stevens M, Johnstone EC, Crow TJ. Skin conductance responsivity during acute episodes of schizophrenia as a predictor of symptomatic improvement. *Psychol Med.* 1979;9:101–106.
62. Flament MF, Koby E, Rapoport JL, Berg CJ, Zahn T, Cox C, Denckla M, Lenane M. Childhood obsessive-compulsive disorder: a prospective follow-up study. *J Child Psychol Psychiatry.* 1990;31:363–380.
63. Loeber R, Trembalay RE, Gagnon L, Charlebois P. Continuity and desistance in disruptive boys: early fighting in school. *Dev Psychopathology.* 1989;1:39–50.
64. Garralda ME, Connell J, Taylor DC. Psychophysiological anomalies in children with emotional and conduct disorders. *Psychol Med.* 1991;21:947–957.

Part V

OTHER CLINICAL ISSUES

The papers in this section address a range of issues important to investigators and clinicians concerned with the diagnosis and treatment of psychiatric disorders in children and adolescents. In the first paper, Rogeness, Javors, and Pliszka provide a thorough review of the neurochemistry and neurophysiology of three neurotransmitters: dopamine (DA), norepinephrine (NE), and serotonin (5HT). Selection was guided by fact that the DA, NE, and 5HT systems appear to be important in the interaction and regulation of an individual's behavior with the external environment. The anatomical distribution of the biogenic amines, each having their cell bodies located in a few centers from which they innervate many common areas of the brain, is consistent with the biogenic amines having a modulatory or regulatory role on brain systems. Dysregulation or imbalances in the biogenic amine systems could be important in the pathophysiology of several child psychiatric disorders. The authors review neurochemical studies of childhood major depression, ADHD, conduct disorder, and Tourette's disorder. The methodology available to measure neurotransmitter function in children is many steps removed from the processes taking place in vivo, making interpretation of results difficult. The evidence for neurochemical dysregulation in Tourette's disorder currently is greater and perhaps better understood than in other child psychiatric disorders. However, technical advances are being made at a rapid rate. This clear and thoughtful review provides not only a summary of the status of the field to date, but a sound basis for assessing and integrating new knowledge.

The impetus for the second paper in this section derives from the observation that fathers are dramatically underrepresented in research on developmental psychopathology. Phares and Compas provide a useful summary of the relationship between paternal factors and the emergence of psychopathological conditions during childhood and adolescence. It should come as no surprise that findings from studies of clinically referred children, clinically referred fathers, as well as nonreferred samples of children and their fathers all indicate that paternal behaviors, personality characteristics, and psychopathology are significant sources of risk for child and adolescent psychopathology. The evidence from studies of clinically referred or diagnosed fathers and of nonreferred fathers and children indicates that paternal factors are related to a wide range of both externalizing and internalizing disorders in their children. In studies of clinically referred children and their fathers, however, paternal factors were more strongly associated with externalizing problems. The authors interpret the evidence as indicating that the

301

presence of paternal psychopathology is a sufficient, but not a necessary condition for the emergence of symptoms of behavioral and/or emotional disorder during the developmental period, and suggest that future research be directed towards clarifying the mechanisms through which characteristics of fathers exert their effects.

Leonard and colleagues report the results of a systematic investigation of tics and Tourette's disorder among children with obsessive-compulsive disorder and their families. Fifty-four children who had participated in treatment protocols for obsessive-compulsive disorder were reassessed two to seven years later. Children with Tourette's disorder were excluded from the initial study, but those with chronic vocal or motor tics were not. The presence or absence of tics and Tourette's disorder at follow-up was established in the course of a structured psychiatric interview and neurologic examination. A total of 171 first-degree relatives were also screened for tic disorders. At follow-up 59% (N = 32) had lifetime histories of tics, and eight of these met criteria for Tourette's disorder. The rate of obsessive-compulsive disorder as well as tics in first-degree relatives was higher than published estimates, and was independent of the proband's tic status. The findings are interpreted as supporting the hypothesis that in some cases, obsessive-compulsive disorder and Tourette's disorder may be alternative manifestations of the same underlying genetically transmitted illness. Patients with Tourette's disorder had an earlier age of onset of obsessive-compulsive symptoms than those who were without tics, but the nature of their obsessions and compulsions were essentially no different from those of the remainder of the sample. However, a few patients exhibited behavior that was difficult to categorize as a ritual or tic. Typically a ritual is performed in response to a specific thought and a tic in response to an urge. Examples of behaviors that were difficult to classify included that of a boy who spit after the thought his mouth was contaminated, and that of another boy who "compulsively" bounced a ball and touched his fingers rhythmically because his "bones made him do it." These observations suggest the possibility that there may be a spectrum of behaviors ranging from the classical tics of patients with Tourette's disorder to a mixed picture of tics and rituals to clear-cut rituals.

In the final paper in this section, Caplan, Guthrie, and Foy compare the discourse characteristics (use of linguistic devices that tie speech together) of 31 schizophrenic children whose mean CA was 10.2 ± 1.5 and whose mean MA was 9.1 ± 2.0 with those of MA matched normal controls. In addition, relations between discourse characteristics and formal thought disorder were examined within the schizophrenic group. The patients all met DSM-III criteria for schizophrenia, and children with a history of neurological, language, or hearing disorder were excluded from both the patient and control groups. Speech samples were elicited in the course of the administration of the Kiddie Formal Thought Disorder

Game. At the time of testing 52% of the schizophrenic children were receiving neuroleptic medication. Reliable ratings of videotapes yielded frequency counts of the following signs of thought disorder: illogical thinking, loose associations, incoherence, and poverty of content of speech. Frequency counts of discourse characteristics including cohesive ties, referential cohesion, conjunction, and lexical cohesion were also obtained. As has been reported in studies of schizophrenic adults, schizophrenic children speak less than normal mental age matched subjects, and their speech does not provide the listener with as many links (cohesive ties) to previous utterances or with as many references (referential cohesion) to people, objects, or events. As do thought-disordered adults, schizophrenic children with loose associations also confuse the listener by the unclear and ambiguous way they refer to people, objects and events in their speech. While these discourse similarities provide evidence for the comparability of adult and childhood onset schizophrenia, the schizophrenic children of the present study were found to have additional discourse deficits that distinguish their speech from that of adult patients. They provide the listener with fewer connectives, repeat words or word roots less often, and exhibit more frequent deletions than do normal children—abnormalities that can be interpreted as reflecting developmental delays. Comparison of the speech of medicated and nonmedicated children suggests that neuroleptics might have two contrasting effects on the communication skills of schizophrenic children. On the one hand, medication appears to decrease some psychotic aspects of the schizophrenic child's speech; medicated children had lower loose association scores. On the other hand, neuroleptics also appear to impinge upon such nonpsychotic aspects of speech as verbal productivity and cohesive devices.

14

Neurochemistry and Child and Adolescent Psychiatry

Graham A. Rogeness, Martin A. Javors, and Steven R. Pliszka
University of Texas Health Science Center, San Antonio

This article reviews some of the neurochemistry and neurophysiology of three neurotransmitters: dopamine, norepinephrine, and serotonin. These neurotransmitters are selected because they appear to be involved in the regulation of several important behavioral systems that help regulate the interaction of the organism with its external environment, because many of the psychotropic drugs' modes of action may result from their effects on these neurotransmitter systems, and because the majority of neurochemical studies in child psychiatry have focused on these three neurotransmitters. After the review of the neurotransmitter systems, neurochemical studies in several child psychiatric disorders are reviewed to illustrate possible biochemical/ behavioral relationships in child psychiatry.

There are at least 30 neurotransmitters (NTs) in the CNS (Coyle, 1985), most or all of which may have varying roles in behavioral patterns seen in psychiatric disorders. In this article, we will be reviewing three NTs: norepinephrine (NE), dopamine (DA), and serotonin (5HT), and ways in which their function may be important in child psychiatric disorders. These three are selected because 1) they appear to be involved in the regulation of several important behavioral systems that help regulate the interaction of the organism with its external environment, 2) many of the psychotropic drugs' modes of action may be due to their effects on these NTs, and 3) the majority of neurochemical studies in child psychiatry

Reprinted with permission from *Journal of the American Academy of Child and Adolescent Psychiatry*, 1992, Vol. 31(5), 765–781. Copyright © 1992 by the American Academy of Child and Adolescent Psychiatry.

This work was supported by grants from the Meadows Foundation and the San Antonio Area Foundation.

have focused on these three NTs. Limiting this review to these three NTs and not discussing some of their interactions with and regulation by other NTs is an over-simplification, but one that facilitates the presentation and understanding of the information.

In this report, we will describe some of the ways in which these three NTs are regulated neurochemically, and how they theoretically may be involved in the function and/or regulation of several behavioral systems. Based on these theories, we will make hypotheses regarding how different relationships among these three NT systems may affect behavior and relate to psychiatric disorders in children. We will then summarize neurochemical methods currently used to try to obtain a measure of the functioning of these NT systems and review neurochemical studies in several child psychiatric disorders, examining whether or not the data provide any support for the proposed hypotheses.

REGULATION OF NEUROTRANSMITTER FUNCTION

The activity of a neurotransmitter at a synapse is regulated in multiple ways. These ways suggest that there are many safeguards within the brain to keep systems in balance. For the sake of description, we will divide regulation into "within system" regulation and "outside system" regulation.

Within system regulation. NTs have mechanisms for self-regulation. For example, availability and effectiveness of 5HT at a synapse would be influenced by precursor availability, synthesizing enzymes, metabolic enzymes, release and reuptake of 5HT at the synapse, and pre- and postsynaptic receptor function. Table 1 shows these steps for DA, NE, and 5HT, and Table 2 shows steps in chemical transmission at the synapse. There are pharmacological agents that alter function at each of these steps. For example, reserpine interferes with storage of NTs in synaptic vesicles, MAO inhibitors inhibit their degradation by MAO, tricyclic antidepressants inhibit the reuptake by nerve terminals, clonidine stimulates presynaptic $\alpha 2$ receptors to inhibit release of NE, neuroleptics block postsynaptic DA receptors, and lithium affects the second messenger phosphatidylinositol system. One can look at the many steps in regulation as either many possible ways for a system to get out of balance or many ways in which a system may compensate if one part of the system gets out of balance. The system may also be able to be in balance at normal activity, but be unable to stay in balance during increased activity (when stressed). For example, sufficient precursor may be available to maintain balance during normal activity, but not during increased activity, therefore depleting the availability of NT and interfering with the optimum functioning of the system.

Outside system regulation. A neuron using a specific NT connects with neurons using other NTs. For example, serotonergic neurons connect with nonserotonergic

TABLE 1
Neurotransmitter Metabolic and Receptor Chacteristics

	Dopamine	Norepinephrine	Serotonin
Precursors	Phenylalanine, tyrosine	Phenylalanine, tyrosine	Tryptophan
Synthetic enzymes (rate-limiting)	Tyrosine hydroxylase	Tyrosine hydroxylase Dopamine-β-hydroxylase	Tryptophan hydroxylase
Storage	Synaptic vesicles	Synaptic vesicles	Synaptic vesicles
Catabolic enzymes			
Intracellular	MAO	MAO	MAO
Extracellular	COMT	COMT	
Receptors			
Presynaptic	D_2, D_3	α_2	5HT1A, 5HT1D
Postsynaptic	D_1, D_2, D_3	α_1, α_2, β_1, β_2	5HT1A, 5HT1C, 5H1D, 5HT2, 5HT3
Second messengers	cAMP, Ca++, DAG, IP3, K+	cAMP, Ca+, IP3, arachadonic acid, phosphatidic acid	cAMP, Ca++, IP3, DAG, K+

cAMP = adenosine 3', 5'-cyclic phosphate, COMT = erthrocyte catecho-O-methyltransferase, MAO = monoamine oxidase.

TABLE 2
Chemical Transmission

Initiation of transmission
  Release of presynaptic NT
  Binding of NT to postsynaptic receptors
  Activation of receptors
  Regulation of second messengers
Termination of transmission
  Excitation of presynaptic terminal ended, therefore no further NT being released
  Depletion of NT and no more available for release
  Binding of NT to presynaptic receptors turns off the release of NT
  Reuptake of NT by the presynaptic terminal
  Metabolism by extracellular enzymes such as COMT; intracellular metabolism by MAO depleting NT available for release or rerelease

neurons. The neuron has autoreceptors at different sites that assist in self-regulation as well as postsynaptic receptors receiving signals from other neurons. The activity of that neuron is therefore dependent on regulation from other neurons as well as regulation within its own NT system. This outside regulation also works to maintain the system in balance and to respond optimally when needed.

In the next section, we will describe the location of the three NT systems in the brain and the subtypes of receptors for the three NTs. Major advances have been made in the classification of receptors and in the understanding of how they function when activated. It is likely that advances in this area will lead to new pharmacological treatments and a better understanding of brain-behavior relationships. For more details regarding the synthesis and metabolism of DA, NE, and 5HT, see Cooper et al. (1986a, 1986b).

NEUROCHEMISTRY AND NEUROANATOMY

Location of Neurotransmitter Systems and Description of Receptors

Location of CNS biogenic amine neuronal systems. The dopaminergic, noradrenergic, and serotonergic systems are shown schematically in Figure 1 (Bjorklund and Lindvall, 1984; Cooper et al., 1986a). Dopamine cell bodies are present in two midbrain regions: the substantia nigra and ventral tegmental area. Noradrenergic cell bodies occur in the locus coeruleus and the lateral tegmental areas of the brain. Serotonergic cell bodies are located in the midline or raphe regions of the pons and upper brain stem. As shown in Figure 2, the axons from the cell bodies project to virtually all areas of the brain, and the three NT systems innervate many common areas of the brain. In addition, direct interaction among these three neuronal systems has been demonstrated. Although the regulation of the balance among these systems requires more study, the common areas of innervation and their direct interconnection support the hypothesis that the balance among the three NT systems may be important in the regulation and expression of behavior.

Classification and subtypes for DA, NE, and 5HT receptors. A receptor is a protein or glycoprotein in the plasma membrane whose exposed surface can specifically bind various types of chemical compounds or ligands. A receptor is classified in a variety of ways. First, a receptor is classified according to the NTs that bind to it. For example, receptors that bind the DA, NE, and 5HT with high affinity are called dopaminergic, adrenergic, and serotonergic receptors, respectively. These types of receptors have been more specifically classified into subtypes based on the differences discovered in: 1) their affinity for their particular NT and the affinity of drugs for the receptor (pharmacology), 2) the location of the receptors (tissue distribution), 3) the gene(s) that encodes for the receptor pro-

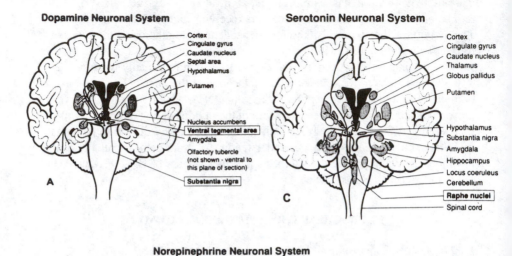

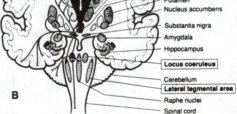

Figure 1. *(Left)* Schematic drawings of neuronal systems in coronal section of human brain. Brain structures are shown on both sides of the drawing. On the right side are listed the names of the brain structures. On the left side the solid lines represent axonal projections from cell bodies *(solid circles)* to the innervated brain structures. *A*, Dopaminergic neuronal system. *B*, Adrenergic (norepinephrine) neuronal system. *C*, Serotonergic neuronal system.

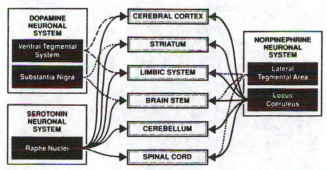

Figure 2. Schematic drawing showing projections of dopaminergic, adrenergic, and serotonergic systems into common areas of the brain.

tein (molecular biology), and 4) the intracellular activity that the receptor can activate (transduction system).

The subtypes of the receptors for the three NTs and their pre-and postsynaptic location are shown in Table 1. The activation of presynaptic receptors (called autoreceptors) inhibits the release of NT, and the activation of postsynaptic receptors alters the cellular activity of postsynaptic neurons. The presence and/or density of the receptor subtypes varies in different brain regions. For example, D3 receptors are mostly present in discrete brain areas belonging to or related to the limbic system (Sokoloff et al., 1990).

In addition to the receptor subtypes having different locations and different affinities for NTs and affinities for drugs, there are differences in the transduction system that the receptor subtypes activate to produce an intracellular effect.

Membrane transducing systems for DA, NE, and 5HT neuronal systems in the CNS. A membrane transducing system is a cluster of proteins and lipids that usually consists of a receptor, a G protein, and a catalytic subunit (enzyme) or ion channel (Fig. 3). The receptor is embedded in the plasma membrane and is exposed on both the extracellular and intracellular sides of the plasma membrane. Specific agonists for a receptor bind to its extracellular surface with high specificity and activate the G protein that associates with a specific receptor. G proteins can activate (Gs) or inhibit (Gi) enzymes or ion channels to which they are coupled. This physiological action results in an increase or decrease of intracellular second messengers. The level of second messengers in the cell cytoplasm or membrane dictate the biochemical activity of the cell.

All of the NE, DA, and 5HT receptor types interact with G proteins. Recent studies (Gilman, 1989) have revealed that G proteins are made up of three protein subunits (α, β, and τ). The α subunit of Gs and Gi proteins binds either GDP

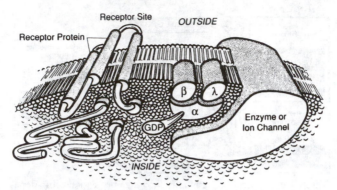

Figure 3. Schematic drawing of a plasma membrane transduction system. The plasma membrane consists of a double layer of phospholipids *(ball and stick models)* in which are embedded various types of proteins. The receptor component of the transduction system is a protein comprised of seven membrane spanning sections with inner and outer membrane loops. This general receptor structure is identical for dopaminergic, adrenergic, and serotonergic receptors. The regulatory G protein, which can be inhibitory or stimulatory, consists of α, β, and τ subunits. GDP is bound to the G protein on the α subunit. When an agonist binds to the receptor, GDP is replaced by GTP, and the activated α subunit stimulates or inhibits the activity of an ion channel or enzyme associated with the particular receptor. Only a general structure is drawn for the functional component of the transduction system, which can be an enzyme or an ion channel. A wide variety of functions are associated with this structure.

(inactive form) or GTP (active form). When the agonist (NE, DA, 5HT) binds to the receptor protein on the outside of the membrane, the G protein on the inside of the membrane is activated. This activation results in the separation of the α subunit from the β and τ subunit of the G protein. The separated active α subunit either stimulates or inhibits the functional activity of the transducing system (Brown and Birnbaummer, 1988; Gilman, 1989). This activity could be an ion channel or enzyme function that regulates the levels of second messengers inside the cell. It is the interaction of second messengers in the cytosolic compartment that determines cellular neuronal function.

There is additional diversity of function between cell types at the level of second messenger function. Second messengers are intracellular atoms or molecules that produce the activation or inactivation of some intracellular biochemical or physiological activity as a function of second messenger concentration. In general, adenosine $3',5'$-cyclic phosphate (cAMP) as a second messenger will cause the phosphorylation of several proteins (usually protein kinases that activate or inactivate other enzymes) within a given cell type. These kinases will vary with cell type, conferring additional specificity for cAMP function. Ca^{++} (calcium ion), also an important and well-studied second messenger, will bind to an intracellular protein called calmodulin in a ratio of 4:1. The resulting Ca* calmodulin complex will also cause the phosphorylation of several proteins, probably enzymes. Although the scope of this report does not allow a detailed discussion of second messenger induced cellular changes, second messenger action includes effects on membrane ion channels, intracellular enzymes, protein kinases, and transcription and translation processes.

Coexistence of peptide NTs with amine NTs. We will only note, but not discuss, the recent discovery that peptide NTs coexist in nerve terminals previously thought to contain only NE, 5HT, or DA. These peptides may be coreleased with the traditional NTs on activation of a neuron. The consideration of the relative effects of the two NTs presents a whole new level of complexity in the CNS that may have significance at the physiological and behavioral level.

Methods of Measurement of NT Function

Strategies to examine for NT differences in child psychiatric disorders have included the measurement of NTs and their metabolites in urine, blood, and cerebrospinal fluid (CSF), measurement of enzymes, studies on platelets, and pharmacological probes. The use of positive emission tomography imaging is a new technique to study NT function, but its use is in its infancy in child psychiatry (Kuperman et al., 1990). Newer molecular biology techniques involving gene expression may add significantly to our knowledge of child psychiatric disorders but are beyond the scope of this review. Some of the advantages and disadvantages of the above techniques are shown in Table 3. For more details regarding the measurement of NT function in child disorders, see Rasmusson et al. (1990).

Integrating Neurochemistry and Neuroanatomy

Increasingly, understanding hypotheses about the neurobiology of psychiatric disorders requires that the clinician take an integrated view of NT function, neurochemical pathways, and neuroanatomical structures. Increasingly, more sophisticated views of the interrelationships of the basal ganglia, cerebral cortex, and limbic system are emerging from basic science studies, leading to new thoughts on their involvement in mental illness.

Recent advances in basal ganglia research indicate that the basal ganglia collect signals from a large part of the cerebral cortex, redistribute these cortical inputs both with respect to one another and with respect to inputs from the limbic system, and then focus the output of these signals to particular regions of the frontal

TABLE 3
Neurochemical Measures

A. Body fluids

The majority of neurochemical studies in child psychiatry have measured NTS and their metabolites in cerebrospinal fluid (CSF), blood, or urine. Some advantages and disadvantages of each are outlined below. The metabolites commonly measured for norepinephrine are 3-methoxy-4-hydroxyphenylglycol (MHPG), vanillymandelic acid (VMA), and normetanephrine (NMET); for dopamine are homovanilic acid (HVA) and dihydroxyphenylacetic acid (DOPAC); and 5-hydroxyindoleacetic acid (5-HIAA) for serotonin.

	Advantages	Disadvantages
CSF	More directly measures brain metabolism of NTs	1. Cannot differentiate from what functional site metabolites are produced 2. Invasive 3. Measures at only one point in time. Hard to do repeated spinal taps 4. Exchange takes place between CSF and plasma for some metabolites such as MHPG
Plasma	(a) Relatively noninvasive (b) Can obtain repeated samples (c) Significant percentage of HVA and MHPG are from CNS metabolism	(a) Reflects more peripheral than CNS metabolism
Urine	(a) Noninvasive (b) Large quantities enable one to measure all the metabolites and look at relationships among NTs and metabolites (c) Can obtain quantitative measure of production of NTs and metabolites in 24-hour production	(a) More reflective of peripheral metabolism (b) More difficult to collect accurate and complete samples

B. Enzymes

Enzymes such as DβH, COMT, and MAO can be measured from blood samples. Advantages are that samples are easily obtainable and the enzyme activities are genetically determined and tend to be relatively constant over time. A disadvantage is that the activity of the enzyme may bear no direct relationship to the functional activity of the NTs.

C. Platelet as a model of the synapse

The platelet functionally resembles the serotonin nerve ending. It has therefore been used for a variety of studies including NT content, NT uptake, NT receptors, and NT transducing systems.

Advantages	Disadvantages
1. Accessible	1. Technically difficult
2. Able to measure a variety of functions that are necessary for synaptic function	2. May not be a direct relationship between platelet function and synaptic function in the CNS

D. Probes

Certain drugs stimulate receptors for a specific NT. For example, clonidine stimulates the α_2 receptor. By using these agents and then evaluating functional or chemical responses to the agent, one may learn how the particular NT system is functional in an individual. Disadvantages are that it may be a relatively invasive procedure in children and that the probes may affect more than one system making the results difficult to interpret.

E. Brain imaging

Brain imaging will allow for evaluation of specific neurotransmitter systems in the CNS. This use of these procedures have recently been reviewed in the *Journal of the American Academy of Child and Adolescent Psychiatry* (Kuperman et al., 1990).

lobes and brain stem (Graybiel, 1990). The organization and function of the basal ganglia suggest it is important to learning and/or maintaining motor, behavioral, and emotional sets. Because of this role of the basal ganglia, investigators have suggested that dysfunction in the basal ganglia may be involved in the pathophysiology of schizophrenia (Carlsson and Carlsson, 1990), obsessive-compulsive disorder (Chappell et al., 1990; Modell et al., 1989; Swedo and Rapoport, 1990), Tourette's disorder (Chappell et al., 1990; Leckman et al., 1991), and attention deficit hyperactivity disorder (Lou et al., 1989; Heilman et al., 1991).

Basal ganglia research indicates that there are a series of parallel cortico-striato-nigropallidal-thalamocortical circuits (Goldman-Rakic and Selemon, 1990). It is as if each cell or functional group of cells in the cerebral cortex sends a private line through the basal ganglia and back to the cortex. Figure 4 is a simplified diagram of the path of these circuits.

The circuits from each cortical area appear to consist of both a direct circuit and an indirect circuit (Alexander and Crutcher, 1990). Increased output through the direct circuit results in increased excitation of cortical neurons, whereas increased output through the indirect circuit results in a decrease in excitation of cortical neurons. The direct and indirect pathways therefore have opposite effects.

The function of the circuits is best understood in terms of motor functions. The basal ganglia appear to participate in enabling particular movements and controlling sequencing of these movements, rather than directly causing them to occur. Disinhibition of the basal ganglia alone is not sufficient to trigger a coordinated movement. A command signal from other sources is also necessary (Chevalier and Deniau, 1990).

DA neurons reside in the substantia nigra compacta, which receives input from the striatum. The DA neurons of the substantia nigra compacta terminate primarily on neurons in the dorsal striatum. The function of the DA input to the striatum may be to reinforce any cortically initiated activation of a particular circuit, perhaps by having contrasting effects on the direct and indirect circuit (Alexander and Crutcher, 1990). Therefore, in Parkinson's disease, where DA neurons are lost in the substantia nigra compacta and DA input to the striatum is decreased, the basal ganglia would be less responsive in enabling particular movements and their sequencing. The commands for action would be sent to basal ganglia, but the response of the basal ganglia circuits would be slowed, and the motor action would be initiated more slowly with poorer control over sequencing. The response to signals to stop the motor action would also be slowed. One of the characteristics of Parkinsonism is difficulty in initiating movements, and once the movement is started, stopping it. The command center gives the orders, but because of the DA deficiency, the responses to the orders are overly slow. By analogy, one could hypothesize that excessive nigrostriatal DA input or tone would lead to the basal ganglia circuits being overly responsive and responding too quickly to commands

BASAL GANGLIA CIRCUITS

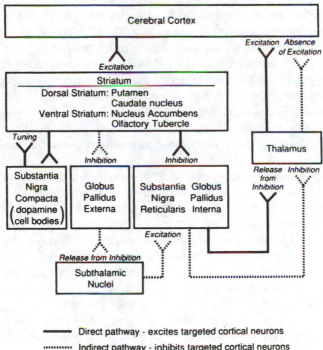

_____ Direct pathway - excites targeted cortical neurons

··········· Indirect pathway - inhibits targeted cortical neurons

Figure 4. Schematic drawing of direct and indirect cortico-striato-nigro pallidal-thalamocortical circuits. Each functional group of cortical cells appears to send private lines (direct and indirect circuits) through the basal ganglia to the thalamus and back to the cortex.

or perhaps even responding spontaneously. Such a condition could occur in Tourette's disorder, resulting in tics and vocalizations. Even if the basal ganglia disinhibition in Tourette's was not due to excessive DA tone, blocking of DA input to the striatum by neuroleptics would decrease the responsiveness of the basal ganglia circuits and have the beneficial effect of decreasing the tics and vocalizations.

The basal ganglia participate in a number of functions, including cognitive and limbic processes. There are cognitive (Brown and Marsden, 1990) and affective changes in Parkinsonism (Wilner, 1983a), and these changes could be due, in part, to the decreased dopaminergic input to the cognitive and limbic portion of the striatum. Similarly, some of the obsessive-compulsive symptoms in the form of obsessive-compulsive disorder associated with Tourette's disorder could relate to an increased dopaminergic tone in cognitive striatal circuits, with a resultant tendency to repetitive, intrusive thoughts and behaviors.

The limbic or ventral striatum (nucleus accumbens and olfactory tubercle) receives input from the limbic cortex, the amygdala and hippocampus, which are structures critical in learning, memory, and affective behavior.

The nucleus accumbens projects to the globus pallidus ventralis and to the substantia nigra compacta. The projections to the substantia nigra compacta influence DA input to the sensorimotor striatum (Smith and Bolan, 1991). Thus activation of the nucleus accumbens by the limbic cortex results in disinhibition of the limbic-striatal-pallidal-thalamos-cortical loop as well as influencing dopaminergic input to the sensorimotor striatum from the substantia nigra compacta.

DA input to the nucleus accumbens is from a group of cells in the mesencephalon, termed the *ventral tegmental area*. These cells project to the nucleus accumbens in a manner analogous to the way substantia nigra compacta neurons project to the sensorimotor striatum. DA input to the nucleus accumbens may therefore "tune" the circuits leading from the nucleus accumbens, influencing sensorimotor responses as well as affective and cognitive responses.

Together with the endogenous opiates, the ventral tegmental area to the nucleus accumbens dopamine pathway may be critical in the experience of reward (Petit et al., 1984; Wise, 1983; Wise and Rompre, 1989; Zito et al., 1985). Cloninger (1987) hypothesized that individuals with a highly active dopaminergic system (possibly on a genetic basis) were more likely to seek novelty and reward and would be predisposed to abuse alcohol and other drugs. Such individuals might derive a greater sense of pleasure from commonly abused drugs (due to more active "reward pathways") and would be more vulnerable to addiction.

Another brain system important in the modulation of affective behavior is the Papez circuit. This circuit begins in the limbic cortex (the cingulate gyrus) and projects to the entorhinal cortex (a part of the temporal lobe). The hippocampal formation forms the next part. From here the circuit flows to the mamillary bodies, on to the thalamus, and back to the limbic cortex. Neuronal activity through the circuit is modulated by NE neurons from the locus coerulus and by 5HT neurons from the raphe nucleus.

Gray (1982) describes the input to the entorhinal area. Essentially, there is convergent input from all major areas of the neo and limbic cortex, such that the hippocampus must have access to nearly all ongoing stimuli, albeit in a highly processed form. Furthermore, the locus coerulus and raphe constantly modulate the activity of the septohippocampal system. In live animals, correlations can be found between the rhythm of the hippocampal cells and certain types of behavior (for reviews, see Gray, 1982; O'Keefe and Nadel, 1978). Thus the hippocampus is well situated to examine the current state of the organism's world, and send information back to the limbic cortex, septal region and hypothalamus to guide behavior. The hypothalamus, as the "head ganglion" of the autonomic nervous system, can control the output of the autonomic nervous system in "fight or flight" situations. The septohippocampal system outlined above plays an essential role in Gray's (1982) theory of anxiety.

In general, DA, NE, and 5HT appear to have modulatory effects on the above systems: "tuning" the systems, and/or increasing or decreasing the responsiveness of the system. The anatomy of the three NT systems is consistent with such a tuning role, with each of the biogenic amines sending projections to widespread areas of the brain from only a few centers (Figs. 1 and 2). An important function of these three biogenic amines may therefore be to assist the organism in keeping different brain systems in proper tune to meet the changing demands of the environment and learn more effectively from the environment. In the next sections we will discuss further how this interaction or tuning of the three biogenic amine systems may play a part in child psychiatric disorders, followed by a review of some of the neurochemical studies in child psychiatry. It should be borne in mind, however, that while these theories have great heuristic value, it is very difficult to test these hypotheses in humans, and at present there are no direct clinical applications of this work.

BEHAVIORAL SYSTEMS AND CHILD PSYCHIATRIC DISORDERS

Behavioral Systems

NE, DA, and 5HT systems appear to be important in the interaction and regulation of an individual's behavior with the external environment (Antelman and Caggiula, 1977; Depue and Spoont, 1986). DA appears to be the NT most involved in the expression of active behavioral patterns that include motor activity, aggressive behavior, and sexual behavior. NE and 5HT appear to be involved in regulating the DA dependent behavior. NE, with support from 5HT, appears important in attending to and assessing the environment. These systems have been defined primarily in nonhumans, but appear applicable to humans as well. In the descriptions that follow, we will take some liberty by giving hypothetical human examples that will make it easier to see how these systems may affect learning and behavior in humans and may therefore apply to child psychiatry. Based on the function of these systems, we will then make hypotheses about dysregulation in these systems and resulting behavior patterns.

Gray (1982; 1987) has described a behavioral facilitatory system (BFS) and a behavioral inhibitory system (BIS). Quay (1988a, b) has elaborated on Gray's work and hypothesized how these systems may relate to child psychiatric disorders. The BFS is a generalized behavioral system that functions to mobilize behavior so that active engagement with the environment occurs. Examples of such behaviors include extraversion, sexual behavior, and aggressive behavior. The components of the BFS are thought to be integrated in the mesolimbic dopaminergic system (Depue and Spoont, 1986; Gray, 1982). The BFS is activated primarily by rewarding stimuli or by aversive stimuli when escape or avoidance is possible. For example, a child sees a candy bar in a store. The BFS is stimulated by this environmental stimuli and sets off the behavioral sequence to get the candy bar and eat it. The BFS is action with no restraint. The restraint is provided externally by the mother who prevents the action. Escape/avoidance is also considered rewarding. The boy, after taking candy, sees the store clerk coming and escapes/avoids the aversive consequences by running from the store and/or lying about what he did. The BFS responds to signals from the environment with action. If its action is blocked (prevention from taking the candy or running away), frustration occurs, and an aggressive response may occur that may also be dependent on a dopaminergic system.

Without an internal system to provide restraint, the individual would be completely dependent on the external environment for restraint. The BIS is the internal system to provide restraint.

The BIS acts as a comparator and an inhibitor of behavior (Gray, 1982; 1987; Depue and Spoont, 1986). The BIS continuously compares actual environmental circumstances with concepts of expected outcome of behavior. When mismatches occur, the BIS stops behavior by inhibiting the BFS. The neurobiological foundation of the BIS appears to be the septohippocampal system. The regulation of the septohippocampal system appears to be noradrenergic, with additional regulation from serotonergic projections from the median raphe. The conditions to which the BIS responds are nonreward, punishment, and uncertainty. Affectively, frustration may be associated with nonreward, and fear and/or anxiety with punishment and uncertainty. Returning to the example of the boy in the candy store, the BFS would be activated by the reward of candy. The BIS would then evaluate the situation. If the evaluation suggested that punishment would occur, then the BIS would be activated and the behavior inhibited. The BFS is inhibited internally by the BIS rather than relying on external restraint to control the BFS.

The relative strengths of the BFS (dopaminergic system) and BIS (noradrenergic/serotonergic systems) would theoretically influence behavior at a given point in time. For example, an individual with a strong BFS and a weak BIS would be overly responsive to rewarding stimuli in his environment and tend to ignore the negative consequences that might occur when he sought the reward. Because the individual would be "messing up" frequently, even when he did not intend to, there would be a strong tendency for him to be demoralized and have a poor self-esteem. In addition, the relative strengths of the system would also influence the development of behavioral patterns in an individual over time through the influence on learning in the individual. For example, a child with a strong BIS would show good attention to and discriminating ability to the environment. When punished for stealing he would respond to the punishment with fear/ anxiety. The next time he would respond with fear and anxiety to signals of punishment (the thought of stealing) and the stealing behavior would be inhibited. Eventually, the thought of stealing would not even occur, and the child could be trusted without supervision. The child would quickly internalize societal rules and would do well with minimal supervision. In contrast, a child with a strong BFS relative to his BIS, would internalize poorly and be much more dependent on environmental controls to maintain socially appropriate behavior. In addition, since this child is conditioning poorly to signals of punishment, he would have less insight into the reasons for his being punished and be more likely to blame others for his problems.

NE (Antelman and Caggiula, 1977; Plaznik and Kostowski, 1983) and 5HT (Coccaro, 1989) have been shown to inhibit, and DA to facilitate, irritable aggression. Serotonergic mechanisms appear stronger in inhibiting irritable, aggressive behavior than do noradrenergic systems, and there is extensive animal and human literature showing 5HT's role in inhibiting aggressive behavior (Coccaro, 1989). Some of the inhibition of aggressive behavior by 5HT appears mediated from the median raphe through the BIS (Depue and Spoont, 1986). The serotonergic projections from the dorsal raphe to the amygdala appear to play a larger role in inhibiting aggression (Pucilowski and Kostowski, 1983) than the projections from the median raphe to the septohippocampus.

Antelman and Caggiula (1977) have elegantly described NE-DA interactions. Among their conclusions are that NE regulates DA dependent behaviors and that when both NE and DA are depressed equally, one may not see the changes in behavior that occur when either one or the other is depressed. The implications of this latter point are that it may be the balance between the regulatory systems, i.e., BFS and BIS, rather than the absolute strength of the systems that determines normal behavior. If the systems are in balance, the intensity of the normal behavior may be different, but it might not deviate from the norm. Dysfunctional behavior may occur when the regulatory systems are out of balance. In this paper, the regulatory systems of interest are the dopaminergic (BFS), noradrenergic (BIS), and serotonergic (BIS, dorsal raphe-amygdala).

The development of and balance among these three systems may be influenced by environmental factors as well as being genetically determined. Environmental factors include psychosocial factors as well as physical factors. The three biogenic amine systems continue their active development after birth, and developmental factors may have permanent effects on these systems.

Developmental Factors

Developmental changes in the dopaminergic and serotonergic systems are reflected in a decline of CSF HVA and CSF 5HIAA with age (Gillberg and Svennerholm, 1987; Kruesi et al., 1990; Langlais et al., 1985; Seifert et al., 1980; Shaywitz et al., 1980; Silverstein et al., 1985). These studies do not show that CSF 3-methoxy-4-hydroxyphenylglycol (MHPG), a metabolite of NE, changes with age after the first 8 or 9 months of age, suggesting that the relative activity of the noradrenergic system in relationship to the dopaminergic and serotonergic systems may be increasing with age, perhaps increasing internal restraint.

Receptor density also changes with age. Seeman et al. (1987) quantified binding to D1 and D2 receptors in human postmortem brains from birth to 104 years of age. The density of both receptors rose sharply between birth and 2 years of age and then dropped sharply from age 3 to age 10. From age 10 through adulthood, there was a slow but steady decline. The ratio between D1 and D2 receptors also changed with age.

The ongoing development of the NT systems after birth suggest that factors that alter their development may affect the behavior of the subject and that the affect on behavior may be different given the different developmental age of the subject. A well known natural experiment that illustrates this is Von Economono's encephalitis, which affects the DA system and produces Parkinsonism in adults and hyperactivity in children (Grinker and Saks, 1966). Shaywitz et al. (1976a) repeated this natural experiment by depleting DA in infant rats. The young rats showed an increase in activity (hyperactivity) that was responsive to amphetamine (Shaywitz et al., 1976b).

Primate studies suggest that psychosocial factors can affect the development of NT systems and that these changes may be permanent and may affect behavior in adulthood. Kraemer et al. (1989) made repeated measures of CSF amines on mother-deprived and mother-reared infants. Mother-deprived infants had lower levels of CSF NE than mother-reared infants. The intercorrelations between measures of 5HT, NE, and DA also differed, suggesting that either the balance between these systems was altered or that one or more of these systems had become less stable. In an earlier study, Kraemer et al. (1984) had shown that adult monkeys who had been maternally deprived were hypersensitive to D-amphetamine, suggesting that the psychosocially induced changes during early development had caused permanent changes in the NT systems affected by D-amphetamine. CSF NE was significantly higher in mother-deprived infants following D-amphetamine administration, suggesting that the NE system was the one that had been affected most by early deprivation.

Hypothetical Relationships among Biogenic Amine Systems and Behavior

Gray (1987) has hypothesized that the relative strengths of the BFS and BIS may be important in the development of personality characteristics, such as extraversion and intraversion, as well as deviant characteristics such as antisocial disorder and anxiety disorders. Cloninger (1987) has hypothesized that excessive mesolimbic dopaminergic activity may make an individual reward driven and subject to the development of addictions. Based on the hypothesized role of NE, DA, and 5HT in the development of the above behaviors and the likelihood that the balance between the three systems is important, one can make hypotheses regarding possible behaviors that could be associated with high or low functioning in each of the NT systems (Table 4), and symptom groups that might occur with different balances among the three systems (Table 5). The information in Tables 4 and 5 is speculative and is an oversimplification based on current information but is helpful in conceptualizing possible biochemical-behavioral relationships.

If relationships between behavior and the three systems hold as shown in Table 5, it has important implications for design of biochemical studies and the interpretation of results. For example, if subjects whose three systems are in balance all fall into the normal behavioral spectrum, a control group of subjects will have a full range of NT measures and frequently not differ from a patient sample. Measuring only one NT system might give misleading results, because the functional effect of that NT system being high or low would be dependent, in part, on the functional activity of another NT system. Because obtaining measures on a single NT system may give misleading results, the most effective strategy for identifying relationships between NT systems and behavior would be to obtain measures of all three systems in an individual. Also, one may wish to select comparison groups that are theoretically quite different biologically. Using "normal" controls as a comparison group may be misleading since a normal control group could have a full range of values, but be in balance. Two groups that would lead to a best comparison might be a conduct disorder (CD) group without anxiety or depression versus an anxiety/depressed group without CD. Based on the theoretical function and relationship between the three NT systems, one can make testable hypotheses about behavior patterns in children based both on the strength of one of these systems and on the balance between the three systems.

The child psychiatric disorders that have been studied most are infantile autism, attention deficit hyperactivity disorder (ADHD), CD, major depressive disorder, and Tourette's disorder. All of these disorders, except for infantile autism, could be seen as disorders secondary to dysregulation or imbalance of the three NT systems. In the next section, we will review neurochemical studies in

TABLE 4

Possible Characteristics Associated with Level of NT System Functional Activity

	High	Low
Dopamine	Increased motor activity, aggressive, extroverted, reward driven	Decreased motor activity, nonaggressive, low interest in others, poor motivation
Norepinephrine	Good concentration and selective attention, conditions easily, internalizes values, easily becomes anxious, overly inhibited, introverted	Inattentive, conditions poorly, internalizes poorly, low anxiety, under inhibited
Serotonin	Good impulse control, low aggression	Poor impulse control, high aggression, increased motor activity

TABLE 5

Hypothetical Characteristics Associated with Functional Balance among NT Systems

	High DA	Low DA
Low NE, Low 5HT	Aggressive CD, ADD with hyperactivity, irritable, no anxiety or depression	Generally "normal," low motivation, schizoid, possible attentional problems
High NE, low 5HT	Aggressive, anxious/depressed CD, mild hyperactivity, adequate concentration	Overly inhibited and anxious, tendency to withdraw
Low NE, high 5HT	Nonaggressive CD, mild ADD with mild hyperactivity	ADD without hyperactivity, inhibited
High NE, high 5HT	Normal, extroverted and anxious, high energy, obsessive compulsive traits	Anxious, inhibited, depressed

ADD = attention deficit disorder, CD = conduct disorder.

these four disorders to see if the data provide any support for the above hypotheses.

NEUROCHEMICAL STUDIES IN CHILD PSYCHIATRIC DISORDERS

Major Depression

Major depression, anxiety disorder, and behavioral inhibition may be associated with high NE and 5HT function and normal to low DA function.

The dexamethasone suppression test is positive more frequently in children and adolescents with major depressive disorder than in children and adolescents with other psychiatric diagnoses (Casat et al., 1989). The increased hypothalamic-pituitary-adrenal axis activity, suggested by the nonsuppression of serum cortisol, may be related to either decreased noradrenergic activity (Sachar et al., 1981; Schlesser et al., 1980) or increased noradrenergic activity (Jimerson et al., 1983; Rosenbaum et al., 1983; Rubin et al., 1985).

The growth hormone response to stimulation by several different biological probes has been shown to be blunted in major depressive disorder in children (Jensen and Garfinkel, 1990; Puig-Antich et al., 1984a; 1984b). Jensen and Garfinkel (1990) suggest that this blunted response may be due to dysregulation in postsynaptic alpha adrenergic receptors and in postsynaptic DA receptor sites.

Twenty-four-hour urine MHPG, a metabolite of NE, was lower in hospitalized depressed children than in healthy outpatient controls; however, children on an orthopedic unit had significantly lower levels of MHPG than the depressed children. There were no differences in NE or vanillylmandelic acid (VMA), another metabolite of NE (McKnew and Cytryn, 1979). Khan (1987) found no differences in MHPG between depressed and control adolescents. De Villiers et al. (1989) measured plasma NE and MHPG in depressed adolescents and found no difference in comparison with healthy adolescents. These studies suggest no change in the excretion of NE in depression.

Carstens et al. (1988) measured α_2-adrenoceptors on platelets and β-adrenoceptors on lymphocytes. The number of α_2 and β binding sites was increased in major depressive disorder. Since α_2 receptors on platelets may be representative of postsynaptic α_2 receptors and β receptors are postsynaptic, this finding would be consistent with up regulation of postsynaptic NE receptors.

Kagan et al. (1987) have compared children with behavioral inhibition to those without. Children with behavioral inhibition had increased urinary NE and increased heart rate. The increased heart rate was thought to be due to increased noradrenergic tone. Rogeness et al. (1990a) found higher systolic blood pressure in major depressive disorder and higher heart rate in anxiety disorder. Behavioral inhibition in children was associated with a family history of major depressive disorder and panic disorder (Rosenbaum et al., 1988).

Rogeness et al. (1990b) measured NE and its metabolites in urine. A possible measure of increased NE function was higher in major depression and separation anxiety disorder in comparison to subjects with conduct disorder. Plasma MHPG correlated positively with anxiety symptoms in a study by Pliszka et al. (1988a), although there were no differences between diagnostic groups. Possible measures of DA function were not different between groups in the Rogeness et al. study (1988; 1990). It is interesting that in adult studies, one of the more consistent findings is low CSF HVA in major depression (Potter et al., 1987; Wilner, 1983a, b). Wilner (1983a, b) has hypothesized low DA function as an etiological factor in some forms of depression.

Measures of 5HT function have been less frequent in major depression and anxiety disorders in children. Modai et al. (1989) measured 5HT uptake into platelets in adolescents. Vmax values were lower in adolescents with affective disorder. The authors suggested the presence of fewer uptake binding sites in the platelets from membranes of depressed adolescents. In contrast, Carstens et al. (1988) measured imipramine binding sites on platelets and showed an increased number in subjects with major depressive disorder, suggesting an increased number of 5HT uptake sites on platelets. Whole blood 5HT, which is essentially a measure of platelet 5HT, has been measured in child psychiatric disorders. 5HT is not synthesized in the platelet, but is actively taken up and stored by the platelet. The measure of platelet or whole blood 5HT is therefore reflective of the platelet's ability to take up and store 5HT and is not a measure of 5HT production or excretion. One study showed a negative correlation between whole blood 5HT and CSF 5HT, suggesting that whole blood 5HT may be inversely related to serotonergic activity (McBride et al., 1989). Therefore, low whole blood 5HT could be associated with increased serotonergic functioning. Rogeness et al. (1985) found decreased whole blood 5HT in subjects with major depressive disorder.

In summary, there is evidence for dysregulation of noradrenergic function in major depressive disorder in children, with the evidence more consistent with increased noradrenergic function than with decreased noradrenergic function. The few biological studies on serotonergic measures can be interpreted as consistent with either increased or decreased serotonergic function. There appear to be no studies in children implicating dysregulated DA function.

Attention Deficit Disorder

Studies of catecholamine function have been extensively reviewed (Zametkin and Rapoport, 1987) and are summarized in Table 6. Investigators have focused on 24-hour collections of urine that are then assayed for NE, epineph-

TABLE 6
Summary of Studies of Urinary Catecholamine Excretion ADHD

Study	Urinary Catecholamines and Their Metabolites						Differences Relative to Controls		
	NE	NM	VMA	MHPG	E	M	DA	DOPAC	HVA
Rapoport et al. (1970)	None	—	—	—	None	None	—	—	—
Wender et al. (1971)	None	None	None	None	None	None	—	—	None
Shekim et al. (1977)	—	Low	—	Low	—	None	—	—	None
Rapoport et al. (1978)	High	—	—	None	—	None	—	None	None
Shekim et al. (1979)	—	None	—	Low	—	None	—	—	—
Shekim et al. (1982)	—	—	—	Low	—	—	—	—	None
Yu-cun and Yu-feng (1984)	—	—	—	Low	—	—	—	—	—
Khan and Dekirmenjian (1981)	—	None	None	High	—	None	—	—	—
Shekim et al. (1987)	—	—	—	Low	—	—	—	—	Low

The Effect of Drug Treatment on Urinary Catecholamine Excretion in ADHD. Differences Relative to Baseline

Study	Drug	NE	NM	VMA	MHPG	E	M	DA	DOPAC	HVA
snekim et al. (1977; 1982)	AMP	—	Down	—	Down	—	Down	—	—	None
Shekim et al. (1983)	AMP	—	—	—	Down	—	—	—	—	Up
Brown and Ebert (1985)	AMP	None	None	None	Down	—	—	None	None	None
Zametkin et al. (1985a)	AMP	None	None	None	Down	—	—	None	None	None
Elia et al. (1990)	AMP	None	None	Down	Down	Up	Up	—	None	None
Zametkin et al. (1985a)	METH	Up	Up	None	None	—	—	None	None	None
Zametkin and Hamburger (1988)	METH	None	None	None	None	Up	—	—	—	—
Elia et al. (1990)	METH	None	None	None	None	—	Up	None	None	None
Zametkin et al. (1985b)	MAOI	None	Up	Down	Down	Up	Up	None	Down	Down
Donnelly et al. (1986)	DMI	Down	—	Down	Down	—	—	—	—	—

AMP = d-amphetamine, METH = methylphenidate, MAOI = Monoamine oxidase inhibitor, DMI = desipramine.

rine (E), DA, and all the principal metabolites of these NTs. The top part of Table 6 summarizes studies that have compared children with ADHD with controls on these variables. As can be seen, no pattern of urinary catecholamine excretion clearly differentiates controls from ADHD children, though a number of laboratories (Shekim et al., 1979; 1982; 1987; Yu-cun and Yu-feng, 1984) have found decreased urinary MHPG relative to controls. It is difficult from this fact alone to make any statement about the baseline noradrenergic functioning in ADHD relative to controls.

Attempts have been made to elucidate the mechanism of stimulant drugs by comparing 24-hour urine catecholamines before and after drug treatment. The bottom of Table 6 summarizes these studies. A relatively consistent finding is that D-amphetamine, monoamine oxidase inhibitors, and desipramine all lower urinary MHPG after 2 to 4 weeks of treatment. In some studies, this decline in urinary MHPG is correlated with changes on behavior rating scales. Methylphenidate, although equally efficacious, does not cause a decline in urinary MHPG. Zametkin et al. (1985) initially found that methylphenidate increases excretion of urinary NE and normetanephrine as well as total body NE turnover, but a subsequent study (Zametkin and Hamburger, 1988) did not confirm this. D-amphetamine is a potent reuptake blocker and inhibitor of monoamine oxidase inhibitor. Because most MHPG is produced intraneuronally, D-amphetamine, by preventing reuptake, decreases the amount of NE available to be metabolized into MHPG. The greater amount of NE in the cleft probably results in greater stimulation of postsynaptic receptors, as well as presynaptic autoreceptors. Methylphenidate, on the other hand, may increase impulse-mediated release of NE, such that total body turnover of NE is increased. Thus, both drugs may increase NE availability in the synaptic cleft through different mechanisms, although it is unclear if this is the principal therapeutic effect of stimulants in ADHD. Rogeness et al. (1986) found an increase in attention deficit symptoms in subjects with low dopamine-β-hydroxylase activity, a condition that could be associated with lower NE activity.

Shekim et al. (1983) showed that urinary DA increases with D-amphetamine treatment, but because drugs with primary DA agonism do not have therapeutic effects in ADHD (Zametkin and Rapoport, 1987), it is unclear to what degree the changes in the dopaminergic system are critical in reducing the symptoms of ADHD.

Studies of 5HT function have not differentiated controls from ADHD (Irwin et al., 1981; Rapoport et al., 1974; Weizman et al., 1988). Fenfluramine, a 5HT agonist, was not therapeutic in the treatment of ADHD (Donnelly et al., 1989).

Psychopharmacological evidence suggests alterations in noradrenergic function are associated with ADHD (Zametkin and Rapoport, 1987). Neurochemical evidence does not permit a clear implication of a single neurotransmitter system. It is hoped that future studies using imaging of brain metabolism via positron emission tomography will yield more specific results. Zametkin et al. (1990) have shown decreased glucose metabolism in the brain of adult subjects with ADHD, suggesting that this methodology may be helpful in developing more understanding of the pathophysiology of ADHD.

Conduct Disorder

Dopaminergic function would be relatively high compared with NE function and/or 5HT function. Aggressive symptoms would be related more to level of 5HT function than to DA level. Associated anxiety/depressive symptoms would be more related to level of NE function.

DSM-III had subtyped CD into conduct disorder undersocialized aggressive (CDUA), conduct disorder socialized aggressive (CDSA), and conduct disorder socialized nonaggressive (CDSNA). From the theoretical framework in this report, CDUA would be associated with low NE and low 5HT function, CDSA with normal to high NE function and low 5HT function, and CDSNA with low NE function and high 5HT function.

Rogeness et al. (1982) found that subjects with CDUA had lower plasma DβH activity. DβH is an enzyme involved in the conversion of DA to NE. Its activity in plasma is genetically determined and relatively constant in an individual over time (Ciaranello and Boehme, 1981; Weinshilboum, 1983). The findings of lower DβH activity in CDUA was replicated in a study of outpatients (Bowden et al., 1988) but not in another (Pliszka et al., 1988b). Lower DβH activity could be consistent with decreased noradrenergic activity. When subjects with high DβH activity were compared with subjects with low DβH activity, the low DβH subjects had urinary catecholamine measures consistent with decreased NE function (Rogeness et al., 1990b). When subjects with low DβH activity were compared with subjects with high DβH activity, subjects with low activity had more conduct and attention deficit symptoms and fewer anxiety and depressive symptoms (Rogeness et al., 1986; 1988; 1990b).

Correlations have been shown between possible measures of noradrenergic function and conduct symptoms. Plasma MHPG correlated negatively with conduct symptoms in one study (Rogeness et al., 1987), and CSF MHPG correlated negatively with one measure of aggressive symptoms in another (Kruesi et al., 1990). The ratio of MHPG/VMA in urine, a possible measure of the ratio of intracellular to extracellular metabolism of NE, also correlated significantly with conduct symptoms (Rogeness et al., 1990b). The above data are consistent with decreased noradrenergic activity being associated with an increase in conduct symptoms.

In the above mentioned studies, there was no difference in DA and its metabolite HVA between subjects with and without CD and no correlation between HVA and conduct symptoms. Interestingly, subjects with low DβH activity had decreased plasma HVA, a finding opposite to what one might predict (Rogeness et al., 1987).

Measures of 5HT function have been consistent with decreased serotonergic function being associated with CD symptoms. Kruesi et al. (1990) found that children and adolescents with disruptive behavior disorders had lower CSF 5HIAA than comparison subjects with obsessive-compulsive disorder. CSF 5HIAA correlated inversely with several measures of aggressiveness. Stoff et al. (1987) measured imipramine binding to platelets in boys and found fewer binding sites in conduct disorder boys. Externalizing behavior and aggression were inversely correlated with imipramine binding in another study (Birmaher et al., 1990). Whole blood 5HT may be inversely related to CSF-5HIAA (McBride et al., 1989) and therefore higher whole blood 5HT may be related to decreased serotonergic function. Pliszka et al. (1988b) found higher whole blood 5HT in aggressive delinquents, and the higher levels correlated positively with aggressive symptoms. In our population of emotionally disturbed inpatients, boys with aggressive CD had significantly higher whole blood 5HT than boys without CD, consistent with the finding of Pliszka et al. (1988b).

Theoretically, a group with low noradrenergic and low serotonergic function should have more aggressive symptoms than a group with low noradrenergic function and high serotonergic function. In one study, subjects with plasma DβH ≤ 6 with whole blood 5HT above the median (low 5HT function) were compared with subjects with DβH ≤ 6 with whole blood 5HT below the median. Fire setting was used as a measure of aggressive/impulsive behavior. There were significantly more subjects with a history of fire setting in the group with whole blood 5HT above the median (Rogeness, 1990). Interestingly, Virkkunen et al. (1987) showed that adult fire setters had both low CSF 5HIAA and low CSF MHPG.

In summary, current data is consistent with decreased noradrenergic and serotonergic functioning being associated with CD. Current neurochemical data does not show an association between increased dopaminergic function and CD.

Tourette's Disorder

Dysregulation of the dopaminergic system has been considered to play a role in the pathogenesis of Tourette's disorder. This is based on data showing that the pharmacological agents that decrease dopaminergic function decrease symptomatology and those that increase dopaminergic function tend to increase symptoms (Leckman et al., 1988b). Neurochemical studies have been consistent with the dopaminergic system being involved in Tourette's disorder. Cohen et al. (1978; 1979), Butler et al. (1979), Singer et al. (1982), Leckman et al. (1988a, b) found decreased turnover and/or basal levels of CSF HVA in Tourette's disorder. Cohen et al. (1979) hypothesized that Tourette's subjects had supersensitivity of DA receptors with feedback inhibition of presynaptic DA release. Plasma HVA has also been shown to be low in Tourette's subjects with a negative correlation between plasma HVA and severity of symptoms (Riddle et al., 1988).

Neurochemical evidence has not shown a relationship between noradrenergic function and Tourette's disorder. CSF-MHPG (Butler et al., 1979; Cohen et al., 1979; Leckman et al., 1988b; Singer et al., 1982) and plasma MHPG (Riddle et al., 1988) were not different between Tourette's subjects and controls. Clonidine, an alpha-2 adrenergic agonist, is helpful in the treatment of Tourette's disorder. However, studies do not support changes in $\alpha2$ receptor function in Tourette's disorder (Leckman et al., 1990; Silverstein et al., 1985). Responsiveness to clonidine in Tourette's disorder is predicted by responsiveness to haloperidol (Borison et al., 1982) and clonidine also affects the dopaminergic system and serotonergic system as well as the noradrenergic system (Leckman et al., 1984; 1986; Silverstein et al., 1985). Bornstein and Baker (1990) in a study showing that urinary phenylethylamine was lower in a subset of Tourette's subjects found lower urinary normetanephrine, a metabolite of NE, in Tourette's subjects in comparison to controls. Interestingly, 24-hour urine normetanephrine correlated positively with plasma HVA ($r = 0.57$, $N = 39$, $p < 0.001$) but not to plasma MHPG ($r = 0.001$) in our studies on emotionally disturbed children, suggesting that the low urinary normetanephrine in the above study may be consistent with the low plasma HVA and CSF HVA in the studies cited earlier.

Studies suggest that serotonergic function may be decreased in some subjects with Tourette's. CSF 5HIAA was low in several studies (Butler et al., 1979; Cohen et al., 1979; Leckman et al., 1988a, b), and plasma tryptophan was low in another (Leckman et al., 1984). Cohen et al. (1979) hypothesized that decreased serotonergic function could lead to decreased inhibitory function in the median raphe neurons as well as oversensitive serotonergic receptors on motor neurons where 5HT is excitatory. Bornstein and Baker (1988) found that urinary 5HIAA and HVA correlated with neuropsychological measures in Tourette's subjects, providing additional support for dysregulation of dopaminergic and serotonergic function in Tourette's subjects.

Shapiro et al. (1984) measured plasma DβH, erythrocyte catechol-0-methyltransferase (COMT) and platelet and plasma MAO—enzymes involved in the metabolism of DA, NE, and 5HT. There were no differences in DβH or COMT in Tourette's subjects, but platelet and plasma MAO were higher.

Two postmortem studies have suggested that dysregulation in the dopaminergic and/or other transmitter systems may be due to an abnormality within a second messenger system (Singer et al., 1990) or in an endogenous opioid system (Haber et al., 1986). In the study by Singer et al. (1990), four Tourette's subjects at postmortem examination had decreased concentrations of cyclic adenosine monophosphate. There were no differences in concentrations of DA, NE, or 5HIAA. Cyclic adenosine monophosphate is a second messenger for several receptors including the D2 receptor for which haloperidol is an antagonist.

Haber et al. (1986) found a decreased concentration of dynorphin, an endogenous opioid in a postmortem study of a single subject with Tourette's. Additional evidence for the possible involvement of dynorphin is the finding of increased CSF dynorphin in subjects with Tourette's (Leckman et al., 1988a). Endogenous opioids interact with dopaminergic neurons (Gillman and Sandyk, 1986; Broderick, 1987), raising the possibility that dysfunction in the dopaminergic system in Tourette's is secondary to dysfunction in the endogenous opioid system. Sandyk (1989) reviewed evidence suggesting abnormal opiate receptor function in Tourette's subjects.

In summary, pharmacological and neurochemical evidence is consistent with dysregulation of the dopaminergic system. This dysregulation may be secondary to dysfunction in other systems that regulate dopaminergic function. It is interesting that the most consistent finding to date is decreased CSF and plasma HVA (the metabolite of DA), when the evidence indicates an overly sensitive dopaminergic system. Earlier, we had discussed how a system has multiple ways to regulate itself, and the decrease in DA turnover in Tourette's may be such an attempt at internal regulation as a compensation for supersensitive DA receptors (Cohen et al., 1979); a dysfunction in a second messenger system (Singer et al., 1990); or in another system that interacts with the dopaminergic system, the endogenous opioid system.

The neurochemical studies suggest decreased serotonergic function in Tourette's, but the evidence is weaker than it is for increased dopaminergic function. Because serotonergic function appears to have an inhibitory and modulating role on dopaminergic function, increased serotonergic activity might be able to compensate for some of the dysregulation in the dopaminergic system. Therefore, decreased serotonergic activity could reflect a decreased ability to compensate for increased dopaminergic activity and therefore a more severe expression of the Tourette's symptomatology. The neurochemical evidence for a role of NE in Tourette's disorder is weak.

SUMMARY

In this article, we reviewed some of the neurochemistry of the biogenic amines, NE, DA, and 5HT. The anatomical distribution of the biogenic amines, each of the three having their cell bodies located in a few centers from which they innervate many common areas of the brain, is consistent with the biogenic amines having a modulatory or regulatory role on brain systems. This modulatory or regulatory role may assist the organism in interacting with and adjusting to his environment. The effect of 5HT and NE in the septohippocampal system and of DA in the basal ganglia system illustrates this role of keeping the systems in proper tune to respond most effectively to environmental demands.

Cloninger (1987) and Gray (1982; 1987) have hypothesized, based on studies in animals, that genetic or constitutional differences in the activity of these amine systems may affect the way that humans interact with and respond to their environment. In certain cases, this might lead to the development of psychiatric disorders.

Based on the above hypotheses, dysregulation or imbalances in the biogenic amine systems could be important in the pathophysiology of several child psychiatric disorders. We reviewed neurochemical studies in four child psychiatric disorders to determine if there were data on biogenic amine metabolism that were consistent with the hypothesized role of the biogenic amine systems in these disorders.

The methodology that has been available to measure neurotransmitter function in children is many steps removed from the processes taking place in brain systems and makes interpretation of results difficult. The evidence for neurochemical dysregulation in Tourette's disorder is greater and perhaps better understood than in other child psychiatric disorders. Studies on Tourette's disorder illustrate some of the difficulty in interpreting neurochemical results as well as illustrate one of the points in this report regarding imbalances and dysregulation in biogenic amine systems and compensatory mechanisms to keep a system in balance.

The expression of symptoms in Tourette's disorder may be viewed as secondary to dysregulation in the dopaminergic system. The neurochemical defect causing the disorder could be due to a problem within the dopaminergic system (within system dysregulation) or with a system that interacts with the DA system (outside system dysregulation). One can then look at the neurochemical findings in Tourette's from several different perspectives.

As reviewed earlier, one of the most consistent findings in Tourette's is decreased CSF HVA, suggesting decreased turnover (production) of DA in Tourette's. This is in conflict with evidence suggesting that symptoms are secondary to increased activity. Comings and Comings (1987b) have suggested that Tourette's disorder is due to hypofunctioning in the mesocortical pathway together with hypersensitivity of subcortical DA pathways. In this model, the decreased turnover in the mesocortical DA system would be greater than the increased turnover in the subcortical pathways, resulting in a net decrease in HVA turnover when measured peripherally. This illustrates one of the problems of peripheral neurochemical measures because the NTS and their metabolites that are measured come from more than one anatomical or physiological system.

Cohen et al. (1979) offered a different explanation, suggesting that the decreased HVA turnover was due to decreased release of presynaptic DA as a way to compensate for overly sensitive postsynaptic receptors. For the purpose of illustration, we will assume that one genetic form of Tourette's is due to an overly sensitive postsynaptic receptor system. The decrease in DA release would then be a "within system" compensation to maintain the DA system within balance. If this within system adjustment was not adequate, "outside system" adjustments would also occur such as increased activity in noradrenergic and serotonergic systems. If these within system and "outside system" adjustments were adequate to compensate for the defect in the postsynaptic dopaminergic system, the individual, even though he had the genetic defect, might be free or relatively free of Tourette's symptoms. However, because of the compensatory changes in other NT systems, i.e., increased noradrenergic and/or serotonergic function, he may be at risk to have symptoms associated with dysregulation in these systems such as anxiety/depressive disorder or obsessive-compulsive disorder. An inability of these systems to compensate because of genetic factors or of a developmental/environmental nature might lead to a situation of high dopaminergic activity with relatively low or decreased noradrenergic and/or serotonergic function with resulting attentional and impulse control problems. The low CSF 5-HIAA found in some subjects with Tourette's (Butler et al., 1979; Cohen et al., 1979; Leckman et al., 1988b) may represent a lack of adequate compensation in the serotonergic system, leading to greater symptomatic expression in these subjects. Comings and Comings (1987a, c, d, e, f) have shown that Tourette's disorder is associated with an increased frequency of other psychiatric disorders. It is possible that the increased frequency of symptoms of these other disorders in Tourette's is related in part to dysregulation in the noradrenergic and serotonergic systems that are compensating for a defect or dysregulation in the dopaminergic system.

In summary, Tourette's symptoms appear to be expressed through dysregulation of the dopaminergic system. One could have more than one genetic defect causing the dysregulation, such as a within system defect in the postsynaptic receptor system, or an outside system defect such as in the endogenous opioid system. Environmental factors (physical and psychosocial) pre- and postnatally would affect the development of the NT systems and their ability to compensate for a genetic defect. The compensation or lack of compensation in these systems would relate to the degree of expression of the Tourette's symptoms and may result in symptoms of other psychiatric disorders not specifically related to Tourette's.

Given the complexity of the neurochemistry and neurophysiology of the CNS, one may wonder how the neurochemical measures at our disposal can help us understand the pathogenesis of psychiatric disorders. As primitive as our methods have been, some light has already been shed. The hypotheses and understanding developed to date as well as newer study techniques that have been or are being developed are likely to lead to further advances. Study techniques include not only new neurochemical/neurophysiological techniques, such as positron emission tomography, but also methods of classifying subjects that may rely on neurochemical measures in addition to or instead of clinical measures. A disorder like ADHD may have multiple etiologies just as pneumonia has multiple etiologies. By relying solely on clinical classification, we may group all subjects with pneumonia into one group, and therefore be unable to identify the different etiological factors in the development of the disorder.

REFERENCES

Alexander, G. E. & Crutcher, M. D. (1990), Functional architecture of basal ganglia circuits: neural substrates of parallel processing. *Trends in Neurosciences* 13:266–271.

Antelman, S. M. & Caggiula, A. R. (1977), Norepinephrine-dopamine interactions and behavior. *Science* 195:646–653.

Birmaher, B., Stanley, M., Greenhill, L., Twomey, J., Gavrilescu, A. & Rabinovich, H. (1990), Platelet imipramine binding in children and adolescents with impulsive behavior. *J. Am. Acad. Child Adolesc. Psychiatry* 29:914–918.

Bjorklund, A. & Lindvall, O. (1984), Dopamine-containing systems in the CNS. In: *Handbook of Chemical Neuroanatomy. Vol. 2: Classical Transmitters in the CNS, Part I,* eds. A. Bjorkland & T. Hokfelt. Amsterdam: Elsevier Science Publishers, B. V., pp. 55–122.

Borison, R. L., Ang, L., Chang, S., Dysken, M., Comatz, J. E. & Davis, J. M. (1982), New pharmacological approaches in the treatment of Tourette syndrome. In: *Gilles de la Tourette Syndrome,* eds. A. J. Friedhoff & T. N. Chase. New York: Raven Press, pp. 377–382.

Bornstein, R. A. & Baker, G. B. (1988), Neuropsychological correlates of urinary amine metabolites in Tourette's syndrome. *Int. J. Neurosci.* 42:113–120.

————(1990), Urinary amines in Tourette's syndrome patients with and without phenylethylamine abnormality. *Psychiatry Res.* 31:279–286.

Bowden, C. L., Deutsch, C. K. & Swanson, J. M. (1988), Plasma dopamine-β-hydroxylase and platelet monoamine oxidase in attention deficit disorder and conduct disorder. *J. Am. Acad. Child Adolesc. Psychiatry,* 27:171–174.

Broderick, P. A. (1987), Striatal neurochemistry of dynorphin-(1-13): *in vivo* electrochemical semidifferential analyses. *Neuropeptides,* 10:369–386.

Brown, A. M. & Birnbaumer, L. (1988), Direct G protein gating of ion channels. *Am. J. Physiol.,* 254:H401–H410.

Brown, G. L. & Ebert, M. H. (1985), Catecholamine metabolism in hyperactive children. In: *The Catecholamines in Psychiatric and Neurologic Disorders,* eds. C. R. Lake & M. G. Ziegler. Boston: Butterworth, p. 185.

Brown, R. G. & Marsden, C. D. (1990), Cognitive function in Parkinson's disease from description to theory. *Trends in Neurosciences,* 13:21–28.

Butler, I. J., Koslow, S. H., Seifert, W. E., Caprioli, R. M. & Singer, H. S. (1979), Biogenic amine metabolism in Tourette syndrome. *Ann. Neurol.*, 6:37–39.

Carlsson, M. & Carlsson, A. (1990), Interactions between glutamatergic and monoaminergic systems within the basal ganglia—implications for schizophrenia and Parkinson's disease. *Trends in Neurosciences*, 13:272–276.

Carstens, M. E., Engelbrecht, A. H., Russell, V. A., van Zyl, A. M. & Taljaard, J. J. F. (1988), Biological markers in juvenile depression. *Psychiatry Res.*, 23:77–88.

Casat, C. D., Arana, G. W. & Powell, K. (1989), The DST in children and adolescents with major depressive disorder. *Am. J. Psychiatry*, 146:503–507.

Chappell, P. B., Leckman, J. F., Pauls, D. & Cohen, D. J. (1990), Biochemical and genetic studies of Tourette's Syndrome: implications for treatment and future research. In: *Application of Basic Neuroscience to Child Psychiatry*, eds. S. I. Deutsch, A. Weizman & R. Weizman. New York: Plenum Press, pp. 241–260.

Chevalier, G. & Deniau, J. M. (1990), Disinhibition as a basic process in the expression of striatal functions. *Trends in Neurosciences*, 13:277–280.

Ciaranello, R. D. & Boehme, R. E. (1981), Biochemical genetics of neurotransmitter enzymes and receptors: relationships to schizophrenia and other major psychiatric disorders. *Clin. Genet.*, 19:358–372.

Cloninger, C. R. (1987), Neurologic adaptive mechanisms in alcoholism. *Science*, 236:410–416.

Coccaro, E. F. (1989), Central serotonin and impulsive aggression. *Br. J. Psychiatry*, 155:52–62.

Cohen, D. J., Shaywitz, B. A., Caparulo, B. K., Young, J. G. & Bowers, M. B., Jr. (1978), Chronic, multiple tics of Gilles de la Tourette's disease. *Arch. Gen. Psychiatry*, 35:245–250.

——————Young, J. G. et al. (1979), Central biogenic amine metabolism in children with the syndrome of chronic multiple tics of Gilles de la Tourette: norepinephrine, serotonin and dopamine. *J. Am. Acad. Child Psychiatry*, 18:320–342.

Comings, D. E. & Comings, B. G. (1987a), A controlled study of Tourette syndrome. IV. Obsessions, compulsions, and schizoid behaviors. *Am. J. Hum. Genet.*, 41:782–803.

——————(1987b), A controlled study of Tourette syndrome. VII. Summary: a common genetic disorder causing disinhibition of the limbic system. *Am. J. Hum. Genet.*, 41:839–866.

——————(1987c), A controlled study of Tourette syndrome. I. Attention-deficit disorder, learning disorders, and school problems. *Am. J. Hum. Genet.*, 41:701–741.

——————(1987d), A controlled study of Tourette syndrome. II. Conduct. *Am. J. Hum. Genet.*, 41:742–760.

——————(1987e), A controlled study of Tourette syndrome. III. Phobias and panic attacks. *Am. J. Hum. Genet.*, 41:761–781.

——————(1987f), A controlled study of Tourette syndrome. V. Depression and mania. *Am. J. Hum. Genet.*, 41:804–821.

——————(1987g), A controlled study of Tourette syndrome. VI. Early development. *Am. J. Hum. Genet.*, 41:822–838.

Cooper, J. R., Bloom, F. E. & Roth, R. H. (1986a), Catecholamines II: CNS aspects. In: *The Biochemical Basis of Neuropharmacology*, eds. J. R. Cooper, F. E. Bloom & R. H. Roth. New York: Oxford University Press, pp. 259–314.

————————(1986b), Serotonin (5-hydrotryptamine) and histamine. In: *The Biochemical Basis of Neuropharmacology*, eds. J. R. Cooper, F. E. Bloom & R. H. Roth. New York: Oxford University Press, pp. 315–351.

Coyle, J. T. (1985), Introduction to the pharmacology of the synapse. In: *American Psychiatric Association Annual Review*, eds. R. E. Hales & A. J. Frances. Washington, D.C.: American Psychiatric Press, Inc., pp. 6–16.

De Villiers, A. S., Russell, V. A., Carstens, M. E. et al. (1989), Noradrenergic function and hypothalamic-pituitary-adrenal axis activity in adolescents with major depressive disorder. *Psychiatry Res.*, 27:101–109.

Depue, R. A. & Spoont, M. R. (1986), Conceptualizing a serotonin trait. A behavioral dimension of constraint. *Ann. N.Y. Acad. Sci.*, 487:47–62.

Donnelly, M., Rapoport, J. L., Potter, W. Z., Oliver, J., Keysor, C. S. & Murphy, D. L. (1989), Fenfluramine and dextramphetamine treatment of childhood hyperactivity. *Arch. Gen. Psychiatry*, 46:205–212.

Elia, J., Borcherding, B. G., Potter, W. Z., Mefford, I. N., Rapoport, J. L. & Keysor, C. S. (1990), Stimulant drug treatment of hyperactivity: biochemical correlates. *Clin. Pharmacol. Ther.*, 48:57–66.

Gillberg, C. & Svennerholm, L. (1987), CSF monoamines in autistic syndromes and other pervasive developmental disorders of early childhood. *Br. J. Psychiatry*, 151:89–94.

Gillman, M. A. & Sandyk, R. (1986), The endogenous opioid system in Gilles de la Tourette syndrome. *Med. Hypotheses*, 19:371–378.

Gilman, A. G. (1989), G proteins and regulation of adenylyl cyclase. *JAMA*, 262:1819–1825.

Goldman-Rakic, P. S. & Selemon, L. D. (1990), New frontiers in basal ganglia research. *Trends in Neurosciences.*, 13:241–244.

Gray, J. A. (1982), *The Neuropsychology of Anxiety: An Inquiry Into the Functions of the Septo-Hippocampal System*. Oxford: Oxford University Press.

————(1987), *The Psychology of Fear and Stress*. Cambridge: Cambridge University Press.

Graybiel, A. M. (1990), Neurotransmitters and neuromodulators in the basal ganglia. *Trends in Neurosciences*, 13:244–254.

Grinker, R. R. & Saks, A. L. (1966), *Neurology*. Springfield, IL: Charles C. Thomas, p. 642.

Haber, S. N., Kowall, N. W., Vonsattel, J. P., Bird, E. D. & Richardson, E. P., Jr. (1986), Gilles de la Tourette's syndrome. A postmortem neuropathological and immunohistochemical study. *J. Neurol. Sci.*, 75:225–241.

Heilman, K. M., Voeller, K. K. S. & Nadeau, S. E. (1991), A possible pathophysiologic substrate of attention deficit hyperactivity disorder. *J. Child Neurol.*, 6:S76–S81.

Irwin, M., Belendink, K., McCloskay, K. & Freedman, D. X. (1981), Tryptophan metabolism in children with attention deficit disorder. *Am. J. Psychiatry*, 138:1082–1085.

Jensen, J. B. & Garfinkel, B. D. (1990), Growth hormone dysregulation in children with major depressive disorder. *J. Am. Acad. Child Adolesc. Psychiatry,* 29:259–301.

Jimerson, D. C., Insel, T. R., Reus, V. I. & Kopin, I. J. QA(1983), Increased plasma MHPG in dexamethasone-resistant depressed patients. *Arch. Gen. Psychiatry,* 40:173–176.

Kagan, J., Reznik, J. S. & Snidman, N. (1987), The physiology and psychology of behavioral inhibition in young children. *Child Dev.,* 58:1459–1473.

Khan, A. U. (1987), Biochemical profile of depressed adolescents. *J. Am. Acad. Child Adolesc. Psychiatry,* 26:873–878.

————Dekirmenjian, H. (1981), Urinary excretion of catecholamine metabolites in hyperkinetic child syndrome. *Am. J. Psychiatry,* 138:108–112.

Kraemer, G. W., Ebert, M. H., Lake, C. R. & McKinney, W. T. (1984), Cerebrospinal fluid changes associated with pharmacological alteration of the despair response to social separation in rhesus monkeys. *Psychiatry Res.,* 11:303–315.

—————————Schmidt, D. E. & McKinney, W. T. (1989), A longitudinal study of the effect of different social rearing conditions on cerebrospinal fluid norepinephrine and biogenic amine metabolites in rhesus monkeys. *Neuropsychopharmacology,* 2:175–189.

Kruesi, M. J. P., Rapoport, J. L., Hamburger, S. et al. (1990), Cerebrospinal fluid monoamine metabolites, aggression, and impulsivity in disruptive behavior disorders of children and adolescents. *Arch. Gen. Psychiatry,* 47:419–426.

Kuperman, S., Gaffney, G. R., Hamden-Allen, G., Preston, D. F. & Venkatesh, L. (1990), Neuroimaging in child and adolescent psychiatry. *J. Am. Acad. Child Adolesc. Psychiatry,* 29:159–172.

Langlais, P. J., Walsh, F. Y., Bird, E. D. & Levy, H. C. (1985), Cerebrospinal fluid neurotransmitter metabolites in neurologically normal infants and children. *Pediatrics,* 75:580–586.

Leckman, J. F., Anderson, G. M., Cohen, D. J., et al. (1984), Whole blood serotonin and tryptophan levels in Tourette's disorder: effects of acute and chronic clonidine treatment. *Life Sci.,* 35:2497–2503.

————Ort, S., Caruso, K. A., Anderson, G. M., Riddle, M. A. & Cohen, D. J. (1986), Rebound phenomena in Tourette's syndrome after abrupt withdrawal of clonidine. Behavioral, cardiovascular, and neurochemical effects. *Arch. Gen. Psychiatry,* 43:1168–1176.

————Riddle, M. A., Berrettini, W. H. et al. (1988a), Elevated CSF dynorphin A [1–8] in Tourette's syndrome. *Life Sci.,* 43:2015–2023.

—————————Cohen, D. J. (1988b), Pathobiology of Tourette's syndrome. In: *Tourette's Syndrome and Tic Disorders: Clinical Understanding and Treatment,* eds. D. J. Cohen, R. D. Bruun & J. F. Leckman. New York: John Wiley & Sons, pp. 103–118.

————Detlor, J., Harcherik, D. F. et al. (1990), Acute and chronic clonidine treatment in Tourette's syndrome: a preliminary report on clinical response and effect on plasma and urinary catecholamine metabolites, growth hormone, and blood pressure. *J. Am. Acad. Child Psychiatry,* 22:433–440.

————Knorr, A. M., Rasmusson, A. M. & Cohen, D. J. (1991), Basal ganglia research and Tourette's syndrome. *Trends in Neurosciences*, 14:94.

Lou, H. C., Hendriksen, L., Bruhn, P., Borner, H. & Nielsen, B. (1989), Striatal dysfunction in attention deficit and hyperkinetic disorder. *Arch. Neurol.*, 46:48–52.

McBride, P. A., Anderson, G. M., Hertzig, M. E. et al. (1989), Serotonergic responsivity in male young adults with autistic disorder. *Arch. Gen. Psychiatry*, 46:213–221.

McKnew, D. H., Jr. & Cytryn, L. (1979), Urinary metabolites in chemically depressed children. *J. Am. Acad. Child Psychiatry*, 18:608–615.

Modai, I., Apter, A., Meltzer, M., Tyano, S., Walevski, A. & Jerushalmy, Z. (1989), Serotonin uptake by platelets of suicidal and aggressive adolescent psychiatric inpatients. *Neuropsychobiology*, 21:9–13.

Modell, J. G., Mounty, J. M., Curtis, G. C. & Griden, J. F. (1989), Neurophysiologic dysfunction in basal ganglia/limbic striatal and thalamocortical circuits as a pathogenetic mechanism of obsessive-compulsive disorder. *J. Neuropsychiatry*, 1:27–36.

O'Keefe, J. & Nadel, L. (1978), *The Hippocampus as a Cognitive Map*. Oxford: Clarendon Press.

Petit, H. O., Ettenberg, A., Bloom, F. E. & Koob, G. F. (1984), Destruction of dopamine in the nucleus accumbens selectively attentuates cocaine but not heroin self administration. *Psychopharmacology* (Berlin), 84:167–173.

Plaznik, A. & Kostowski, W. (1983), The interrelationship between brain noradrenergic and dopaminergic neuronal systems in regulating animal behavior: possible clinical implications. *Psychopharmacol. Bull.*, 19:5–11.

Pliszka, S. R., Rogeness, G. A. & Medrano, M. A. (1988a), DβH, MHPG, and MAO in children with depressive, anxiety, and conduct disorders: relationship to diagnosis and symptom ratings. *Psychiatry Res.*, 24:35–44.

————————Renner, P., Sherman, J. & Broussard, T. (1988b), Plasma neurochemistry in juvenile offenders. *J. Am. Acad. Child Adolesc. Psychiatry*, 27:588–594.

Potter, W. Z., Rudorfer, M. V. & Pickar, D. (1987), Effects of psychotropic drugs on neurotransmitters in man. *Life Sci.*, 41:817–820.

Pucilowski, O. & Kostowski, W. (1983), Aggressive behavior and the central serotonergic system. *Behav. Brain Res.*, 9:33–48.

Puig-Antich, J., Novacenko, H., Davies, M. et al. (1984a), Growth hormone secretion in prepubertal children with major depression. I: Final report on response to insulin-induced hypoglycemia during a depressive episode. *Arch. Gen. Psychiatry*, 41:455–460.

————————————et al. (1984b), Growth hormone secretion in prepubertal children with major depression: III. Response to insulin-induced hypoglycemia after recovery from a depressive episode and in a drug-free state. *Arch. Gen. Psychiatry*, 41:471–475.

Quay, H. C. (1988a), Attention deficit disorder and the behavioral inhibition system: the relevance of the neuropsychological theory of Jeffrey A. Gray. In: *Attention Deficit Disorder: Criteria, Cognition, Intervention*, eds. L. M. Bloomingdale & J. Sergeant. Oxford: Pergammon Press, pp. 117–125.

————(1988b), The behavioral reward and inhibition system in childhood behavior disorder. In: *Attention Deficit Disorder, Vol III*, ed. L. M. Bloomingdale. New York: Pergammon Press, pp. 177–186.

Rapoport, J. L., Lott, I., Alexander, D. & Abramson, A. (1970), Urinary noradrenaline and playroom behavior in hyperactive boys. *Lancet*, 2:1141.

—————————Quinn, P. O., Scribanic, N. & Murphy, D. L. (1974), Platelet serotonin of hyperactive school age boys. *Br. J. Psychiatry*, 125:138–140.

——————Mikkelsen, E. J., Ebert, M. H., Brown, G. L., Weise, V. K. & Kopin, I. J. (1978), Urinary catecholamines and amphetamine excretion in hyperactive and normal boys. *J. Nerv. Ment. Dis.*, 166:731–737.

Rasmusson, A. M., Riddle, M. A., Leckman, J. F., Anderson, G. M. & Cohen, D. J. (1990), Neurotransmitter assessment in neuropsychiatric disorders of childhood. In: *Applications of Basic Neuroscience to Child Psychiatry*, eds. S. I. Deutsch, A. Weizman & R. Weizman. New York: Plenum Press, pp. 33–60.

Riddle, M. A., Leckman, J. F., Anderson, G. M. et al. (1988), Tourette's syndrome: clinical and neurochemical correlates. *J. Am. Acad. Child Adolesc. Psychiatry*, 27:409–412.

Rogeness, G. A. (1990), Norepinephrine and aggressive behavior. *Proceedings of the Annual Meeting of the American Academy of Child and Adolescent Psychiatry*, Chicago.

————Hernandez, J. M., Macedo, C. A. & Mitchell, E. L. (1982), Biochemical differences in children with conduct disorder socialized and undersocialized. *Am. J. Psychiatry*, 139:307–311.

————Mitchell, E. L., Custer, G. J. & Harris, W. R. (1985), Comparison of whole blood serotonin and platelet MAO in children with schizophrenia and major depressive disorder. *Biol. Psychiatry*, 20:270–275.

————Hernandez, J. M., Macedo, C. A., Amrung, S. A. & Hoppe, S. K. (1986), Near-zero plasma dopamine-β-hydroxylase and conduct disorder in emotionally disturbed boys. *J. Am. Acad. Child Psychiatry*, 25:521–527.

————Javors, M. A., Maas, J. W., Macedo, C. A. & Fischer, C. (1987), Plasma dopamine-β-hydroxylase, HVA, MHPG and conduct disorder in emotionally disturbed boys. *Biol. Psychiatry*, 22:1158–1162.

————Maas, J. W., Javors, M. A., Macedo, C. A., Harris, W. R. & Hoppe, S. K. (1988), Diagnoses, catecholamine metabolism, and plasma dopamine-β-hydroxylase. *J. Am. Acad. Child Adolesc. Psychiatry*, 27:121–125.

————Cepeda, C., Macedo, C. A., Fischer, C. & Harris, W. R. (1990a), Differences in heart rate and blood pressure in children with conduct disorder, major depression, and separation anxiety. *Psychiatry Res.*, 33:199–206.

————Javors, M. A., Maas, J. W., & Macedo, C. A. (1990b), Catecholamines and diagnosis in children. *J. Am. Acad. Child Adolesc. Psychiatry*, 29:234–241.

Rosenbaum, A. H., Maruta, T., Schatzberg, A. F. et al. (1983), Toward a biochemical classification of depressive disorders: VII. Urinary free cortisol and urinary MHPG in depressions. *Am. J. Psychiatry*, 140:314–318.

Rosenbaum, J. F., Biederman, J., Gersten, M., et al. (1988), Behavioral inhibition in children of parents with panic disorder and agoraphobia. *Arch. Gen. Psychiatry*, 45:463–470.

Rubin, A. L., Price, L. H. & Charney, D. S. (1985), Noradrenergic function and the cortisol response to dexamethasone in depression. *Psychiatry Res.*, 15:5–15.

Sachar, E. J., Halbreich, U., Asnis, G. M., Nathan, R. S., Halpern, F. S. & Ostrow, L. (1981), Dextroamphetamine and cortisol in depression: morning plasma cortisol levels suppressed. *Arch. Gen. Psychiatry*, 38:1113–1117.

Sandyk, R. (1989), Abnormal opiate receptor functions in Tourette's syndrome. *Int. J. Neurosci.*, 44:209–214.

Schlesser, M. A., Winokur, G. & Sherman, B. M. (1980), Hypothalamic-pituitary-adrenal axis activity in depressive illness. *Arch. Gen. Psychiatry*, 37:737–743.

Seeman, P., Bzowej, N. H., Guan, H. C. et al. (1987), Human brain dopamine receptors in children and aging adults. *Synapse*, 1:399–404.

Seifert, W. E., Foxx, J. L. & Butler, I. J. (1980), Age effect on dopamine and serotonin metabolite levels in CSF. *Ann. Neurol.*, 8:38–42.

Shapiro, A. K., Baron, M., Shapiro, E. & Levitt, M. (1984), Enzyme activity in Tourette's syndrome. *Arch. Neurol.*, 41:282–285.

————Yager, R. D. & Klopper, J. H. (1976a), Selective brain dopamine depletions in developing rats: an experimental model of minimal brain dysfunction. *Science*, 191:305–308.

————Klopper, J. H., Yager, R. D. & Gordon, J. W. (1976b), Paradoxical response to amphetamine in developing rats treated with 6-hydroxydopamine. *Nature*, 261:153–155.

Shaywitz, B. A., Cohen, D. J., Leckman, J. F., Young, J. G. & Bowers, M. B., Jr. (1980), Ontogeny of dopamine and serotonin metabolites in the cerebrospinal fluid of children with neurological disorders. *Dev. Med. Child Neurol.*, 22:748–754.

Skekim, W. O., Dekirmenjian, H. & Chapel, J. L. (1977), Urinary catecholamine metabolites in hyperkinetic boys treated with d-amphetamine. *Am. J. Psychiatry*, 134:1276–1279.

————————————(1979), Urinary catecholamine MHPG excretion in minimal brain dysfunction and its modification by d-amphetamine. *Am. J. Psychiatry*, 136:667–671.

————Javaid, J., Dekirmenjian, H., Chapel, J. L. & Davis, J. M. (1982), Effects of d-amphetamine on urinary metabolites of dopamine and norepinephrine in hyperactive boys. *Am. J. Psychiatry*, 139:485–488.

————————Davis, J. M. & Bylund, D. B. (1983), Urinary MHPG and HVA excretion in boys with attention deficit disorder and hyperactivity treated with d-amphetamine. *Biol. Psychiatry*, 18:707–714.

————Sinclair, E., Glaser, R., Horwitz, E., Javaid, J. & Bylund, D. B. (1987), Norepinephrine and dopamine metabolites and educational variables in boys with attention deficit disorder and hyperactivity. *J. Child Neurol.*, 2:50–56.

Silverstein, F., Smith, C. B. & Johnston, M. V. (1985), Effect of clonidine on platelet alpha 2-adrenoreceptors and plasma norepinephrine of children with Tourette syndrome. *Dev. Med. Child Neurol.*, 27:793–799.

Silverstein, F. S., Johnston, M. V., Hutchinson, R. J. & Edwards, N. L. (1985), Lesch-Nyhan syndrome: CSF neurotransmitter abnormalities. *Neurology*, 35:907–911.

Singer, H. S., Butler, I. J., Tune, L. E., Seifert, W. E. & Coyle, J. T. (1982), Dopaminergic dysfunction in Tourette syndrome. *Ann. Neurol.*, 12:361–366.

———Hahn, I. H., Krowiak, E., Nelson, E. & Moran, T. (1990), Tourette's syndrome: a neurochemical analysis of postmortem cortical brain tissue. *Ann. Neurol.*, 27:443–446.

Smith, A. D. & Bolam, J. P. (1991), The neural network of the basal ganglia as revealed by the study of synaptic connections of identified neurones. *Trends in Neurosciences*, 13:259–265.

Sokoloff, P., Giros, B., Martres, M. P., Bouthenet, M. L. & Schwartz, J. C. (1990), Molecular cloning and characterization of a novel dopamine receptor (D3) as a target for neuroleptics. *Nature*, 347:146–151.

Stoff, D. M., Pollock, L., Vitiello, B., Behar, D. & Bridger. W. H. (1987), Reduction of (T3YH)-imipramine binding sites on platelets of conduct-disordered children. *Neuropsychopharmacology*, 1:55–62.

Swedo, S. E. & Rapoport, J. L. (1990), Neurochemical and neuroendocrine considerations of obsessive-compulsive disorders in childhood. In: *Application of Basic Neuroscience to Child Psychiatry*, eds. S. I. Deutsch, A. Weizman & R. Weizman, New York: Plenum Press, pp. 275–284.

Virkkunen, M., Nuutila, A., Goodwin, F. K. & Linnoila, M. (1987), Cerebrospinal fluid monoamine metabolite levels in male arsonists. *Arch. Gen. Psychiatry*, 44:241–247.

Weinshilboum, R. M. (1983), Biochemical genetics of catecholamines in man. *Mayo Clin. Proc.*, 58:319–330.

Weizman, A., Bernhout, E., Weitz, R., Tyano, S. & Rehavi, M. (1988), Imipramine binding to platelets of children with attention deficit disorder with hyperactivity. *Biol. Psychiatry*, 23:491–496.

Wender, P., Epstein, R. S., Kopin, I. J. & Gordon, E. K. (1971), Urinary monoamine metabolites in children with minimal brain dysfunction. *Am. J. Psychiatry*, 127:1411–1415.

Wilner, P. (1983a), Dopamine and depression: a review of recent evidence. II. Theoretical approaches. *Brain Research Reviews*, 6:225–236.

———(1983b), Dopamine and depression: a review of recent evidence. I. Empirical studies. *Brain Research Reviews*, 6:211–224.

Wise, R. A. (1983), Actions of drugs of abuse on brain reward systems. *Pharmacol. Biochem. Behav.*, 13:213–223.

———& Rompre, P. P. (1989), Brain dopamine and reward. *Annu. Rev. Psychol.*, 40:191–225.

Yu-cun, A. & Yu-feng, W., (1984), Urinary 3-methoxy-4-hydroxyphenylglycol sulfate excretion in seventy-three school children with minimal brain dysfunction syndrome. *Biol. Psychiatry*, 19:861–870.

Zametkin, A. J. & Hamburger, S. D. (1988), The effect of methylphenidate on urinary catecholamine excretion in hyperactivity: a partial replication. *Biol. Psychiatry*, 23:350–356.

———& Rapoport, J. L. (1987), Neurobiology of attention deficit disorder with hyperactivity: where have we come in 50 years? *J. Am. Acad. Child Psychiatry*, 26:676–686.

———Karoum, F., Linnoila, M. et al. (1985a), Stimulants, urinary catecholamines, and indoleamines in hyperactivity: a comparison of methylphenidate and dextroamphetamine. *Arch. Gen. Psychiatry*, 42:251–255.

———Rapoport, J. L., Murphy, D. L., Linnoila, M., Karoum, F., Potter, W. Z., & Ismond, D. (1985b), Treatment of hyperactive children with monoamine oxidase inhibitors: II. plasma and urinary monoamine findings after treatment. *Arch. Gen. Psychiatry*, 42:969–973.

———Nordahl, T. E., Gross, M. et al. (1990), Cerebral glucose metabolism in adults with hyperactivity of childhood onset. *N. Engl. J. Med.*, 323:1361–1366.

Zito, A., Vickers, G. & Roberts, D. C. S. (1985), Disruption of cocaine and heroin self administration following kainic acid lesions of nucleus accumbens. *Pharmacol. Biochem. Behav.*, 23:1029.

15

The Role of Fathers in Child and Adolescent Psychopathology: Make Room for Daddy

Vicky Phares
University of Connecticut, Storrs

Bruce E. Compas
University of Vermont, Burlington

This review summarizes research concerning the relation between paternal factors and child and adolescent psychopathology. When compared with mothers, fathers continue to be dramatically underrepresented in developmental research on psychopathology. However, findings from studies of children of clinically referred fathers and nonreferred samples of children and their fathers indicate that there is substantial association between paternal characteristics and child and adolescent psychopathology. Findings from studies of fathers of clinically referred children are stronger for fathers' effects on children's externalizing than internalizing problems. In most cases the degree of risk associated with paternal psychopathology is comparable to that associated with maternal psychopathology. Evidence indicates that the presence of paternal psychopathology is a sufficient but not necessary condition for child or adolescent psychopathology.

A cornerstone of the field of developmental psychopathology involves the identification of factors associated with increased risk for emotional and behavioral maladjustment in children and adolescents. Numerous personal and environmental factors have been identified as correlates of child and adolescent psychopathology, including childhood temperament (e.g., Chess & Thomas, 1984), marital

Reprinted with permission from *Psychological Bulletin*, 1992, Vol. III (3), 387–412. Copyright © 1992 by the American Psychiatric Association.

Preparation of this manuscript was supported in part by National Institute of Mental Health Grant MH43819. We are grateful to Tom Achenbach, Harold Leitenberg, and three anonymous reviewers for their comments on a draft of this article.

divorce and discord (e.g., Emery, 1982), exposure to stress and adversity (e.g., Compas, 1987; Garmezy & Rutter, 1983), deprivation of adequate care (e.g., Rutter, 1981), and maternal psychopathology (e.g., Downey & Coyne, 1990). However, characteristics of fathers, including paternal psychopathology, have received relatively little attention in the investigation of child and adolescent psychopathology.

The impetus for studying fathers' contributions to maladjustment and psychopathology in their children comes from at least two sources. The first involves the study of the role of fathers in normal child development. In a 1975 article entitled "Fathers: Forgotten Contributors to Child Development," Lamb argued that there was an urgent need to pay more attention, in both theory and research, to the role of fathers in the socialization of children (Lamb, 1975). Since that time, substantial advances have been made in research on the role of the father in child development (for reviews see Bronstein & Cowan, 1988; Earls, 1976; Lamb, 1976, 1981, 1986, 1987; Lamb, Pleck, & Levine, 1985). However, most of this research has been concerned with normative developmental processes, such as attachment and social development. The increased knowledge that is now available about the role of fathers in normal child development provides a basis for the investigation of the role of paternal factors in deviant or dysfunctional developmental paths.

A second impetus for investigating the role of fathers in developmental psychopathology emanates from concerns regarding a possible sexist bias toward studying mothers' contributions to child and adolescent maladjustment while ignoring similar contributions by fathers. Caplan and colleagues have noted that there has been a pervasive tendency to blame mothers for causes of maladjustment in their children (Caplan, 1986, 1989; Caplan & Hall-McCorquodale, 1985). Caplan and Hall-McCorquodale reviewed publications from 3 different years (1970, 1976, 1982) in nine clinical journals and found that 72 different kinds of child psychopathology were attributed to mothers, whereas none were attributed to fathers. They also found that mothers were mentioned in specific examples of child problems at a rate of 5:1 compared with fathers. Whereas mother–child interactions were investigated in 77% of the studies, only 49% of the studies investigated father–child interactions. Overall, they noted that mothers were never described in solely positive terms, whereas fathers were often mentioned as a solely positive influence on the child (Caplan & Hall-McCorquodale, 1985).

The failure to include fathers in these studies may be the result of several factors (for discussion, see Phares, 1992). For example, researchers may assume that many children do not have contact with their father because of parental divorce. However, although only 67% of U.S. children under 18 years old live with both biological parents, most of the remaining 33% of children have some contact with their biological fathers (Seltzer & Bianchi, 1988). Alternatively, the failure to include fathers in clinical child studies may be due to an assumption that fathers are less willing or able to participate in research. However, in a review of child development studies involving fathers, it was found that fathers were no more difficult to recruit than mothers, and subject refusal was more related to factors such as time involvement and number of data collections than to parent gender (Woollett, White, & Lyon, 1982).

How might fathers contribute to child and adolescent psychopathology? The evidence is clear that maternal psychopathology, most notably depression, is strongly associated with child and adolescent psychopathology (Downey & Coyne, 1990; Gelfand & Teti, 1990). The effects of maternal psychopathology appear to be determined by multiple processes and pathways, including (a) genetic transmission of disorder or risk for disorder, (b) dyadic interactions between mothers and children, (c) maternal parenting practices (e.g., managing and structuring the child's social environment, coaching and teaching practices), and (d) marital conflict between parents (e.g., Dodge, 1990; Downey & Coyne, 1990; Rutter, 1990). Which of these processes are involved in the transmission of specific disorders is unclear. For example, although recent research has shed considerable light on the maladaptive patterns of parent–child interactions in families of depressed mothers, it is not clear that all types of maladjustment that have been observed in these children are directly attributable to interactions with their mother. Downey and Coyne suggest that the high rates of depression in these children may be a direct consequence of maternal depression but that externalizing problems in these children may be a consequence of the high levels of marital conflict that are present in families of depressed mothers.

Although fathers interact with their children in somewhat different ways than do mothers (Siegal, 1987), it is likely that these same basic mechanisms underlie any impact that fathers may have on maladjustment in their children. Thus, the contribution of fathers to child and adolescent psychopathology may be the result of fathers' direct interactions with their children as well as through more indirect processes involving marital conflict and family stress. However, before these possible mechanisms can be considered, Dodge (1990) has noted a more fundamental question that must be addressed regarding the role of fathers in their children's adjustment, "Just what difference do fathers make?" (p. 5).

Our purpose is to review recent research on paternal effects on child and adolescent psychopathology and to discuss conceptual and methodological issues related to this research. The following five questions are addressed: (1) Have fathers been included in studies of child and adolescent psychopathology? (2) Is there evidence that fathers contribute to child and adolescent psychopathology, and if so, do paternal factors represent necessary or sufficient conditions for child and adolescent dysfunction? (3) Are paternal effects limited to certain types of problems in children and adolescents? (4) Are paternal effects limited to certain behaviors or disorders of fathers, especially those that are more prone to occur in men (e.g., alcohol abuse and antisocial personality)? (5) What mechanisms are responsible for any paternal effects that are found? To pursue these questions, publications from 1984 to 1991 concerned with parents and child and adolescent psychopathology are analyzed to determine whether there has been a continued tendency to include mothers more than fathers in this research. This is followed by a review of empirical studies during this period that have provided data on the role of fathers in child and adolescent psychopathology.

ARE FATHERS INCLUDED IN STUDIES OF DEVELOPMENTAL PSYCHOPATHOLOGY, 1984–1991?

To determine whether fathers continue to be underrepresented in this literature, we examined the inclusion of fathers and mothers in clinical child and adolescent research. We reviewed the following eight clinical and developmental journals from January 1984 through January 1991: *Child Development, Developmental Psychology, Journal of Abnormal Child Psychology, Journal of Abnormal Psychology, Journal of the American Academy of Child and Adolescent Psychiatry, Journal of Child Psychology and Psychiatry and Allied Disciplines, Journal of Clinical Child Psychology*, and *Journal of Consulting and Clinical Psychology*. In addition to the articles found through the review of these eight journals, a computer-based literature review (PsycLIT) was completed to identify any articles that investigated paternal characteristics (with or without maternal characteristics) in relation to child or adolescent psychopathology. The following criteria were used for inclusion in the tally of articles: the research was empirical (not solely theoretical or a case study), it investigated issues related to child or parental psychopathology or both (not solely normative developmental processes), and it analyzed some characteristic of the parents (other than use of the parent solely as an informant on the child's behavior). Because we were interested in parental characteristics and child psychopathology, studies that examined parental characteristics but did not include the parents themselves as participants (e.g., analyses of paternal or maternal psychiatric history from hospital chart review) were included in the tally.

Of the 577 articles identified, 277 studies (48%) involved mothers only, 151 studies (26%) involved both fathers and mothers and analyzed them separately, 141 studies (25%) either included both fathers and mothers but did not analyze them separately or more frequently involved "parents" and did not specify parents' gender, and only 8 studies (1%) involved fathers only. This distribution differed significantly from chance $\chi^2(3, N = 577) = 251.24; p < .001$. Furthermore, these rates indicate no improvement in the inclusion of fathers in this literature since the Caplan and Hall-McCorquodale (1985) review.

This analysis suggests that clinical child research continues to use mothers more than fathers. The difference in numbers (48% of the studies included mothers only; 1% of the studies included fathers only) is quite striking and would not be expected unless there was not some type of bias operating in the research process (whether because of theoretical framework or presumed availability of fathers and mothers as participants). The 25% of the studies that did not specify whether the parents were fathers or mothers is especially difficult to use to establish paternal versus maternal effects on child psychopathology. The 26% of the studies that included both paternal and maternal characteristics and analyzed the variables separately are included in the current review, as are the studies that included fathers but not mothers.

An important methodological issue in developmental psychopathology concerns the nature of the target population that is sampled (e.g., children receiving outpatient services, children of parents in inpatient settings, nonreferred schoolchildren). The current review is organized by target population as follows: (a) clinically referred or diagnosed children and characteristics of their fathers, (b) clinically referred or diagnosed fathers and characteristics of their children, and (c) nonreferred children and fathers and characteristics of both. Within each section, the reviews are organized by diagnosis or type of problem addressed. The diagnostic terminology used throughout the review reflects the nomenclature found in these studies.

FATHERS OF DIAGNOSED OR CLINICALLY REFERRED CHILDREN

The first research methodology has involved the investigation of characteristics of fathers whose children have been referred for clinical services. Studies have used one or more of the following three analyses: comparison of fathers of clinically referred children with fathers of nonreferred control children, comparison of fathers and mothers of clinically referred children, and comparison of fathers of children with one disorder with fathers of children with a different disorder. Each type of study is discussed separately in reference to different types of child psychopathology. Many paternal characteristics have been investigated in relation to a wide range of childhood disorders, with most studies using a cross-sectional design. The studies are grouped by type of child psychopathology, with the primary problem areas being attention-deficit hyperactivity disorder, conduct disorder, delinquency, substance abuse, unspecified behavior problems, depression, suicidal behavior, anxiety disorders, schizophrenia, autism, and eating disorders.

Attention-Deficit Hyperactivity Disorder

Fathers of children with attention-deficit hyperactivity disorder (ADHD) have been found to differ from fathers of normal control children on a variety of characteristics, such as attention span (Alberts-Corush, Firestone, & Goodman, 1986), behavioral interactions (Tallmadge & Barkley, 1983), perceptions of parenting behavior and parental self-esteem (Margalit, 1985; Mash & Johnston, 1983), and expectations for future complaint child behavior (Sobol, Ashbourne, Earn, & Cunningham, 1989). For example, Alberts-Corush et al. (1986) found that biological fathers of ADHD children performed significantly more poorly on several measures of attention and reaction times than adoptive fathers of ADHD children and both biological and adoptive fathers of normal children. With regard to expectations about their children's behavior, Sobol et al. (1989) found that fathers had lower expectations for future compliant behavior from their ADHD children than did fathers of non-ADHD control children. Taken together, these studies suggest that there are consistent differences between fathers of ADHD children and fathers of normal children on a variety of characteristics including attention span, perceptions, and expectations.

In contrast, few differences in emotional functioning and psychological symptoms have been found between fathers of ADHD children and fathers of normal control children. For example, fathers of ADHD children did not differ from fathers of nonclinical children in their perceptions of family affective functioning (Cunningham, Benness, & Siegel, 1988). Although fathers of ADHD children reported significantly more drinks per week than did fathers of nonclinical children (Cunningham et al., 1988), fathers of ADHD children did not differ in the rates of alcoholism or antisocial personality disorder (Reeves, Werry, Elkind, & Zametkin, 1987) or in the level of depressive symptoms (Cunningham et al., 1988) when compared with fathers of normal control children. These studies suggest that although fathers of ADHD children differ from fathers of normal control children on various nonclinical variables (such as attention span and perceptions of parenting behavior), they do not differ on most measures of paternal psychopathology.

A similar pattern was found for mothers of ADHD children when compared with mothers of nonreferred children on nearly all of the variables discussed above (Alberts-Corush et al., 1986; Lahey et al., 1988; Margalit, 1985; Mash & Johnston, 1983; Reeves et al., 1987; Sobol et al., 1989; Stewart, deBlois, & Cummings, 1980; Tallmadge & Barkley, 1983). The only difference was that although fathers of ADHD children did not differ from fathers of normal control children in their level of depressive symptoms, mothers of ADHD children did report significantly more depressive symptoms than mothers of normal control children (Cunningham et al., 1988).

When comparing fathers and mothers of ADHD children, almost no significant differences have emerged on a variety of characteristics, such as attention span (Alberts-Corush et al., 1986), behavioral interactions (Tallmadge & Barkley, 1983), perceptions of parenting behavior and parental self-esteem (Margalit, 1985; Mash & Johnston, 1983), and perceptions of family affective functioning (Cunningham et al., 1988). In a sample of ADHD twins, high paternal and maternal criticism, high paternal and maternal malaise, and low maternal warmth were all associated with fathers' and mothers' ratings of their children's hyperactive behavior (Goodman & Stevenson, 1989). Additionally, Margalit found that ADHD children's life satisfaction in the family was most strongly predicted by paternal support, followed by paternal discipline, paternal indulgence, and maternal support. Note also that the majority of these studies have primarily used boys, and there were no comparisons of ADHD boys and ADHD girls in relation to paternal and maternal characteristics because of the small number of girls involved in these studies.

Two studies have found differences between fathers and mothers of ADHD children (Cunningham et al., 1988; Sobol et al., 1989). Fathers rated attributions of their ADHD children's noncompliant behavior as less external than did mothers (Sobol et al., 1989), and fathers of ADHD children reported fewer depressive symptoms but more drinks per week than did mothers of ADHD children (Cunningham et al., 1988). Taken together, these studies suggest that there may be more similarities than differences between the fathers and mothers of ADHD children.

Two studies have investigated fathers of ADHD children in comparison with fathers of other clinically referred children (Lahey et al., 1988; Stewart et al., 1980). However, because rates of comorbidity between ADHD and conduct disorder have been found to be high, with estimates of the overlap ranging from 41% to 75% (Lahey et al., 1988; for review see Hinshaw, 1987), it is important to focus on comparisons of children diagnosed with ADHD alone and not in combination with other psychiatric disorders such as conduct disorder. Both of these studies of fathers of ADHD children investigated that distinction. In a study comparing ADHD (without conduct disorder) boys with other clinically referred boys (such as conduct disorder, depression), Stewart et al. found that fathers of ADHD boys did not differ from the fathers of other clinically referred boys in their rates of antisocial personality disorder, substance abuse, or affective disorders. Similarly, in a sample of primarily boys (72% of the sample), Lahey et al. found that rates of paternal and maternal antisocial personality disorder, substance abuse, and affective disorders did not differ between the ADHD (without conduct disorder) group and the other clinically referred group. These studies suggest that fathers of ADHD children did not differ from fathers of other clinically referred children in their rates of psychopathology.

In summary, when compared with the fathers of normal control children, fathers of ADHD children have shown many differences, including shorter attention span (Alberts-Corush et al., 1986), poor behavioral interactions (Tallmadge & Barkley, 1983), and less favorable perceptions of parenting behavior and parenting self-esteem (Margalit, 1985; Mash & Johnston, 1983). However, fathers of ADHD children have shown almost no differences in rates of psychopathology when compared with fathers of normal control children or with fathers of other clinically referred children. Finally, fathers of ADHD children have shown almost no differences from mothers of ADHD children, and there appear to be more similarities than differences between fathers and mothers of ADHD children.

Conduct Disorder

Only one study was found that investigated fathers of conduct disorder (CD) children in comparison with fathers of normal control children. In a sample of primarily boys (89% of the CD sample), Reeves et al. (1987) found that fathers of children in the CD group (89% of whom also had an ADHD diagnosis) were more likely to be alcoholic or to have antisocial personality disorder, or both, than fathers of normal control children.

Only one study was found that compared fathers and mothers of CD children, and the study was designed to look specifically at girls with the CD diagnosis. P. L. Johnson and O'Leary (1987) found that the associations between CD girls' characteristics and paternal characteristics were fewer and smaller in magnitude than the corresponding associations between girls' and mothers' characteristics. Of the 10 correlations between parental and children's behavior, none of the paternal correlations were significant (maternal overt hostility and aggression were positively related to children's conduct problems; maternal marital satisfaction, positive behavior, and low negative behavior were positively related to children's social competence; P. L. Johnson & O'Leary, 1987). This suggests that the relation between the psychopathology of fathers and their CD sons may be stronger than between fathers and their CD daughters, although this has not been directly compared within a single study.

The majority of studies that included fathers of CD children compared these fathers with fathers of other clinically referred or diagnosed children (e.g., Dean & Jacobson, 1982; Hamdan-Allen, Stewart, & Beeghly, 1989; Jary & Stewart, 1985; Lahey et al., 1988; Reeves et al., 1987; Stewart et al., 1980). Reeves et al. found that fathers of children with a dual diagnosis of CD and ADHD were more likely to be alcoholic or to have antisocial personality disorder, or both, than fathers of ADHD children and anxious children. Fathers of CD/ADHD children were also more likely to have a history of aggression, arrest, and imprisonment than fathers of other clinically referred children (Lahey et al., 1988). Fathers of children with CD alone showed higher rates of antisocial personality disorder and substance abuse, and mothers showed higher rates of antisocial personality disorder and depression than fathers and mothers of other clinically referred children (Lahey et al., 1988). Fathers of CD children were found to be more depressed than fathers of children with either a learning disability or a personality disorder (Dean & Jacobson, 1982). Additionally, Stewart et al. (1980) and Jary and Stewart (1985) found that the fathers of aggressive CD boys were more likely to be alcoholics or to have an antisocial personality disorder when compared with fathers of other clinically referred boys (such as ADHD or depression). In a comparison of pervasive aggressive conduct disorder boys (PACD) with situational aggressive conduct disorder boys (SACD), paternal antisocial personality disorder, maternal alcoholism, and maternal drug abuse were all significantly higher for the PACD group than the SACD and non-CD clinical control groups, and paternal alcoholism was higher in both CD groups than in the non-CD clinical control group (Hamdan-Allen et al., 1989). Overall, a strong link was found between children's (primarily boys') CD and paternal psychiatric disorders and to a lesser extent maternal psychiatric disorders, including antisocial personality disorder, alcoholism, and substance abuse.

A related behavior problem that is not necessarily exclusive to CD children is that of assaultive and aggressive behavior in a comparison of four groups of adolescent inpatients (nonassaultive–nonsuicidal, assaultive only, assaultive–suicidal, suicidal only), no significant differences were found in paternal or maternal alcohol abuse or affective disorder (Pfeffer, Newcorn, Kaplan, Mizruchi, & Plutchik, 1989). Paternal and maternal assaultiveness, depression, suicidal behavior, psychiatric hospitalization, and alcoholism were also not significantly correlated with the assaultiveness ratings of their children who were psychiatric inpatients (Pfeffer, Solomon, Plutchik, Mizruchi, & Weiner, 1985). A similar study again found that the assaultive behavior of child psychiatric inpatients was not significantly related to paternal or maternal assaultiveness; however, paternal and maternal assaultiveness were significantly related to child assaultive behavior for a group of outpatients and nonpatients (Pfeffer, Plutchik, Mizruchi, & Lipkins, 1987). Stewart and DeBlois (1983) found that the aggressive and antisocial behaviors of boys seen at a child psychiatry clinic were significantly related to their father's aggressive and antisocial behaviors. They also found that the boys' noncompliant behavior was associated with both their father's aggressive behavior and their father's antisocial behavior (Stewart & deBlois, 1983). In a sample of psychiatrically hospitalized children, Lewis, Shanok, Grant, and Ritvo (1983) found that fathers of homicidally aggressive children were more likely to be physically violent and alcoholic than the fathers of nonhomicidal children and that mothers of homicidally aggressive children were more likely to have a history of psychiatric hospitalization than the mothers of nonhomicidal children.

In summary, children's conduct disorders have been found to be strongly linked to fathers' antisocial and aggressive behavior. This link appears to be stronger between fathers and sons than between fathers and daughters, although this has not been directly compared in a single study. This research suggests the need for investigation into the differential effects of fathers and mothers with their CD sons and daughters.

Delinquency

A variety of paternal and maternal factors have been found to be associated with adolescent delinquency, including lack of paternal and maternal supervision and discipline along with a history of parental criminality (for review see Loeber, 1990; Loeber & Dishion, 1983); inconsistent family communication patterns (Lessin & Jacob, 1984); high amounts of paternal and maternal defensive communication in a competitive context (Alexander, Waldron, Barton, & Mas, 1989); conflictual, unaffectionate father–son relations and conflictual, unsupportive mother–son relations (Borduin, Pruitt, & Henggeler, 1986; Hanson, Henggeler, Haefele, & Rodick, 1984); poor relationships with parents regarding paternal and maternal affection and autonomy (Atwood, Gold, & Taylor, 1989); high paternal social desirability and high maternal social desirability and neuroticism (Borduin, Henggeler, & Pruitt, 1985); and high levels of paternal deviance, parental aggressiveness, parental conflict, and low levels of maternal self-confidence, maternal affection, and supervision (McCord, 1979).

In a comparison of a group of delinquents with a nondelinquent control group, families of delinquents showed lower rates of facilitative information exchange, fathers of delinquents were more dominant toward their wife, and delinquent adolescents were more dominant toward their mothers (Henggeler, Edwards, & Borduin, 1987). Additionally, Lewis, Pincus, Lovely, Spitzer, and Moy (1987) found that when compared with nondelinquents, delinquents were significantly more likely to have been physically abused by their fathers and mothers, to have witnessed severe family violence, and to have a mother with a history of psychiatric hospitalization. The groups did not differ significantly in fathers' psychiatric hospitalizations, paternal alcoholism, or maternal alcoholism (Lewis et al., 1987). However, paternal alcohol use was found to be associated with the delinquents' attentional problems at 11 years old and number of arrests at the age of 18 (Wallander, 1988). Alcohol abuse was also found to be more prevalent among the fathers and mothers of delinquents who had been physically abused when compared with the fathers and mothers of delinquents who had not been physically abused (Tarter, Hegedus, Winsten, & Alterman, 1984).

As was true of the ADHD and CD literature, the majority of research on juvenile delinquency also used samples of primarily male delinquents. In an exception, Henggeler et al. (1987) compared the fathers and mothers of female and male delinquents and found that fathers of female delinquents were significantly more neurotic than fathers of male delinquents and that fathers and mothers of female delinquents showed significantly more conflict toward each other than fathers and mothers of male delinquents (Henggeler et al., 1987).

Two studies have investigated paternal factors related to adolescent runaway behavior. Englander (1984) found that adolescent female runaways felt that their fathers and mothers showed less positive feelings toward them and showed less family harmony than did nonrunaways. Fry (1982) investigated paternal correlates of runaway behavior of both male and female delinquents and found that father attributes of detachment, less child-centeredness and less communicativeness, and adolescent attributes of rebelliousness and irresponsibility were the most significant predictors of adolescent runaway behavior. Taken together, these studies suggest that adolescent runaways perceived their fathers as unsupportive and as being in an adversarial role.

In summary, numerous studies have shown a link between paternal factors and delinquency. Furthermore, paternal and maternal effects apparently are comparable, although this has not been directly tested in any of these studies.

Alcohol and Substance Abuse

Very few studies have investigated adolescent alcohol and substance abuse and paternal characteristics in clinically referred samples of adolescents, and the findings have been equivocal. For example, Klinge and Piggott (1986) found that fathers' and mothers' alcohol and drug use were not significantly related to their adolescents' alcohol and drug use. Significant relations were found, however, for fathers' and mothers' scapegoating of their drug-abusing adolescents (Gantman, 1978) and in heroin-abusing adolescents' perceptions of paternal, but not maternal, ineffectiveness and inability to communicate (Jiloha, 1986). These findings point to the need for further investigation into the relation between paternal characteristics and adolescent alcohol and substance abuse, both through cross-sectional and prospective designs.

Nonspecific Behavior Problems

In contrast to the work with ADHD, CD, delinquent, and substance-abusing children, some researchers have investigated paternal and maternal correlates of child behavior problems of clinically referred children without specifying diagnostic categories. For example, Roehling and Robin (1986) compared unrealistic beliefs regarding parent–adolescent relationships in distressed families referred for therapy and nondistressed control families from the community. On the basis of the Family Beliefs Inventory, they found that distressed fathers adhered to more unreasonable beliefs concerning perfectionism, ruination, obedience, and malicious intent of their adolescents than did fathers in nondistressed families (Roehling & Robin, 1986). There were no significant differences between mothers in distressed and nondistressed families.

In comparing the personal adjustment of fathers and mothers of children referred for unspecified conduct problems, Webster-Stratton (1988) found that fathers reported significantly less parenting stress, depression, and negative life events than mothers. Additionally, Webster-Stratton found that although fathers' personal adjustment measures were unrelated to fathers' behavior with their children, maternal personal adjustment measures (parenting stress, depression, poor marital adjustment, and negative life events) were significantly related to a high number of maternal criticisms and physically negative behaviors with their children. Similarly, Schaughency and Lahey (1985) found that fathers' ratings of their children's conduct problems and externalizing problems were unrelated to their self-reported depression, although mothers' ratings of their children's behavior problems were significantly related to their self-reported depression. Christensen, Phillips, Glasgow, and Johnson (1983) found that both fathers' and mothers' depression was associated with poor marital adjustment and less likelihood of a positive approach with their children referred for behavior problems. These authors also found that fathers' personal discomfort was negatively related to a positive approach with children and positively related to intolerance of their children's negative behaviors (Christensen et al., 1983).

Two intriguing studies have compared perceived paternal and maternal responsibility for children's behavior problems (Penfold, 1985; Watson, 1986). In a sample of children referred for treatment of unspecified emotional/behavioral problems, parents differed in their perceived responsibility for their children's problems in much the same way that responsibility has been attributed in the psychological literature. Fathers tended not to attribute responsibility for their children's problems to themselves, but mothers were significantly more likely to attribute the responsibility of their children's problems to themselves rather than to external sources (Penfold, 1985; Watson, 1986). In fact, fathers were much more likely to blame the mothers for their children's behavioral problems (Penfold, 1985).

In summary, these studies provide conflicting evidence of the effect of paternal characteristics on characteristics of their children referred for nonspecific behavior problems. Schaughency and Lahey (1985) found no relation between paternal depression and paternal reports of child behavior, and Webster-Stratton (1988) found no relation between paternal adjustment and fathers' interactions with their children. However, Christensen et al. (1983) found that fathers' depression and personal discomfort were related to their interactions with their children. These relations need to be clarified in further research on paternal characteristics and children's emotional/behavioral problems. Consistent evidence was found, however, in the perception of responsibility for children's emotional/behavioral problems. Both fathers and mothers tended to feel that mothers were responsible for their children's emotional/behavioral problems. Note that the "mother blaming" that exists in the literature parallels the mother blaming that exists in the community.

Depression

In a review of parent–child relations and depression, Burbach and Borduin (1986) noted that in comparison with the amount of research on retrospective reports of parent–child relations of depressed adults, few studies have investigated the parent–child relations of depressed children. However, a few studies have directly investigated the fathers of depressed children. In a study comparing depressed children and normal control children, John, Gammon, Prusoff, and Warner (1987) found that children's self-reported relationships with their fathers, but not their mothers, were significantly more maladaptive for children with major depression than for normal control children. In contrast, Cole and Rehm (1986) found no differences in father–child interactions but found that mothers of depressed children rewarded their children less than mothers of normal control children (and clinic-nondepressed children). Kaslow, Rehm, Pollack, and Siegel (1988) found that there were no differences in rates of fathers' depression between three groups (depressed clinic, nondepressed clinic, and nonclinic children) but that there were significantly more depressed mothers in the two clinic-referred groups. Additionally, children with dysthymia perceived their relationships with both their father and their mother to be more maladaptive than did normal control children (John et al., 1987).

A few studies have compared the relations of paternal and maternal psychopathology with children's depression. In studies of depressed children, paternal–child interactions were not significantly related to childhood depression, but poor maternal communication and low maternal affection were associated with increased childhood depression (Puig-Antich et al., 1985a, 1985b). Paternal psychological symptoms were related to children's anxiety but not depression, whereas maternal psychological symptoms were significantly related to children's self-reported depression and anxiety (Jensen, Bloedau, Degroot, Ussery, & Davis, 1990). Fathers' depressive symptoms were, however, related to clinician–father discrepancies of child depressive symptoms, but there was no relation between mothers' depressive symptoms and clinician–mother discrepancies (Ivens & Rehm, 1988). This indicated that depressed fathers rated their children as having more depressive symptoms in a structured diagnostic interview than did clinicians. Fathers were less likely than mothers to have a history of depression, and fathers were more likely than mothers to have a history of substance abuse and antisocial pathology in a sample of depressed children (Mitchell, McCauley, Burke, Calderon, & Schloredt, 1989).

In a sample comparing depressed and nondepressed psychiatrically disturbed children and adolescents, neither paternal nor maternal depression alone distinguished between the two groups, but depressed children and adolescents were significantly more likely to have two parents with a history of depression than the nondepressed group (Mitchell et al., 1989). Additionally, rates of paternal psychopathology did not distinguish between the two groups, although rates of maternal anxiety disorders, alcoholism, drug abuse, and suicidality were significantly higher in the depressed group (Mitchell et al., 1989). In an analysis of children with coexisting depression and anxiety disorders, fathers and mothers were no more likely to have an anxiety disorder than the fathers and mothers of children with only depression (Mitchell, McCauley, Burke, & Moss, 1988). Similarly, fathers and mothers of children with coexisting depression and CD were no more likely to have a history of substance abuse or antisocial personality than fathers and mothers of children with depression only. In regard to bipolar affective disorder, no significant differences were found in paternal or maternal care or protection (Joyce, 1984) nor in fathers' and mothers' rates of psychiatric disturbance (Dwyer & DeLong, 1987).

Overall, there does not appear to be a strong link between paternal factors and childhood depression. Instead, there appears to be a somewhat stronger association between maternal characteristics and childhood depression than between paternal characteristics and childhood depression. Only in the study by John et al. (1987) did father effects emerge where no mother effects were found, but in five studies maternal effects were found in the absence of paternal effects (Cole & Rehm, 1986; Jensen et al., 1990; Kaslow et al., 1988; Puig-Antich et al., 1985a, 1985b). However, there were important paternal correlates to child depression, such as children's self-reported paternal–child relationships, that require further investigation.

Suicidal Behavior

Three studies were found that investigated the fathers and mothers of suicidal children and adolescents. McKenry, Tishler, and Kelley (1982) compared adolescents who had attempted suicide with nonsuicidal adolescents admitted to an emergency room with minor injuries. They found that the attempters and nonattempter controls did not differ in their perceptions of their fathers' interest in them, although attempters perceived their mothers to be significantly less interested in them than did the nonattempter controls. Attempters and their fathers, but not their mothers, rated the parents' marriage as less well adjusted than did the nonattempters and their fathers. All three members in the attempters' family (father, mother, and adolescent) viewed time spent with the family as significantly less enjoyable than the three corresponding members of the nonattempters' family. Fathers of attempters perceived their spouses' parenting skills as significantly lower than did the fathers of nonattempters. Fathers of attempters were significantly more depressed than fathers of nonattempters, and mothers of attempters were significantly more anxious and had more prior suicidal ideation than mothers of nonattempters (McKenry et al., 1982).

In a comparison of fathers of suicidal children with fathers of children with other psychiatric disorders, Myers, Burke, and McCauley (1985) examined suicidal and nonsuicidal preadolescents on an inpatient psychiatric unit and found that the suicidal preadolescents were significantly more likely to have a physically abusive biological father and a physically abused mother than nonsuicidal preadolescents. They also found that the suicidal and nonsuicidal inpatients did not differ significantly in family history of alcoholism, depression, antisocial activities, personality disorder, or psychosis, although they did not investigate these disorders separately for fathers and mothers (Myers et al., 1985). These results are consistent with a previously mentioned study that found that paternal and maternal alcohol abuse and affective disorder did not distinguish between adolescent inpatients who were either nonassaultive–nonsuicidal, suicidal only, assaultive only, or assaultive–suicidal (Pfeffer et al., 1989). None of these studies directly compared fathers and mothers of suicidal children and adolescents.

In summary, fathers of suicidal children and adolescents appear more distressed than fathers of normal control children with regard to increased depression and decreased enjoyment of time in the family and in the marriage. Fathers of suicidal children do not appear different from fathers of nonsuicidal, psychiatrically disturbed children except for a higher incidence of physical abuse toward their children and spouse. Although fathers and mothers of suicidal children were not directly compared, the pattern of findings for fathers and mothers appears relatively comparable.

Anxiety Disorders

A few studies have examined fathers of children with diagnosed anxiety disorders. Both fathers and mothers of anxious and obsessive–compulsive adolescents were found to have more obsessional characteristics than fathers and mothers in a nonclinical control sample (Clark & Bolton, 1985). However, fathers of anxious children were not found to have any greater likelihood of antisocial personality disorder or alcoholism compared with fathers of normal control children, but mothers of children with anxiety disorders were found to have increased rates of anxiety disorders themselves when compared with children in a nonclinical sample (Reeves et al., 1987). In a sample of school phobic children, fathers reported clinically significant levels of family dysfunction in the father–child relationship in the areas of role performance, values, and norms (Bernstein, Svingen, & Garfinkel, 1990). Mothers' reports were also clinically significant in the same areas for the mother–child relationship. Overall, fathers and mothers rated their relationships with their school phobic child in a very similar manner (Bernstein et al., 1990). Taken together, these studies provide some evidence for greater disturbance in fathers of children with anxiety disorders when compared with fathers in nonclinical control samples, although the findings are somewhat equivocal.

Schizophrenia

The study of schizophrenia has had a long history of focusing on mother–child interactions in the etiology of the disorder. Still, there has been some research investigating fathers' interactions with children who eventually develop schizophrenia. As long ago as 1956, Lidz, Parker, and Cornelison used clinical observations and interviews to investigate the role of the father in the development of schizophrenia. More recently, harsh paternal discipline has been found to be associated with schizophrenic inpatient assaults and dangerousness (Yesavage et al., 1983), and paternal outward-directed hostility and maternal inward-directed hostility have been associated with readmittance to a psychiatric inpatient unit (Angermeyer, 1982).

Family communication style, such as expressed emotion (EE) and communication deviance, has been linked to the onset and course of schizophrenic disorders (e.g., Hahlweg et al., 1989; Miklowitz, Goldstein, et al., 1989; Miklowitz, Strachan, et al., 1986; Strachan, Feingold, Goldstein, Miklowitz, & Nuechterlein, 1989). Although most of these studies included both fathers and mothers of schizophrenic offspring, differences between fathers and mothers were rarely evaluated. In a sample of relatives of schizophrenics that were combined for the analyses (36% fathers, 56% mothers, and 8% other relatives), Miklowitz et al. (1986) found that high-EE relatives showed significantly higher communication deviance than low-EE relatives. Additionally, they found that high-EE critical attitudes were more evident in fathers and nonparent relatives than mothers, whereas high-EE overinvolvement and critical overinvolvement attitudes were more evident in mothers than fathers and nonparent relatives (Miklowitz et al., 1986). They also found that relatives with high-EE overinvolvement attitudes (represented primarily by mothers rather than fathers) showed the highest levels of communication deviance; however, the direct comparison was not completed for fathers and mothers.

Autism

In a comprehensive review, Sanua (1986) reviewed 20 years of research on autistic children and concluded that fathers and mothers of autistic children were no different than fathers and mothers of normal control children. Sanua also concluded that fathers and mothers of autistic children were no different than fathers and mothers of nonautistic clinically referred children and children with organic damage. Although some studies have found differences between fathers of autistic children and nonautistic children (e.g., Wolff, Narayan, & Moyes, 1988), the overriding evidence has suggested that there were no differences between fathers and mothers of autistic children and parents of nonautistic children.

Eating Disorders

Numerous studies have investigated family interaction patterns in families of anorexic, bulimic, and nonreferred adolescents (e.g., Garfinkel et al., 1983; Humphrey, 1986, 1987, 1989; Humphrey, Apple, & Kirschenbaum, 1986; Leon, Lucas, Colligan, Ferdinande, & Kamp, 1985). The eating-disordered and non-eating-disordered families are usually found to differ in observations or perceptions of family interactions; however, there are notable examples in which no differences were found. For example, fathers of anorexics did not differ from fathers of nonreferred control adolescents on a measure of family relationships, but mothers and their anorexic daughters reported more difficulty with task accomplishment, role performance, communication, and affective expression than did controls (Garfinkel et al., 1983). Additionally, Garfinkel and colleagues (1983) found that fathers and mothers of anorexics did not differ from controls in ratings of their own body size or body satisfaction. Fathers of anorexics showed higher levels of conscientiousness than fathers of nonreferred adolescent controls on the Sixteen Personality Factor Questionnaire (16PF), but mothers of anorexics did not differ from mothers of controls in rates of psychopathology (Garfinkel et al., 1983).

Leon et al. (1985) also investigated perceptions of family interactions with anorexic adolescents and their fathers and mothers. When compared with their counterparts in a normal-weight control group, fathers and mothers of anorexic girls perceived the family environment to be less conducive to the expression of feelings and as less cohesive. The anorexic and normal-weight adolescents did not differ significantly in their perceptions of the family environment (Leon et al., 1985). Humphrey and her colleagues (Humphrey, 1986, 1987, 1989; Humphrey et al., 1986) did, however, find differences between anorexic adolescents (as well as bulimics and bulimic–anorexics) and normal control adolescents in their perceptions of parent–child relationships. For example, Humphrey (1986) found that bulimics and bulimic–anorexics perceived their parents to be less affirming, understanding, nurturing, and comforting toward them than did nonclinical adolescents. Bulimic adolescents also perceived greater deficits in parental nurturance than the bulimic–anorexic, anorexic, and nonclinical adolescents. These findings were most consistent for the bulimic daughter–father relationship (e.g., significant findings on eight out of eight clusters) and less consistent for the bulimic daughter–mother relationship (e.g., significant findings on only two of the eight clusters).

In a related study of observed family interactions, Humphrey (1989) found that both fathers and mothers of anorexics gave a double message of nurturance and affection combined with neglect of their daughter's needs. Fathers and mothers of bulimics were hostilely enmeshed with their daughter and appeared to undermine their daughter's attempts at separation and self-assertion. In contrast, the fathers and mothers of nonreferred adolescents showed higher levels of helping, protecting, trusting, approaching, and enjoying one another. Although these different patterns were found for both fathers and mothers in the three groups, fathers showed less unique differences across the groups than mothers (Humphrey, 1989).

Taken together these studies suggest that investigation of perceptions of paternal and maternal relationships may be helpful in distinguishing subtypes of eating disorders as well as elucidating different patterns of involvement of fathers and mothers of adolescents with eating disorders and normal-weight non-eating-disordered adolescents.

Summary

Overall, fathers of children who have received a psychiatric diagnosis or who have been referred for psychological treatment show increased levels of psychopathology when compared with fathers of children who have not been diagnosed or referred for psychological treatment. The results of these studies are summarized in Table 1. Paternal characteristics are more consistently related to externalizing problems (ADHD, conduct disorder, delinquent behaviors) than internalizing problems (depression, anxiety disorders) in their children.

CHILDREN OF DIAGNOSED OR CLINICALLY REFERRED FATHERS

A second research methodology has involved studies of children whose fathers have sought or been referred for clinical services or have received a psychiatric diagnosis. The behavioral and psychological adjustment of these children has been examined in cross-sectional, retrospective, and—more rarely—prospective longitudinal studies. Fathers with a variety of diagnoses have been included. Furthermore, children's adjustment has been measured using a variety of methods

TABLE 1
Findings From Studies of Paternal Factors in Child and Adolescent Psychopathology:
Studies of Referred/Diagnosed Children

Problem type	Referred children
Attention-deficit hyperactivity disorder (ADHD)	Fathers of ADHD children higher on nonclincal measures than fathers of controls (5 studies); no differences from fathers of controls on paternal psychopathology (2 studies)
	No differences reported between mothers and fathers (6 studies); mixed findings on paternal–maternal differences in 2 studies
	No differences in comparisons with children from other diagnostic categories (2 studies)
Conduct disorder (CD)	Fathers of CD children higher in alcoholism and antisocial personality disorder than fathers of controls (1 study)
	Greater associations bewteen mothers and CD daughters than fathers and CD daughters (1 study)
	Fathers of CD sons higher in disturbance than fathers of sons with other disorders (6 studies)
Delinquency	Equivocal findings comparing fathers of delinquent adolescents with controls (2 studies)
	Fathers and mothers of delinquent daughters show more conflict than fathers and mothers of delinquent sons (1 study)
	No comparisons with other disorders
	Multiple paternal characteristics correlated with delinquency in adolescents (6 studies)
Alcohol/substance abuse	Equivocal findings regarding paternal correlates and adolescents' substance abuse (3 studies)
	No other studies
Nonspecific behavior problems	Fathers had more unrealistic beliefs than in control families (1 study)
	Equivocal findings comparing fathers and mothers (3 studies)
	No comparisons with other disorders
Depression	No differences from controls in family interactions and paternal depressive symptoms (2 studies)
	Greater evidence for child depression associated with maternal than paternal depression (4 studies)
	No differences in paternal psychopathology compared with other diagnostic groups of children (3 studies)
Suicidal behavior	Fathers of attempters more depressed than controls (1 study)
	No studies comparing fathers and mothers
	Fathers of suicidal children more physically abusive than clinical comparison (1 study)
Anxiety disorders	Fathers higher in obsessional characteritics than fathers of controls (1 study)
	No differences between fathers and mothers of school phobics (1 study)
	No studies with other diagnostic groups
Schizophrenia	No studies with control groups, father–mother comparisons, or with other diagnostic groups
	Harsh paternal discipline and hostility correlated with schizophrenia in offspring (2 studies)
Autism	See Sanua (1986) for review of studies
Eating disorders	More maladaptive family interactions and environments, including fathers, than controls (5 studies); no differences from controls (1 study)
	Equivocal findings comparing fathers and mothers (1 study)
	No studies with other diagnostic groups

(behavior checklists, self-report questionnaires, diagnostic interviews) and from a variety of informants (children, parents, teachers, clinicians). The studies are grouped by type of paternal psychopathology, with the major diagnostic groups being antisocial personality/criminality, alcoholism and substance abuse, depression, anxiety disorders, schizophrenia, perpetrators of child physical and sexual abuse, and physical illness.

Paternal Antisocial Personality Disorder and Criminality

Paternal criminality and antisocial behavior have been identified as significant risk factors for delinquent behavior in offspring in a number of studies (see reviews by Loeber & Dishion, 1983, 1987). In spite of the importance of this area of research, we were able to identify only one study that examined the functioning of children whose parents had committed criminal or antisocial acts (Kandel et al., 1988). This study focused on the role of IQ as a protective factor for offspring at high risk for antisocial behavior. Offspring of fathers with serious criminal offenses who were able to avoid criminal behavior themselves were found to have higher IQs than those offspring of criminal fathers who had been identified for serious criminal behavior.

The apparent absence of research in this area may be the result of reliance on an alternative research methodology to pursue the relation between paternal criminality/antisocial behavior and child functioning. That is, the more typical research design has been to identify a sample of youth who have committed delinquent acts and then to examine the criminal status of their father. Although this has been a productive approach to understanding the link between parental and offspring criminality and delinquency, it may have led to a somewhat distorted picture of the effects of paternal criminality. By focusing on identified populations of delinquent youth, other problems of the offspring of criminal fathers may have been overlooked. Thus, studies that examine a broad range of factors related to the adjustment and functioning of children of fathers who are identified for antisocial or criminal behaviors are still much needed.

Paternal Alcoholism and Substance Abuse

Substantial research indicates that children of alcoholic fathers, or more generally fathers who abuse alcohol, are at increased risk for a wide range of emotional and behavioral difficulties. In fact, the literature on the relation between parental alcoholism and children's maladjustment is rare in that fathers with this disorder have been studied more often than mothers. In a comprehensive review of this literature from 1975 to 1985, West and Prinz (1987) noted, "nearly all of the samples in studies reviewed contained more male than female alcoholics, and many consisted entirely of men. Consequently, less is known about the impact of maternal alcoholism on children's risk for psychopathology" (p. 205). This is not surprising in light of the higher rate of alcoholism in men as opposed to women (Helzer, 1987).

The findings of studies between 1975 and 1985 reviewed by West and Prinz (1987) indicate that paternal alcoholism is related to a host of problems in children, including externalizing behavior problems such as hyperactivity and conduct disorder (e.g., Fine, Yudin, Holmes, & Heinemann, 1976; Knop, Teasdale, Schulsinger, & Goodwin, 1985), alcohol/substance abuse (e.g., Herjanic, Herjanic, Penick, Tomelleri, & Armbruster, 1977; Merikangas, Weissman, Prusoff, Pauls, & Leckman, 1985), and delinquency (e.g., Offord, Allen, & Abrams, 1978; Rimmer, 1982) and symptoms of internalizing problems such as depression and anxiety (e.g., Herjanic et al., 1977).

Studies that have appeared after those reviewed by West and Prinz (i.e., after 1985) have continued to report that children of alcoholic fathers evidence a wide range of emotional and behavioral difficulties. When compared with control samples, children of alcoholic fathers have been found to have higher rates of alcoholism (Goodwin, 1986); to have a greater tendency for self-deprecation (Berkowitz & Perkins, 1988); to be less happy (Callan & Jackson, 1986); to perceive their family environment as less happy, trusting, secure, cohesive, and affectionate (Callan & Jackson, 1986); to be higher in the *impatience–aggressive* dimension of Type A behavior (Manning, Balson, & Xenakis, 1986); and to display more symptoms of neuroticism (Benson & Heller, 1987) and acting out problems (Benson & Heller, 1987).

Perhaps because of the lower incidence of alcoholism in women, studies comparing children of alcoholic mothers and children of alcoholic fathers have been rare. Those data that are available offer mixed results. In a study of responsivity to stress, Levenson, Oyama, and Meek (1987) found that paternal alcoholism was associated with increased children's responsivity to stress after consuming alcohol, whereas maternal alcoholism was not related to stress responsivity in children. In contrast, Werner (1986) found that children with an alcoholic mother were more likely to develop high levels of psychosocial problems compared with children of alcoholic fathers. Steinhausen, Gobel, and Nestler (1984) compared children with either an alcoholic mother, an alcoholic father, or two alcoholic parents and did not find differences on a series of questionnaires and psychiatric symptom scores related to children's adjustment. An earlier study by El-Guebaly, Offord, Sullivan, and Lynch (1978) is noteworthy in this regard. They compared groups of children who were identified on the basis of either paternal or maternal alcoholism, depression, or schizophrenia and did not find differences in parents' reports of their children's behavior problems in families with alcoholic fathers as compared with families with alcoholic mothers.

Only a few studies have compared children whose fathers are alcoholic with children whose fathers suffer from other forms of psychiatric disturbance. However, these studies indicate that this is an important area for further research. For example, Jacob and Leonard (1986) found that children of alcoholic fathers and children of depressed fathers did not differ from one another but were both rated higher than normal controls on combined ratings by both parents on the Child Behavior Checklist (CBCL; Achenbach & Edelbrock, 1983); however, no differences were found among children of depressed fathers, alcoholic fathers, and normal control fathers on teacher ratings of behavior problems. El-Guebaly et al. (1978) found some evidence that parents' reports of child behavior problems were higher in families of depressed fathers and schizophrenic fathers than in families of alcoholic fathers. However, these differences were no longer significant after controlling for differences between families in number of children.

In summary, children of alcoholic fathers have been consistently found to be at risk for a wide variety of emotional and behavioral difficulties. Findings have been more limited and equivocal when comparing the effects of paternal alcoholism and maternal alcoholism and when comparing the effects of alcoholic fathers with other psychiatrically disturbed fathers.

Paternal Depression

Depression is perhaps the most extensively researched form of parental psychopathology as a source of risk for child maladjustment. Given the substantially higher rate of depression in adult women than in adult men, it is not surprising that the vast majority of this research has examined the functioning of children of depressed mothers. In fact, in several recent reviews of studies of children of depressed parents, no mention is made of depression in fathers (e.g., Beardslee, 1986; Beardslee, Bemporad, Keller, & Klerman, 1983; Cytryn, McKnew, Zahn-Waxler, & Gershon, 1986; Orvaschel, Weissman, & Kidd, 1980; Weintraub, Winters, & Neale, 1986). However, findings from a number of recent studies indicate that failure to consider the impact of paternal depression represents an important omission.

At least 11 recent studies have examined the functioning of children of depressed fathers (Atkinson & Rickel, 1984; Beardslee, Schultz, & Selman, 1987; Billings & Moos, 1983, 1985; El-Guebaly et al., 1978; Jacob & Leonard, 1986; D. N. Klein, Clark, Dansky, & Margolis, 1988; D. N. Klein, Depue, & Slater, 1985; Orvaschel, Walsh-Allis, & Ye, 1988; Radke-Yarrow, Cummings, Kuczynski, & Chapman, 1985; Zahn-Waxler, Cummings, McKnew, & Radke-Yarrow, 1984). In 8 of these studies, children of depressed fathers were found to be at increased risk for behavioral and psychological maladjustment when compared with control children (Atkinson & Rickel, 1984; Beardslee et al., 1987;

Billings & Moos, 1983, 1985; El-Guebaly et al., 1978; Jacob & Leonard, 1986; D. N. Klein et al., 1988; Orvaschel et al., 1988). For example, Jacob and Leonard found that children of depressed fathers (and children of alcoholic fathers) were rated by their parents as higher in behavior problems than children of control fathers. These authors also noted that there was considerable heterogeneity among the children with alcoholic and depressed fathers, with only a minority of these children exceeding the clinical cutoffs suggested by Achenbach and Edelbrock (1983) for the CBCL. Orvaschel et al. (1988) used structured clinical interviews to assess psychopathology in children of parents with recurrent major depression and found that children of depressed fathers (and mothers) had higher rates of psychopathology than children of nondepressed control parents. Data reported by Billings and Moos (1983, 1985) are particularly important because they provide the only follow-up data on children of depressed fathers. Both at the initial assessment (Billings & Moos, 1983) and at a 1-year follow-up (Billings & Moos, 1985), children of depressed parents, including depressed fathers, were found to be rated as more impaired than controls.

Samples of depressed fathers are most often included in studies along with samples of depressed mothers, and the majority of these studies have failed to find any differences in children's risk for maladjustment as a function of which parent is identified as depressed (Atkinson & Rickel, 1984; Beardslee et al., 1987; Billings & Moos, 1983, 1985; D. N. Klein et al., 1988; Orvaschel et al., 1988). For example, Orvaschel et al. (1988) examined the rates of psychopathology in children of 8 fathers and 26 mothers diagnosed for major depression. They found that the rates of psychopathology in children of depressed parents were consistently higher when compared with control children, but the association between sex of the diagnosed parent and children's diagnostic status was not significant. Children of depressed parents in this study were found to have higher rates of diagnoses of not only affective disorders but also attention-deficit disorder (ADD) and anxiety disorders. Similarly, Billings and Moos (1983) reported on parents' ratings of the functioning of their children in a sample of 90 depressed mothers, 43 depressed fathers, and 135 controls. They found that the gender of the depressed parent was not related to children's functioning, with children of depressed parents being rated as having more physical, emotional, behavioral, school, and peer problems than control children. These findings held up at a subsequent follow-up with this sample (Billings & Moos, 1985). Finally, the earlier study by El-Guebaly et al. (1978) reported evidence indicating that children of depressed fathers were rated by their parents as having more behavior problems than were children of depressed mothers. However, this difference was no longer significant after the investigators controlled for differences in family size between the two samples.

Two studies by D. N. Klein and colleagues suggest that the effects of unipolar and bipolar depression may differ for fathers and mothers. D. N. Klein et al. (1988) compared children of 5 fathers and 19 mothers with unipolar depression, 8 fathers and 11 mothers with medical illnesses, and 18 controls. The rate of dysthymia was greater in the offspring of depressed parents than in controls but was not related to the sex of the depressed parent. In contrast, D. N. Klein et al. (1985) examined the adolescent children of 11 fathers and 13 mothers diagnosed with bipolar depression. They found that a significantly greater number of children of bipolar mothers received a psychiatric diagnosis (69%) than did children of bipolar fathers (27%).

In summary, although samples of depressed fathers have been small, the findings of recent studies indicate that children of depressed fathers are at increased risk for a variety of emotional and behavioral problems. Furthermore, at least with regard to unipolar depression in parents, children of depressed fathers appear to exhibit a similar level of problems as children of depressed mothers.

Paternal Anxiety Disorders

As indicated by findings from the Epidemiological Catchment Area (ECA) study, anxiety disorders may be the most frequent psychiatric disorder among adults (Regier et al., 1984). Although rates of all types of anxiety disorders are higher among women than among men, data from the ECA study and other surveys of adult samples indicate that some forms of anxiety have surprisingly high rates of prevalence among adult men (Barlow, 1988). For example, estimates of prevalence rates of simple phobias in men range from 2.3% to 7.3% of men, and social phobia is estimated at approximately 1.7% in men. These high rates of anxiety disorders among men make it especially important to examine the relation between anxiety disorders in fathers and the adjustment of their children.

In light of these statistics, it is distressing that we were able to identify only one study of the functioning of children whose fathers have anxiety disorders (reported in Weissman, Gershon, et al., 1984; Weissman, Leckman, Merikangas, Gammon, & Prusoff, 1984). Furthermore, this study was designed to examine the functioning of children whose parents were diagnosed for depression in a sample of 60 probands (43% fathers, 57% mothers), and the effects of parental anxiety were only studied when anxiety disorders were present in addition to parental depression. The presence of an anxiety disorder (agoraphobia, panic disorder, generalized anxiety disorder) in a parent increased the risk for disorder in children when compared with children of normal control parents and children whose parents were diagnosed with only depression. There were no differences in the rates of psychiatric disorders in children when examined as a function of gender of the diagnosed parent. However, the authors urge caution in interpreting this failure to find a difference as a function of sex of parent because of the small samples of children in some of the groups.

The high base rates of the prevalence of some forms of anxiety disorders in men, combined with the virtual absence of data on the functioning of children of fathers with anxiety disorders, make this an area of high priority for future research.

Paternal Schizophrenia

Similar to research on parental depression, studies of the adjustment and development of children of schizophrenic parents have focused predominantly on children whose mothers have been diagnosed with the disorder. The absence of investigations of children of schizophrenic fathers may be the result of two factors. First, many of the children in these studies have mothers who were schizophrenic and unmarried, and typically little or no information is available to researchers on the psychiatric status of the biological father (Walker & Emory, 1983). Second, schizophrenic men are said to be unlikely to marry and have children and therefore are considered atypical and are not often available for study (Watt, 1986).

Note that several ongoing longitudinal projects concerned with children at risk for schizophrenia have included samples of offspring of both fathers and mothers who were diagnosed as schizophrenic (see Watt, 1986; and Watt, Anthony, Wynne, & Rolf, 1984, for reviews of these studies). For example, the St. Louis High-Risk Research Project (Worland, Janes, Anthony, McGinnis, & Cass, 1984), the New York High-Risk Project (Erlenmeyer-Kimling et al., 1984), and the Stony Brook High-Risk Project (Weintraub & Neale, 1984) all included both schizophrenic fathers and mothers in the selection of their original samples. Unfortunately, most of the reports of analyses of the data from these comprehensive studies have not included parental gender as an independent variable.

The few reports of analyses that distinguish schizophrenic fathers and mothers have produced mixed results regarding the development, adjustment, and presence of psychopathology in their children. Silverton, Mednick, Schulsinger, Parnas, and Harrington (1988) studied the relation between low birth weight and cerebral ventricular enlargement in individuals whose mothers were schizophrenic, some of whom had fathers who were also schizophrenic and some of whom had fathers who did not receive this diagnosis. They found that the association between birth weight and ventricular enlargement was greater in those individuals whose father was schizophrenic and interpreted this as an indicator of increased genetic risk for the disorder when the father was also schizophrenic. In contrast, Itil, Huque, Shapiro, Mednick, and Schulsinger (1983) compared the electroencephalogram (EEG) functioning of 21 children of schizophrenic fathers, 43 children with schizophrenic mothers, 7 children whose father and mother were schizophrenic, and 71 children whose parents had no psychiatric diagnosis. Children of schizophrenic fathers differed from controls on only 4 of 22 EEG measures, whereas children of schizophrenic mothers differed from controls on 13 of 22 measures. Furthermore, children of schizophrenic fathers were found to differ from children of schizophrenic mothers on 11 of these measures. The authors concluded that "it appears that schizophrenic mothers have a more dominating effect on the brain function of their offspring than do schizophrenic fathers" (Itil et al., 1983, p. 74).

With regard to children's social and psychological functioning, an early study described above (El-Guebaly et al., 1978) compared the functioning of children whose father as opposed to mother was diagnosed as schizophrenic. They found that children of schizophrenic fathers were rated by their parents as having more behavioral and emotional problems than were children of schizophrenic mothers. However, these effects were no longer significant after controlling for differences in family size. In analyses of data from the New York High-Risk Project, Erlenmeyer-Kimling et al. (1984) reported on the adjustment of 23 children of schizophrenic fathers, 44 children of schizophrenic mothers, 13 children with two schizophrenic parents, 25 children of psychiatric control parents, and 100 children of parents who received no psychiatric diagnosis. Specifically, they examined the proportion of each group who had been hospitalized or received treatment for psychological problems. With regard to children of schizophrenic parents, 3 of 23 (13%) of schizophrenic fathers, 10 of 44 (22.7%) of schizophrenic mothers, and 3 of 13 (23%) of two schizophrenic parents had been hospitalized or received treatment. Although the authors did not report any statistical analyses of these data, we conducted a chi-square analysis, and this failed to reveal a significant difference as a function of gender of the diagnosed parent. Weintraub and Neale (1984) reported that schizophrenic fathers were perceived more negatively (i.e., unaccepting and uninvolved) by their children than were fathers who received no psychiatric diagnosis. In contrast, schizophrenic mothers were perceived by their children as more involved, more child-centered, and more lax in discipline than were nondiagnosed mothers. Finally, findings from the University of Rochester Child and Family Study provided information on the interactions of schizophrenic fathers and mothers as well as their spouse with their children in a free-play situation (Baldwin, Baldwin, Cole, & Kokes, 1984). Fathers were more active than mothers with their children regardless of their status as patient or spouse, and nonschizophrenic spouses were more active than patients with their children regardless of their gender.

In summary, the literature to this point on the degree of risk for children of schizophrenic fathers is unclear. These children may be at increased risk for neurological, psychological, and behavioral difficulties. However, in at least some areas of functioning, children of schizophrenic fathers may be less impaired than are children of schizophrenic mothers. Several ongoing longitudinal studies of children of schizophrenic mothers and fathers may shed more light on these issues.

Fathers Who Physically and Sexually Abuse Their Children

The literature on fathers who are identified for abuse of their children encompasses sexual, physical, and emotional abuse. Research into these various types of abuse has taken very different forms. Because most intrafamilial sexual abuse of children is perpetrated by fathers, this literature has concentrated primarily on this population. In contrast, studies of physical and emotional abuse have involved mothers almost exclusively (Wolfe, 1985).

In a review of the literature on childhood sexual abuse, Browne and Finkelhor (1986) concluded that in those studies in which the relationship of the victim and the perpetrator was examined, there was evidence of greater psychological trauma in victims from experiences involving fathers or father figures compared with all other types of perpetrators. However, at the time of their review this evidence was based on only two studies that found more severe maladjustment in children victimized by their father (Finkelhor, 1979; Russell, 1987), one study that found a greater effect for sexual abuse by stepfathers but not biological fathers (Tufts' New England Medical Center, Division of Child Psychiatry, 1984), and one study that found small but nonsignificant differences in victims' maladjustment as a result of being abused by their father.

Since this review, several more recent studies have found increasing evidence for greater levels of psychological maladjustment associated with sexual abuse by fathers or father figures as opposed to other perpetrators (Harter, Alexander, & Neimeyer, 1988; Scott & Stone, 1986; Sirles, Smith, & Kusama, 1989). Scott and Stone (1986) compared adolescents who had been victims of father–daughter incest with a control sample with no history of sexual abuse and found that incest victims were more elevated than controls on all clinical scales of the Minnesota Multiphasic Personality Inventory (MMPI), and these victims were in the clinical range on the Validity (F), Psychasthenia, and Schizophrenia Scales. In a comparison of 29 college women with a history of sexual abuse by a family member and 59 controls, Harter et al. (1988) found that abuse in general was not related to victims' maladjustment after controlling for a set of family and social cognitive variables. However, abuse by a paternal figure was related to poorer adjustment even after accounting for these other factors. Sirles et al. (1989) examined the initial psychiatric profiles of a sample of sexually abused children who were evaluated at an outpatient child psychiatry clinic. Children abused by a paternal figure were significantly more likely to receive a psychiatric diagnosis (45% of those abused by their biological father and 44% of those abused by their stepfather) than children who had been abused by another relative (25.7%). In summary, these more recent studies underscore the adverse outcomes associated with childhood sexual abuse and underscore the increased risk when this abuse has been perpetrated by the biological father or other father figure.

The picture with regard to the effects of physical abuse by fathers is much less clear. In a previous review of this literature, Wolfe (1985) reported that studies to that point in time had been based almost entirely on samples of mothers only. Although the majority of research with parents of physically abused children has continued to involve primarily mothers, some recent studies have investigated paternal correlates of child physical abuse. For example, Garbarino, Sebes, and Schellenbach (1984) found that families at high risk for physical abuse were more chaotic and enmeshed, with low paternal supportive behavior and high maternal punitiveness. Rogeness, Amrung, Macedo, Harris, and Fisher (1986) also found higher rates of psychopathology in parents, especially fathers, of physically abused and neglected children. More specifically, they found mothers of neglected children had higher rates of psychiatric disturbance, but not alcoholism or antisocial personalities, than mothers of children who were not abused or neglected. Fathers of abused or neglected children had higher rates of psychiatric disturbance and antisocial personality than fathers of nonabused or neglected children. Additionally, fathers of abused or neglected boys, but not girls, were found to have significantly higher rates of alcoholism (Rogeness et al., 1986).

Mothers and fathers who have physically abused their children were also found to report more psychological symptoms than mothers and fathers of nonabused children (Reid, Kavanagh, & Baldwin, 1987). Mothers of abused children reported higher rates than controls on all self-reported psychological symptoms that were measured (disposition, hostile–withdrawn, aggression, intellectual inefficiency, and conduct problems), but fathers of abused children self-reported higher rates of only conduct problems compared with fathers of nonabused children. Mothers and fathers of abused children also reported significantly more child conduct problems than controls; however, independent observations showed few differences in child, maternal, or paternal behavior between the two groups (Reid et al., 1987).

Taken together, these studies suggest the importance of including both mothers and fathers, as well as observers, in the investigation of parental correlates to child physical abuse, because different patterns of results have been found with the use of different informants.

Paternal Physical Illness

The presence of a chronic or acute illness in fathers may have an impact on the psychological adjustment of their children. However, this possibility has not been examined to any great extent in the literature. We identified only one study that directly examined the psychological adjustment of children whose father was physically ill. Rickard (1988) assessed the level of behavior problems in children of fathers with chronic low-back pain (CLBP), children of diabetic fathers, and children of fathers with no identifiable physical illness. Children of fathers with CLBP were higher than children in either of the comparison groups on teacher-reported and self-reported behavioral and emotional problems, including external-izing behavior problems, physical complaints, crying/whining, avoidance, dependency, greater external health locus of control, days absent from school, and visits to the school nurse.

A second study examined parent–child interactions in families of fathers with hypertension (Baer, 1983). Families with hypertensive fathers showed higher rates of negative nonverbal behaviors in laboratory interactions than control families. These differences were not accounted for by fathers' behavior but rather were attributable to differences in the actions of mothers and children in these families. When the authors examined a specific nonverbal behavior, gaze aversion, during family interactions, they found that mothers—but not fathers or children—in families with hypertensive fathers showed higher rates of gaze aversion before and after but not during negative and critical remarks by the father.

These studies suggest the need for more research on the possible effects of paternal physical illness on children. Furthermore, they suggest that the mecha-nisms by which paternal illness might affect children may be rooted in complex forms of family interactions, especially when associated with chronic illness.

Summary

As summarized in Table 2, children whose father has been referred for psycho-logical treatment or has received a psychiatric diagnosis are at increased risk for a variety of different types of psychopathology as compared with children whose father has not been referred or diagnosed. In many cases, the level of maladjust-ment is similar in children whether their father or mother has received a diagnosis or been referred for treatment.

STUDIES OF NONREFERRED SAMPLES OF FATHERS AND CHILDREN

A third methodology has involved studies of indicators of maladjustment and psychopathology in children in samples in which neither the father nor the child has been diagnosed or referred for clinical services. The majority of these studies are correlational, examining the degree of association between an index of psy-chological symptoms in the father and a comparable measure for the child.

TABLE 2
Findings From Studies of Paternal Factors in Child and Adolescent Psychopathology:
Studies of Referred/Diagnosed Fathers

Problem type	Referred fathers
Antisocial personality disorder (APD)	No studies comparing APD fathers to controls, mothers, or other diagnostic groups
Alcohol/substance abuse	Children of alcoholic fathers more disturbed than children of control fathers (7 studies)
	No differences between children of alcoholic fathers and mothers (4 studies)
	No differences between children of alcoholic fathers and children of fathers with other disorders (2 studies)
Depression	Children of depressed fathers more disturbed than controls (8 studies); no differences from controls (3 studies)
	No differences between children of depressed fathers and children of depressed mothers (6 studies)
	No differences from other disorders (1 study)
Anxiety disorders	No differences between children of anxious/depressed fathers and children of controls (1 study)
	No differences between children of anxious/depressed fathers and children of anxious/depressed mothers (1 study)
	No studies with other diagnostic groups
Schizophrenia	Children of schizophrenic fathers more disturbed than children of controls (2 studies)
	No difference between children of schizophrenic fathers and children of schizophrenic mothers (2 studies); children of schizophrenic mothers more distrubed than children of schizophrenic fathers (1 study)
	No studies with other diagnostic groups
Physical and sexual abuse	Children sexually abused by fathers more disturbed than children abused by nonfathers (3 studies)
	Children physically abused by fathers or mothers more disturbed than controls (2 studies)
	No studies with other diagnostic groups
Physical illness	Children of physically ill fathers more disturbed than controls (3 studies); no differences from controls (2 studies)
	No other studies

Delinquency

Several delinquent-type behaviors in children and adolescents have been investigated in relation to parental characteristics, and similar patterns tend to emerge for fathers and mothers. For example, rejection by father or by mother was associated with lying in a sample of fourth- and seventh-grade boys (Stouthamer-Loeber & Loeber, 1986), and low levels of paternal and maternal acceptance were associated with boys' fighting in both school and home (Loeber & Dishion, 1984). Decreased perceptions of love by their father and mother and increased amounts of anger toward their father and mother were associated with increased levels of self-reported delinquency in a sample of male and female adolescents (R. E. Johnson, 1987), and both fathers' and mothers' support for aggression was associated with self-reported aggressive delinquency in male and female adolescents (Neapolitan, 1981). Additionally, in a study that only investigated fathers and sons, boys who share their future plans, thoughts, and feelings with their father were less likely to exhibit violent behavior (Brownfield, 1987). Overall, paternal and maternal correlates of delinquent behavior are similar and quite evident in nonreferred samples.

Alcohol and Substance Use

Several studies with nonreferred samples of adolescents have found an association between paternal characteristics and the use of alcohol and marijuana by their offspring. Forney et al. (1984), in a study of alcohol use by sixth and eighth graders, found that children who were heavy drinkers tended to have fathers who were heavy drinkers. Barnes and colleagues (Barnes, 1984; Barnes, Farrell, & Cairns, 1986) did not find a significant relation between paternal alcohol use and drinking by adolescents, but they did find an association between paternal socialization practices and child alcohol use. Specifically, adolescents who drank more heavily had fathers who were rated as low in providing support and nurturance to their children. Lack of support and nurturance from mothers was also found to be positively related to adolescent alcohol use in both of these studies (Barnes, 1984; Barnes et al., 1986).

A series of papers by J. S. Brook and colleagues have reported on the association between paternal characteristics and marijuana use in a sample of college men and women (Brook, Whiteman, Brook, & Gordon, 1982; Brook, Whiteman, Gordon, & Brook, 1983, 1984a, 1984b, 1986). Participants in this study were 403 female and 246 male college students and their fathers. A very similar picture was obtained of the role of paternal factors in marijuana use by both sons and daughters. Fathers' personality characteristics and child-rearing practices were directly and indirectly related to their sons' and daughters' marijuana use, with the nature of the effects depending on which other predictor variables were included in the analyses. For example, fathers' personality and child-rearing practices were directly related to their sons' marijuana use even after controlling for characteristics of the mother–son relationship (Brook et al., 1983), but these paternal characteristics interacted with sons' peer relationships in predicting marijuana use (Brook et al., 1982). A similar pattern of findings was found in analyses of father–daughter effects (Brook et al., 1984b, 1986).

These studies indicate that the relations between paternal characteristics and child behaviors, alcohol use, and drug use found in studies of referred samples of fathers and children (reported above) are also evident in samples of nonreferred fathers and children. Thus, paternal factors are important in understanding children's alcohol and drug use even in the absence of clinically significant levels of substance abuse.

Nonspecific Behavior Problems

A wide variety of paternal and maternal characteristics have been investigated in relation to children's emotional/behavioral problems in nonreferred samples. Four areas will be summarized in this section: parental behavior and child sociometric status, parental behavior and child adjustment, parental psychological symptoms and child emotional/behavioral problems, and marital conflict and child adjustment.

In analyses of children's sociometric status, fathers of neglected boys engaged in less affectively arousing physical play than fathers of rejected and popular boys, and mothers of rejected boys were more directive than mothers of neglected or popular boys (MacDonald, 1987). Additionally, fathers and mothers of unpopular and moderately popular children used fewer explanations to aid their children than fathers and mothers of popular children (Roopnarine & Adams, 1987), and fathers and mothers of rejected or isolated children reported more patriarchal child-rearing attitudes, had lower self-confidence, and used praise more infrequently than fathers and mothers of amiable or popular children (Peery, Jensen, & Adams, 1985).

With regard to parental behavior and child adjustment, fathers' but not mothers' perceptions of their child were related to teachers' and peers' reports of psychosocial adjustment (Stollak et al., 1982), but fathers' and mothers' problem solving skills were not related to their children's emotional/behavioral problems (Kendall & Fischler, 1984). Fathers' but not mothers' parenting behavior was associated with children's temperament, where paternal involvement, reasoning guidance, limit setting, responsiveness, and intimacy were associated with children's increased behavioral adaptability and decreased emotional intensity (Nelson & Simmerer, 1984).

Paternal and maternal psychological symptoms have been investigated in a variety of nonreferred samples where both fathers' and mothers' symptoms were generally associated with their children's symptoms. For example, both fathers' and mothers' self-reported psychological symptoms were associated with their children's emotional/behavioral problems (e.g., Jensen, Traylor, Xenakis, & Davis, 1988; Phares, Compas, & Howell, 1989). However, Forehand, Long, Brody, and Fauber (1986) found that mothers' but not fathers' self-reported depressive symptoms were related to children's CD problems, although both fathers' and mothers' levels of conflict with their children were related to children's CD problems.

Additionally, in a community-based sample in Puerto Rico, maternal psychiatric history but not paternal psychiatric history was associated with a child having a *Diagnostic and Statistical Manual of Mental Disorders* (American Psychiatric Association, 1980) diagnosis and impairment in adaptive functioning (Bird, Gould, Yager, Staghezza, & Canino, 1989). When controlling for socioeconomic status and the other parent's psychiatric history, paternal psychiatric history was related to children's diagnoses of overanxious disorder, and maternal psychiatric history was related to children's diagnoses of oppositional disorder and major depression (Velez, Johnson, & Cohen, 1989). Overall, these studies suggest that both fathers' and mothers' psychological symptoms are risk factors for children's problems in adjustment.

Fathers' and mothers' reports of interparental conflict and poor marital quality have been associated with a number of adverse effects on children, including increased behavior problems (M. M. Klein & Shulman, 1980) and poor cognitive and social functioning (Wierson, Forehand, & McCombs, 1988). Father–child and mother–child teaching interactions were also influenced by poor marital quality but in opposite directions: Fathers in distressed marriages used effective and involved teaching practices (Brody, Pillegrini, & Sigel, 1986). In both good and poor marriages, poor father–child relationships and poor mother–child relationships were associated with children's increased psychological symptoms (Jenkins & Smith, 1990). These authors argued that good father–child and mother–child relationships can serve as protective factors against the deleterious effects of interparental conflict (Jenkins & Smith, 1990).

Depression

Seven recent studies have examined the relation between paternal factors and symptoms of depression in nonreferred children. Father characteristics were related to their children's depressive symptoms in five of the seven studies. Three of the studies were cross-sectional in design and examined depressive symptoms (Forehand & Smith, 1986), suicidal thoughts (Wright, 1985), and self-criticism and dependency as sources of vulnerability to depression (McCranie & Bass, 1984). Forehand and Smith (1986) found that adolescent daughters' reports of depressive symptoms on the Children's Depression Inventory were related to fathers' reports of depressive symptoms on the Beck Depression Inventory (BDI) but not to mothers' BDI scores. Wright (1985) examined the incidence of suicidal ideation in high school seniors and college students and found that fathers' problems with alcohol and a poor relationship with the father distinguished those with and without suicidal thoughts in the high school sample, whereas a poor relationship with the father distinguished the groups in the college sample. No maternal variables distinguished the groups in either sample. McCranie and Bass (1984) studied the relation between retrospective reports of parental behavior in child-hood and current levels of dependency and self-criticism in a sample of young women. Self-criticism was correlated with reports of fathers' use of strict control, inconsistency of love, and achievement control; none of the father variables were related to dependency. Reports of mothers' parenting behaviors were correlated to both self-criticism and dependency.

Two longitudinal studies found a relation between paternal characteristics and their children's depressive symptoms. Lefkowitz and Tesiny (1984) found that fathers' rejection of the children at age 8 was a significant predictor of their chil-dren's depressive symptoms at age 19. This relation held even after controlling for characteristics of the mother–child relationship. Unfortunately, in two additional cross-sectional studies reported in this article, the authors obtained data concern-ing mothers but not fathers. Richman and Flaherty (1987) examined reports of depressive symptoms and recollections of parental behavior during childhood in a sample of 1st-year medical students. Data were collected at the beginning and end of the academic year to allow for prospective analyses of the data. Reports of low levels of paternal affection and paternal overprotection were related to depressive symptoms at follow-up after controlling for initial levels of depressive symptoms; only overprotection by the mother was a significant predictor.

Two studies failed to find an association between paternal factors and children's depression. Seligman et al. (1984) did not find a relation between fathers' depres-sive symptoms or attributional style and children's depressive symptoms. Both depressive symptoms and attributional style of mothers were related to children's depressive symptoms. Kashani, Burbach, and Rosenberg (1988) failed to find an association between fathers' methods of conflict resolution in the family and depressive symptoms in their adolescent children. In contrast, both adolescents' and their mother's methods of conflict resolution were related to adolescents' depressive symptoms.

In summary, there is relatively strong support for the link between paternal fac-tors and child depressive symptoms in nonreferred samples. This is in contrast to the lack of association between paternal factors and the level of depression in clin-ically referred depressed children reported above.

Paternal Unemployment

The acute and chronic stressful experiences associated with paternal economic loss and unemployment have received sufficient attention in the literature that they warrant a separate comment here. In an excellent recent review of this area of research, McLoyd (1989) reported that significant effects of paternal job and eco-nomic loss on children have been found in numerous studies. However, rather than indicating a direct effect of paternal unemployment on children's adjustment, the evidence supports an indirect model in which paternal economic loss leads to greater negativity and pessimism in the father, which in turn leads to deterioration in the father–child relationship, which results in children's sociemotional problems, somatic symptoms, and reduced personal expectations and aspirations.

McLoyd (1989) identified several moderating variables that affect the relation between paternal economic loss and child maladjustment, including the child's gender, temperament, relationship with the mother, degree of contact with the father, and the child's attractiveness as rated by the father. For example, in their analyses of data on fathers and their children during the Great Depression, Elder, Nguyen, and Caspi (1985) found that adolescent girls' behavior was strongly adversely influenced by the fathers' rejecting behavior but that no such effect was found for adolescent boys.

Paternal Stressful Events

Although personally experienced stressful life events have been shown to be related to psychological maladjustment in numerous studies involving adults, adolescents, and children, considerably less research has examined the association between psychological maladjustment and stressful events experienced by others. Along this line, a few studies have investigated the association between fathers' stressful events and levels of maladjustment in their children and have provided moderate support for this relation. A strength of research in this area is that five of the six recent studies were longitudinal in design.

Two studies have examined fathers' reactions to and coping with specific stressful events. Handford et al. (1986) studied the reactions of 35 children and their parents to the Three Mile Island nuclear accident over a period of 1½ years. Children's anxiety about the event was not directly related to fathers' or mothers' reactions but was related to the discrepancy between parents' reactions. That is, children reported higher anxiety in families in which fathers and mothers differed in their mood and reaction to the accident compared with families in which parents reacted similarly. Elizur (1986) examined the coping responses of parents of children who were experiencing difficulties in adjusting to the transition to elementary school. Improvements in children's adjustment over the first 2 years of school were related to fathers' coping behavior, efforts by the mothers to stimulate fathers' coping behavior, parental cooperation regarding coping behaviors, and supportive parental attitudes toward the child.

Four studies examined the association of a variety of unspecified major and minor stressful events in parents' life with levels of psychological adjustment in their children. Using prospective designs in which parent and child stress and psychological adjustment were assessed at two points in time, Cohen, Burt, and Bjork (1987) and Holahan and Moos (1987) reported some evidence that fathers' stress and their children's maladjustment were correlated cross-sectionally but no evidence that they were associated in prospective or longitudinal analyses.

In cross-sectional analyses (Compas, Howell, Phares, Williams, & Ledoux, 1989) and longitudinal analyses (Compas, Howell, Phares, Williams, & Giunta, 1989) with a sample of parents and their young adolescent children, it was hypothesized that the relation between parental stress and their children's emotional/ behavioral problems would be mediated by the parents' psychological symptoms. Structural equation analyses with the cross-sectional data indicated that fathers' stressful events led to increases in their psychological symptoms and that fathers' (but not mothers') psychological symptoms were related to their children's self-reports of maladjustment (Compas, Howell, Phares, Williams, & Ledoux, 1989). In longitudinal analyses (Compas, Howell, Phares, Williams, & Giunta, 1989), fathers' symptoms were also associated with their children's self-reports of maladjustment at follow-up, but similar to the findings of Cohen et al. (1987) and Holahan and Moos (1987), fathers' symptoms did not predict their children's maladjustment in prospective or longitudinal analyses. When mothers' reports of their children's maladjustment were used as the criterion, fathers' psychological symptoms were not a significant predictor, but mothers' symptoms were significant in these analyses. Additional analyses of these data were conducted to determine the effect of including as opposed to excluding fathers from the analyses. Using children's self-reports of their maladjustment as the criterion, when fathers were excluded from the analyses, mothers' psychological symptoms were a significant predictor of their children's symptoms in cross-sectional analyses at the first point in time, although this effect was not replicated at follow-up. These additional analyses suggest that including as opposed to excluding fathers from studies such as this can change the picture that is obtained of the association between mothers' and children's psychological symptoms.

Summary

Consistent with studies of referred or diagnosed children and studies of referred or diagnosed fathers, studies with nonreferred samples of fathers and children indicate that there is a substantial association between paternal factors and child and adolescent maladjustment (see Table 3).

DISCUSSION

We now return to the five questions that we outlined in the introduction to guide our interpretation of this literature.

1. Have fathers been included in studies of child and adolescent psychopathology? Evidence for the role of paternal factors in child and adolescent psychopa-

TABLE 3

Findings From Studies of Paternal Factors in Child and Adolescent Psychopathology:
Studies of Nonreferred Fathers and Children

Problem type	Nonreferred fathers and children
Delinquency	Consistent correlations of paternal factors with delinquent behaviors in children (5 studies)
Alcohol/substance use	Consistent correlations between paternal factors and adolescent alcohol and substance use (5 studies)
Nonspecific behavior problems	Significant correlations between paternal factors and child adjustment, symptoms, and behavior (12 studies); no association between paternal factors and child adjustment or symptoms (3 studies)
Depression	Significant correlations between paternal factors and children's depressive symptoms (5 studies); no association between paternal factors and children's depressive symptoms (2 studies)
Paternal unemployment	See McLoyd (1989) for review of recent studies
Paternal stress	Consistent correlations between paternal stress or psychological symptoms and children's adjustment and symptoms (6 studies)

thology has accumulated in spite of a strong tendency to include mothers but not fathers in recent investigations of developmental psychopathology. Specifically, of the studies reviewed between 1984 and 1991, 48% included only mothers, whereas only 1% included only fathers. Although it is encouraging that 26% of studies during this time period obtained and analyzed data separately for fathers and mothers, this bias toward studying mothers and therefore implicitly blaming mothers for problems in their children has continued unabated.

2. Is there evidence that fathers contribute to child and adolescent psychopathology, and if so, do paternal factors represent necessary or sufficient conditions for child and adolescent dysfunction? It is clear from the studies described in this review that fathers play a significant and substantial role in the occurrence of psychopathology in their children. Findings from studies of children who have been referred for clinical services or who have received a psychiatric diagnosis, studies of fathers who have been referred for services or who have received a psychiatric diagnosis, and studies of nonreferred or nondiagnosed samples of fathers and children all lead to the same conclusion: Paternal behaviors, personality characteristics, and psychopathology are significant sources of risk for child and adolescent psychopathology.

The evidence for the contribution of paternal factors differed somewhat in studies of referred or diagnosed children, as opposed to studies of referred or diagnosed fathers or nonreferred samples. In studies of referred children, there were clear differences between fathers of children with externalizing problems (ADHD, CD, delinquent behaviors) and fathers of control children without identified clinical problems. However, the evidence was either weak or equivocal in comparisons of fathers of children with internalizing problems (depression, anxiety disorders) and fathers of children in control samples. On the basis of only studies of diagnosed or referred children, paternal factors apparently are more clearly implicated in children's externalizing than internalizing problems. However, the picture is different when one examines the studies of diagnosed or referred fathers and studies of nonreferred samples. Children of referred or diagnosed fathers were found to function more poorly than control children regardless of the type of problem identified in the father.

This pattern of findings indicates that child and adolescent psychopathology is the result of a variety of different factors, of which paternal characteristics are but one. When researchers identify a sample of referred or diagnosed children, the sample may be quite diverse with regard to the etiological factors that have contributed to maladjustment in these samples. Paternal factors may be implicated in the onset and maintenance of problems for some of these children and adolescents but not for others. On the other hand, when researchers have identified samples of fathers who are characterized by substantial levels of psychopathology, the majority of children of these fathers may be at risk for maladjustment. As such, paternal psychopathology may represent a sufficient condition for the development of maladjustment in children, but it may not be a necessary condition for child or adolescent psychopathology.

3. Are paternal effects limited to certain types of problems in children and adolescents? The answer appears to depend somewhat on the type of methodology used. The evidence from studies of clinically referred or diagnosed fathers and of nonreferred fathers and children indicates that paternal factors are related to symptoms of a wide range of both externalizing (e.g., ADHD, CD, delinquency) and internalizing (e.g., depression, anxiety) disorders in children. However, in studies that included samples of clinically referred or diagnosed children, paternal factors were more strongly implicated in child and adolescent externalizing than internalizing problems. Thus, the correlates of child and adolescent internalizing appear to be more heterogenous than correlates of externalizing problems.

4. Are paternal effects limited to certain behaviors or disorders of fathers, especially those that are more prone to occur in men (e.g., alcohol abuse and antisocial personality)? We found no evidence that risk for child maladjustment was limited to any particular type of paternal psychopathology. It is not surprising to find that problems that have high rates of occurrence in adult men (e.g., alcoholism and antisocial personality) and problems that have similarly high rates of problems in boys (e.g., conduct disorder and delinquency) showed a strong father–child association. Surprisingly strong evidence was found for increased levels of maladjustment in children of fathers with problems more typically associated with adult women (and therefore with mothers). Most noteworthy was the evidence for the

adverse effects of paternal unipolar depression on children. Other areas, such as paternal anxiety disorders, have received relatively little attention and are important topics for future research. Furthermore, we found no evidence of specificity in risk for particular disorders. For example, children of alcoholic fathers and children of depressed fathers have been found to have increased rates of a wide variety of internalizing and externalizing behavior problems. Similarly, children with a particular type of clinical problem cannot be distinguished by the presence of a specified problem in their fathers.

5. What mechanisms are responsible for any paternal effects that are found? Although it is clear that fathers do make a difference in child and adolescent maladjustment, the mechanisms for these effects have not been clearly identified. However, direct comparisons of different diagnostic groups of both fathers and of children have provided data that have been useful in two ways in this regard. First, comparative studies allow for the determination of the differential effects of various types of paternal disorders on child adjustment and of the role of paternal factors in different childhood disorders. Second, comparative data allow researchers to determine which effects are attributable to a specific disorder and which are associated with nonspecific effects of paternal psychopathology. For example, Jacob and colleagues have found that most effects of paternal alcoholism and paternal depression on child and adolescent functioning are common to the two disorders (e.g., Jacob, Krahn, & Leonard, 1991). This indicates that the adverse effects associated with paternal alcoholism and depression are the result of characteristics and processes that are common to the families of both of these diagnostic groups.

The paucity of data on the mechanisms underlying paternal effects is perhaps not surprising in light of the relative absence of studies of fathers and child and adolescent maladjustment. By contrast, in spite of considerably more research on maternal factors in this area, the mechanisms underlying maternal contributions remain unclear as well (Downey & Coyne, 1990; Rutter, 1990). Downey and Coyne (1990) point out the importance of considering both proximal characteristics of the parent–child relationship as well as more distal features of the family environment and stressors impacting on the family when attempting to explain the processes through which parents contribute to child and adolescent maladjustment. Their reminder to consider "third variables" that may lead to both parental and child maladjustment will be important to consider in the identification of mechanisms for paternal effects.

Implications for Future Research

The studies we have reviewed strongly suggest an agenda for future research in the field of developmental psychopathology. Although studies to date provide a clear affirmative answer to the question of whether fathers make a significant contribution to the occurrence of psychopathology in their children, these investigations have not clarified the mechanisms through which these effects are exerted. It will not be sufficient to merely increase the amount of evidence that is accumulated concerning fathers and child psychopathology; there need to be substantial changes in the types of evidence that are gathered as well. We now discuss six broad issues that need to be addressed in future research. Throughout this discussion we draw on two exemplary research programs in this area as illustrations of the types of research that are needed. These are the research programs of Jacob and colleagues on children of alcoholic and depressed fathers (e.g., Jacob et al., 1991; Jacob & Leonard, 1986; Jacob, Seilhamer, & Rushe, 1989) and Humphrey and associates on paternal characteristics associated with adolescent eating disorders (e.g., Humphrey, 1986, 1987, 1989; Humphrey et al., 1986).

Separate analysis of maternal and paternal factors. An essential first step in further clarifying the role of fathers in child and adolescent psychopathology is the acquisition of data that can be uniquely attributed to characteristics of fathers. Although this may seem to be a straightforward point, it is problematic that 25% of the studies reviewed between 1984 and 1991 obtained data concerning both fathers and mothers but aggregated the data in such a way that it was not possible to determine the separate contributions of fathers and mothers to child maladjustment. When data are aggregated in this way, we can consider only the effects of parental factors on child psychopathology without identifying the separate contributions of fathers and mothers, or the interaction of paternal and maternal variables. Along this line, in their investigations of eating disorders Humphrey and colleagues have used discriminant function analysis to distinguish maternal and paternal effects (Humphrey, 1986, 1987, 1989; Humphrey et al., 1986). Jacob et al. (1991) have conducted direct observation studies of depressed fathers and alcoholic fathers and their wives interacting with their adolescent children, both in dyad and triad patterns. These authors note that in the future their sample will include depressed and alcoholic mothers as well, allowing for direct comparisons of mothers and fathers matched for type of disorder (Jacob et al., 1991).

It is only by separating the data pertaining to fathers and mothers that we can discern when and under what circumstances paternal and maternal factors have similar or different effects on child psychopathology. Many of the studies we reviewed made direct comparisons of the effects of paternal and maternal factors. The findings were quite mixed, and no simple conclusions can be drawn from these comparisons at present except to say that in general, little evidence could be found distinguishing the contributions of fathers and mothers. However, this remains an important target of future research, as the degree of maternal and paternal differences may vary across different types of problems. For example, evidence suggests that unipolar and bipolar depression may have different effects on children when manifested by mothers as opposed to fathers (D. N. Klein, Clark, et al., 1988; D. N. Klein, Depue, & Slater, 1985). Furthermore, patterns of assortative mating associated with certain disorders may lead to substantial numbers of families in which there is evidence of significant psychopathology in both parents (e.g., Merikangas & Spiker, 1982). This highlights the need for careful analysis of the diagnostic status of both parents within families.

Variables that may moderate paternal effects. Although main effects of father characteristics on child maladjustment are certainly of interest, paternal factors more likely affect child psychopathology through interactions with other variables that serve as moderators of these associations. Although findings from prior studies have suggested a number of potential moderators of paternal effects, no clear and replicable evidence has accumulated to support conclusions regarding the role of any specific variables as yet. Several factors warrant systematic attention in future research. First, the gender of the child will be important to consider and may be of greater consequence for some types of problems than for others. Jacob et al. (1991) report separate analyses of the interactions of sons and daughters with depressed and alcoholic fathers in laboratory conditions involving parental access to alcohol. Father–daughter interactions varied as a function of the consumption of alcohol by the father during the observation session, whereas father–son interactions did not. Humphrey and colleagues have not investigated gender differences in their studies of eating disorders, most likely because of the dramatically higher prevalence of these disorders in adolescent girls as compared with boys.

A second potential moderator variable is the developmental level of the child. Paternal personality characteristics, parenting practices, or the onset of paternal psychopathology may exert different effects on the child or adolescent as a function of the period of development in which the potential disruption occurs. For example, the onset or recurrence of severe symptoms of paternal alcoholism and associated disruptions in parenting and parent–child relationships may have very different implications when this occurs during infancy as opposed to early adolescence. Furthermore, exposure to problems associated with chronic alcoholism, depression, or other disorders over long periods of development may have a substantially different effect than exposure to paternal symptoms in an acute episode of disorder during a specific developmental period. Unfortunately, children's developmental level has not been systematically investigated.

Third, nonshared environmental factors may play an important role in determining which children within a family may be adversely affected by paternal factors. That is, it cannot be assumed that all children within a single family will experience the same environment—including their interactions with, perceptions of, and response to their father. The importance of understanding nonshared environmental factors has been shown in studies of a variety of different developmental processes in the field of behavioral genetics (e.g., Plomin & Daniels, 1987). These processes need to be studied in relation to paternal factors in developmental psychopathology. This requires that researchers study all children within a family, rather than the traditional design of randomly selecting one child within a family for study, and that they analyze within-family as well as between-families differences. Note that very few of the studies reviewed above obtained data concerning more than one child per family.

Nonshared experiences within the family may relate to other moderating factors, such as child gender. Research has shown that fathers treat boys and girls more differently than do mothers (Siegal, 1987). This suggests that paternal factors may contribute substantially to different experiences within the family for boys and girls. These effects may be magnified in families in which the father displays dysfunctional patterns of parenting.

Mechanisms through which paternal factors exert their influence. As noted above, now that associations between paternal factors and child psychopathology have been documented, it is essential for researchers to discern *how* characteristics of fathers exert their effects. Potential mechanisms of the transmission of father effects could include but are not limited to (a) genetic effects and gene–environment interactions, (b) dyadic interactions between parent and child, including modeling and related social learning processes, (c) parenting practices and behaviors, including coaching and teaching and providing a guiding and nurturing social environment, (d) patterns of disrupted or dysfunctional family interactions, and (e) mutual or reciprocal processes of father–child and child–father effects (cf. Parke, MacDonald, Beitel, & Bhavnagri, 1988). For example, Humphrey and colleagues have included analyses of reciprocal processes of father–daughter, daughter–father, mother–daughter, and daughter–mother effects in their observations of adolescents with eating disorders and their parents (Humphrey, 1986, 1989; Humphrey et al., 1986).

The study of possible mechanisms through which paternal factors exert their influence on child psychopathology involves distinguishing mediating variables from the moderating factors described above. That is, mediating factors involve variables that could account for the association between paternal and child characteristics without altering this relation. In contrast, moderating factors are variables that statistically alter the association between paternal and child factors. The distinction between mediating and moderating factors will be important to retain in future research in this area (for more extended discussions of this distinction, see Baron & Kenny, 1986; Finney, Mitchell, Cronkite, & Moos, 1984).

Paternal and maternal protective factors. In the interest of understanding factors that contribute to child and adolescent psychopathology, research with fathers has concentrated on those variables that are associated with increased *risk* for child and adolescent maladjustment. However, it is equally important to understand those characteristics of fathers and aspects of the father–child relationship that could protect children from psychopathology. This approach requires the investigation of family processes of both risk and protection, including paternal factors that could protect children from the adverse effects of maternal psychopathology and maternal characteristics that could protect children from paternal psychopathology.

Explicit acknowledgement of conceptual models to guide future research. In the pursuit of understanding factors that may moderate paternal effects and the mechanisms through which paternal factors exert their effects, large and complex sets of variables quite likely will emerge as important in this research area. Therefore, it is imperative that future research be guided by clearly defined and conceptually sound models of parent–child relationships and family functioning. Without the conceptual clarity offered by sound theoretical models, investigations of paternal contributions to child and adolescent psychopathology are likely to offer little more than a hodgepodge of complex statistical findings.

At the most general level, models for studying parent–child relationships and interactions can be categorized as (a) noninteractive models, (b) unidirectional models, (c) dyadic models that include bidirectional processes, (d) dyadic models that include the impact of third parties, and (e) family network models (Sigel & Parke, 1987). More specifically, research can be guided by particular theories of the etiology of psychopathology. For example, in a review of research concerned with children of depressed mothers, Gelfand and Teti (1990) noted the influence of cognitive theories, coercive family process models, interactional models of depression, social cognitive theories, mutual regulation models, and attachment theories. Research on paternal factors in developmental psychopathology has often lacked a specified model to guide the selection of measures and interpretation of findings. The field will benefit from more careful attention to the conceptual basis of future research.

The work of Humphrey and of Jacob are instructive in this regard. A strength of Humphrey's research has been the investigation of the structural analysis of social behavior model, a circumplex model of interpersonal dyadic relationships and their intrapsychic representations (Humphrey, 1986, 1987, 1989). Similarly, Jacob and colleagues have been explicit about the family systems model that provides the basis for their investigations of families of depressed and alcoholic fathers (Jacob et al., 1989).

Methodological problems. As we have noted throughout this review, four important methodological issues that need to be addressed in future research are (a) the use of different forms of measurement and informants to assess child and adolescent maladjustment, (b) the use of different methods of assessment and different criteria in the identification of paternal psychopathology and the identification of correlates of various paternal diagnoses, (c) the need for longitudinal as opposed to cross-sectional research designs, and (d) concerns regarding the representativeness of samples of fathers and children.

The importance of taking account of differences in reports on child and adolescent psychopathology obtained from different informants has been well documented (Achenbach, McConaughy, & Howell, 1987). However, differences in reports from parents, teachers, clinicians, and children have not been systematically dealt with by studies of paternal effects on child maladjustment. The use of fathers as sources of information on their own functioning as well as the adjustment of their children may be especially problematic, as both measures may be subject to similar sources of error and bias. This problem has been discussed extensively in regard to research on maternal factors in developmental psychopathology (e.g., Brody & Forehand, 1986; for review see Forehand, 1987), but the problem has not been addressed in studies of fathers. Fathers' psychological symptoms have been found to be associated with their reports of their children's maladjustment in the same manner as mothers' reports, which highlights the need to attend to this possible confound (Phares et al., 1989).

A similar concern needs to be addressed regarding the assessment and identification of paternal psychopathology. Most studies have relied on fathers' self-reports of symptoms or of clinical interviews, although other studies have also used mothers' reports on their husband's functioning. In addition to concerns about the source of information, there has also been variability in the criteria used to define the diagnostic status of fathers. Concerns about the use of diagnostic interviews as opposed to questionnaires and problems resulting from the use of differing diagnostic criteria have been outlined by Downey and Coyne (1990) in their review of studies of children of depressed mothers. The concerns that they describe should be taken to heart by researchers examining paternal psychopathology as well.

Virtually all of the research in this area has been cross-sectional and retrospective. As such, it has been aimed at describing the association between paternal and child characteristics but has not provided information on the predictive relations between these variables or on generating explanations for the relations that have been found. Prospective longitudinal data are needed to clarify the direction of influence (father to child, child to father, bidirectional) and the nature of these relations.

Finally, attention needs to be paid to the sample characteristics of those fathers, children, and families who are recruited to participate in research. Although no selective bias has been identified in fathers who consent to participate in psychological research versus those who decline participation, researchers need to remain vigilant in their attempts to discern possible biases not only in fathers but also in children and families who consent versus decline to participate in research. Attention to selection criteria for fathers and children should facilitate comparisons of fathers with different disorders and children with different disorders who are carefully matched on other variables to determine the specific and nonspecific effects associated with different forms of psychopathology.

SUMMARY

Fathers continue to be dramatically underrepresented compared with mothers in research on developmental psychopathology. However, this review has shown that fathers play a significant role in the development of child and adolescent psychopathology. Specifically, paternal psychopathology appears to be a sufficient but not necessary condition for child and adolescent maladjustment. The role of paternal factors does not appear to be limited to any particular type of paternal or child disorder. Although previous studies have established the importance of fathers' contribution to child and adolescent maladjustment in general, an important agenda for future research is to generate data that will allow for more specific predictions of when and how fathers are involved in the development and maintenance of psychological disorders in their children.

REFERENCES

Achenbach, T. M., & Edelbrock, C. (1983). *Manual for the Child Behavior Checklist and Revised Child Behavior Profile.* Burlington, VT: University Associates in Psychiatry, University of Vermont.

Achenbach, T. M., McConaughy, S. H., & Howell, C. T. (1987). Child/adolescent behavioral and emotional problems: Implications of cross-informant correlations for situational specificity. *Psychological Bulletin,* 101, 213–232.

Alberts-Corush, J., Firestone, P., & Goodman, J. T. (1986). Attention and impulsivity characteristics of the biological and adoptive parents of hyperactive and normal control children. *American Journal of Orthopsychiatry,* 56, 413–423.

Alexander, J. F., Waldron, H. B., Barton, C., & Mas, C. H. (1989). The minimizing of blaming attributions and behaviors in delinquent families. *Journal of Consulting and Clinical Psychology,* 57, 19–24.

American Psychiatric Association. (1980.) *Diagnostic and statistical manual of mental disorders* (3rd ed.). Washington, DC: Author.

Angermeyer, M. C. (1982). The association between family atmosphere and hospital career of schizophrenic patients. *British Journal of Psychiatry,* 141, 1–11.

Atkinson, A. K., & Rickel, A. U. (1984). Postpartum depression in primiparous parents. *Journal of Abnormal Psychology,* 93, 115–119.

Atwood, R., Gold, M., & Taylor, R. (1989). Two types of delinquents and their institutional adjustment. *Journal of Consulting and Clinical Psychology,* 57, 68–75.

Baer, P. E. (1983). Conflict management in the family: The impact of paternal hypertension. *Advances in Family Intervention, Assessment and Theory,* 3, 161–184.

Baldwin, C. P., Baldwin, A. L., Cole, R. E., & Kokes, R. F. (1984). Free play family interaction and the behavior of the patient in free play. In N. F. Watt, E. J. Anthony, L. C. Wynne, & J. E. Rolf (Eds.), *Children at risk for schizophrenia: A longitudinal perspective* (pp. 376–387). New York: Cambridge University Press.

Barlow, D. H. (1988). *Anxiety and its disorders: The nature and treatment of anxiety and panic*. New York: Guilford Press.

Barnes, G. M. (1984). Adolescent alcohol abuse and other problem behaviors: Their relationships and common parental influences. *Journal of Youth and Adolescence*, 13, 329–348.

Barnes, G. M., Farrell, M. P., & Cairns, A. (1986). Parental socialization factors and adolescent drinking behaviors. *Journal of Marriage and the Family*, 48, 27–36.

Baron, R. M., & Kenny, D. A. (1986). The moderator–mediator variable distinction in social psychological research: Conceptual, strategic, and statistical considerations. *Journal of Personality and Social Psychology*, 51, 1173–1182.

Beardslee, W. R. (1986). The need for the study of adaptation in the children of parents with affective disorders. In M. Rutter, C. E. Izard, & P. B. Read (Eds.), *Depression in young people: Developmental and clinical perspectives* (pp. 189–204). New York: Guilford Press.

Beardslee, W. R., Bemporad, J., Keller, M. B., & Klerman, G. L. (1983). Children of parents with major affective disorder: A review. *American Journal of Psychiatry*, 140, 825–832.

Beardslee, W. R., Schultz, L. H., & Selman, R. L. (1987). Level of social cognitive development, adaptive functioning, and *DSM-III* diagnoses in adolescent offspring of parents with affective disorders: Implications of the development of the capacity for mutuality. *Developmental Psychology*, 23, 807–815.

Benson, C. S., & Heller, K. (1987). Factors in the current adjustment of young adult daughters of alcoholic and problem drinking fathers. *Journal of Abnormal Psychology*, 96, 305–312.

Berkowitz, A., & Perkins, H. W. (1988). Personality characteristics of children of alcoholics. *Journal of Consulting and Clinical Psychology*, 56, 206–209.

Bernstein, G. A., Svingen, P. H., & Garfinkel, B. D. (1990). School phobia: Patterns of family functioning. *Journal of the American Academy of Child and Adolescent Psychiatry*, 29, 24–30.

Billings, A. G., & Moos, R. H. (1983). Comparisons of children of depressed and nondepressed parents: A social-environmental perspective. *Journal of Abnormal Child Psychology*, 11, 463–486.

Billings, A. G., & Moos, R. H. (1985). Children of parents with unipolar depression: A controlled 1-year follow-up. *Journal of Abnormal Child Psychology*, 14, 149–166.

Bird, H. R., Gould, M. S., Yager, T., Staghezza, B., & Canino, G. (1989). Risk factors for maladjustment in Puerto Rican children. *Journal of the American Academy of Child and Adolescent Psychiatry*, 28, 847–850.

Borduin, C. M., Henggeler, S. W., & Pruitt, J. A. (1985). The relationship between juvenile delinquency and personality dimensions of family members. *The Journal of Genetic Psychology*, 146, 563–565.

Borduin, C. M., Pruitt, J. A., & Henggeler, S. W. (1986). Family interactions in Black, lower-class families with delinquent and nondelinquent adolescent boys. *The Journal of Genetic Psychology*, 147, 333–342.

Brody, G. H., & Forehand, R. (1986). Maternal perceptions of child adjustment as a function of the combined influence of child behavior and maternal depression. *Journal of Consulting and Clinical Psychology*, 54, 237–240.

Brody, G. H., Pillegrini, A. D., & Sigel, I. E. (1986). Marital quality and mother–child and father–child interactions with school-aged children. *Developmental Psychology*, 22, 291–296.

Bronstein, P., & Cowan, C. P. (Eds.). (1988.) *Fatherhood today: Men's changing role in the family*. New York: Wiley.

Brook, J. S., Whiteman, M., Brook, D. W., & Gordon, A. S. (1982). Paternal and peer characteristics: Interactions and association with male college students' marijuana use. *Psychological Reports*, 51, 1319–1330.

Brook, J. S., Whiteman, M., Gordon, A. S., & Brook, D. W. (1983). Paternal correlates of adolescent marijuana use in the context of the mother–son and parental dyads. *Genetic Psychology Monographs*, 108, 197–213.

Brook, J. S., Whiteman, M., Gordon, A. S., & Brook, D. W. (1984a). Identification with paternal attributes and its relationship to the son's personality and drug use. *Developmental Psychology*, 20, 1111–1119.

Brook, J. S., Whiteman, M., Gordon, A. S., & Brook, D. W. (1984b). Paternal determinants of female adolescent's marijuana use. *Developmental Psychology*, 20, 1032–1043.

Brook, J. S., Whiteman, M., Gordon, A. S., & Brook, D. W. (1986). Father–daughter identification and its impact on her personality and drug use. *Developmental Psychology*, 22, 743–748.

Browne, A., & Finkelhor, D. (1986). Impact of child sexual abuse: A review of the literature. *Psychological Bulletin*, 99, 66–77.

Brownfield, D. (1987). Father–son relationships and violent behavior. *Deviant Behavior*, 8, 65–78.

Burbach, D. J., & Borduin, C. M. (1986). Parent–child relations and the etiology of depression: A review of methods and findings. *Clinical Psychology Review*, 6, 133–153.

Callan, V. J., & Jackson, D. (1986). Children of alcoholic fathers and recovered alcoholic fathers: Personal and family functioning. *Journal of Studies on Alcohol*, 47, 180–182.

Caplan, P. J. (1986, October). Take the blame off mother. *Psychology Today*, pp. 70–71.

Caplan, P. J. (1989). *Don't blame mother: Mending the mother–daughter relationship*. New York: Harper & Row.

Caplan, P. J., & Hall-McCorquodale, I. (1985). Mother-blaming in major clinical journals. *American Journal of Orthopsychiatry*, 55, 345–353.

Chess, S., & Thomas, A. (1984). *Origins and evolution of behavior disorders: From infancy to early adult life*. New York: Brunner/Mazel.

Christensen, A., Phillips, S., Glasgow, R. E., & Johnson, S. M. (1983). Parental characteristics and interactional dysfunction in families with child behavior problems: A preliminary investigation. *Journal of Abnormal Child Psychology*, 11, 153–166.

Clark, D. A., & Bolton, D. (1985). Obsessive–compulsive adolescents and their parents: A psychometric study. *Journal of Child Psychology and Psychiatry*, 26, 267–276.

Cohen, L. H., Burt, C. E., & Bjork, J. P. (1987). Effects of life events experienced by young adolescents and their parents. *Developmental Psychology*, 23, 583–592.

Cole, D. A., & Rehm, L. P. (1986). Family interaction patterns and childhood depression. *Journal of Abnormal Child Psychology*, 14, 297–314.

Compas, B. E. (1987). Stress and life events during childhood and adolescence. *Clinical Psychology Review*, 7, 275–302.

Compas, B. E., Howell, D. C., Phares, V., Williams, R. A., & Giunta, C. T. (1989). Risk factors for emotional/behavioral problems in young adolescents: A prospective analysis of adolescent and parental stress and symptoms. *Journal of Consulting and Clinical Psychology*, 57, 732–740.

Compas, B. E., Howell, D. C., Phares, V., Williams, R. A., & Ledoux, N. (1989). Parent and child stress and symptoms: An integrative analysis. *Developmental Psychology*, 25, 550–559.

Cunningham, C. E., Benness, B. B., & Siegel, L. S. (1988). Family functioning, time allocation, and parental depression in the families of normal and ADDH children. *Journal of Clinical Child Psychology*, 17, 169–177.

Cytryn, L., McKnew, D. H., Zahn-Waxler, C., & Gershon, E. S. (1986). Developmental issues in risk research: The offspring of affectively ill parents. In M. Rutter, C. E. Izard, & P. B. Read (Eds.), *Depression in young people: Developmental and clinical perspectives* (pp. 163–188). New York: Guilford Press.

Dean, R. S., & Jacobson, B. P. (1982). MMPI characteristics for parents of emotionally disturbed and learning-disabled children. *Journal of Consulting and Clinical Psychology*, 50, 775–777.

Dodge, K. (Ed.). (1990). Developmental psychopathology in children of depressed mothers. *Developmental Psychology*, 26, 3–6.

Downey, G., & Coyne, J. C. (1990). Children of depressed parents: An integrative review. *Psychological Bulletin*, 108, 50–76.

Dwyer, J. T., & DeLong, G. R. (1987). A family history study of twenty probands with childhood manic-depressive illness. *Journal of the American Academy of Child and Adolescent Psychiatry*, 26, 176–180.

Earls, F. (1976). The fathers (not the mothers): Their importance and influence with infants and young children. *Psychiatry*, 39, 209–226.

Elder, G., Nguyen, T., & Caspi, A. (1985). Linking family hardship to children's lives. *Child Development*, 56, 361–375.

El-Guebaly, N., Offord, D. R., Sullivan, K. T., & Lynch, G. W. (1978). Psychosocial adjustment of the offspring of psychiatric inpatients: The effect of alcoholic, depressive and schizophrenic parentage. *Canadian Psychiatric Association Journal*, 23, 281–289.

Elizur, J. (1986). The stress of school entry: Parental coping behaviors and children's adjustment to school. *Journal of Child Psychology and Psychiatry*, 27, 625–638.

Emery, R. (1982). Interparental conflict and the children of discord and divorce. *Psychological Bulletin*, 92, 310–330.

Englander, S. W. (1984). Some self-reported correlates of runaway behavior in adolescent females. *Journal of Consulting and Clinical Psychology*, 52, 484–485.

Erlenmeyer-Kimling, L., Marcuse, Y., Cornblatt, B., Friedman, D., Rainer, J. D., & Rutschmann, J. (1984). The New York High-Risk Project. In N. F. Watt, E. J. Anthony, L. C. Wynne, & J. E. Rolf (Eds.), *Children at risk for schizophrenia: A longitudinal perspective* (pp. 169–189). New York: Cambridge University Press.

Fine, E., Yudin, L., Holmes, J., & Heinemann, S. (1976). Behavioral disorders in children with parental alcoholism. *Annals of the New York Academy of Sciences*, 273, 507–517.

Finkelhor, D. (1979). *Sexually victimized children*. New York: Free Press.

Finney, J. W., Mitchell, R. E., Cronkite, R., & Moos, R. H. (1984). Methodological issues in estimating main and interactive effects: Examples from the coping/social support and stress field. *Journal of Health and Social Behavior*, 10, 85–98.

Forehand, R. (1987). Parental roles in childhood psychopathology. In C. L. Frame & J. L. Matson (Eds.), *Handbook of assessment in childhood psychopathology* (pp. 489–507). New York: Plenum Press.

Forehand, R., Long, N., Brody, G. H., & Fauber, R. (1986). Home predictors of young adolescents' school behavior and academic performance. *Child Development*, 57, 1528–1533.

Forehand, R., & Smith, K. A. (1986). Who depresses whom? A look at the relationship of adolescent mood to maternal and paternal mood. *Child Study Journal*, 16, 19–23.

Forney, M. A., Forney, P. D., Davis, H., Van Hoose, J., Cafferty, T., & Allen, H. (1984). A discriminant analysis of adolescent problem drinking. *Journal of Drug Education*, 14, 347–355.

Fry, P. S. (1982). Paternal correlates of adolescents' running away behaviors: Implications for adolescent development and considerations for intervention and treatment of adolescent runaways. *Journal of Applied Developmental Psychology*, 3, 347–360.

Gantman, C. A. (1978). Family interaction patterns among families with normal, disturbed, and drug-abusing adolescents. *Journal of Youth and Adolescence*, 7, 429–440.

Garbarino, J., Sebes, J., & Schellenbach, D. (1984). Families at risk for destructive parent–child relations in adolescents. *Child Development*, 55, 174–183.

Garfinkel, P. E., Garner, D. M., Rose, J., Darby, P. L., Brandes, J. S., O'Hanlon, J., & Walsh, N. (1983). A comparison of characteristics in the families of patients with anorexia nervosa and normal controls. *Psychological Medicine*, 13, 821–828.

Garmezy, N., & Rutter, M. (Eds.). (1983). *Stress, coping and development in children*. New York: McGraw-Hill.

Gelfand, D. M., & Teti, D. M. (1990). The effects of maternal depression on children. *Clinical Psychology Review*, 10, 329–354.

Goodman, R., & Stevenson, J. (1989). A twin study of hyperactivity: II. The aetiological role of genes, family relationships and perinatal adversity. *Journal of Child Psychology and Psychiatry*, 30, 691–709.

Goodwin, D. W. (1986). Heredity and alcoholism. *Annals of Behavioral Medicine*, 8, 3–6.

Hahlweg, K., Goldstein, M. J., Nuechterlein, K. H., Magana, A. B., Mintz, J., Doane, J. A., Miklowitz, D. J., & Snyder, K. S. (1989). Expressed emotion and patient–relative interaction in families of recent onset schizophrenics. *Journal of Consulting and Clinical Psychology*, 57, 11–18.

Hamdan-Allen, G., Stewart, M. A., & Beeghly, J. H. (1989). Subgrouping conduct disorder by psychiatric family history. *Journal of Child Psychology and Psychiatry*, 30, 889–897.

Handford, H. A., Mayes, S. D., Mattison, R. E., Humphrey, F. J., Bagnato, S., Bixler, E. O., & Kales, J. D. (1986). Child and parent reaction to the Three Mile Island nuclear accident. *Journal of the American Academy of Child Psychiatry*, 25, 346–356.

Hanson, C. L., Henggeler, S. W., Haefele, W. F., & Rodick, J. D. (1984). Demographic, individual, and family relationship correlates of serious and repeated crime among adolescents and their siblings. *Journal of Consulting and Clinical Psychology*, 52, 528–538.

Harter, S., Alexander, P. C., & Neimeyer, R. A. (1988). Long-term effects of incestuous child abuse in college women: Social adjustment, social cognition, and family characteristics. *Journal of Consulting and Clinical Psychology*, 56, 5–8.

Helzer, J. E. (1987). Epidemiology of alcoholism. *Journal of Consulting and Clinical Psychology*, 55, 284–292.

Henggeler, S. W., Edwards, J., & Borduin, C. M. (1987). The family relations of female juvenile delinquents. *Journal of Abnormal Child Psychology*, 15, 199–209.

Herjanic, B., Herjanic, M., Penick, E., Tomelleri, C., & Armbruster, R. (1977). Children of alcoholics. In F. A. Seixas (Ed.), *Currents in alcoholism* (Vol. 2, pp. 445–455). New York: Grune & Stratton.

Hinshaw, S. P. (1987). On the distinction between attention deficits/hyperactivity and conduct problems/aggression in child psychopathology. *Psychological Bulletin*, 101, 443–463.

Holahan, C. J., & Moos, R. H. (1987). Risk, resistance, and psychological distress: A longitudinal analysis with adults and children. *Journal of Abnormal Psychology*, 96, 3–13.

Humphrey, L. L. (1986). Structural analysis of parent–child relationships in eating disorders. *Journal of Abnormal Psychology*, 95, 394–402.

Humphrey, L. L. (1987). Comparison of bulimic–anorexic and nondistressed families using structural analysis of social behavior. *Journal of the American Academy of Child and Adolescent Psychiatry*, 26, 248–255.

Humphrey, L. L. (1989). Observed family interactions among subtypes of eating disorders using structural analysis of social behavior. *Journal of Consulting and Clinical Psychology*, 57, 206–214.

Humphrey, L. L., Apple, R. F., & Kirschenbaum, D. S. (1986). Differentiating bulimic–

anorexic from normal families using interpersonal and behavioral observational systems. *Journal of Consulting and Clinical Psychology,* 54, 190–195.

Itil, T. M., Huque, M. F., Shapiro, D. M., Mednick, S. A., & Schulsinger, F. (1983). Computer-analyzed EEG findings in children of schizophrenic parents ("high risk" children). *Integrative Psychiatry,* 1, 71–79.

Ivens, C., & Rehm, L. P. (1988). Assessment of childhood depression: Correspondence between reports by child, mother, and father. *Journal of the American Academy of Child and Adolescent Psychiatry,* 27, 738–741.

Jacob, T., Krahn, G. L., & Leonard, K. (1991). Parent–child interactions in families with alcoholic fathers. *Journal of Consulting and Clinical Psychology,* 59, 176–181.

Jacob, T., & Leonard, K. (1986). Psychosocial functioning in children of alcoholic fathers, depressed fathers and control fathers. *Journal of Studies of Alcohol,* 47, 373–380.

Jacob, T., Seilhamer, R. A., & Rushe, R. (1989). Alcoholism and family interactions: A research paradigm. *American Journal of Drug and Alcohol Abuse,* 15, 73–91.

Jary, M. L., & Stewart, M. A. (1985). Psychiatric disorder in the parents of adopted children with aggressive conduct disorder. *Neuropsychobiology,* 13, 7–11.

Jenkins, J. M., & Smith, M. A. (1990). Factors protecting children living in disharmonious homes: Maternal reports. *Journal of the American Academy of Child and Adolescent Psychiatry,* 29, 60–69.

Jensen, P. S., Bloedau, L., Degroot, J., Ussery, T., & Davis, H. (1990). Children at risk: I. Risk factors and child symptomatology. *Journal of the American Academy of Child and Adolescent Psychiatry,* 29, 51–59.

Jensen, P. S., Traylor, J., Xenakis, S. N., & Davis, H. (1988). Child psychopathology rating scales and interrater agreement: I. Parents' gender and psychiatric symptoms. *Journal of the American Academy of Child and Adolescent Psychiatry,* 27, 442–450.

Jiloha, R. C. (1986). Psycho-social factors in adolescent heroin addicts. *Child Psychiatry Quarterly,* 19, 138–142.

John, K., Gammon, G. D., Prusoff, B. A., & Warner, V. (1987). The Social Adjustment Inventory for Children and Adolescents (SAICA): Testing of a new semistructured interview. *Journal of the American Academy of Child and Adolescent Psychiatry,* 26, 898–911.

Johnson, P. L., & O'Leary, K. D. (1987). Parental behavior patterns and conduct disorders in girls. *Journal of Abnormal Child Psychology,* 15, 573–581.

Johnson, R. E. (1987). Mother's versus father's role in causing delinquency. *Adolescence,* 22, 305–315.

Joyce, P. R. (1984). Parental bonding in Bipolar Affective Disorder. *Journal of Affective Disorders,* 1, 319–324.

Kandel, E., Mednick, S. A., Kirkegaard-Sorensen, L., Hutchings, B., Knop, J., Rosenberg, R., & Schulsinger, F. (1988). IQ as a protective factor for subjects at high risk for antisocial behavior. *Journal of Consulting and Clinical Psychology,* 56, 224–226.

Kashani, J. H., Burbach, D. J., & Rosenberg, T. K. (1988). Perception of family conflict resolution and depressive symptomatology in adolescents. *Journal of the American Academy of Child and Adolescent Psychiatry,* 27, 42–48.

Kaslow, N. J., Rehm, L. P., Pollack, S. L., & Siegel, A. W. (1988). Attributional style and self-control behavior in depressed and nondepressed children and their parents. *Journal of Abnormal Child Psychology*, 16, 163–175.

Kendall, P. C., & Fischler, G. L. (1984). Behavioral and adjustment correlates of problem solving: Validational analyses of interpersonal cognitive problem-solving measures. *Child Development*, 55, 879–892.

Klein, D. N., Clark, D. C., Dansky, L., & Margolis, E. T. (1988). Dysthymia in the off-spring of parents with primary unipolar affective disorder. *Journal of Abnormal Psychology*, 97, 265–274.

Klein, D. N., Depue, R. A., & Slater, J. F. (1985). Cyclothymia in the adolescent offspring of parents with bipolar affective disorder. *Journal of Abnormal Psychology*, 94, 115–127.

Klein, M. M., & Shulman, S. (1980). Behavior problems of children in relation to parental instrumentality–expressivity and marital adjustment. *Psychological Reports*, 47, 11–14.

Klinge, V., & Piggott, L. R. (1986). Substance use by adolescent psychiatric inpatients and their parents. *Adolescence*, 21, 323–331.

Knop, J., Teasdale, T., Schulsinger, F., & Goodwin, D. (1985). A prospective study of young men at high risk for alcoholism: School behavior and achievement. *Journal of Studies of Alcohol*, 46, 273–278.

Lahey, B. B., Piacentini, J. C., McBurnett, K., Stone, P., Hartdagen, S., & Hynd, G. (1988). Psychopathology in the parents of children with conduct disorder and hyperactivity. *Journal of the American Academy of Child and Adolescent Psychiatry*, 27, 163–170.

Lamb, M. E. (1975). Fathers: Forgotten contributors to child development. *Human Development*, 18, 245–266.

Lamb, M. E. (Ed.). (1976). *The role of the father in child development*. New York: Wiley.

Lamb, M. E. (Ed.). (1981). *The role of the father in child development* (Rev. ed.). New York: Wiley.

Lamb, M. E. (Ed.). (1986). *The father's role: Applied perspectives*. New York: Wiley.

Lamb, M. E. (Ed.). (1987). *The father's role: Cross-cultural perspectives*. New York: Wiley.

Lamb, M. E., Pleck, J. H., & Levine, J. A. (1985). The role of the father in child development: The effects of increased paternal involvement. In B. B. Lahey & A. E. Kazdin (Eds.), *Advances in clinical child psychology* (Vol. 8, pp. 229–266). New York: Plenum Press.

Lefkowitz, M. M., & Tesiny, E. P. (1984). Rejection and depression: Prospective and con-temporaneous analyses. *Developmental Psychology*, 20, 776–785.

Leon, G. R., Lucas, A. R., Colligan, R. C., Ferdinande, R. J., & Kamp, J. (1985). Sexual, body-image, and personality attitudes in anorexia nervosa. *Journal of Abnormal Child Psychology*, 13, 245–258.

Lessin, S., & Jacob, T. (1984). Multichannel communication in normal and delinquent families. *Journal of Abnormal Child Psychology*, 12, 369–384.

Levenson, R. W., Oyama, O. N., & Meek, P. S. (1987). Greater reinforcement from alcohol for those at risk: Parental risk, personality risk, and sex. *Journal of Abnormal Psychology*, 96, 242–253.

Lewis, D. O., Pincus, J. H., Lovely, R., Spitzer, E., & Moy, E. (1987). Biopsychosocial characteristics of matched samples of delinquents and nondelinquents. *Journal of the American Academy of Child and Adolescent Psychiatry*, 26, 744–752.

Lewis, D. O., Shanok, S. S., Grant, M., & Ritvo, E. (1983). Homicidally aggressive young children: Neuropsychiatric and experiential correlates. *American Journal of Psychiatry*, 140, 148–153.

Lidz, T., Parker, B., & Cornelison, A. (1956). The role of the father in the family environment of the schizophrenic patient. *American Journal of Psychiatry*, 113, 126–132.

Loeber, R. (1990). Development and risk factors of juvenile antisocial behavior and delinquency. *Clinical Psychology Review*, 10, 1–41.

Loeber, R., & Dishion, T. J. (1983). Early predictors of male delinquency: A review. *Psychological Bulletin*, 94, 68–99.

Loeber, R., & Dishion, T. J. (1984). Boys who fight at home and school: Family conditions influencing cross-setting consistency. *Journal of Consulting and Clinical Psychology*, 52, 759–768.

Loeber, R., & Dishion, T. J. (1987). Antisocial and delinquent youths: Methods for their early identification. In J. D. Burchard & S. N. Burchard (Eds.), *Prevention of delinquent behavior* (pp. 75–89). Newbury Park, CA: Sage.

MacDonald, K. (1987). Parent–child physical play with rejected, neglected, and popular boys. *Developmental Psychology*, 23, 705–711.

Manning, D. T., Balson, P. M., & Xenakis, S. (1986). The prevalence of Type A personality in the children of alcoholics. *Alcoholism: Clinical and Experimental Research*, 10, 184–189.

Margalit, M. (1985). Perception of parents' behavior, familial satisfaction, and sense of coherence in hyperactive children. *Journal of School Psychology*, 23, 355–364.

Mash, E. J., & Johnston, C. (1983). Parental perceptions of child behavior problems, parenting self-esteem, and mothers' reported stress in younger and older hyperactive and normal children. *Journal of Consulting and Clinical Psychology*, 51, 86–99.

McCord, J. (1979). Some child-rearing antecedents of criminal behavior in adult men. *Journal of Personality and Social Psychology*, 37, 1477–1486.

McCranie, E. W., & Bass, J. D. (1984). Childhood family antecedents of dependency and self-criticism: Implications for depression. *Journal of Abnormal Psychology*, 93, 3–8.

McKenry, P. C., Tishler, C. L., & Kelley, C. (1982). Adolescent suicide: A comparison of attempters and nonattempters in an emergency room population. *Clinical Pediatrics*, 21, 266–270.

McLoyd, V. C. (1989). Socialization and development in a changing economy: The effects of paternal job and income loss on children. *American Psychologist*, 44, 293–302.

Merikangas, K., & Spiker, D. G. (1982). Assortative mating among inpatients with primary affective disorder. *Psychological Medicine*, 12, 753–764.

Merikangas, K., Weissman, M., Prusoff, B., Pauls, D., & Leckman, J. (1985). Depressives with secondary alcoholism: Psychiatric disorders in offspring. *Journal of Studies on Alcohol*, 46, 199–204.

Miklowitz, D. J., Goldstein, M. J., Doane, J. A., Nuechterlein, K. H., Strachan, A. M., Snyder, K. S., & Magana-Amato, A. (1989). Is expressed emotion an index of a transactional process? I. Parents' affective style. *Family Process*, 28, 153–167.

Miklowitz, D. J., Strachan, A. M., Goldstein, M. J., Doane, J. A., Snyder, K. S., Hogarty, G. E., & Falloon, I. R. H. (1986). Expressed emotion and communication deviance in the families of schizophrenics. *Journal of Abnormal Psychology*, 95, 60–66.

Mitchell, J., McCauley, E., Burke, P., Calderon, R., & Schloredt, K. (1989). Psychopathology in parents of depressed children and adolescents. *Journal of the American Academy of Child and Adolescent Psychiatry*, 28, 352–357.

Mitchell, J., McCauley, E., Burke, P., & Moss, S. J. (1988). Phenomenology of depression in children and adolescents. *Journal of the American Academy of Child and Adolescent Psychiatry*, 27, 12–20.

Myers, K. M., Burke, P., & McCauley, E. (1985). Suicidal behavior by hospitalized preadolescent children on a psychiatric unit. *Journal of the American Academy of Child and Adolescent Psychiatry*, 24, 474–480.

Neapolitan, J. (1981). Parental influences on aggressive behavior: A social learning approach. *Adolescence*, 16, 831–840.

Nelson, J. N., & Simmerer, N. J. (1984). A correlational study of children's temperament and parent behavior. *Early Child Development and Care*, 16, 231–250.

Offord, D., Allen, N., & Abrams, N. (1978). Parental psychiatric illness, broken homes, and delinquency. *Journal of the American Academy of Child Psychiatry*, 17, 224–238.

Orvaschel, H., Walsh-Allis, G., & Ye, W. (1988). Psychopathology in children of parents with recurrent depression. *Journal of Abnormal Child Psychology*, 16, 17–28.

Orvaschel, H., Weissman, M. M., & Kidd, K. K. (1980). Children and depression: The children of depressed parents; the childhood of depressed patients; depression in children. *Journal of Affective Disorders*, 2, 1–16.

Parke, R. D., MacDonald, K. B., Beitel, A., & Bhavnagri, N. (1988). The role of the family in the development of peer relationships. In R. Peters & R. J. McMahan (Eds.), *Social learning systems: Approaches to marriage and the family* (pp. 17–44). New York: Brunner/Mazel.

Peery, J. C., Jensen, L., & Adams, G. R. (1985). The relationship between parents' attitudes toward child rearing and the sociometric status of their preschool children. *The Journal of Psychology*, 119, 567–574.

Penfold, P. S. (1985). Parent's perceived responsibility for children's problems. *Canadian Journal of Psychiatry*, 30, 255–258.

Pfeffer, C. R., Newcorn, J., Kaplan, G., Mizruchi, M. S., & Plutchik, R. (1989). Subtypes of suicidal and assaultive behaviors in adolescent psychiatric inpatients: A research note. *Journal of Child Psychology and Psychiatry*, 30, 151–163.

Pfeffer, C. R., Plutchik, R., Mizruchi, M. S., & Lipkins, R. (1987). Assaultive behavior in child psychiatric inpatients, outpatients, and nonpatients. *Journal of the American Academy of Child and Adolescent Psychiatry*, 26, 256–261.

Pfeffer, C. R., Solomon, G., Plutchik, R., Mizruchi, M. S., & Weiner, A. (1985). Variables that predict assaultiveness in child psychiatric inpatients. *Journal of the American Academy of Child Psychiatry*, 26, 775–780.

Phares, V. (1992). Where's Poppa?: The relative lack of attention to the role of fathers in child and adolescent psychopathology. *American Psychologist*, 47, 656–664.

Phares, V., Compas, B. E., & Howell, D. C. (1989). Perspectives on child behavior problems: Comparisons of children's self-reports with parent and teacher reports. *Psychological Assessment: A Journal of Consulting and Clinical Psychology*, 1, 68–71.

Plomin, R., & Daniels, D. (1987). Why are children in the same family so different from one another? *Behavioral and Brain Sciences*, 10, 1–60.

Puig-Antich, J., Lukens, E., Davies, M., Goetz, D., Brennan-Quattrock, J., & Todak, G. (1985a). Psychosocial functioning in prepubertal major depressive disorders: I. Interpersonal relationships during the depressive episode. *Archives of General Psychiatry*, 42, 500–507.

Puig-Antich, J., Lukens, E., Davies, M., Goetz, D., Brennan-Quattrock, J., & Todak, G. (1985b). Psychosocial functioning in prepubertal major depressive disorders: II. Interpersonal relationships after sustained recovery from affective episode. *Archives of General Psychiatry*, 42, 511–517.

Radke-Yarrow, M., Cummings, E. M., Kuczynski, L., & Chapman, M. (1985). Patterns of attachment in two- and three-year-olds in normal families and families with parental depression. *Child Development*, 56, 884–893.

Reeves, J. C., Werry, J. S., Elkind, G. S., & Zametkin, A. (1987). Attention deficit, conduct, oppositional, and anxiety disorders in children: II. Clinical characteristics. *Journal of the American Academy of Child and Adolescent Psychiatry*, 26, 144–155.

Regier, D. A., Meyers, J. K., Kramer, M., Robins, L. N., Blazer, D. G., Hough, R. L., Eaton, W. W., & Locke, B. Z. (1984). The NIMH epidemiologic catchment area program. *Archives of General Psychiatry*, 41, 934–941.

Reid, J. B., Kavanagh, K., & Baldwin, D. V. (1987). Abusive parents' perceptions of child problem behaviors: An example of parental bias. *Journal of Abnormal Child Psychology*, 15, 457–466.

Richman, J. A., & Flaherty, J. A. (1987). Adult psychosocial assets and depressive mood over time: Effects of internalized childhood attachments. *Journal of Nervous and Mental Disease*, 175, 703–712.

Rickard, K. (1988). The occurrence of maladaptive health-related behaviors and teacher-rated conduct problems in children of chronic low back pain patients. *Journal of Behavioral Medicine*, 11, 107–116.

Rimmer, J. (1982). The children of alcoholics: An exploratory study. *Children and Youth Services Review*, 4, 365–373.

Roehling, P. V., & Robin, A. L. (1986). Development and validation of the Family Beliefs Inventory: A measure of unrealistic beliefs among parents and adolescents. *Journal of Consulting and Clinical Psychology*, 54, 693–697.

Rogeness, G. A., Amrung, S. A., Macedo, C. A., Harris, W. R., & Fisher, C. (1986).

Psychopathology in abused or neglected children. *Journal of the American Academy of Child Psychiatry*, 25, 659–665.

Roopnarine, J. L., & Adams, G. R. (1987). The interactional teaching patterns of mothers and fathers with their popular, moderately popular, or unpopular children. *Journal of Abnormal Child Psychology*, 15, 125–136.

Russell, D. E. H. (1987). *The secret trauma: Incest in the lives of girls and women*. New York: Basic Books.

Rutter, M. (1981). *Maternal deprivation reassessed* (2nd ed.). Harmonsworth, Middlesex, England: Penguin Books.

Rutter, M. (1990). Commentary: Some focus and process considerations regarding the effects of parental depression on children. *Developmental Psychology*, 26, 60–67.

Sanua, V. D. (1986). The personality and psychological adjustment of family members of autistic children: II. A critical review of the literature research in the United States. *International Journal of Family Psychiatry*, 1, 331–358.

Schaughency, E. A., & Lahey, B. B. (1985). Mothers' and fathers' perceptions of child deviance: Roles of child behavior, parental depression, and marital satisfaction. *Journal of Consulting and Clinical Psychology*, 53, 718–723.

Scott, R. L., & Stone, D. A. (1986). MMPI profile constellations in incest families. *Journal of Consulting and Clinical Psychology*, 54, 364–368.

Seligman, M. E. P., Peterson, C., Kaslow, N. J., Tanenbaum, R. L., Alloy, L. B., & Abramson, L. Y. (1984). Attributional style and depressive symptoms among children. *Journal of Abnormal Psychology*, 93, 235–238.

Seltzer, J. A., & Bianchi, S. M. (1988). Children's contact with absent parents. *Journal of Marriage and the Family*, 50, 663–677.

Siegal, M. (1987). Are sons and daughters treated more differently by fathers than by mothers? *Developmental Review*, 7, 183–209.

Sigel, I. E., & Parke, R. D. (1987). Structural analysis of parent–child research models. *Journal of Applied Developmental Psychology*, 8, 123–137.

Silverton, L., Mednick, S. A., Schulsinger, F., Parnas, J., & Harrington, M. E. (1988). Genetic risk for schizophrenia, birthweight, and cerebral ventricular enlargement. *Journal of Abnormal Psychology*, 97, 496–498.

Sirles, E. A., Smith, J. A., & Kusama, H. (1989). Psychiatric status of intrafamilial sexual abuse victims. *Journal of the American Academy of Child and Adolescent Psychiatry*, 28, 225–229.

Sobol, M. P., Ashbourne, D. T., Earn, B. M., & Cunningham, C. E. (1989). Parents' attributions for achieving compliance from attention-deficit-disordered children. *Journal of Abnormal Child Psychology*, 17, 359–369.

Steinhausen, H. C., Gobel, D., & Nestler, V. (1984). Psychopathology in the offspring of alcoholic parents. *Journal of the American Academy of Child Psychiatry*, 23, 465–471.

Stewart, M. A., & deBlois, C. S. (1983). Father–son resemblances in aggressive and antisocial behaviour. *British Journal of Psychiatry*, 142, 78–84.

Stewart, M. A., deBlois, C. S., & Cummings, C. (1980). Psychiatric disorder in the parents of hyperactive boys and those with conduct disorder. *Journal of Child Psychology and Psychiatry*, 21, 283–292.

Stollak, G. E., Messe, L. A., Michaels, G. Y., Buldain, R., Catlin, R. T., & Paritee, F. (1982). Parental interpersonal perceptual style, child adjustment, and parent–child interactions. *Journal of Abnormal Child Psychology*, 10, 61–76.

Stouthamer-Loeber, M., & Loeber, R. (1986). Boys who lie. *Journal of Abnormal Child Psychology*, 14, 551–564.

Strachan, A. M., Feingold, D., Goldstein, M. J., Miklowitz, D. J., & Nuechterlein, K. H. (1989). Is expressed emotion an index of a transactional process? II. Patient's coping style. *Family Process*, 28, 169–181.

Tallmadge, J., & Barkley, R. A. (1983). The interactions of hyperactive and normal boys with their fathers and mothers. *Journal of Abnormal Child Psychology*, 11, 565–579.

Tarter, R. E., Hegedus, A. M., Winsten, N. E., & Alterman, A. I. (1984). Neuropsychological, personality, and familial characteristics of physically abused delinquents. *Journal of the American Academy of Child Psychiatry*, 23, 668–674.

Tufts' New England Medical Center, Division of Child Psychiatry. (1984.) *Sexually exploited children: Service and research project.* Final report for the Office of Juvenile Justice and Delinquency Prevention. Washington, DC: U.S. Department of Justice.

Velez, C. N., Johnson, J., & Cohen, P. (1989). A longitudinal analysis of selected risk factors for childhood psychopathology. *Journal of the American Academy of Child and Adolescent Psychiatry*, 28, 861–864.

Walker, E., & Emory, E. (1983). Infants at risk for psychopathology: Offspring of schizophrenic parents. *Child Development*, 54, 1269–1285.

Wallander, J. L. (1988). The relationship between attention problems in childhood and antisocial behavior eight years later. *Journal of Child Psychology and Psychiatry*, 29, 53–61.

Watson, J. (1986). Parental attributions of emotional disturbance and their relation to the outcome of therapy: Preliminary findings. *Australian Psychologist*, 21, 271–282.

Watt, N. F. (1986). Risk research in schizophrenia and other major psychological disorders. In M. Kessler & S. E. Goldston (Eds.), *A decade of progress in primary prevention* (pp. 115–153). Hanover, NH: University Press of New England.

Watt, N. F., Anthony, E. J., Wynne, L. C., & Rolf, J. E. (Eds.). (1984). *Children at risk for schizophrenia: A longitudinal perspective.* New York: Cambridge University Press.

Webster-Stratton, C. (1988). Mothers' and fathers' perceptions of child deviance: Roles of parent and child behaviors and parent adjustment. *Journal of Consulting and Clinical Psychology*, 56, 909–915.

Weintraub, S., & Neale, J. M. (1984). The Stony Brook High-Risk Project. In N. F. Watt, E. J. Anthony, L. C. Wynne, & J. E. Rolf (Eds.), *Children at risk for schizophrenia: A longitudinal perspective* (pp. 243–263). New York: Cambridge University Press.

Weintraub, S., Winters, K. C., & Neale, J. M. (1986). Competence and vulnerability in children with an affectively disordered parent. In M. Rutter, C. E. Izard, & P. B. Read

(Eds.), *Depression in young people: Developmental and clinical perspectives* (pp. 205–220). New York: Guilford Press.

Weissman, M. M., Gershon, E. S., Kidd, K. K., Prusoff, B. A., Leckman, J. F., Dibble, E., Hamovit, J., Thompson, D., Pauls, D. L., & Guroff, J. J. (1984). Psychiatric disorders in the relatives of probands with affective disorders. *Archives of General Psychiatry*, 41, 13–21.

Weissman, M. M., Leckman, J. F., Merikangas, K. R., Gammon, G. D., & Prusoff, B. A. (1984). Depression and anxiety disorders in parents and children. *Archives of General Psychiatry*, 41, 845–852.

Werner, E. E. (1986). Resilient offspring of alcoholics: A longitudinal study from birth to age 18. *Journal of Studies on Alcohol*, 47, 34–40.

West, M. O., & Prinz, R. J. (1987). Parental alcoholism and childhood psychopathology. *Psychological Bulletin*, 102, 204–218.

Wierson, M., Forehand, R., & McCombs, A. (1988). The relationship of early adolescent functioning to parent-reported and adolescent-perceived interparental conflict. *Journal of Abnormal Child Psychology*, 16, 707–718.

Wolfe, D. A. (1985). Child-abusive parents: An empirical review and analysis. *Psychological Bulletin*, 97, 462–482.

Wolff, S., Narayan, S., & Moyes, B. (1988). Personality characteristics of parents of autistic children: A controlled study. *Journal of Child Psychology and Psychiatry*, 29, 143–153.

Woollett, A., White, D. G., & Lyon, M. L. (1982). Studies involving fathers: Subject refusal, attrition and sampling bias. *Current Psychological Reviews*, 2, 193–212.

Worland, J., Janes, C. L., Anthony, E. J., McGinnis, M., & Cass, L. (1984). St. Louis High Risk Research Project: Comprehensive progress report of experimental studies. In N. F. Watt, E. J. Anthony, L. C. Wynne, & J. E. Rolf (Eds.), *Children at risk for schizophrenia: A longitudinal perspective* (pp. 105–147). New York: Cambridge University Press.

Wright, L. S. (1985). Suicidal thoughts and their relationship to family stress and personal problems among high school seniors and college undergraduates. *Adolescence*, 20, 575–580.

Yesavage, J. A., Becker, J. M. T., Werner, P. D., Patton, M. J., Seeman, K., Brunsting, D. W., & Mills, M. J. (1983). Family conflict, psychopathology, and dangerous behavior by schizophrenic inpatients. *Psychiatry Research*, 8, 271–280.

Zahn-Waxler, C., Cummings, E. M., McKnew, D. H., & Radke-Yarrow, M. (1984). Altruism, aggression, and social interactions in young children with a manic-depressive parent. *Child Development*, 55, 112–122.

16

Tics and Tourette's Disorder: A 2- to 7-Year Follow-up of 54 Obsessive-Compulsive Children

Henrietta L. Leonard, Marge C. Lenane, Susan E. Swedo,
David C. Rettew, Elliott S. Gershon, and Judith L. Rapoport
National Institute of Mental Health, Bethesda, Maryland

Objective: *This study examined a hypothesized etiologic relationship between Tourette's disorder and obsessive-compulsive disorder.* Method: *Fifty-four children who had initially participated in treatment protocols for obsessive-compulsive disorder (Tourette's disorder was an exclusionary criterion) were reevaluated 2–7 years later with a neurological examination and a structured interview to establish the presence or absence of tics and Tourette's disorder. The children's first-degree relatives (N = 171) were also screened for tic disorders.* Results: *At baseline, 57% (N = 31) of the patients had lifetime histories of tics. At follow-up, 59% (N = 32) had lifetime histories of tics; eight of these (all males) met the criteria for Tourette's disorder (six had developed the disorder, and two, it could be argued in retrospect, might have met the criteria at baseline). The patients with lifetime histories of tics had greater anxiety, a higher ratio of CSF 5-hydroxyindoleacetic acid to homovanillic acid, and a younger age at onset of obsessive-compulsive disorder than those without tics. The patients with Tourette's disorder differed from other male patients only in having an earlier age at onset of obsessive-compulsive disorder. Of the first-degree relatives, 1.8% (N = 3) had Tourette's disorder, and 14% (N = 24) had a tic disorder.* Conclusions: *Except for their earlier age at onset of obsessive-compulsive disorder, the patients with*

Reprinted with permission from *American Journal of Psychiatry*, 1992, Vol. 149(9), 1244–1251. Copyright © 1992 by the American Psychiatric Association.

Preliminary data from this study were presented in part at the Second International Scientific Symposium on Tourette Syndrome, Boston, June 17, 1991.

Tourette's disorder were indistinguishable from those without. The apparent high rate of tics and Tourette's disorder in the subjects and their relatives is consistent with the hypothesis that in some cases, obsessive-compulsive disorder and Tourette's disorder may be alternative manifestations of the same underlying illness.

Obsessive-compulsive disorder has been reported in association with a number of basal ganglia disorders, specifically, Sydenham's chorea,[1] post-encephalitic Parkinson's disease,[2] Huntington's chorea (S. Folstein, personal communication), and Tourette's disorder.[3] Of these, obsessive-compulsive disorder has been noted most often in Tourette's disorder; the more recent systematic studies have reported that one-third to one-half of adult[3-5] and child[6] patients with Tourette's disorder are afflicted. Studies of patients with obsessive-compulsive disorder also suggest a relationship between Tourette's disorder and obsessive-compulsive disorder; an increased prevalence of chronic tics has been noted by several observers.[5,7,8]

Other compelling evidence for a relationship between Tourette's disorder and obsessive-compulsive disorder comes from family studies of probands with Tourette's disorder.[3,5,9,10] Pauls et al.[3] reported that the rate of obsessive-compulsive disorder among 45 first-degree biologic relatives of 13 probands with Tourette's disorder without obsessive-compulsive disorder was 26%. This was higher than the expected rate in the general population and was similar to the rate for relatives of probands who had Tourette's disorder with obsessive-compulsive disorder. The mode of transmission of Tourette's disorder and chronic tics is consistent with autosomal dominant inheritance with incomplete penetrance and sex-influenced expressivity.[10] Pauls et al.[3,10] hypothesized that at least some forms of obsessive-compulsive disorder are etiologically related to Tourette's disorder and chronic tics and that obsessive-compulsive disorder may be an alternative phenotypic manifestation of the gene(s) responsible for Tourette's disorder. At present, however, the exact relationship between Tourette's disorder and obsessive-compulsive disorder is unknown, and there are no systematic studies of Tourette's disorder in family members of probands with obsessive-compulsive disorder.

The actual prevalences of Tourette's disorder and chronic tics are unknown, as no large general population samples have been systematically screened for tics. The prevalence of Tourette's disorder in selected populations has been estimated to be 2.9,[11] 5.2,[12] and 40[13] per 10,000, but the studies have been limited by their sampling techniques. Tic disorders are more common than Tourette's disorder in the general population, and estimates have ranged from 4% to 6%[14-16] to 12%.[17,18] Sampling techniques and varied diagnostic criteria for tics limited these studies, and in several samples nonspecific nervous or unusual movements were included, which may have inflated the estimates.

This report concerns tics and Tourette's disorder at 2- to 7-year follow-up in 54 children and adolescents with severe primary obsessive-compulsive disorder for whom a diagnosis of Tourette's disorder, but not chronic tics, had initially been ruled out. We hypothesized that despite the initial exclusion of Tourette's disorder, some of the patients with obsessive-compulsive disorder would "develop" Tourette's disorder, given the reported association between the two disorders, the presence of tics at baseline among many patients, and the hypothesis that within families of probands with Tourette's disorder the two disorders are etiologically related. The study addressed the following questions. 1) What are the lifetime and current rates of Tourette's disorder and tics at follow-up in child probands with obsessive-compulsive disorder and their first-degree relatives? 2) Is there a characteristic demographic, clinical, laboratory, or familial pattern among probands with obsessive-compulsive disorder and Tourette's disorder or chronic tics that might elucidate a relationship between the conditions?

METHOD

Fifty-four children and adolescents with severe primary obsessive-compulsive disorder who had been consecutively admitted to clomipramine treatment trials conducted between 1985 and 1988[19,20] were contacted for follow-up evaluation. At baseline, these 36 boys and 18 girls had a mean age of 13.6 years (SD = 2.0, range = 7–19) and a mean age at onset of obsessive-compulsive disorder of 9.9 years (SD = 3.3, range = 2–16). A diagnosis of Tourette's disorder was an exclusionary criterion for these studies, but a chronic vocal or motor tic was not.

At follow-up, the 54 subjects with obsessive-compulsive disorder had a mean age of 17.4 years (SD = 3.0, range = 10–24). They were reevaluated 2–7 years (mean = 3.4 years, SD = 1.0) after baseline. Information was obtained for all 54 subjects, and 48 (89%) of the patients were seen in person. Information on the remaining six (11%) was available from at least two of the following sources: telephone interview with the patient (N = 3), family report (N = 6), current private physician's report (N = 2), and medical records (N = 3).

At baseline evaluation, assessment of lifetime and current *DSM-III-R* tic diagnoses consisted of clinical interviews and administration of the Diagnostic Interview for Children and Adolescents[21] (including the tic section of the parent interview) to a parent and child, review of available medical records, and a neurological examination. Demographic measures, associated comorbidity, and scores on severity rating scales, including the National Institute of Mental Health (NIMH) global scales for obsessive-compulsive disorder, anxiety, depression, and functioning,[22] have been reported by Leonard et al.[20] Interrater reliability (kappa) between the two raters (H.L.L. and S.E.S.) ranged from 0.91 to 0.97 and is detailed elsewhere.[23] Forty-three (80%) of the patients underwent lumbar puncture.[24]

At follow-up, the measures were repeated, and the NIMH global obsessive-compulsive disorder score[22] was used as the follow-up rating of the severity of that disorder. Additionally, the Tourette syndrome/tics section-modified of the Yale Schedule for Tourette and Other Behavioral Syndromes[25] was administered to either the parent (about the proband) or the proband, and the Children's Global Assessment Scale[26] was completed. Twenty-two patients had a repeat lumbar puncture; however, those results have not yet been analyzed.

With the use of the Diagnostic Interview for Children and Adolescents[21] or the Schedule for Affective Disorders and Schizophrenia (SADS)[27] (according to the age of the person being interviewed), 170 of the probands' 173 first-degree relatives over 6 years of age were interviewed in person when the probands entered the study. In addition, a forensic psychiatric evaluation of one father was available. Thus, diagnoses were made for 52 mothers (mean age = 44.7 years, SD = 4.2), 51 fathers (mean age = 47.6 years, SD = 5.3), 30 sisters (mean age = 17.2 years, SD = 4.6), and 38 brothers (mean age = 15.9 years, SD = 5.4). (Because two sets of brothers were included among the 54 subjects, for the family data one brother was randomly assigned as the proband and one as the sibling for each family. Thus, 52 probands are referred to for the family data. It should be noted that none of the four brothers had a tic disorder.) Lenane et al.[28] previously reported that among the first-degree relatives of 46 of these 54 probands, 15 parents (17%) and three siblings (5%; age corrected, 35%) had lifetime histories of obsessive-compulsive disorder at baseline. Three additional cases were diagnosed subsequently, at the time of this follow-up. (Two fathers had not acknowledged obsessive-compulsive symptoms at the first evaluation, and one sibling developed them in the interim.) All relatives had been observed for tics and had been asked during the baseline clinical interview about the presence of motor and vocal tics; however, no formal neurological examinations or structured ratings of tics were obtained, other than the Diagnostic Interview for Children and Adolescents— Parent Version[21] for the siblings. At follow-up, the Yale Schedule for Tourette and Other Behavioral Syndromes (Tourette syndrome/tics section-modified)[25] was administered to at least one parent of every family, who reported on all family members, in order to confirm the original tic status and to assess any changes. Forty-eight mothers, 12 fathers, four siblings, and 28 probands were reinterviewed directly about family members, and 27 families had more than one family member interviewed.

BMDP stepwise discriminant analyses with jackknife validation[29] were used to determine which baseline and follow-up variables best discriminated 1) between patients with and without tics and 2) among males with Tourette's disorder, chronic/transient tics, and no tics. This procedure controlled for an otherwise inflated error rate that would have occurred with the use of a large number of univariate tests. Comparisons of specific obsessive-compulsive disorder symptoms between patients with and without tics were made with chi-square tests.

Since not all first-degree relatives had passed through the risk period for developing illness, the rates of tics and obsessive-compulsive disorder were age corrected using known cumulative data on age at onset.[30,31] We used a modified Stromberg method[32] to correct for each person's age according to the percentage of the risk period for each disorder through which he or she had passed. Statistical comparisons of age-corrected rates of illness between different groups were made with chi-square and Fisher's exact tests. The age of 15 years was arbitrarily assigned to adults who recalled an onset of tics in adolescence but could not be more specific (N = 11).

Life table survival analyses that used BMDP program P1L were performed to compute the cumulative hazard function (probability of developing an illness by a certain age) for tics and obsessive-compulsive disorder in the first-degree relatives.[29,33,34] This procedure yields more information than simple lifetime prevalence estimates, as it allows for the estimation of the risk of an illness at a given age within a given population. To assess the relative effects of several variables simultaneously on the relatives' survival function (not developing illness), the Cox proportional hazards model was used with BMDP program P2L.[29,34] Comparisons between male and female relatives on this hazard function could then be made using the Mantel-Cox statistic.[33-35]

RESULTS

The Patients

At baseline, 16 (30%) of the 54 patients with obsessive-compulsive disorder had a current transient or chronic tic, and 31 (57%) had lifetime histories of tics (including the current status). At follow-up, 22 subjects (12 male and 10 female) had no lifetime history of tics, and 32 subjects (24 male and eight female) (59%) had lifetime histories of transient/chronic tics or Tourette's disorder; 17 (31%) had current diagnoses of tics. Of the 32 with lifetime tic diagnoses, eight (15% of the total of 54 patients) met lifetime diagnostic criteria for Tourette's disorder, 12 (22% of the 54) for chronic tics, and 12 for transient tics. At follow-up, from rereview of initial medical records and from additional information obtained from structured interview, it could be argued that two of the eight subjects with Tourette's disorder (all male) might have met the diagnostic criteria for Tourette's disorder at baseline. Thus, six (11%) of 54 subjects who did not meet criteria for Tourette's disorder at baseline "developed" Tourette's disorder in the interim.

Of the 32 patients with lifetime histories of tics, at baseline 17 (53%) also had lifetime histories of an anxiety disorder, seven (22%) had attention deficit hyperactivity disorder, and seven had oppositional/conduct disorder. Of the 22 patients without a lifetime history of tics, 10 (45%) had an anxiety disorder, five

(23%) had attention deficit hyperactivity disorder, and four (18%) had oppositional/conduct disorder at baseline.

Among the 32 patients with lifetime histories of tics, nine (28%) had relatives with obsessive-compulsive disorder, and 13 (41%) had relatives with tics. Among the 22 patients with no lifetime history of tics, seven (32%) had relatives with obsessive-compulsive disorder, and 11 (50%) had relatives with tics.

The sex of the subject, a family history of obsessive-compulsive disorder, a family history of tics, and all variables shown in Table 1 were entered into the discriminant analysis. The statistically significant variables best able to distinguish the 32 patients with lifetime histories of tics from the 22 without were, in order of significance, a higher score (more symptoms) on the NIMH global anxiety scale at baseline, a greater baseline ratio of CSF 5-hydroxyindoleacetic acid (5-HIAA) to homovanillic acid (HVA), and a younger age at onset of obsessive-compulsive disorder. Together, these three variables correctly classified 81% of the patients with tics and 57% of the patients without tics, for an overall ability of 69%. There was no difference (by chi-square test) between the presenting major obsessive-compulsive symptoms of patients with and patients without lifetime histories of tics. Washing compulsions were the most frequently reported for both groups, followed by checking and repeating.

At follow-up, although all of the eight patients with Tourette's disorder met the *DSM-III-R* diagnostic criteria, the symptoms were mild. Only four patients were aware that they had a tic disorder, and only two had had a previous medication trial for the tics. All but one of the Tourette's disorder patients had lifetime histories of tics at baseline. Three had attention deficit hyperactivity disorder, one had learning disabilities (visual perceptual), and one had oppositional and conduct disorder. Three patients with Tourette's disorder had a first-degree relative with obsessive-compulsive disorder, and four had a family history of tics (one relative met criteria for Tourette's disorder). The primary presenting symptoms were typical for obsessive-compulsive disorder—specifically, washing rituals (N = 5), hoarding (N = 1), repeating (N = 1), and scrupulosity (N = 1).

To see whether the patients with Tourette's disorder differed on any measure (in the previous discriminant analysis) from those with chronic/transient tics and from those without any tic diagnosis, a second discriminant analysis was performed. Only males were chosen for these comparisons in order to control for any confounding influence of gender. Only a younger age at onset of obsessive-compulsive disorder distinguished the group of patients with Tourette's disorder from the other two groups. Age at onset of obsessive-compulsive disorder distinguished 50% of the patients with Tourette's disorder, 80% of those with tics, and 0% of the patients without tics, for an overall rate of 46%. The mean ages at onset of obsessive-compulsive disorder for the eight boys with Tourette's disorder, the chronic/transient tic group, and the group without tics were 6.5 years (SD = 3.5),

TABLE 1
Baseline and 2- to 7-Year Follow-Up Data on 54 Male and Female
Patients With Obsessive-Compulsive Disorder With and Without a
Lifetime History of Tics at Follow-Up

Item	Patients With Lifetime History of Tics (N=32)		Patients Without Lifetime History of Tics (N=22)	
	Mean	SD	Mean	SD
Age at onset of obsessive-compulsive disorder (years)[a]	9.2	3.3	10.8	3.1
Age at follow-up (years)	17.5	3.3	17.4	2.4
IQ	109.7	14.7	104.8	9.4
Baseline CSF measure[b]				
5-HIAA level (age corrected; pmol/ml)	117.2	35.8	108.1	26.4
HVA level (age corrected; pmol/ml)	268.2	93.9	273.3	66.6
5-HIAA/HVA ratio[c]	0.45	0.11	0.40	0.05
MHPG level (pmol/ml)	48.8	11.5	42.0	10.4
Baseline serotonin level (ng/10^8 platelets)	55.5	26.1	50.0	17.6
NIMH global scale rating at baseline				
Obsessive-compulsive disorder	8.5	1.4	8.6	1.4
Depression	4.7	2.1	4.4	2.1
Anxiety[c]	6.5	2.1	4.9	1.7
Functioning	7.6	1.7	7.5	2.1
Response to clomipramine at 5 weeks (%)	27	21	27	28
NIMH global obsessive-compulsive disorder rating at follow-up	5.7	2.9	4.1	2.3
Children's Global Assessment Scale score at follow-up	61.9	20.8	73.7	19.4

[a]From discriminant analysis, partial R^2=0.08, $p<0.05$.
[b]N=22 for patients with lifetime history of tics; N=21 for patients without lifetime history of tics.
[c]From discriminant analysis, partial R^2=0.15, $p<0.05$.

10.4 years (SD = 2.9), and 11.3 years (SD = 3.1), respectively. No significant differences between the three groups were found for the CSF measures: 5-HIAA/HVA ratios for the Tourette's disorder group, the transient/chronic tic group, and the group without tics were, respectively, 0.53 (SD = 0.12) (N = 3), 0.45 (SD = 0.12) (N = 11), and 0.40 (SD = 0.05) (N = 12).

The Families

At follow-up, three (1.8%) of the first-degree relatives (one father and two male siblings) met criteria for a lifetime diagnosis of Tourette's disorder. All three were evaluated in person to confirm the diagnosis. The three different probands whose family members had Tourette's disorder were in three separate patient diagnostic subgroups: obsessive-compulsive disorder and Tourette's disorder, obsessive-compulsive disorder with chronic tics, and obsessive-compulsive disorder without tics.

The age-corrected lifetime prevalence rates of obsessive-compulsive disorder and tic disorders (including chronic, transient, and Tourette's disorder) among the 171 first-degree relatives are presented in Table 2. The most striking findings were the apparent high rates of tics (14%) and obsessive-compulsive disorder (17%) among the first-degree relatives of the probands and the fact that illness in relatives was unrelated to the sex of the probands. There were significantly more male relatives than female relatives with tics and significantly more male relatives than female relatives with obsessive-compulsive disorder. As shown in Table 3, the rates of illness (obsessive-compulsive disorder, tics, or Tourette's disorder) in first-degree relatives did not differ significantly according to proband status (no tics, tics, and Tourette's disorder) by chi-square test.

The Cox proportional hazards model was used to test simultaneously the effects of the probands' sex, age at onset of obsessive-compulsive disorder, comorbid attention deficit hyperactivity disorder, severity of obsessive-compulsive disorder, and severity of tics and the effects of the sex of the relative on the survival function (not having a diagnosis) of the relative. Testing each variable alone on this cumulative hazard function, we found that the only covariate with a significant impact on illness in the relative was the sex of the relative (obsessive-compulsive disorder, $\chi^2 = 4.67$, df $= 1$, p<0.03; tics, $\chi^2 = 13.46$, df $= 1$, p $= 0.002$; obsessive-compulsive disorder or tics, $\chi^2 = 12.73$, df $= 1$, p $= 0.0004$). The cumulative effect of the five *proband* variables combined failed as an overall regression model to make a statistically significant contribution to the hazard function (illness in the relative). Thus, of the six variables tested, only the sex of the relative was important in predicting the relative's possible development of tics and/or obsessive-compulsive disorder.

As a further confirmation, the Mantel-Cox statistic in life table analyses was used to compare male and female relatives on the cumulative hazard function (probability of developing tics or obsessive-compulsive disorder by a certain age). Male relatives were found to have a greater risk of both tics (Mantel-Cox statistic $= 13.83$, df $= 1$, p $= 0.0002$) and obsessive-compulsive disorder (Mantel-Cox statistic $= 4.91$, df $= 1$, p $= 0.03$) (Figure 1). Similar results were obtained for developing either tics or obsessive-compulsive disorder when these were combined into a single analysis.

TABLE 2
Lifetime Histories of Obsessive-Compulsive Disorder and Tic Disorder Among First-Degree Relatives of 52 Probands with Obsessive-Compulsive Disorder

	Relatives of 34 Male Probands						Relatives of 18 Female Probands						Relatives of All 52 Probands					
	Male (N=62)		Female (N=52)		Total (N=114)		Male (N=27)		Female (N=30)		Total (N=57)		Male (N=89)		Female (N=82)		Total (N=171)	
Measure	N	%	N	%	N	%	N	%	N	%	N	%	N	%	N	%	N	%
Tics	17	27[a]	2	4	19	17	4	15	1	3	5	9	21	24[a]	3	4	24	14
Age corrected		28		4		17		15		3		9		24		4		14
Obsessive-compulsive disorder	11	18	5	10	16	14	5	19	1	3	6	11	16	18[b]	6	7	22	13
Age corrected		25		12		19		23		4		13		23		10		17
Total relatives affected	22	35[c]	6	12	28	25	7	26	2	7	9	16	29	33[a]	8	10	37	22
Age corrected		35		12		25		26		7		16		33		10		22

[a]Rate of illness significantly greater in male relatives than in female relatives (p<0.005, Fisher's exact test).
[b]Rate of illness significantly greater in male relatives than in female relatives (p<0.05, Fisher's exact test).
[c]Rate of illness significantly greater in male relatives than in female relatives (p<0.01, Fisher's exact test).

TABLE 3

Lifetime Prevalence of Obsessive-Compulsive Disorder, Tics, and Tourette's Disorder in 171 First-Degree Relatives of 52 Probands with Primary Obsessive-Compulsive Disorder[a]

Proband Diagnosis	Relatives With Obsessive-Compulsive Disorder[b]		Relatives With Tics[b,c]		Relatives With Tourette's Disorder[b]		Total Relatives Affected[d]	
	N	%	N	%	N	%	N	%
Obsessive-compulsive disorder, no tics	12	16	9	12	1	1	17	23
Age corrected		22		12		1		23
Obsessive-compulsive disorder and tics	7	10	11	15	1	1	14	28
Age corrected		13		15		1		20
Obsessive-compulsive disorder and Tourette's disorder	3	12	4	16	1	4	6	25
Age corrected		16		16		1		24
Total	22	13	24	14	3	6	37	22
Age corrected		17		14		6		22

[a] There were no significant differences in rates of illness in relatives by diagnosis of probands (chi-square or Fisher's exact test).
[b] Obsessive-compulsive disorder, tic, and Tourette's disorder diagnoses are not mutually exclusive.
[c] Category includes transient and chronic tics and Tourette's disorder.
[d] Age-correction factor of tics was used for this category; two age corrections could not be made, and the conservative correction (that of illness with earlier onset) was chosen.

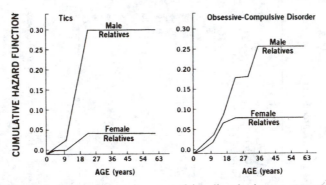

Figure 1. Tics and obsessive-compulsive disorder by age at onset in 171 first-degree relatives of 52 probands with obsessive-compulsive disorder

DISCUSSION

In this study, which addressed the question of the prevalence of Tourette's disorder and tics in child patients with obsessive-compulsive disorder and in their first-degree relatives, 59% ($N = 32$) of the 54 subjects had lifetime histories of tics when evaluated at follow-up, although only one-third ($N = 17$) actually had a current diagnosis. Methodological difficulties have led to widely varying estimates of the rate of tics and Tourette's disorder in the general population,[11-18] so without systematic population studies, direct comparisons of our study group's rates with expected rates are not possible. However, the 11%–15% lifetime prevalence of Tourette's disorder in the patients with obsessive-compulsive disorder and the 1.8% rate in their first-degree relatives is higher than the published estimates of 0.03%–0.40%.[11-13] Similarly, the lifetime rates of tics in the patients with obsessive-compulsive disorder (59%) and their first-degree relatives (14%) are outside the reported range of 4%–12%.[14-18] This seemingly high rate of tics and Tourette's disorder among the probands and their first-degree relatives lends support to the hypothesis that some cases of obsessive-compulsive disorder and Tourette's disorder may be etiologically related.

Illness (obsessive-compulsive disorder, Tourette's disorder, and/or tics) in the first-degree relatives was not related to either the sex or the tic status of the obsessive-compulsive disorder probands. This finding is consistent with that of Pauls et al.[10] among families of probands with Tourette's disorder; these authors reported that obsessive-compulsive disorder in the relatives was independent of the sex and diagnosis (with or without obsessive-compulsive disorder) of the proband with Tourette's disorder. In our current study, the male first-degree relatives had a higher rate of tics and of obsessive-compulsive disorder than did the female relatives. In contrast, Pauls et al.[10] reported that male relatives were more likely to have Tourette's disorder, and female relatives were more likely to have obsessive-compulsive disorder without tics, suggesting that obsessive-compulsive disorder could represent the part of the Tourette's disorder spectrum that is more frequently expressed in females. This difference between studies might be explained by the smaller number of families evaluated in our study or by the difference in proband status (obsessive-compulsive disorder versus Tourette's disorder).

A major limitation of the family portion of this report is that our data may underestimate the rate of tics. Although all relatives were seen in person and assessed for the presence/absence of tics, the reevaluation in person with a structured instrument was not done with every relative. Childhood tics that had subsequently resolved may not have been remembered by adults. Thus, if tics were not reported by the patient or family members and had gone "unnoticed" by the interviewer, they would not have been included.

It was hypothesized that at follow-up, some of the probands with obsessive-compulsive disorder might have "developed" Tourette's disorder, given the reported association between Tourette's disorder and obsessive-compulsive disorder and the presence of tics at baseline. Indeed, six males (11%) of 54 patients with obsessive-compulsive disorder who did not meet diagnostic criteria for Tourette's disorder at baseline did so at follow-up. Although it is not surprising that children with tics (who had not passed through their risk period) might subsequently develop Tourette's disorder, the presence of Tourette's disorder in 11% of the subjects seems high, particularly in light of the initial exclusionary criteria.

What distinguished the patients with obsessive-compulsive disorder and Tourette's disorder from those without Tourette's disorder? Only early age at onset of obsessive-compulsive disorder and male sex predicted who might develop Tourette's disorder. This is in keeping with the known predominance in males and the postulated sex-influenced genetic expressivity.[3] Although we previously reported that the age at onset of obsessive-compulsive disorder was lower for boys than for girls,[36] the significance of the earlier onset of obsessive-compulsive disorder in the patients with Tourette's disorder is not clear and has not been previously reported.

The patients with obsessive-compulsive disorder and Tourette's disorder were not distinguishable by the nature of their obsessions or compulsions. In general, the obsessive-compulsive symptoms were those typically seen, but a few patients exhibited behavior that was difficult to categorize as a ritual or tic. The categorization of the behavior was based on its complexity and the presence/absence of cognition preceding the action. Typically, a ritual is performed in response to a specific thought and a tic in response to an urge. Behaviors which remained difficult to classify clearly included that of a boy who would spit after the thought that his mouth had become contaminated by human body fluids and that of another patient who "compulsively" bounced a ball and touched his fingers in a rhythmic fashion because his "bones made him do it." Even if obsessive-compulsive disorder and Tourette's disorder are different manifestations of the same underlying illness, it appears that tics and rituals are for the most part clinically distinct and distinguishable. There may be a spectrum of behaviors, ranging from the classical tics of patients with Tourette's disorder to a mixed picture of tics and rituals to clear-cut rituals. Although this set of data does not help us truly address the distinction between tics and rituals, the clinical picture of obsessive-compulsive disorder was essentially not different among the probands with obsessive-compulsive disorder with and without Tourette's disorder.

An earlier age at onset of obsessive-compulsive disorder, a higher baseline anxiety rating (although not a *DSM-III-R* anxiety diagnosis), and a higher CSF 5-HIAA/HVA ratio distinguished the patients with obsessive-compulsive disorder and tic disorders from those without such a comorbid diagnosis. The meaning of the association between anxiety and tics is unclear, as the relation between anxiety and Tourette's disorder has not been systematically studied, and there was no increase in the number of individuals with anxiety disorders—just an increase in the anxiety rating. Perhaps anxiety and tics exacerbate each other or, less likely, they could both be manifestations of the underlying illness.

The increased CSF 5-HIAA/HVA ratio in the patients with obsessive-compulsive disorder and tics is consistent with hypotheses of altered neurotransmitters in Tourette's disorder and obsessive-compulsive disorder.[24,37-39] The present findings are in the same direction as those reported by Cohen et al.[37] for a group of six patients with Tourette's disorder who had a (nonsignificantly) higher 5-HIAA/HVA ratio than did a comparison group of eight patients with medical disorders. Although our patients with Tourette's disorder had a higher CSF 5-HIAA/HVA ratio than that of the male chronic and transient tic group (N = 11), which in turn was higher than that of the group without tics (N = 12), none of these differences was significant. Only three of our eight patients with Tourette's disorder had lumbar punctures, so the small size of the study group may have contributed to the lack of a significant difference. Although no conclusions can be drawn from these nonsignificant results from a small number of subjects, it is tempting to speculate that tics and Tourette's disorder may be associated with disturbances of the serotonin/dopamine ratio.

This is the first large, systematic family study of tics and Tourette's disorder among probands with obsessive-compulsive disorder and their first-degree relatives. The high rate of tics and Tourette's disorder in the 54 patients with obsessive-compulsive disorder is consistent with the previously reported frequent association of these disorders. The apparent high rate of obsessive-compulsive disorder and tics in the first-degree relatives of the probands, independent of the probands' tic status, supports the hypothesis[3,10] that in some cases, obsessive-compulsive disorder and Tourette's disorder may be alternative manifestations of the same underlying (genetic) illness. Even if the same etiologic mechanism may be responsible for some cases of Tourette's disorder and obsessive-compulsive disorder, the clinical picture of obsessive-compulsive disorder was indistinguishable among those with and without a comorbid tic diagnosis.

REFERENCES

1. Swedo SE, Rapoport JL, Cheslow DL, Leonard HL, Ayoub EM, Hosier DM, Wald ER: High prevalence of obsessive-compulsive symptoms in patients with Sydenham's chorea. Am J Psychiatry 1989; 146:246–249

2. von Economo C (ed): Encephalitis Lethargic, Its Sequelae and Treatment. New York, Oxford University Press, 1931

3. Pauls DL, Towbin KE, Leckman JF, Zahner GEP, Cohen DJ: Gilles de la Tourette's syndrome and obsessive-compulsive disorder: evidence supporting a genetic relationship. Arch Gen Psychiatry 1986; 43:1180–1182

4. Frankel M, Cummings JL, Robertson MM, Trimble MR, Hill MA, Benson DF: Obsessions and compulsions in Gilles de la Tourette syndrome. Neurology 1986; 36:379–382

5. Pitman RK, Green RC, Jenike MA, Mesulam MM: Clinical comparison of Tourette's disorder and obsessive-compulsive disorder. Am J Psychiatry 1987; 144:1166–1171

6. Grad LR, Pelcovitz D, Olson M, Matthews M, Grad GJ: Obsessive-compulsive symptomatology in children with Tourette's syndrome. J Am Acad Child Adolesc Psychiatry 1987; 26:69–73

7. Swedo SE, Rapoport JL, Leonard HL, Lenane M, Cheslow D: Obsessive-compulsive disorder in children and adolescents. Arch Gen Psychiatry 1989; 46:335–341

8. Riddle MA, Scahill L, King R, Hardin MT, Towbin KE, Ort SI, Leckman JF, Cohen DJ: Obsessive compulsive disorder in children and adolescents: phenomonology and family history. J Am Acad Child Adolesc Psychiatry 1990; 29:766–772

9. Robertson MM, Gourdie A: Familial Tourette's syndrome in a large British pedigree: associated psychopathology, severity, and potential for linkage analysis. Br J Psychiatry 1990; 156:515–521

10. Pauls DL, Raymond CL, Stevenson JM, Leckman JF: A family study of Gilles de la Tourette syndrome. Hum Genet 1991; 48:154–163

11. Caine ED, McBride MC, Chiverton P, Bamford KA, Rediess S, Shiao J: Tourette's syndrome in Monroe County school children. Neurology 1988; 38:472–475

12. Burd L, Kerbeshian J, Wikenheiser M, Fisher W: Prevalence of Gilles de la Tourette's syndrome in North Dakota adults. Am J Psychiatry 1986; 143:787–788

13. Comings DE, Himes JA, Comings BG: An epidemiologic study of Tourette's syndrome in a single school district. J Clin Psychiatry 1990; 51:463–469

14. Rutter M, Tizard J, Whitmore K: Education, Health and Behavior. London, Longman, 1970

15. Pringle ML, Butler NR, Davie R: 11,000 Seven Year Olds. London, National Bureau for Cooperation in Child Care, 1967

16. Rutter M, Yule W, Berger M, Yule B, Morton J, Bagley C: Children of West Indian immigrants, I: rates of behavioral deviance and psychiatric disorder. J Child Psychol Psychiatry 1974; 15:241–262

17. Verhulst FC, Akkerhuis GW, Althaus M: Mental Health in Dutch Children, I: A Cross-Cultural Comparison. Acta Psychiatr Scand (Suppl) 1985; 323

18. Lapouse R, Monk MA: Behavior deviations in a representative sample of children: variation between sex, age, race, social class, and family size. Am J Orthopsychiatry, 1964; 34:436–446

19. Flament MF, Rapoport JL, Berg CJ, Sceery W, Kilts C, Mellstrom B, Linnoila M: Clomipramine treatment of childhood obsessive-compulsive disorder. Arch Gen Psychiatry 1985; 42:977–983

20. Leonard HL, Swedo SE, Rapoport JL, Koby EV, Lenane MC, Cheslow DL, Hamburger SD: Treatment of obsessive-compulsive disorder with clomipramine and desipramine in children and adolescents: a double-blind crossover comparison. Arch Gen Psychiatry 1989; 46:1088–1092

21. Herjanic B, Campbell W: Differentiating psychiatrically disturbed children on the basis of a structured psychiatric interview. J Abnorm Child Psychol 1977; 5:127–135

22. Murphy DL, Pickar D, Alterman IS: Methods for the quantitative assessment of depressive and manic behavior, in The Behavior of Psychiatric Patients. Edited by Burdock EI, Sudilovsky A, Gershon S. New York, Marcel Dekker, 1982

23. Swedo SE, Schapiro MB, Grady CL, Cheslow DL, Leonard HL, Kumar A, Friedland R, Rapoport SI, Rapoport JL: Cerebral glucose metabolism in childhood-onset obsessive-compulsive disorder. Arch Gen Psychiatry 1989; 46:518–523

24. Swedo SE, Leonard HL, Kruesi MJ, Rettew DC, Listwak SJ, Berrettini W, Stipetic M, Hamburger S, Gold PW, Potter WZ, Rapoport JL: Cerebrospinal fluid neurochemistry of children and adolescents with obsessive-compulsive disorder. Arch Gen Psychiatry 1992; 49:29–36

25. Pauls DL, Hurst CR: Schedule for Tourette and Other Behavioral Syndromes. New Haven, Conn, Child Study Center, Yale University School of Medicine, 1981

26. Shaffer D, Gould MS, Brasic J, Ambrosini P, Fisher P, Bird H, Aluwahlia S: A children's global assessment scale (CGAS). Arch Gen Psychiatry 1983; 40:1228–1231

27. Spitzer RL, Endicott J: Schedule for Affective Disorders and Schizophrenia (SADS), 3rd ed. New York, New York State Psychiatric Institute, Biometrics Research, 1978

28. Lenane MC, Swedo SE, Leonard H, Pauls DL, Sceery W, Rapoport JL: Psychiatric disorders in first degree relatives of children and adolescents with obsessive compulsive disorder. J Am Acad Child Adolesc Psychiatry 1990; 29:407–412

29. Dixon WJ (ed): BMDP Statistical Software. Berkeley, University of California Press, 1983

30. Shapiro AK, Shapiro ES, Bruun RD: Gilles de la Tourette Syndrome. New York, Raven Press, 1978

31. Black A: The natural history of obsessional neurosis, in Obsessional States. Edited by Beech HR. London, Methuen, 1974, p 38

32. Stromberg E: Zum Ersatz des Weinbergschen "abgekurzten Verfahrens": zugleich ein Beitrag zur Frage von der Erblichkeit des Erkrankungsalters bei der Schizophrenie. Zentralbl Gesamte Neurol Psychiatrie 1935; 153:764–797

33. Kalbfleisch JD, Prentice RL: The Statistical Analysis of Failure Time Data. New York, John Wiley & Sons, 1980

34. Gershon ES, Hamovit JH, Guroff JJ, Nurnberger JI: Birth-cohort changes in manic and depressive disorders in relatives of bipolar and schizoaffective patients. Arch Gen Psychiatry 1987; 44:314–319

35. Lawless JF: Statistical Models and Methods for Lifetime Data. New York, John Wiley & Sons, 1982

36. Swedo SE, Rapoport JL, Leonard H, Lenane M, Cheslow D: Obsessive-compulsive disorder in children and adolescents: clinical phenomenology of 70 consecutive cases. Arch Gen Psychiatry 1989; 46:335–341

37. Cohen DJ, Shaywitz BA, Caparulo B, Young JG, Bowers MB: Chronic, multiple tics of Gilles de la Tourette's disease. Arch Gen Psychiatry 1978; 35:245–250

38. Butler IJ, Koslow SH, Seifert WE, Caprioli RM, Singer HS: Biogenic amine metabolism in Tourette syndrome. Ann Neurol 1979; 6:37–39

39. Goodman WK, McDougle CJ, Price LH, Riddle MA, Pauls DL, Leckman JF: Beyond the serotonin hypothesis: a role for dopamine in some forms of obsessive compulsive disorders? J Clin Psychiatry 1990; 51(suppl 8):36–43

17

Communication Deficits and Formal Thought Disorder in Schizophrenic Children

Rochelle Caplan and Donald Guthrie

University of California, Los Angeles

Judith G. Foy

Loyola Marymount University, Los Angeles

This study examined 31 schizophrenic children to determine if they used discourse devices that make speech coherence differently from sex and mental age matched normal children. It also investigated whether the discourse deficits of the schizophrenic children were related to clinical measures of formal thought disorder. Using Halliday and Hassan's analysis of cohesion, the authors found that schizophrenic children underutilize some discourse devices and overutilize others. Several of their discourse deficits were similar to those described in schizophrenic adults. The schizophrenic children, however, also had additional discourse deficits, which probably reflect developmental delays. The authors also demonstrated that the schizophrenic children with loose associations had different discourse deficits and discourse/IQ correlates than schizophrenic children without loose associations. The schizophrenic children receiving neuroleptic medication had lower loose associations scores than the

Reprinted with permission from *Journal of the American Academy of Child and Adolescent Psychiatry*, 1992, Vol. 31(1), 151–159. Copyright © 1992 by the American Academy of Child and Adolescent Psychiatry.

Presented at the Annual Meeting of the Academy of Child and Adolescent Psychiatry, Chicago, 1990.

This study was supported by National Institute of Mental Health Grant KO1-MH00538, MH-30897, and MH16381 from the National Institute of Mental Health and by the UCLA Women's Hospital Auxiliary. We thank Barbara Fish, Susan Curtiss, and Peter Tanguay for their comments on earlier versions of this paper as well as Amy Mo and Andrew Degas for their technical assistance.

unmedicated subjects. The authors discuss the possible confounding effect of medication and loose associations, as well as the developmental, cognitive, and clinical implications of the study's findings.

The speech of schizophrenic patients has been regarded as a hallmark of schizophrenia since Kraepelin first described dementia precox (Kraepelin, 1896). Formal thought disorder involves a number of clinical signs that describe the form or manner in which the schizophrenic patient presents his or her thoughts to the listener. These include the signs of formal thought disorder in the *DSM-III-R*, loose associations and incoherence, as well as those signs that have been used traditionally to describe formal thought disorder, such as derailment, digressive speech, tangentiality, circumstantiality, echolalia, and perseveration (Andreasen, 1979).

Rochester and Martin (1979) investigated the difficulty professionals and laymen encounter when following the speech of schizophrenics. They examined if this difficulty could be explained by the patient's impaired use of linguistic devices that tie the spoken text together. They presented two hypotheses. First, schizophrenic adults would either underutilize or overutilize cohesive devices. Second, schizophrenic speakers would make implicit reference to people, objects, and events on the erroneous assumption that the listener already had sufficient information to follow the train of thought.

Using Halliday and Hassan's (1976) analysis of cohesion, Rochester and Martin (1979) found that schizophrenic adults with formal thought disorder linked their sentences (clauses) primarily through repetition of the same word, word root, or related words, such as synonyms, antonyms, or superordinates (lexical cohesion) (see Table 1). When this lexical cohesion is used in excess, the connections between the speaker's ideas could appear to be tenuous and idiosyncratic because their link is primarily semantic and not ideational. Rochester and Martin (1979) also reported that thought-disordered schizophrenics used less pronouns, demonstratives, definite articles, and comparatives than normal subjects to refer to people, objects, or events (referential cohesion). These patients also frequently referred to themselves and the immediate environment (situation exophora). Under these circumstances, listeners have difficulty in piecing together what the speaker is saying. In terms of the nonthought-disordered adult patients, Rochester and Martin (1979) found that their speech was less discursive. These patients spoke less and used fewer cohesive links compared with nonthought-disordered and normal subjects.

Harvey (1983) also demonstrated that thought-disordered schizophrenic adults used lexical cohesion as their predominant cohesion pattern. They also provided the listener with little linguistic information by using less pronouns, articles, demonstratives, and comparatives during their conversation. When they used

TABLE 1

Cohesion Categories, Reference, Patterns, and Examples[a]

Category	Type	Examples[b]
Referential cohesion	Pronominal	A boy called Peter saw a ghost. He was scared.
	Demonstrative	The boy was crying and then this boy called his mother.
	Comparative	I don't like this story. I like the first one more.
Conjunction	Additive	The witch gets burned and that's the end of the story.
	Adversative	I don't know how, but he makes me be bad, bad.
	Causal	I have nightmares because I start to laugh.
	Temporal	I'll go play when I'm done eating.
	Continuative	I: Do you have scary dreams? S: Well, last night I saw this big monster in my closet.
Lexical cohesion	Same root	The kids were bad. Tim was bad, too.
	Synonym	The kids were mean to Tim. They were always nasty to him.
	Superordinate	I don't mind spaniels. But really, I don't like dogs.
Substitution	Nominal	I: Why did you say that was a true story? S: 'Cause it's a made up one.
	Verbal	That boy says "Hi," and so does the other one.
	Clausal	That's the only thing magic does. I know it's so.
Ellipsis	Nominal	He was mean, John also.
	Verbal	I: Do you think a child could have a dream like this about a ghost? S: Maybe he could.
	Clausal	I: Did you like telling stories? S: No, I don't.
Reference patterns	Unclear	Uh, I went and looked at the guy to see what they were doing.
	Ambiguous	And —and —and so when Halloween came her Dad made a hat and then her mother made a witch costume and she was happy.
	Exophora	I: Did you like that story? S: How does this tape recorder work? (Situational) This is a story about a witch. One upon a time there was an old ugly witch. I don't like witches to come to my house (Self).

[a] Adapted from Halliday and Hassan (1976), Rochester and Martin (1979), and Harvey (1983).
[b] Referant and referring/presumed item.

these linguistic devices to refer to people and events, thought-disordered schizo-phrenics had not previously identified the referents for the listener (unclear refer-ence), and they referred to more than one possible referent (ambiguous reference) (Table 1). In addition, Harvey and Brault (1986) found a significant association between unclear reference and ambiguous reference and Andreasen's (1979) pos-itive (derailment, incoherence, and tangentiality) and negative signs of formal thought disorder (poverty of content of speech).

In contrast to the extensive literature on schizophrenic adults, few studies have been conducted on the clinical assessment of formal thought disorder (Arboleda and Holzman, 1985; Caplan et al., 1989) or the discourse deficits (Foy and Caplan, 1988; Leaper and Emmory, 1985) of schizophrenic children. There are also no reports on the relationship between formal thought disorder and discourse deficits in schizophrenic children.

Using the Kiddie Formal Thought Disorder Rating Scale (K-FTDS), Caplan demonstrated that two of the four *DSM-III* formal thought disorder signs, loose associations and illogical thinking, were reliable and valid measures of childhood onset schizophrenia (Caplan et al., 1989, 1990a). The two remaining *DSM-III* signs, incoherence and poverty of content of speech, however, occurred infre-quently in schizophrenic children and were, therefore, not reliable measures. She also found that the absence of loose associations correctly classified 97% of the normal children, and its presence correctly identified only 71% of the schizo-phrenic children (Caplan et al., 1989, 1990a). As defined in the K-FTDS (Caplan et al., 1989), a child with loose associations unpredictably changes the topic of conversation to an unrelated topic. Applying Rochester and Martin's (1979) find-ings to schizophrenic children, Caplan postulated that this clinical measure would reflect the schizophrenic child's difficulty in adequately using linguistic devices to tie his or her clauses together (Caplan et al., 1990a).

Regarding discourse studies of schizophrenic children, a pilot study demon-strated that, like schizophrenic adults, 15 schizophrenic children employed signif-icantly less referential cohesion to established antecedents than a group of normal, mental age matched children (Foy and Caplan, 1988). Unlike their adult counter-parts, this small group of schizophrenic children did not differ from the normal group in their use of lexical cohesion, unclear reference, or ambiguous reference. They did, however, use fewer conjunctions to link contiguous clauses (sentences) than the normal children. Leaper and Emmory (1985) described two schizo-phrenic children who presented with the discourse deficits described by Rochester and Martin (1979) and Harvey (1983) in schizophrenic adults. The findings of these studies are, however, inconclusive because of their small sample size.

Using a representative sample size, Harvey et al. (1982) found that children of parents with schizophrenia, like schizophrenic adults, used fewer words and cohe-sive ties, but they used more lexical cohesion, unclear reference, and ambiguous reference than children of parents with no psychiatric disturbance. Because of the wide range of diagnoses encountered in children at risk for schizophrenia, one cannot conclude from this study that schizophrenic children and adults have similar discourse deficits.

The goal of the study presented here was to determine the discourse deficits of a representative sample of schizophrenic children and the relationship of these deficits to loose associations and illogical thinking. It was predicted that schizophrenic children would have some discourse deficits in common with schizophrenic adults as well as deficits peculiar to childhood onset schizophrenia. The authors expected the latter findings to reflect developmental factors. Based on Rochester and Martin's (1979) and Harvey's (1983) studies, the authors also predicted that schizophrenic children with and without loose associations would have different discourse patterns. No association was anticipated between illogical thinking and these linguistic devices because illogical thinking is primarily related to deficits in the development of reasoning skills, as measured by conservation (Caplan et al., 1990b).

METHOD

Subjects

As shown in Table 2, this study was conducted on 31 (25 boys and 6 girls) schizophrenic subjects, with a mean chronological age of 10.2 years (SD = 1.5) and mental age of 9.1 years (SD = 2.0). Each schizophrenic child was matched by sex and mental age with a normal child. The 31 normal subjects were younger children whose chronological ages were matched to the mental age of the individual patients (Table 2). The IQ differences between the patient ($\overline{X}_{FULLSCALE\ IQ}$ = 91, SD = 15.7) and normal groups ($\overline{X}_{FULLSCALE\ IQ}$ = 112, SD = 13.8) are addressed in the data analysis section of this paper.

The schizophrenic subjects were recruited from the University of California-Los Angeles (UCLA) Neuropsychiatric Institute's Inpatient and Outpatient Child Services as well as from two Los Angeles schools for emotionally disturbed children. The majority of the schizophrenic subjects were Anglo-Americans (67%), 4% were bilingual Asians, 18% were bilingual Hispanics, and 11% were Afro-Americans. At the time of testing, 62% of the schizophrenic children were inpatients and 52% were receiving neuroleptic medication. The remaining schizophrenic children had not received neuroleptics or other psychoactive medications for at least 2 weeks before their participation in the study.

The patients were diagnosed independent of the research team by the Diagnostic Unit of UCLA's Childhood Psychoses Clinical Research Center with the Interview for Childhood Disorders and Schizophrenia by a research team blind

TABLE 2

Age, IQ, Formal Thought Disorder Scores, and Medication Status of Schizophrenic and Normal Children

Mean Values	Schizophrenic			Normal
	LA[a] >0	LA[c] = 0	Total	
N	20	11	31	31
Mental age	8.7	10.3	9.3	9.1
	SD = 1.9	SD = 1.99	SD = 2.00	SD = 2.10
Chronological age	9.9	10.7	10.3	9.1
	SD = 1.6	SD = 1.4	SD = 1.51	SD = 2.10
Full-scale IQ (WISC-R)	87	96	91	112
	SD = 11.25	SD = 12.73	SD = 12.4	SD = 13.8
Verbal IQ	84	97	89	108
	SD = 15.4	SD = 12.95	SD = 15.7	SD = 24.4
Performance IQ	93	96	94	111
	SD = 16.74	SD = 15.37	SD = 16.10	SD = 15.3
Illogical thinking	0.29	0.40	0.33	0.14[b]
	SD = 0.24	SD = 0.36	SD = 0.29	SD = 0.18
Loose associations	0.21	0.00	0.13	0.00[c]
	SD = 0.17	SD = 0.00	SD = 0.17	SD = 0.00
Medication status				
On	8	9	17	NA
Off	12	2	14	NA

[a] LA = loose associations.

[b] Two-way ANOVA (Diagnosis, Age) between all schizophrenic and normal children significant at 0.001 level.

[c] Chi-square analysis ($\chi^2 = 26.95$, $df = 1$, $p < .0001$) between all schizophrenic and normal children was done on the incidence of scores above zero because of the zero variance of LA in the normal subjects.

to the discourse and formal thought disorder scores of each subject. The chance corrected interrater agreement on diagnosis with the Interview for Childhood Disorders and Schizophrenia was 0.89 (Russell et al., 1989). In addition to questions from the Schedule for Affective Disorders and Schizophrenia for School-Age Children (Puig-Antich and Chambers, 1978) and the Diagnostic Interview Schedule for Children (Herjanic and Campbell, 1977), this interview includes questions that ensure an adequate assessment of schizophrenia and schizotypal personality disorder. Children who did not meet *DSM-III* criteria for schizophrenia were excluded from the study.

The normal subjects were recruited from four Los Angeles schools and from the community via newspaper advertisements. Like the patients (83%), most of the normal children were from middle-class families (81%). Unlike the patient sample, fewer of the normal children were Anglo-Americans (41%), and more were bilingual Asians (34%) and bilingual Hispanics (25%).

Children with a history of a neurological, language, or hearing disorder were excluded from the patient and normal samples. The normal children were also screened for psychiatric disorders by phone conversation with their parents. If a child manifested psychiatric symptoms either at the time of the study or in the past, he or she was not included in the study. Parents and children were advised on the study's procedures to obtain their informed consent.

Procedures

Speech samples were elicited from the children with the Kiddie Formal Thought Disorder Story Game (Caplan et al., 1989). To eliminate variability, videotapes of the 20- to 25-minute-long Story Game were rated for formal thought disorder and transcribed for coding cohesion and reference patterns.

The Kiddie Formal Thought Disorder Story Game. Caplan's standardized Story Game, modelled after Gardner's (1971) clinical instrument, yields speech samples that provide reliable and valid ratings of formal thought disorder in children (Caplan et al., 1989, 1990a). It was administered by a trained clinician. The child listened to two audiotaped stories, one about a ghost, the other about an ostracized boy, respectively. After each story, the child retold the tale and answered open-ended standardized questions about the story. The child also made up a story chosen from several topics: the Incredible Hulk, a witch, an unhappy child, or a good or bad child.

The Kiddie Formal Thought Disorder Rating Scale. Detailed guidelines for rating the four K-FTDS signs (Caplan et al., 1989) can be obtained from the senior author. Table 3 presents a synopsis of the definitions of the four K-FTDS signs with examples.

According to the K-FTDS, the unit of speech, the clause, is defined as a noun

TABLE 3

Synopsis of the Kiddie Formal Thought Disorder Rating Scale

Kiddie Formal Thought Disorder Rating Scale	Definition	Example
Illogical thinking	Inappropriate and immature use of causal utterances.	"I left my hat in her room because her name is Mary."
	Unfounded and inappropriate reasoning in noncausal utterances.	Sometimes I'll go to bed and when I'm done laughing, I start wheezing and that's when I relax."
	Utterances in which statements are simultaneously made and refuted.	"I don't like that story, but I liked it as a story."
Loose associations	The child changes the topic of conversation to a new unrelated topic without preparing the listener for the topic change.	Interviewer: "Why do you think that's a reason not to like Tim?" Child: "And I call my mom sweetie."
Incoherence	The contents of an utterance are not understood by the listener because of scrambled syntax.	Interviewer: "What happened next in your story?" Child: "The day witches no day goes."
Poverty of content of speech	In the presence of at least two utterances, the child does not elaborate on the topic.	"I suppose—What? Maybe—Well yes, I see. I suppose that's all."

phrase and a verbal phrase followed by a pause (Rochester et al., 1977). To be rated as having illogical thinking, the child's speech must meet one of three criteria. First, the child uses causal clauses inappropriately. Second, the child presents the listener with unfounded and inappropriate reasoning in noncausal clauses. Third, the child contradicts him or herself within one to two clauses by simultaneously making and refuting statements. Loose associations are rated when the child says something that is off topic without having previously prepared the listener for the topic change. A clause is rated as incoherent if the rater cannot comprehend its contents because of scrambled syntax. Poverty of content of speech is rated if, in the presence of at least two clauses, the child does not elaborate on the topic of conversation.

Videotapes of the Story Game were independently rated with the K-FTDS by two trained raters who had no previous knowledge of the individual child's diagnosis. The scores derived from the K-FTDS ratings were frequency counts of the scale's four signs—illogical thinking, loose associations, incoherence, and poverty of content of speech—divided by the number of clauses made by the child.

The chance corrected κ reliability statistic (Fleiss, 1973) was calculated for the K-FTDS scores of a subsample of 17 schizophrenic, four schizotypal, and 10 normal children (Caplan et al., 1989). Incoherence and poverty of content of speech occurred in only two children in the sample studied. Interrater reliability was, therefore, computed only for illogical thinking ($\kappa = 0.78$, SE $= 0.03$) and loose associations ($\kappa = 0.66$, SE $= 0.01$).

Cohesion and Reference Patterns. The cohesion coding guidelines, adapted from Halliday and Hassan (1976), Rochester and Martin (1979), and Harvey (1983) are summarized below. Examples of these measures are presented in Table 1.

Cohesion refers to the linguistic devices that tie together the ideas expressed by the speaker. The unit of speech for the cohesion ratings, the clause, contains at least an implicit or explicit noun phrase and a verb phrase followed by a pause (Rochester et al., 1977). The following types of cohesion were coded: referential cohesion, conjunction, lexical cohesion, ellipsis, and substitution.

Referential cohesion involves use of a pronoun, demonstrative, definite article, or comparative to refer back to people or objects in the preceding spoken text. *Conjunction* ties together contiguous clauses by using additive, contrastive, causal, temporal, and continuative relationships. *Lexical cohesion* entails repetition by using the same word, another word derived from the same root, a synonym, or a superordinate. *Substitution* ties the spoken text together by replacing nominal, verbal, and clausal units with a word or group of words. *Ellipsis* deletes a word, phrase, or clause whose referent is unambiguously located in the previous utterance.

Three *reference patterns* that are known to be impaired in schizophrenic adults

(Harvey, 1983; Rochester and Martin, 1979) and in children at risk for schizo-phrenia (Harvey et al., 1982) were also included: *unclear reference*, ambiguous reference, and reference to the nonverbal context (exophora). The speaker makes an unclear reference when he or she refers to a person or object that has not been previously mentioned in the spoken text. The speaker makes an *ambiguous refer-ence* if he or she uses a referent that can apply to more than one person or object. Reference to the nonverbal context or situational *exophora* included self-reference, reference to the interviewer, or to items in the testing room.

Trained undergraduate students with no knowledge of the children's diagnoses transcribed the Story Game videotapes. Two blind raters coded the transcriptions independently to obtain the frequency of cohesion and reference patterns scores during the entire Story Game. The sum of these frequency scores was the total cohesive ties score. To control for the variation in the number of clauses, cohesive ties, and words elicited from each child during the entire Story Game, each cohe-sion and reference pattern frequency score was divided by the total number of clauses, cohesive ties, and words.

The interrater agreement (Pearson correlation coefficient) of the cohesion and reference pattern scores on 10 schizophrenic and 10 normal children was 0.94 for referential cohesion, 0.99 for conjunction, 0.89 for lexical cohesion, 0.70 for ellipsis, 0.67 for substitution, 0.72 for exophora, and 0.92 for unclear or ambig-uous reference. The ratings of ambiguous and unclear reference were combined because of their low base rate.

Cognitive Testing

A psychometrist, who knew the child's diagnosis, administered the Wechsler Intelligence Test for Children-Revised (WISC-R) (Wechsler, 1976) to all children.

Data Analysis

The cohesion and reference pattern scores, expressed as rate of occurrence per clause and per word, constituted the outcome variables. The mental age matched subject pairs comprised the experimental units for analysis. Because of possible IQ differences between members of the pairs, full-scale IQ was used as a covariate. This analysis was conducted after parallel linear relationships were con-firmed between the dependent variables and full-scale IQ across the subject groups. Three sets of analyses were conducted. Mental age group (age 5.6–9.6 years, age 9.7–12.6 years) was an interpair factor, and diagnosis (schizophrenia versus normal) was an intrapair factor in the three sets. The presence of loose associations, illogical thinking, and neuroleptic medication in the schizophrenic member of the pair formed a crossed interpair factor in the first, second, and third set of analyses, respectively. The authors were unable to include both formal thought disorder measures and medication status in the same analyses because the further crossing of factors reduced the sample size. Because there were bilingual Asian and Hispanic children in the normal group, a descriptive analysis to rule out any effect of ethnicity was used.

The effects of loose associations, illogical thinking, and neuroleptics were examined separately using a three-way analysis of covariance (ANCOVA) on the pairs of schizophrenic and normal children, separate two-way ANCOVAs on the subgroups of patients with and without these variables and their paired normal matches, and a one-way ANCOVA on the schizophrenic children with and without these variables. Global associations were computed among cohesion and reference pattern rates, verbal productivity (i.e., the number of words used by each child), formal thought disorder rates, and IQ scores using Pearson correlations. Using *t*-tests, the authors also examined the effects of the child's neuroleptic status on the formal thought disorder and IQ measures.

RESULTS

Diagnostic Differences (Table 4, See All Patients Column)

With medication status excluded from the analysis of covariance, the schizophrenic children used significantly fewer cohesive ties, referential cohesion, conjunction, and lexical cohesion per clause than their yoked normal matches. There was no significant interaction between diagnosis, full-scale IQ, and mental age. ANCOVA of the per word measures demonstrated that the lower verbal productivity of the schizophrenic children did not account for their lower referential cohesion and conjunction scores. This analysis highlighted that, after adjusting for verbal productivity, the schizophrenic children used more ellipsis and exophora than their paired mental age matches.

Within the schizophrenic group, however, the children who spoke less (i.e., lower mean number of words) had significantly lower referential cohesion ($r = 0.53$, $p < 0.002$), conjunction ($r = 0.50$, $p < 0.003$), lexical cohesion ($r = 0.41$, $p < 0.02$), unclear or ambiguous reference ($r = 0.54$, $p < 0.001$), and exophora ($r = 0.41$, $p < 0.02$), but more ellipsis per word ($r = -0.49$, $p < 0.004$). Similar relationships in the normal group were found for conjunction, unclear or ambiguous reference, exophora, and ellipsis but not for referential and lexical cohesion.

The effects of ethnic heterogeneity on the cohesion and reference score differences between the schizophrenic and normal children were examined. A similar distribution of scores in the Anglo-American, Afro-American, bilingual Asian, and bilingual Hispanic children was found.

TABLE 4

Differences in Mean Discourse Rates of Schizophrenic and Normal Children

Discourse Measures	All Patients[a]	Loose Associations			Neuroleptics	
		Total[b]	Yes[c]	No[c]	Yes[c]	No[c]
N	31	31	20	11	17	14
Words						
Per clause	6.83**	NS	NS	5.97**	7.64**	NS
All cohesive ties						
Per clause	7.41**	NS	6.71**	5.89*	9.06***	4.54*
Referential cohesion						
Per clause	8.85****	NS	6.80*	NS	10.56**	NS
Per word	5.73**	NS	12.85***	NS	6.87**	NS
Conjunction						
Per clause	10.26***	NS	4.05*	8.88**	11.82***	4.40*
Per word	6.76**	NS	NS	7.64**	12.58***	NS
Lexical cohesion						
Per clause	4.20*	6.69**	3.99*	NS	NS	NS
Per word	NS	8.33***	NS	NS	NS	NS
Exophora						
Per clause	NS	NS	NS	NS	NS	NS
Per word	5.87**	NS	4.80**	NS	8.57**	NS
Ellipsis						
Per clause	NS	NS	NS	NS	3.13*	5.01**
Per word	5.87**	NS	4.80**	NS	8.57**	NS
Unclear or ambiguous						
Per clause	NS	5.09**	NS	NS	NS	7.18**
Per word	NS	10.63****	NS	NS	NS	NS
Substitution						
Per clause	NS	NS	NS	NS	NS	8.82**
Per word	NS	NS	NS	NS	NS	4.58*

[a] Two-way ANCOVA (Diagnosis, Mental Age) between schizophrenic and normal pairs ($df = 1, 27$).
[b] Three-way ANCOVA (Diagnosis, Mental Age, Loose Associations or Neuroleptic Status) between schizophrenic and normal pairs ($df = 1, 26$).
[c] Two-way ANCOVA (Diagnosis, Mental Age) for schizophrenic patients subclassified by loose associations and medication status and their yoked normal matches.
* $p < 0.01$, ** $p < 0.001$, *** $p < 0.0001$

Relationship between Discourse and K-FTDS Measures

Separate two-way ANCOVAs comparing the rates per clause and per word of the patients with and without loose associations to their normal matches revealed the following findings (Table 4, see Loose Associations column). First, the patients with loose associations used less referential cohesion and more exophora than their normal matches. Second, the patients without loose associations used fewer words and conjunctions than the normal children. Third, within the schizophrenic group, the children with loose associations used significantly more lexical cohesion, ellipsis, and unclear or ambiguous reference than those without loose associations.

A similar analysis on the dichotomized illogical thinking measures using the 0.1 cutoff, described by Caplan et al. (1989), revealed no significant differences in discourse patterns.

Developmental Factors

A two-way ANCOVA (Diagnosis, Mental Age) with three rather than two age groups (4.4–6.9 years, 7–9.6 years, and 9.7–13 years) revealed that the schizophrenic and normal subjects with a mental age below 7 years used fewer words, $F(2, 28) = 6.04$, $p < 0.006$, cohesive ties, $F(2, 28) = 3.30$, $p < 0.04$, referential cohesion, $F(2, 28) = 3.37$, $p < 0.04$, and conjunctions, $F(2, 28) = 5.03$, $p < 0.01$, per clause than the older schizophrenic and normal subjects.

Cognitive Factors

Although the schizophrenic children with and without loose associations had similar mean full-scale, verbal, and performance IQ values (Table 2), these two subgroups demonstrated different relationships with IQ measures (Table 5). Lexical cohesion correlated negatively with full-scale IQ and performance IQ scores but not with verbal IQ scores in the patients with loose associations. In the schizophrenic children with no loose associations, however, verbal IQ correlated positively with the lexical cohesion, cohesive ties, conjunction, and exophora scores.

Neuroleptic Factors (Table 4, See Neuroleptics Column)

A two-way ANCOVA revealed that the patients receiving neuroleptic medication used significantly fewer words, referential cohesion and conjunction but more exophora and ellipsis than their paired normal matches. The unmedicated patients,

TABLE 5
Correlation between Discourse Rates and IQ[a] Scores in Schizophrenic Children

| | Loose Associations | | | | | |
| | Yes | | | No | | |
Discourse Rate[b]	FSIQ	VIQ	PIQ	FSIQ	VIQ	PIQ
Lexical cohesion	-0.66***	-0.41	-0.46*	0.66*	0.80***	0.22
Cohesive ties	-0.40	-0.24	-0.40	0.55	0.73*	0.03
Conjunction	-0.18	-0.07	-0.30	0.60	0.71**	-0.07
Exophora	-0.32	-0.23	-0.19	0.71**	0.80***	0.36

[a] FSIQ = full-scale IQ, VIQ = verbal IQ, PIQ = performance IQ.
[b] Per clause.
*$p < 0.05$, ** $p < 0.01$, *** $p < 0.001$.

however, differed from their normal matches only in the total number of cohesive ties, ellipsis, unclear or ambiguous reference, and substitutions.

A within group one-way ANCOVA demonstrated that the medicated patients had significantly lower rates per clause of words, $F(1, 28) = 8.78$, $p < 0.006$, cohesive ties, $F(1, 28) = 6.52$, $p < 0.01$, referential cohesion, $F(1, 28) = 4.58$, $p < 0.04$, conjunction, $F(1, 28) = 10.81$, $p < 0.002$, and unclear or ambiguous reference, $F(1, 28) = 4.84$, $p < 0.03$, but higher ellipsis rates than the unmedicated patients. The analyses on the rates per word demonstrated significantly fewer conjunctions, but more ellipsis in the unmedicated patients.

Regarding the relationship between medication status and formal thought disorder scores, approximately half the medicated subjects had loose associations (8 of 17), and half had no loose associations (9 of 17). Most of the unmedicated patients (12 of 14), however, had loose associations. Although the schizophrenic children receiving medication tended to have lower loose association scores than the unmedicated children, this difference did not prove to be significant, $t(29) = 1.5$, $p < 0.2$. There were also no significant differences in the illogical thinking and IQ scores of the medicated and unmedicated subjects.

DISCUSSION

The study's findings suggest that, among schizophrenic children, some discourse deficits are similar to those of schizophrenic adults (Harvey, 1983; Rochester and Martin, 1979). Like schizophrenic adults, schizophrenic children speak less than normal mental age matched subjects, and their speech does not provide the listener with enough links (cohesive ties) to previous utterances or with enough reference (referential cohesion) to people, objects, or events mentioned in earlier utterances. Schizophrenic children also break the flow of speech to refer to people, objects, or events in their immediate surroundings. Like thought-disordered schizophrenic adults (Harvey, 1983; Harvey and Brault, 1986; Rochester and Martin, 1979), schizophrenic children with loose associations confuse the listener by the unclear and ambiguous way they refer to people, objects, and events in their speech. Schizophrenic children with loose associations also prefer to link their clauses with repetition of the same words or word root, synonyms, antonyms, or superordinates. These discourse similarities provide evidence for the comparability of adult and childhood onset schizophrenia and support the findings of recent clinical (Cantor et al., 1982; Green et al., 1984; Russell et al., 1989) and information processing studies (Asarnow and Sherman, 1984).

In comparison to schizophrenic adults (Harvey, 1983; Rochester et al., 1979), schizophrenic children have three discourse deficits that distinguish their speech from the adult patients. They provide the listener with fewer connectives between contiguous clauses (conjunction) and with less repetition of words or word roots (lexical cohesion) than normal children. Finally, they also delete or omit part of a previous clause on the presumption that the listener retains enough information from this clause (ellipsis). By using fewer conjunctions, less lexical cohesion, and more ellipsis than normal children, the conversing schizophrenic child makes it difficult for the listener to piece together the links in his or her speech.

The normal child's ability to linguistically and conceptually process the connections between his or her clauses through conjunctions matures between early childhood and the end of middle childhood (Amidon, 1976; French and Nelson, 1985; Johnson and Chapman, 1980). Normal children also become competent users of lexical cohesion during middle childhood once they are conceptually able to construct semantic hierarchies and to connect their ideas by reiteration or use of synonyms, antonyms, superordinates, or general terms (Gregg, 1986; Karmiloff-Smith, 1985). The conjunction and lexical cohesion deficits of schizophrenic children could, therefore, represent developmental delays.

In support of this hypothesis, children at risk for schizophrenia tend to communicate more like schizophrenic adults than schizophrenic children (Harvey et al., 1982). They use more, not less, lexical cohesion, and they use the same amount of conjunction as normal children. The onset of schizophrenia during middle childhood could, therefore, impair or retard the acquisition of these linguistic skills. A prospective study of children with middle childhood onset of schizophrenia would allow us to determine if they outgrow these earlier deficits and become more similar to schizophrenic adults.

To use ellipsis, one needs to be aware of the grammatical constraints that determine what parts of the clause can be deleted (Table 1). The elevated rates of occurrence of ellipsis in schizophrenic children suggests that, like schizophrenic adults (Grove and Andreasen, 1985), the children are aware of these grammatical constraints. Like schizophrenic children, learning disabled subjects (Gregg, 1985), children with low reading scores (Norris and Bruning, 1988), adults with head injuries (Mentis and Prutting, 1987), and adults with Alzheimer's disease (Ripich and Terrell, 1988) have high rates of ellipsis. Mentis and Prutting (1987) have hypothesized that by using ellipsis, speakers with head injuries decrease the stress involved in retrieving information from a previous clause. If this hypothesis is applicable to schizophrenic children, it is possible that they use more ellipsis than normal children because they have difficulty retrieving the speaker's or their own previous clauses.

This hypothesized difficulty in retrieval could reflect impaired attention or information processing. The authors recently demonstrated that schizophrenic children with loose associations have low WISC-R distractibility factor scores (Caplan et al., 1990c). The present finding that children with loose associations have more ellipsis than their normal yoked matches suggests that overutilization of ellipsis could also be associated with impaired attention. The authors are currently investigating if the hypothesized difficulty in retrieving linguistic information from previous clauses is associated with impaired attention or information processing in schizophrenic children.

Do schizophrenic children have discourse deficits because they talk less? The study demonstrated significant differences between the schizophrenic and normal children for the discourse rates per clause as well as per word. This suggests that the schizophrenic children's discourse deficits were independent of the number of words they used. Grove and Andreasen (1985) have suggested that schizophrenic adults have difficulty generating speech and that this difficulty is related to negative symptoms of schizophrenia. Within the schizophrenic group, the children without loose associations used significantly less words than their yoked normal matches. Rochester and Martin (1979) also reported that schizophrenic adults without formal thought disorder spoke less than those with formal disorder.

Because loose associations are a positive symptom of schizophrenia (Andreasen, 1979), the poor verbal productivity of the children without loose associations could be similar to the impoverished speech of adult schizophrenics with negative symptoms. In addition, the discrete discourse deficits of the children with loose associations and the lack of an association between these deficits and verbal IQ scores suggest that this subgroup of schizophrenic children might resemble adult schizophrenics with positive symptoms (Crow, 1980).

One additional factor could have influenced the discourse findings: neuroleptic medication. To the best of the authors' knowledge, there have been no drug studies on the effects of neuroleptics on the discourse characteristics of schizophrenic subjects. From their extensive review of the studies on the cognitive effects of neuroleptics in schizophrenic adults, Spohn and Strauss (1989) concluded that these drugs reduce disordered thinking, attention or information processing dysfunction, and bizarre verbalizations. There have been no comparable studies in schizophrenic children. In aggressive, nonschizophrenic children, haloperidol reduces reaction time and performance on the Porteus Maze test (Platt et al., 1984). In low doses, it has no adverse effects on discriminant learning in autistic children (Anderson and Campbell, 1989). Acute doses of thiothixene, trifluoperidol, and trifluoperazine have been associated with increased verbal productivity in autistic children (Fish et al., 1972). In high doses, haloperidol might impair cognitive skills, such as short-term memory in retarded children (Aman, 1984).

Although retrospective, the medication findings suggest that neuroleptics could have two contrasting effects on the communication skills of schizophrenic children. On the one hand, as reported in schizophrenic adults (Spohn et al., 1986), they might decrease some psychotic aspects of the schizophrenic child's speech. On the other hand, they also might impinge on nonpsychotic aspects of speech, such as the patient's ability to enrich his or her speech through verbal productivity and cohesive devices. The trend for lower loose associations scores in the medicated schizophrenic children and the high unclear or ambiguous reference rates in the unmedicated patients could support the study's first hypothesis. In support of the second hypothesis, neuroleptics appear to increase the differences between the schizophrenic and normal children for cohesion and reference pattern measures other than unclear or ambiguous reference and substitution. The possible confounding influence of the presence of loose associations in most of the unmedicated schizophrenic children, however, underscores the importance of a prospective drug study on a representative sample of schizophrenic children with and without loose associations.

From the clinical perspective, by examining the relationship between sensitive and specific clinical ratings of formal thought disorder, discourse deficits, and IQ measures, we have begun to delineate two clinical subgroups of childhood onset schizophrenia: with and without loose associations. These two subgroups might represent the childhood version of the positive and negative subgroupings described in schizophrenic adults. The study's findings also highlight the clinical importance of examining the potential therapeutic and adverse effects of neuroleptic medication on the speech characteristics and thought processes of schizophrenic children. Finally, the clinical specificity of these findings for childhood onset schizophrenia should be examined by comparing the communicative deficits of schizophrenic children with those of children with bipolar and unipolar disorders.

REFERENCES

Aman, M. G. (1984), Drugs and learning in mentally retarded persons. In: *Advanced Human Psychopharmacology.*, Vol. 3, eds. G. D. Burrows & J. S. Werry. Greenwich, CN: JAI Press, pp. 121–163.

Amidon, A. (1976), Children's understanding of sentences with contingent relations: why are temporal and conditional connectives so difficult? *J. Exp. Child Psychol.*, 22:423–437.

Anderson, L. T. & Campbell, M. (1989), The effect of haloperidol on discriminant learning and behavioral symptoms in autistic children. *J. Autism Dev. Disord.*, 19:227–239.

Andreasen, N. C. (1979), Thought, language, and communication disorders. I. Clinical assessment, definition of terms, and evaluation of their reliability. *Arch. Gen. Psychiatry*, 36:1315–1323.

Arboleda, C. & Holzman, P. S. (1985), Thought disorder in children at risk for psychosis. *Arch. Gen. Psychiatry*, 42:1004–1013.

Asarnow, R. F. & Sherman, T. (1984), Studies of visual information processing in schizophrenic children. *Child Dev.,* 55:249–261.

Cantor, S., Evans, J., Pearce, J. & Pezzot-Pearce, T. (1982), Childhood schizophrenia: present but not accounted for. *Am. J. Psychiatry,* 139:758–763.

Caplan, R., Guthrie, D., Fish, B., Tanguay, P. E. & David-Lando, G. (1989), The Kiddie Formal Thought Disorder Rating Scale (K-FTDS). Clinical assessment, reliability, and validity. *J. Am. Acad. Child Adolesc. Psychiatry,* 28:208–216.

————Perdue, S., Tanguay, P. E. & Fish, B. (1990a), Formal thought disorder in childhood onset schizophrenia and schizotypal personality disorder. *J. Child. Psychol. Psychiatry,* 31:1103–1114.

————Foy, J. G., Sigman, M. & Perdue, S. (1990b), Conservation and formal thought disorder in schizophrenic and schizotypal children. *Developmental Psychopathology,* 2:183–190.

————Asarnow, R. F. & Sherman, T. L. (1990c), Cognition and formal thought disorder in schizophrenic and schizotypal children. *J. Psychiatr. Res.,* 31:169–177.

Crow, T. J. (1980), Molecular pathology of schizophrenia: More than one disease process. *Br. Med. J. [Clin. Res.],* 280:1–9.

Fish, B., Campbell, M., Shapiro, T. & Floyd, A. (1972), Comparison of trifluperidol, trifluperazine and chlorpromazine in preschool schizophrenic children: the value of less sedative antipsychotic agents. *Current Therapeutic Research,* 14:759–766.

Fleiss, J. (1973), *Statistical Methods for Rates and Proportions.* New York: John Wiley and Sons.

Foy, J. G. & Caplan, R. (1988), Pragmatic language skills in children with schizophrenia. *Soc. Neurosc. Abstr.:* 1171.

French, L. A. & Nelson, K. (1985), Young children's knowledge of relational terms. Some ifs, ors, and buts. In: *Springer Series in Language and Communication* New York: Springer-Verlag.

Gardner, R. A. (1971), *Therapeutic Communication with Children. The Mutual Storytelling Technique.* New York: Science House, Inc.

Green, W. H., Campbell, M., Hardesty, A. S., Grega, D. M., Padron-Gayol, M., Shell, J. & Erlenmeyer-Kimling, L. (1984), A comparison of schizophrenic and autistic children. *J. Am. Acad. Child Psychiatry,* 4:399–409.

Gregg, N. (1985), Cohesion: inter and intra sentence errors. *J. Learn. Disabil.,* 19:338–341.

————(1986), College learning disabled, normal, and basic writers. A comparison of frequency and accuracy of cohesive ties. *Journal of Psychoeducational Assessment,* 3:223–231.

Grove, W. M. & Andreasen, N. C. (1985), Language and thinking in psychosis. Is there an input abnormality? *Arch. Gen. Psychiatry,* 42:26–32.

Halliday, M. A. K. & Hassan, R. (1976), *Cohesion in Spoken and Written English.* London: Longmans.

Harvey, P. D. (1983), Speech competence in manic and schizophrenic psychoses: the association between clinically rated thought disorder and performance. *J. Abnorm. Psychol.,* 92:368–377.

———Brault, J. (1986), Speech performance in mania and schizophrenia: the association of positive and negative thought disorders and reference failure. *J. Commun. Disord.,* 19:161–174.

———Weintraub, S. & Neale, J. M. (1982), Speech competence of children vulnerable to psychopathology. *J. Abnorm. Child Psychol.,* 10:373–388.

Herjanic, B. & Campbell, W. (1977), Differentiating psychiatrically disturbed children on the basis of a structured interview. *J. Abnorm. Child Psychol.,* 5:127–134.

Johnson, H. L. & Chapman, R. S. (1980), Children's judgment and recall of causal connectives: a developmental study of "because," "so," and "and." *J. Psycholinguist Res.,* 9:243–260.

Karmiloff-Smith, A. (1985), Language and cognitive processes from a developmental perspective. *Lang. Cognit. Processes,* 1:61–85.

Kraepelin, E. (1896), *Psychiatrie. Ein Lehrbuch fur studierende und Arzte.* Leipzig: Barth.

Leaper, C. & Emmory, K. (1985), The discourse of thought disordered schizophrenic children. *Brain Lang.,* 25:72–86.

Mentis, M. & Prutting, C. A. (1987), Cohesion in the discourse of normal and head-injured adults. *J. Speech Hear. Res.,* 30:88–98.

Norris, J. A. & Bruning, R. H. (1988), Cohesion in narratives of good and poor readers. *J. Speech Hear. Disord.,* 53:416–424.

Platt, J. E., Campbell, B., Grega, D. M. & Green, W. H. (1984), Cognitive effects of haloperidol and lithium in aggressive conduct-disorder children. *Psychopharmacol. Bull.,* 20:93–97.

Puig-Antich, J. & Chambers, W. (1978), *The Schedule for Affective Disorders and Schizophrenia for School-Age Children (Kiddie-SADS).* New York: New York State Psychiatric Institute.

Ripich, D. N. & Terrell, B. Y. (1988), Patterns of discourse cohesion and coherence in Alzheimer's disease. *J. Speech Hear. Disord.,* 53:8–15.

Rochester, S. R. & Martin, J. R. (1979), *Crazy Talk: A Study of the Discourse of Schizophrenic Speakers.* New York: Plenum Press.

————————Thurston, S. (1977), Thought process disorder in schizophrenia: the listener's task. *Brain Lang.,* 4:95–114.

Russell, A. R., Bott, L. & Sammons, C. (1989), The phenomenology of schizophrenia occurring in childhood. *J. Am. Acad. Child Adolesc. Psychiatry,* 28:399–407.

Spohn, H. E. & Strauss, M. E. (1989), Relation to neuroleptic and anticholinergic medication. *J. Abnorm. Psychol.,* 98:367–380.

———Lolafaye, C., Larson, J., Mittleman, F., Spray, J. & Hayes, K. (1986), Episodic and residual thought pathology in chronic schizophrenics: effect of neuroleptics. *Schizophr. Bull.,* 12:394–407.

Wechsler, D. (1976), *Manual for the Wechsler Intelligence Scale for Children–Revised.* New York: Psychological Corp.

Part VI

TREATMENT AND PREVENTION

As increasing attention comes to be directed to the problem of health care costs, a review of the effectiveness of psychotherapy with children and adolescents is particularly timely. In the first paper in this section Weisz, Weiss, and Donenberg summarize the results of four recent meta-analyses, involving more than 200 controlled outcome studies that have shown consistent evidence of beneficial therapy effects with children and adolescents. However, as these authors point out, most of the studies included in the meta-analyses involved children, interventions, and treatment conditions that were relatively unrepresentative of conventional clinic practice. In the majority of these controlled experimental studies patients were recruited for treatment, not actually clinic referred; samples were selected for homogeneity with all subjects displaying a similar focal problem, and therapy was primarily directed toward these focal problems. Moreover, therapists were often specifically trained in the techniques to be used, with access to a structured manual, and were monitored regularly to ensure adherence.

In contrast, research focused on the treatment of children and adolescents in clinics has shown few if any significant effects. The authors urge caution in interpreting these findings, as such studies are few in number and have a considerable number of methodological problems. Nevertheless, these results do raise questions as to whether positive research findings can be generalized to clinics, where most therapy occurs. As the authors point out, clinic practice differs from research therapy in important ways. Therapists in clinics often carry a large caseload composed of a heterogeneous group of children and adolescents, many of whom have multiple problems. Their work proceeds without the benefit of recent training in specific techniques or close monitoring of their application. The need to develop ways of applying research therapeutic techniques in actual clinical settings is a point well taken.

The second paper in this section by Erickson, Korfmacher, and Egeland describes work in progress. The authors provide a systematic review of attachment research, dividing the growth of interest in parent-child attachment into three distinct waves of influence. The first of these, initiated by Bowlby, defined many of the underlying normative assumptions upon which attachment theory rests. The second was led by Ainsworth, who developed a method for capturing and studying qualitative differences in attachment relationships across individuals. The third wave, recently under way, is focused on the development of models to explain how the attachment relationship extends its influence across time and across generations. Attachment theorists have proposed that an individual internalizes qualitative aspects of the past primary relationship, and that these internalizations result in expectations that in turn influence and guide one's behavior in future relationships, including parenting one's own child. The authors consider the therapeutic implications of the concepts of internal working models that guide the design of Project STEEP (Steps Toward Effective, Enjoyable Parenting). This preventive intervention with new parents employs strategies aimed at increasing the parent's insight into the connection between past and present relationships and enhancing the parent's understanding of the child's needs and feelings; it also employs the therapeutic alliance to help the parent move toward more positive working models of self and others. Although the evaluation of the effectiveness of Project STEEP is not yet complete, this progress report clearly outlines many of the issues involved in the conversion of therapy to practice.

In the final paper in this section, Geller and colleagues report the results of a random assignment, double-blind, placebo-controlled study of nortriptyline in 50 prepubertal 6- to 12-year-old outpatients who met Research Diagnostic Criteria as well as DSM-III criteria for major depressive disorder. The subjects were severely depressed, with a chronic, unremitting course of long duration. They had a high percentage of family histories of affective disorder, alcoholism, and suicidality. Eighty-four percent of the subjects had comorbid separation anxiety disorder, and 18% were comorbid for antisocial behavior. Nortriptyline was administered at dosages sufficient to maintain a plasma level of 80 ± 20 ng/ml. EKG and blood pressure measures were obtained at regular intervals, and side effects were carefully monitored. The rate of response was poor in both groups (active treatment = 30.8%, placebo = 16.7%), which did not differ significantly. Children who received nortriptyline did not report the anticholinergic side effects frequently experienced by adults receiving tricyclic antidepressants. In a carefully reasoned discussion, the authors address factors that may underlie the previously reported poor response of prepubertal children to tricyclic antidepressants, which the findings of this investigation have now replicated. Possible confounding factors including comorbidity, duration and severity of illness, and family history suggest directions for future studies of therapeutic interventions for major depression in children.

18

The Lab Versus the Clinic: Effects of Child and Adolescent Psychotherapy

John R. Weisz

University of California, Los Angeles

Bahr Weiss

Vanderbilt University, Nashville, Tennessee

Geri R. Donenberg

University of California, Los Angeles

Four recent meta-analyses, involving more than 200 controlled outcome studies, have shown consistent evidence of beneficial therapy effects with children and adolescents. However, most of the studies involved experimental procedures, nonreferred subjects, specially trained therapists with small caseloads, and other features that may not represent conventional clinic therapy. Research focused on more representative treatment of referred clients in clinics has shown more modest effects; in fact, most clinic studies have not shown significant effects. Interpretation of these findings requires caution; such studies are few and most could profit from improved methodology. The clinic studies do raise questions as to whether the positive lab findings can be generalized to the clinics where most therapy occurs; however, the lab interventions that have worked so well may point the way to enhanced therapy effects in clinics.

Reprinted with permission from *American Psychologist*, 1992, Vol. 47 (12), 1578–1585. Copyright © 1992 by the American Psychological Association.

Bernadette Gray-Little served as action editor for this article.

The work reported in this article was supported in part through grants from the National Institute of Mental Health (5 RO1 MH38240, 1 RO3 MH34652) to John R. Weisz. For a more detailed treatment of the issues raised here, and a more detailed description of the studies and meta-analyses reviewed, see the book, *Effects of Psychotherapy With Children and Adolescents* (Weisz & Weiss, in press).

At any one time, about 12% of the more than 63 million children and adolescents (referred to in this article as children) in the United States suffer from serious behavioral or emotional problems (Institute of Medicine [IOM], 1989; Saxe, Cross, & Silverman, 1988). Of these children, about 2.5 million receive treatment (Office of Technology Assessment, 1986), at an annual cost of more than $1.5 billion (IOM, 1989). Beyond the financial cost, families of these children invest considerable energy and time, and mental health professionals devote entire careers, to the treatment process. How effective is the therapy provided at such great cost to the youngsters, their families, the therapists, and society? In this article we address that question.

EVIDENCE FROM META-ANALYSES

From the perspective of controlled therapy outcome studies, evidence on the efficacy of child therapy appears to be quite positive. Probably the most efficient and objective means of summarizing the findings of such studies is the technique known as meta-analysis (see Mann, 1990; Smith, Glass, & Miller, 1980; but see also critiques, e.g., Wilson, 1985). Meta-analysis provides a means of quantitatively aggregating the findings of independent studies; it permits summary statements about a body of literature, including statements about the average effect of psychotherapy across studies, expressed in the form of a mean effect size (ES). In this article we briefly review the findings of major child and adolescent meta-analyses; for a more detailed review, see Weisz and Weiss (in press).

Casey and Berman (1985)

In the first child meta-analysis, Casey and Berman (1985) reviewed 75 outcome studies, published between 1952 and 1983, and focused on children aged 12 and younger. The children were treated for such social adjustment difficulties as aggression or withdrawal (40% of the studies), hyperactive or impulsive behavior (13%), and phobias (12%), and such somatic problems as obesity and enuresis (4%). The interventions used included behavioral and cognitive–behavioral methods (56% of the studies) and nonbehavioral methods (48%), including client-centered and psychodynamic approaches. ES values were calculated by computing the mean posttherapy treatment–control group difference on outcome measures and dividing that difference by the pooled within-group standard deviation; ES was thus expressed in standard deviation units, with higher scores indicating more positive therapy effects (as in all the meta-analyses reviewed here). Across the 64 studies that included treatment–control comparisons, the mean ES was 0.71; the average treated child functioned better after treatment than 76% of control group children, averaging across outcome measures.

Weisz, Weiss, Alicke, and Klotz (1987)

In a second meta-analysis, Weisz, Weiss, Alicke, and Klotz (1987) included 105 outcome studies[1] published between 1952 and 1983, focused on children aged 4–18 years. Some 47% of the studies involved treatment of externalizing or *undercontrolled* problems (19% hyperactivity or impulsivity, 12% delinquency, 11% aggressive or undisciplined behavior, and 6% noncompliance); 42% of the studies involved treatment of internalizing or *overcontrolled* problems (24% phobias and anxiety and 17% social withdrawal or isolation); other treated problems included more difficult to classify "adjustment–emotional disturbance" (6%) and underachievement (6%). Across all the treatment groups of all the studies, 77% involved behavioral interventions and 17% nonbehavioral, with the remainder described too vaguely to be classified. ES values were calculated by dividing the posttreatment therapy–control group difference by the control group standard deviation. Across the 105 studies surveyed, the mean ES was 0.79: The average treated child functioned better after treatment than 79% of the control group. Weiss and Weisz (1990) subsequently analyzed the impact of various methodological factors on the ES values obtained in these studies.

Kazdin, Bass, Ayers, and Rodgers (1990)

A third meta-analysis, by Kazdin, Bass, Ayers, and Rodgers (1990), actually began with a broad survey of 223 treatment studies published between 1970 and 1988, involving youngsters aged 4–18 years. Externalizing problems were the focus of treatment in 47% of the studies, internalizing problems in 16%, both externalizing and internalizing in 3%, and learning–academic problems in 15%. The interventions involved some form of behavior modification in 50% of the studies, cognitive–behavioral methods in 22%, group therapy in 9%, client-centered therapy in 5%, play therapy in 5%, and family therapy in 4%. ES values were calculated with procedures similar to those of Casey and Berman (1985) for the subset of 105 studies involving treatment–control comparisons. That subset was further subdivided. For the 64 studies involving comparisons between a treatment group and a *no-treatment* control group, the mean ES was 0.88; after treatment the average treated child was better off than 81% of the no-treatment youngsters. For the 41 studies comparing treatment and *active* control groups, the mean ES was 0.77; after treatment the average treated child was functioning better than 78% of the control group youngsters.

---

[1]In Weisz et al. (1987) we erroneously reported that 108 studies had been included; three studies that had been dropped for failure to meet our methodological criteria were mistakenly retained in our bibliography.

Weisz, Weiss, Morton, Granger, and Han (1992)

We have preliminary data to report from a meta-analysis by Weisz, Weiss, Morton, Granger, and Han (1992), based on 110 studies published between 1967 and 1991. The children, aged 2–18 years, were treated for externalizing problems in 40% of the studies (e.g., 29% self-control problems, 19% aggression, 19% delinquency, 6% noncompliance), for internalizing problems in 30% (e.g., 44% headaches and other somatic problems, 33% phobias and anxiety, 14% depression), and for other problems in 29% (e.g., 31% poor social relationships, 9% personality and self-concept problems). Behavioral treatments were used in 79% of the studies (e.g., 22% cognitive–behavioral, 18% respondent, 10% operant, 7% modeling), nonbehavioral in 15% (e.g., 39% insight-oriented, 39% discussion groups, 17% client-centered), and mixed approaches in 7%. ES, calculated by the same method as in Weisz et al. (1987), averaged 0.71 across the 110 studies; after treatment, the average treated child was functioning better than 76% of control group children.

Specially Focused Meta-Analyses

In addition to the four broad-based child meta-analyses just described, we know of three more narrowly focused contributions. Hazelrigg, Cooper, and Borduin (1987) reviewed outcome studies of *family therapy* involving at least one parent and one child. Focusing on the 10 studies that compared family therapy to no-treatment control groups, Hazelrigg et al. found an ES of 0.45 (average treated case scoring better than 67% of the no-treatment group) on family interaction measures, and 0.50 (average treated case scoring better than 69% of no-treatment group) on behavior rating measures of outcome. Duriak, Fuhrman, and Lampman (1991) reviewed 64 studies of *cognitive–behavioral therapy* with 4–13-year-olds. The mean ES was 0.56; after therapy, the average treated child scored better on outcome measures than 71% of control group peers. Children aged 11–13 years (labeled "formal operational" by the authors) were more positively affected by these cognitive interventions (ES = 0.92) than were children aged 5–7 years (0.57) or 7–11 years (0.55). Finally, Russell, Greenwald, and Shirk (1991) addressed a dimension that is often interwoven with child psychopathology and treatment: *language proficiency*. They reviewed 18 child treatment studies (26 treatment–control group comparisons) that included at least one language measure. Across these studies, the mean ES for language change was 0.32; after therapy the average treated child outscored 63% of the untreated controls on language measures.

Adult and Child Meta-Analytic Findings

Figure 1 summarizes results (in percentile form) of the four broad-based child therapy meta-analyses and of two widely cited meta-analyses of predominantly adult psychotherapy studies (Shapiro & Shapiro, 1982; Smith et al., 1980). The figure shows that the mean effects reported in child meta-analyses are quite comparable to those of adult meta-analyses, and that both sets of findings point to quite positive effects of therapy. ES values ranged from 0.71 to 0.84, hovering near J. Cohen's (1988) threshold of 0.80 for a "large" effect.

LIMITATIONS OF THE META-ANALYTIC DATA: RESEARCH THERAPY VERSUS CLINIC THERAPY

Because the meta-analyses reviewed above indicate consistently positive effects, and because they reflect such a large number of distinct outcome studies

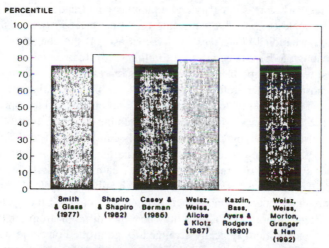

Note. Numbers on the vertical axis reflect the posttherapy percentile standing of treated groups relative to control groups (i.e., the percentage of control group subjects scoring lower than treated subjects, pooling across outcome measures). Smith and Glass (1977) included studies of children, adolescents and adults; Shapiro and Shapiro (1982) included only studies of adults; the four remaining reports focused exclusively on child and adolescent studies. The Kazdin et al. (1990) bar represents our estimate from Kazdin et al's (1990) report. Kazdin et al. actually reported separate effect sizes of 0.88 for 64 treatment vs. no-treatment comparisons, and 0.77 for 41 treatment vs. active control group comparisons; we estimate a pooled effect size of 0.84, with a pooled percentile of 0.80. The bar for Weisz et al. (1992) shows results of a preliminary analysis.

Figure 1. Findings of five meta-analysis of psychotherapy outcome research

($N > 200$) and subjects ($N > 12{,}000$), it may be tempting to conclude that the evidence on child therapy effects is now in, and that the news is very good. Such a conclusion may be premature. To explain why, we need to examine the evidence that forms the basis of the meta-analyses.

Most of the studies included in the meta-analyses (particularly the behavioral studies and studies of the past decade) involved children, interventions, and treatment conditions that were relatively unrepresentative of conventional clinical practice. As noted by Weisz and Weiss (1989), in the majority of these controlled experimental studies, (a) youngsters were recruited for treatment, not actually clinic referred, which suggests that some were not seriously disturbed; (b) samples were selected for homogeneity, with all youngsters displaying a similar focal problem or problems (e.g., a specific phobia, or out-of-seat behavior in school); (c) therapy addressed the focal problems primarily or exclusively; (d) therapists were trained immediately before therapy in the specific techniques they would use; and (e) the therapy involved primary or exclusive reliance on those techniques. Moreover, (f) therapy was often guided by a structured manual and was monitored regularly for its integrity and adherence to a treatment plan. Such features tend to coalesce around a genre that might be termed *research therapy*.

In most conventional *clinic therapy*, by contrast, (a) the clients are seriously disturbed enough to have been referred to clinics; (b) treated youngsters are heterogeneous, with many problems and disorders represented in a therapist's caseload, and most youngsters referred for multiple problems; (c) therapy is usually directed not at one focal problem but at a range of problems; (d) therapists are not likely to have the luxury of intensive recent training in all or most of the techniques they use; (e) therapy cannot be properly limited to a few techniques on which the therapists can concentrate all their energies; and (f) neither treatment manuals nor systematic external monitoring of treatment integrity are common. More generally, therapists typically carry large and diverse caseloads, have heavy paperwork requirements, and face other distractions from their therapeutic work. Thus, conditions in most child clinics may be rather different from (and less optimum than) the conditions typically arranged for controlled outcome studies (see also Persons, 1991).

Other differences between child clinical practice and child therapy outcome research have been noted by Kazdin et al. (1990). In a survey of 223 child outcome studies, Kazdin et al. found that child therapy research, unlike clinical practice, tends to (a) focus on children recruited from and treated in schools; (b) use group approaches rather than individual treatment; (c) use behavioral and cognitive–behavioral methods rather than psychodynamic, eclectic, and family-oriented approaches; (d) emphasize brief interventions averaging 8–10 weeks (vs. 27–55 weeks in clinical practice); (e) deemphasize involvement of parents and other family members; and (f) deemphasize consultation with teachers.

In several respects, then, the procedures and conditions associated with conventional clinic-based therapy for children are different from those typically arranged for outcome research. It is thus unclear whether the findings of meta-analyses, based on that research, can be generalized to the clinic-based therapy that is most often provided to disturbed children in the United States. This suggests that an important transcontextual validity question (Weisz, 1978) remains to be answered: Are the benefits of therapy as demonstrated in controlled outcome studies matched by the benefits of actual clinical practice with children?

Evidence From Clinic-Based Studies

Although answering this question may appear to be a rather straightforward task, a significant obstacle stands in the way of evaluating the effects of clinic-based therapy with referred children: Legal and ethical constraints almost always prevent clinics from randomly assigning treatment applicants to no-treatment control conditions. Thus, the rigorous comparisons of randomly selected treatment and no-treatment control groups that are the forte of controlled, experimental outcome studies are rarely possible in clinic settings.[2]

To address this problem, researchers have tried to develop outcome assessment methods that do not require random assignment of clinic applicants to control groups. An early step in this direction was taken by Eysenck (1952) in a study of adult therapy effects. He compared reported rates of improvement across 19 studies of psychotherapy with "neurotic" adults to estimated base rates of improvement in studies of neurotic adults treated more custodially in state hospitals. Treated adults' rate of improvement fell below the hospital base rate of 72% improvement, leading Eysenck to conclude that "The figures fail to support the hypothesis that psychotherapy facilitates recovery from neurotic disorder" (p. 323; but see critiques of Eysenck's study, e.g., Rosenzweig, 1954).

Levitt's (1957b) cross-study comparison. Levitt (1957b) followed Eysenck's (1952) general procedure to estimate the effects of therapy for "neurotic" children. The base rate of improvement without treatment was estimated from two follow-up studies of children who had dropped out after being accepted for clinic treatment. To this base rate, Levitt compared the improvement rates reported for treated children in 18 published reports of outcome at treatment termination and

---

[2]It is sometimes possible to randomly assign children to receive or not receive *particular* treatments *in addition to* the regular treatment program that *all* clinic children receive; what we refer to here are studies involving random assignment to standard clinic treatment versus no-treatment or active placebo conditions. It is also sometimes possible to quasi-randomly assign clinic applicants to waiting-list control groups. However, this approach has limitations. In most clinics, wait-list assignments cannot be truly random, because children with particularly serious problems receive priority; and wait-list controls usually can only be paired with brief therapy cases, and without follow up, because withholding treatment for long periods simply to match treated cases would violate the clinic mandate.

17 published reports of outcome at follow up. The improvement rate was 72.5% for untreated children, 74% for treated children. These results, Levitt concluded, "fail to support the view that psychotherapy with 'neurotic' children is effective" (p. 195). Levitt's report sparked several critiques (e.g., Barrett, Hampe, & Miller, 1978; Eisenberg & Gruenberg, 1961; Halpern, 1968; Heinicke & Goldman, 1960; Hood-Williams, 1960). Several criticisms were related to the fact that Levitt had estimated base rates of improvement for treated and untreated groups from different studies, and thus different clinic settings and different population bases. Because comparisons were made across (rather than within) studies, it was not possible to assess directly the demographic, developmental, or clinical similarity of the treated and untreated groups being compared. The comparison was thus rather indirect, and the possibility of initial uncontrolled group differences necessarily remained unexamined. Other clinic-based studies, though, have provided more direct and controlled comparisons of treated and untreated groups. We turn now to those studies, reflecting three different research strategies.

Treated children versus matched children in the general population: Shepherd, Oppenheim, and Mitchell (1966). One approach, taken in a British study by Shepherd, Oppenheim, & Mitchell (1966), was to form matched pairs of children treated in clinics and unreferred, untreated children identified through a general population survey. Some 50 pairs, aged 5–15 years, were matched for demographic and clinical characteristics (e.g., problem profiles). Clinician ratings of problem severity showed no reliable differences between the two groups, but a few differences were found among parent variables (e.g., clinic mothers, more than nonclinic mothers, thought their children's problems required professional help). Shepherd et al. compared adjustment in the two groups about two years after the initial assessments. In-home clinical interviews were conducted, and improvement ratings were made by trained judges who were unaware of the clinic–nonclinic status of the children. The ratings indicated that 63% of clinic cases had improved over the two years, and 61% of the nonclinic children had improved. Moreover, among clinic children, number of treatment sessions bore no relation to whether children improved or deteriorated. Neither finding supported the efficacy of clinic treatment.

A limitation of Shepherd et al.'s (1966) study is that the children in their untreated sample had not been referred to clinics. Mothers of these children, compared to the clinic mothers, showed less distress over their children's problems and less interest in professional help; and there may have been other differences between children and families who sought clinic treatment and those who did not. Thus, it is important to complement evidence such as Shepherd et al.'s with evidence on treated and untreated groups who *both* initially sought clinic treatment.

This brings us to another means of fashioning treatment–no-treatment comparisons: comparing treated and untreated children admitted to the same treatment facilities in the same time period, with untreated cases consisting of those who drop out before treatment. This approach addresses the problems associated with the use of nonreferred children (as in Shepherd et al., 1966) and with the use of therapy dropout and completer groups from different clinics and different time periods (as in Levitt, 1957b). Of course, it might be argued that dropouts and therapy completers could differ demographically or clinically (see, e.g., Hood-Williams, 1960). Yet, published studies examining a broad range of child demographic and clinical variables have revealed negligible differences between such groups (see Gould, Shaffer, & Kaplan, 1985; Levitt, 1957a; McAdoo & Roeske, 1973; Weisz, Weiss, & Langmeyer, 1987, 1989); moreover, it is possible to test for differences before comparing groups on outcome measures. Thus, under proper circumstances, children who drop out may be an acceptable (although, of course, not ideal) naturally occurring control group for outcome research in circumstances in which no randomly assigned control group can be constituted. In the following sections we describe four studies that used this approach.[3]

Therapy dropouts versus completers: I. Lehrman, Sirluck, Black, and Glick (1949). In the earliest of these studies (which, incidentally, provided a base rate sample for Levitt, 1957b), Lehrman et al. (1949) focused on 3–20-year-olds seen at Jewish Board of Guardians (JBG) Child Guidance Clinics in New York, before April, 1942; 60% were seen for "primary behavior disorder" (e.g., hostile or impulsive behavior) and 25% for "psychoneurosis," with other problems represented as well. Some 196 cases formed the treatment group; these were deemed "totally treated," through methods that were labeled "transference psychotherapy" (p. 8). An additional 110 cases formed the control group. These had been observed by JBG staff and found eligible for services, but had not received a course of treatment at JBG or elsewhere (usually because parents had declined). Treatment and control groups were compared on a small number of demographic, family, and clinical characteristics early in their clinic contact. Few differences were found; however, the control group had a higher proportion of primary behavior disorder diagnoses than the treatment group (74% vs. 55%), and the reverse was true of the psychoneurosis category (20% vs. 28%).

One year after cases had been closed, outcomes were assessed. Each case was classified as success, partial success, or failure, on the basis of assessments of a JBG evaluation committee. Steps were taken to keep the committee unaware of group membership of the cases, but the interview and case material used by the committee may have been gathered and assembled by JBG staff who knew the

---

[3]We know of two other studies that approximate this methodology. However, both (Jacob, Magnussen, & Kemler, 1972; Witmer & Keller, 1942) have design features that make them not quite appropriate for inclusion here. Witmer and Keller (1942) reported no significant effects of therapy; Jacob et al. (1972) reported mixed findings.

group membership. At follow-up, the percentage classified as success was significantly higher for treated than for control cases (50.5% vs. 31.8%), and the percentage of failure ratings was slightly higher for control than for treated cases (30.0% vs. 26.0%). Given these differences, Lehrman et al. (1949) maintained, "The positive effect of the treatment was established beyond a doubt" (p. 80). This verdict may need to be tempered somewhat by concerns about diagnostic differences between the two groups, and about the degree of "experimental blindness" and impartiality of the staff on whose data outcome assessments were based. Nonetheless, Lehrman et al.'s study stands as an important early methodological and substantive contribution.

Therapy dropouts versus completers: II. Levitt, Beiser, & Robertson (1959). In a second completer versus dropout study, Levitt et al. (1959) studied youngsters averaging about 10 years old when first seen at Chicago's Institute for Juvenile Research. Two groups were compared: 237 treated cases, or *remainers*, and 93 untreated cases, or *defectors*. Defectors had been accepted for treatment but had dropped out before the first therapy session. Remainers had had an average of 18 therapy sessions, with therapy directed to the child alone (10% of the cases), to the child and parent (46%), or to the parent alone (44%). Any child treated elsewhere during the study was excluded. Remainer and defector groups were compared on 61 clinical and background variables assessed at the beginning of their clinic contact (e.g., gender, mental age, nature and severity of problems), with no reliable differences found beyond chance expectancy (Levitt, 1957a).[4]

Outcomes were assessed at an average of about five years after clinic contact. The 26 outcome variables included scores on several psychological tests (e.g., Taylor Anxiety Scale, Minnesota Multiphasic Personality Inventory short form), parent and child ratings (e.g., on current severity of original presenting problems), clinician ratings (e.g., on manifest tension, affective tone of personality), and life adjustment indicators (e.g., completion of schooling, institutional residence). Levitt et al. (1959) found no remainer–defector group differences on outcome measures beyond chance expectancy. As for direction of the group differences, 16 showed more favorable scores for the defector group, whereas only 9 favored the remainer group (sign test $p = .21$). To enhance the possibility of identifying therapy effects, Levitt et al. redefined the remainers to select a *continuer* group, requiring a minimum of 10 therapy sessions, and reanalyzed for continuer–defector differences. The results were essentially the same as in the original analyses, with no reliable evidence of positive treatment effects.

Therapy dropouts versus completers: III. Ashcraft (1971). More than a decade

---

[4]The comparison of remainer and defector groups on clinical and background variables (Levitt, 1957a) appears to have been conducted on groups that overlapped with but were not identical to the remainers and defectors in the treatment outcome study (Levitt et al., 1959). Levitt included 132 remainers and 208 defectors, whereas Levitt et al. included 237 remainers and 93 defectors.

after Levitt et al. (1959), Ashcraft (1971) published another follow-up comparison of clinic-treated youngsters with matched children who had dropped out after intake and had remained untreated. All children in both groups had been seen at one of two clinics in a metropolitan area, at some time during Grades 3–6. The treatment group consisted of 40 children and was 88% male, with a mean age of nine years and seven months, and a mean Wechsler Intelligence Scale for Children (WISC) IQ of 105.8. The dropout group numbered 43 and was 79% male, with a mean age of nine years and four months, and a mean WISC IQ of 104.6. Outcomes were assessed five years after clinic contact. All the children in both groups had been classified as underachievers who had "learning difficulties" that "stemmed from emotional difficulties requiring outpatient treatment" (p. 339). Thus, outcomes were assessed with measures of academic achievement: Stanford Achievement Test Total Achievement Score, Total Language Achievement Score, and Total Quantitative Achievement Score. The treated and untreated groups did not differ reliably on any outcome measure.

Therapy dropouts versus completers: IV. Weisz and Weiss (1989). The clinic-based studies reviewed thus far were all conducted more than two decades ago. One might question whether their findings are relevant to psychotherapy as it is currently practiced in clinics. To address this question, we now turn to a more recent study of clinic treatment, in which Weisz and Weiss (1989) compared treatment completers and dropouts from nine outpatient mental health clinics. The completers were 93 children who had had at least five therapy sessions (average 12.4 sessions) and who had terminated with concurrence of their therapist. The dropouts were 60 children who had attended an intake session, had been judged by clinic staff to be in need of treatment, and had been assigned a therapist, but had not appeared for any sessions after intake. In addition, 14 who had received other mental health services during the period of the study were excluded from the dropout group. Completers averaged 11.0 years of age (at the six-month follow-up) and were 64.5% male; dropouts averaged 10.9 years and were 63.3% male.

Similarity of the groups was assessed on 11 variables that appeared relevant to later outcomes, such as child demographic factors (age, gender, birth order); child clinical measures (Child Behavior Checklist [CBCL; Achenbach & Edelbrock, 1983], internalizing, externalizing, and competence scores, Child Depression Inventory scores, number of therapy sessions prior to this intake); and family factors (socioeconomic status, number of children in the home, miles from home to clinic, and changes in family structure during the six months following intake). No comparison showed a significant group difference.

Weisz and Weiss (1989) collected three measures of adjustment at intake and at six months and one year later. CBCL parent reports were collected to provide information on a broad spectrum of clinically significant behavioral and emotional problems. Parents also gave severity ratings on up to three "major problems for which your child needs help" (identified at intake); this was intended to address specific problems that were a focus of treatment. Finally, Teacher Report Form (TRF; Achenbach & Edelbrock, 1986) reports were collected to provide information on clinically significant behavioral and emotional problems from a source outside the family and not involved in the treatment process. Teachers were not told that the child had been to a clinic; they were asked to fill in the TRF as part of a "youth survey." At six months (for all dropouts and for the 98% of completers who had finished treatment) and at one year, the two groups were compared on the outcome measures described above, with intake scores covaried. On none of the measures was there a significant group difference, at six months or at one year. In other words, the findings revealed no reliable effect of therapy on any of the measures.

For a rough comparison between these results and findings of the four broad-based meta-analyses of experimental studies, effect size estimates were calculated for Weisz and Weiss's (1989) findings. Figure 2 presents all the ES values. As the figure indicates, the six-month CBCL assessment actually showed a trend toward

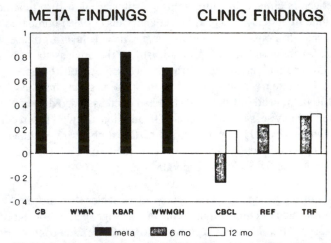

The four bars on the left show results of the meta-analyses: CB = Casey & Berman (1985); WWAK = Weisz, Weiss, Alicke, & Klotz (1987); KBAR = Kazdin, Bass, Ayers, & Rodgers (1990), bar represents our estimate of the pooled effect size, based on Kazdin et al.'s report; WWMGH = Weisz, Weiss, Morton, Granger, & Han (1992), bar represents preliminary findings. The three bars on the right show findings of the Weisz and Weiss (1989) study: CBCL = Child Behavior Checklist findings; REF = findings on severity of primary referral problems, TRF = Teacher Report Form findings.

Figure 2. Effect sizes found in four meta-analyses of child and adolescent psychotherapy outcome studies and in the clinic-based outcome study by Weisz and Weiss (1989)

worse outcomes for treated children than for dropouts; however, for all three measures, at both points of assessment, effect sizes fell well below those found in the meta-analyses. Moreover, none of the clinic effect sizes was significantly different from 0.

Five possible alternative explanations of these null results were analyzed. These included the possibilities of (a) excessive variability in the data causing null findings, (b) biased or defensive reporting by parents of dropout or continuer children, (c) hidden advantages favoring adjustment in the dropout group, (d) immediate postintake improvement in the dropout group leading to their dropping out, and (e) bias caused by the voluntary nature of subject participation in the research. Close scrutiny and data analyses bearing on these explanations raised doubts about their plausibility (see Weisz & Weiss, 1989, pp. 745–746). This further supported a straightforward interpretation of the findings (i.e., that psychotherapy simply had not had a significant effect on the measures used).

Random assignment: De Fries, Jenkins, and Williams (1964). Finally, we turn to the one clinic-based study we have found that involved true random assignment to treatment and control groups. De Fries et al. (1964) studied 6–15-year-olds, all described as seriously disturbed, all having a psychiatric diagnosis, and all in foster care in Westchester County, New York. They formed 27 child pairs, with pair members matched for age, gender, ethnic group, IQ, and psychiatric diagnosis. One member of each pair was randomly assigned to receive usual welfare department services; the other member received psychotherapy, plus enhanced services for the foster family. Before intervention, three clinically experienced judges (unaware of group assignment) rated all the children on (a) relationships in the foster home, (b) adjustment in school and community, (c) symptomatology, and (d) well-being and productivity. Means on each rating were almost identical for the two groups, indicating successful matching.

Therapy appears to have lasted three years and to have been conducted by professional therapists, each supervised by a psychiatrist. After the intervention, outside judges, unaware of group assignment, were asked to use data from opening and closing psychiatric interviews to place each child in an *improved, no change,* or *worsened* category. The judges, working independently, agreed in 81% of their judgments, and were in adjacent categories for the remaining 19%. There were no significant treatment–control differences on this outcome measure. A second goal of intervention had been to prevent institutionalization. This goal was also not achieved; institutionalization occurred somewhat more often among the treated children than among the controls. In summary, this clinic-based study, using random assignment methodology, found no reliable treatment effects.

Implications of the Clinic-Based Findings

The most immediate conclusion suggested by the studies reviewed in this article is that, for clinic-referred children treated by practicing clinicians in clinic settings, the effects of psychotherapy may not be nearly so positive as the findings presented in the meta-analyses indicate. In fact, with the exception of Lehrman et al. (1949), the clinic-based studies have not shown statistically significant effects of psychotherapy. Certainly, the methodologies used in most of these studies fell short of the ideal, with random assignment achieved in only one instance. Moreover, most of the clinic-based studies were conducted decades ago, at a relatively immature stage in the development of therapeutic approaches and standardized assessment of child psychopathology and therapy outcomes. Thus, the need for careful, current replication of the clinic studies is clear. Although it would be a mistake to accept the clinic findings uncritically, it would also be a mistake to ignore or dismiss these findings and the sobering state of affairs with which they confront us: Currently, we lack convincing evidence that the large positive effects of psychotherapy demonstrated in controlled psychotherapy research, and summarized in the meta-analyses, are being replicated in the clinic and community settings where most real-life interventions actually occur.

If the clinic-based findings discussed here are valid and should eventually prove to be well-replicated, they should not be viewed as entirely discouraging. Indeed, they may represent a glass that can be seen as both half empty and half full. From the half-empty perspective, clinic-based therapy for children may not be as effective as one would hope. But from the half-full perspective, the results of the meta-analyses suggest that under proper conditions child therapy may be very effective. When the findings are viewed in this light, a key task for researchers becomes that of identifying those proper conditions under which effects of child therapy may be optimized.

Identifying such conditions may require adapting research therapies to actual clinical conditions with referred clients, then testing the efficacy of research-based therapies in clinic settings. It is possible that research therapy has positive effects because it tends to involve clear delineation of focal problems that will be targets of treatment (i.e., ruling out efforts to treat "the whole child"), precise matching of these problems to treatment methods, and selection of treatment methods that have empirical support. On the other hand, it is also possible that research therapy appears more effective in part because the youngsters being treated are less seriously disturbed or more responsive to intervention than those youngsters typically treated in clinics, or because research therapists are free of constraining conditions (e.g., heavy caseloads) under which clinic therapists often work. Until research therapy is brought into the clinics, it will be difficult to evaluate such possibilities in a definitive way.

Renewing Ties Between Research and Practice

Constructing research of the sort described above will almost certainly require enriched collaboration between researchers and practitioners, a process that may prove healthy for both groups. One of the most widely voiced complaints of practicing clinicians over the years has been that psychotherapy research is of little use to them (see Elliott, 1983; Kupfersmid, 1988; Luborsky, 1972; Orlinsky & Howard, 1978; Parloff, 1980). As Strupp (1989) put it, psychotherapists "have recurrently complained that they can learn but little from psychotherapy research" (p. 717). When clinical psychologists are asked to rank order the usefulness to their practice of various sources of information, research articles and books are generally rated at the bottom of the scale (L. Cohen, 1979; L. Cohen, Sargent, & Sechrest, 1986; Morrow-Bradley & Elliott, 1986). Researchers themselves appear to agree with the concern; as Morrow-Bradley and Elliott noted,

> With virtual unanimity, psychotherapy researchers have argued that (a) psychotherapy research should yield information useful to practicing therapists, (b) such research to date has not done so, and (c) this problem should be remedied. (p. 188)

We suggest that psychotherapy research with children may have considerable relevance to the work of clinicians, and conversely, that the work of clinicians may make important contributions to research. If it is true that child therapy is more effective under research conditions than under clinic conditions, outcome research may well prove useful to practicing clinicians and their young clients by specifying those conditions under which therapeutic gains can be maximized. On the other hand, to achieve this goal, researchers will need to rely heavily on the wisdom and perspective of clinicians whose knowledge about children and treatment has been shaped in the crucible of real life.

REFERENCES

Achenbach, T. M., & Edelbrock, C. S. (1983). *Manual for the child behavior checklist and revised child behavior profile*. Burlington: University of Vermont, Department of Psychiatry.

Achenbach, T. M., & Edelbrock, C. S. (1986). *Manual for the teacher's report form*. Burlington: University of Vermont, Department of Psychiatry.

Ashcraft, C. W. (1971). The later school adjustment of treated and untreated emotionally handicapped children. *Journal of School Psychology: 9*, 338–342.

Barrett, C. L., Hampe, I. E., & Miller, M. C. (1978). Research on child psychotherapy.

In S. L. Garfield & A. E. Bergin (Eds.), *Handbook of psychotherapy and behavior change: An empirical analysis* (2nd ed., pp. 411–435). New York: Wiley.

Casey, R. J., & Berman, J. S. (1985). The outcome of psychotherapy with children. *Psychological Bulletin*, 98, 388–400.

Cohen, J. (1988). *Statistical power analyses for the behavioral sciences* (2nd ed.). Hillsdale, NJ: Erlbaum.

Cohen, L. (1979). The research readership and information source reliance of clinical psychologists. *Professional Psychology*, 10, 780–785.

Cohen, L., Sargent, M., & Sechrest, L. (1986). Use of psychotherapy research by professional psychologists. *American Psychologist*, 41, 198–206.

De Fries, Z., Jenkins, S., & Williams, E. C. (1964). Treatment of disturbed children in foster care. *American Journal of Orthopsychiatry*, 34, 615–624.

Durlak, J. A., Fuhrman, T., & Lampman, C. (1991). Effectiveness of cognitive–behavior therapy for maladapting children: A meta-analysis. *Psychological Bulletin*, 110, 204–214.

Eisenberg, L., & Gruenberg, E. M. (1961). The current status of secondary prevention in child psychiatry. *American Journal of Orthopsychiatry*, 31, 355–367.

Elliott, R. (1983). Fitting process research to the practicing psychotherapist. *Psychotherapy: Theory, Research, and Practice*, 20, 47–55.

Eysenck, H. J. (1952). The effects of psychotherapy: An evaluation. *Journal of Consulting Psychology*, 16, 319–324.

Gould, M. S., Shaffer, D., & Kaplan, D. (1985). The characteristics of dropouts from a child psychiatry clinic. *Journal of the American Academy of Child Psychiatry*, 24, 316–328.

Halpern, W. I. (1968). Do children benefit from psychotherapy? A review of the literature on follow-up studies. *Bulletin of the Rochester Mental Health Center*, 1, 4–12.

Hazelrigg, M. D., Cooper, H. M., & Borduin, C. M. (1987). Evaluating the effectiveness of family therapies: An integrative review and analysis. *Psychological Bulletin*, 101, 428–442.

Heinicke, C. M., & Goldman, A. (1960). Research on psychotherapy with children: A review and suggestions for further study. *American Journal of Orthopsychiatry*, 30, 483–494.

Hood-Williams, J. (1960). The results of psychotherapy with children: A reevaluation. *Journal of Consulting and Clinical Psychology*, 24, 84–88.

Institute of Medicine. (1989.) *Research on children and adolescents with mental, behavioral, and developmental disorders.* Washington, DC: National Academy Press.

Jacob, T., Magnussen, M. G., & Kemler, W. M. (1972). A follow-up of treatment terminators and remainers with short-term and long-term symptom duration. *Psychotherapy: Theory, Research, and Practice*, 9, 139–142.

Kazdin, A. E., Bass, D., Ayers, W. A., & Rodgers, A. (1990). Empirical and clinical focus of child and adolescent psychotherapy research. *Journal of Consulting and Clinical Psychology*, 58, 729–740.

Kupfersmid, J. (1988). Improving what is published: A model in search of an editor. *American Psychologist, 43,* 635–642.

Lehrman, L. J., Sirluck, H., Black, B. J., & Glick, S. J. (1949). Success and failure of treatment of children in the child guidance clinics of the Jewish Board of Guardians, New York City. *Jewish Board of Guardians Research Monographs* (1).

Levitt, E. E. (1957a). A comparison of "remainers" and "defectors" among child clinic patients. *Journal of Consulting Psychology, 21,* 316.

Levitt, E. E. (1957b). The results of psychotherapy with children: An evaluation. *Journal of Consulting Psychology, 21,* 189–196.

Levitt, E. E., Beiser, H. R., & Robertson, R. E. (1959). A follow-up evaluation of cases treated at a community child guidance clinic. *American Journal of Orthopsychiatry, 29,* 337–347.

Luborsky, L. (1972). Research cannot yet influence clinical practice. In A. Bergin & H. H. Strupp (Eds.), *Changing frontiers in the science of psychotherapy* (pp. 120–127). Chicago: Aldine.

Mann, C. (1990). Meta-analysis in the breech. *Science, 249,* 476–480.

McAdoo, W. G., & Roeske, N. A. (1973). A comparison of defectors and continuers in a child guidance clinic. *Journal of Consulting and Clinical Psychology, 40,* 328–334.

Morrow-Bradley, C., & Elliott, R. (1986). Utilization of psychotherapy research by practicing psychotherapists. *American Psychologist, 41,* 188–197.

Office of Technology Assessment. (1986.) *Children's mental health: Problems and services—A background paper* (Publication No. OTA-BP-H-33). Washington, DC: U.S. Government Printing Office.

Orlinsky, D., & Howard, K. (1978). The relation of process to outcome in psychotherapy. In S. Garfield & A. Bergin (Eds.), *Handbook of psychotherapy and behavior change: An empirical analysis* (2nd ed., pp. 283–330). New York: Wiley.

Parloff, M. B. (1980). Psychotherapy and research: An anaclitic depression. *Psychiatry, 43,* 279–293.

Persons, J. B. (1991). Psychotherapy outcome studies do not accurately represent current models of psychotherapy: A proposed remedy. *American Psychologist, 46,* 99–106.

Rosenzweig, S. (1954). A transvaluation of psychotherapy—A reply to Hans Eysenck. *Journal of Abnormal Psychology, 49,* 298–304.

Russell, R. L., Greenwald, S., & Shirk, S. R. (1991). Language change in child psychotherapy: A meta-analytic review. *Journal of Consulting and Clinical Psychology, 59,* 916–919.

Saxe, L., Cross, T., & Silverman, N. (1988). Children's mental health: The gap between what we know and what we do. *American Psychologist, 43,* 800–807.

Shapiro, D. A., & Shapiro, D. (1982). Meta-analysis of comparative therapy outcome studies: A replication and refinement. *Psychological Bulletin, 92,* 581–604.

Shepherd, M., Oppenheim, A. N., & Mitchell, S. (1966). Childhood behaviour disorders and the child-guidance clinic: An epidemiological study. *Journal of Child Psychology and Psychiatry, 7,* 39–52.

Smith, M. L., & Glass, G. V. (1977). Meta-analysis of psychotherapy outcome studies. *American Psychologist*, 32, 752–760.

Smith, M. L., Glass, G. V., & Miller, T. L. (1980). *Benefits of psychotherapy.* Baltimore: Johns Hopkins University Press.

Strupp, H. H. (1989). Psychotherapy: Can the practitioner learn from the researcher? *American Psychologist*, 44, 717–724.

Weiss, B., & Weisz, J. R. (1990). The impact of methodological factors on child psychotherapy outcome research: A meta-analysis for researchers. *Journal of Abnormal Child Psychology*, 18, 639–670.

Weisz, J. R. (1978). Transcontextual validity in developmental research. *Child Development*, 49, 1–12.

Weisz, J. R., & Weiss, B. (1989). Assessing the effects of clinic-based psychotherapy with children and adolescents. *Journal of Consulting and Clinical Psychology*, 57, 741–746.

Weisz, J. R., & Weiss, B. (in press). *Effects of psychotherapy with children and adolescents.* New York: Sage.

Weisz, J. R., Weiss, B., Alicke, M. D., & Klotz, M. L. (1987). Effectiveness of psychotherapy with children and adolescents: A meta-analysis for clinicians. *Journal of Consulting and Clinical Psychology*, 55, 542–549.

Weisz, J. R., Weiss, B., & Langmeyer, D. B. (1987). Giving up on child psychotherapy: Who drops out? *Journal of Consulting and Clinical Psychology*, 55, 916–918.

Weisz, J. R., Weiss, B., & Langmayer, D. B. (1989). On "dropouts" and "refusers" in child psychotherapy: Reply to Garfield. *Journal of Consulting and Clinical Psychology*, 57, 170–171.

Weisz, J. R., Weiss, B., Morton, T., Granger, D., & Han, S. (1992). *Meta-analysis of psychotherapy outcome research with children and adolescents.* Unpublished manuscript, University of California, Los Angeles.

Wilson, G. T. (1985). Limitations of meta-analysis in the evaluation of the effects of psychological therapy. *Clinical Psychology Review*, 5, 35–47.

Witmer, H. L., & Keller, J. (1942). Outgrowing childhood problems: A study in the value of child guidance treatment. *Smith College Studies in Social Work*, 13, 74–90.

19

Attachments Past and Present: Implications for Therapeutic Intervention with Mother– Infant Dyads

Martha Farrell Erickson, Jon Korfmacher, and Byron R. Egeland
Project STEEP, University of Minnesota, Minneapolis

Theory and research on parent–infant attachment and on adult representations of past relationships suggest several possible themes and approaches for therapeutic intervention with parent–infant dyads. These include strategies aimed at increasing the parent's insight into the connection between past and present relationships and enhancing the parent's understanding of the child's needs and feelings, as well as the use of the therapeutic alliance to help the parent move toward more positive working models of self and others. Project STEEP (Steps Toward Effective, Enjoyable Parenting), an ongoing study of the effectiveness of preventive intervention with new mothers, provides one model of therapeutic intervention built on attachment theory and research.

In the past two decades an extensive body of research on parent–child attachment has grown from the theoretical work of John Bowlby and the pioneering assessment strategies developed by Mary Ainsworth. As research continues to clarify the importance of early relationships to human development across the life span, practitioners and applied researchers have demonstrated an increasing interest in sorting out how attachment research can and should inform practice. To date there are more speculations than facts, more questions than answers; yet, we believe it is important to keep the dialogue going, reporting thoughts and work in progress rather than waiting for definitive answers. In that spirit, we use this paper to (a) review key concepts of attachment theory in regard to relation-

---

Reprinted with permission from *Development and Psychopathology*, 1992, Vol. 4, 495–507. Copyright © 1992 by Cambridge University Press.
This research was supported by an NIMH research grant (MH-418792). The authors would like to thank all of the mothers and infants who participated in this study.

ships past and present; (b) explore some possible implications for therapy, particularly therapeutic interventions that target the parent–infant dyad; and (c) describe therapeutic strategies we have used in the STEEP (Steps Toward Effective, Enjoyable Parenting) program as an example of an intervention that builds on attachment theory and research. The effectiveness of interventions of course must be demonstrated through careful, rigorous research, as we currently are undertaking as a part of Project STEEP at the University of Minnesota, but it also is important to identify what we already think and know, based on attachment theory and research, and describe how intervention strategies have been built on that base.

THEORETICAL FOUNDATIONS

Attachment theory was initially offered as an alternative to psychoanalytic and object relations theories. While it retains the importance of the early relationship between infant and caretaker, attachment theory is ethologically based. John Bowlby (1969, 1973, 1980) described a control system defined by infant behaviors with a set goal to keep the child comforted and protected. Infant attachment behaviors, such as seeking and maintaining proximity to the caretaker and resisting and protesting separation, were accorded by Bowlby their own motivation and importance for survival, distinct from feeding (per behavioral theory) and sex (per psychoanalytic theory). More recent formulations have downplayed the behavioral control system and have emphasized internal psychological and emotional aspects to the child–caregiver relationship (see Bretherton, 1985).

The work of Mary Ainsworth and her colleagues did much to popularize attachment theory. They and others showed both that mother–child pairs differ in the quality of their attachment relationship and that it is possible to measure and classify these differences (Ainsworth, Blehar, Waters, & Wall, 1978). More importantly, they shifted some of the attention to the other half of the dyad, demonstrating that maternal behaviors in the early months of the child's life predicted the classification of the relationship of mother and child. For instance, mothers who were sensitive and responsive in interaction with their child at 3 months were more likely to have secure relationships with their child in later months than mothers who were unresponsive or insensitive (Ainsworth et al., 1978; Clarke-Stewart, 1973).

Longitudinal studies, such as the Minnesota Mother–Child Project, have demonstrated the importance of this early relationship for future social development. For example, the project demonstrated that attachment classification at 12 months of age can predict teacher ratings, behavior problems, and quality of relationships with peers in preschool (Erickson, Egeland, & Sroufe, 1985). Attachment also has been shown to relate to social competency in a summer day camp setting when children are 10 and 11 years old (Sroufe & Jacobvitz, 1989; Urban, Carlson,

Egeland, & Sroufe, 1991). These and other studies suggest that the early relationship generalizes to influence relationships with people other than the caretaker.

Although there are no longitudinal data past childhood, several retrospective reports suggest that the first early relationship remains influential in adulthood. Different research groups (Fonagy, Steele, & Steele, 1991; Main & Goldwyn, 1984, in press; Ricks, 1985) have shown that a mother's memory of her early relationship with her own caretaker relates to the classification status of her relationship with her child in the strange situation. For example, Main and Goldwyn (in press) coded responses parents made to the Adult Attachment Interview (AAI), an open-ended interview designed to elicit emotional reactions to early parent–child memories. Parents who could describe positive and negative aspects of their childhood coherently and without defensiveness most often had secure relationships with their children. Parents who were either dismissing of or preoccupied with early attachment issues and who lacked the ability to integrate specific memories with global conceptualization of their early attachments were more likely to have insecure relationships with their children.

Other indirect evidence supports the lasting influence of past attachment relationships. A study on the antecedents of child maltreatment demonstrates that many of the parents who abuse or neglect their children were themselves victims of abuse or neglect when young (Egeland, Jacobvitz, & Sroufe, 1988). Although there has been little research on how early attachment relationships correlate with adult–adult relationships, the preceding studies do suggest that early attachment patterns remain influential across the life span and that this influence may cross generational boundaries. The quality of care a parent receives as a child seems to influence the way the parent responds to and raises his or her own child.

This has been the briefest of introductions to attachment research. Other sources present a more comprehensive picture (Belsky & Nezworski, 1988; Bretherton & Waters, 1985; Greenberg, Cicchetti, & Cummings, 1990), but even with this short overview one can see the distinct waves of influence across the movement's history. The first wave, ushered in by Bowlby, set up many of the underlying normative assumptions upon which the theory operates. The second wave, led by Ainsworth, demonstrated the possibility of capturing and studying the qualitative differences in attachment relationships across individuals. The third wave has focused on the internal mechanisms of the theory and how the attachment relationship manages to extend its influence across time and across generations.

EXPLAINING THE LINK BETWEEN PAST AND
PRESENT ATTACHMENTS

Within this most recent wave, however, there is little consensus on how exactly to explain the intergenerational link between the early childhood experience of parents and the subsequent relationship with their own children. A reasonable assumption, seen in various manifestations, is that an individual internalizes qualitative aspects of the past primary relationship and that these internalizations result in expectations which in turn influence and guide one's behavior in future relationships, including parent–child relationships.

Bowlby (1969, 1973, 1980), borrowing elements from both psychoanalytic and cybernetic theory, described "internal working models" that develop from early attachment experiences. Based on the quality of care received, through continuous experiences with primary attachment figures, an individual builds expectations or models of the world, of relationships, and of people, including the self. These models organize perception and guide behavior in new situations, becoming more stable and more likely to operate outside of conscious awareness as the individual develops.

Selma Fraiberg, an infant mental health specialist, remained closer to psychoanalytic theory in conceptualization than Bowlby did. In her poetic formulation (Fraiberg, Adelson, & Shapiro, 1974), every parent is haunted by "ghosts in the nursery," old spirits "from the unremembered past" that lurk within the parent unseen and influence the caretaking of his or her child. As a clinician, Fraiberg and her writings were mostly concerned with unhealthy or imperiled dyads. Parents are influenced by repressed, unresolved conflicts, where affective components of stressful and anxious childhood experiences with their own caregiver are defended against and unremembered, condemning the parent to repeat these experiences with his or her own child. Similar to Bowlby's formulation, there is a strong emphasis on unconscious processes. Although Fraiberg did not use the term *internal working model*, there are many parallels between her work and attachment theory, and certainly clinical extensions of attachment research have borrowed heavily from Fraiberg (see Lieberman, 1991).

There are several difficulties in discussing internal working models. One is deciding exactly what the cognitive processes are models of, that is, whether they are generalized models of the world, models of relationships, or models of individuals (including self models). The term and concept is general enough to accommodate all these interpretations singly or in different combinations. The type of model may also change as the child develops cognitively and has wider experiences. For example, in the first years of life it may be fair to think of models of the parent–child relationship and of the self as one and the same (Bretherton, 1985; Main, Kaplan, & Cassidy, 1985). As the child develops and forms a separate self-identity, however, separate but complementary models of the self and of significant others may in turn develop.

Sroufe and Fleeson (1986) posited that one may internalize both sides of a relationship, but it is the internalization of the parent's side that influences future parenting. Others place more emphasis on self models. Epstein (1980), although not usually considered an attachment researcher, developed a hierarchical model of self systems that arise from early interaction with caretakers. As Ricks (1985) demonstrated, there are many similarities between the representational models created by Epstein and Bowlby. Constructivists influenced by attachment theory, such as Guidano and Liotti (1985), also proposed models of personality and psychopathology based on emerging theories of self that arise from attachment experiences.

Another difficulty is that the actual cognitive construction of the models is unknown. Although reference to internal working models has become very popular in recent writings on attachment (including this article), the nuts-and-bolts aspect of the models has been mostly neglected. It is possible, as Bretherton (1985) theorized, that models are constructed as a hierarchy of schemas, much like Epstein postulated for self schemas. Basic levels, housing event schemas of specific attachment experiences, are subsumed by higher levels containing increasingly general schemas involving the attachment figure and the self.

Internal working models may also fit constructive theories of cognition, although the orientation proposed by Guidano and Liotti (1985) is too complex to allow an adequate overview here. Briefly, the mind "constructs" models of reality that regulate how we perceive incoming information. The cognitive structures exist in the interaction between "tacit," unconscious levels of processing and "explicit," surface levels of thought representation (such as beliefs or problem-solving behavior). Tacit levels provide a scaffolding or apperceptive framework that constrains explicit processes and conscious attention. They occur very early in life and guide the cognitions of young children before the more abstract explicit processes can develop. For example, in the creation of self-knowledge, Guidano and Liotti (1985) proposed that tacit self-conceptions are created out of early interactions with the caregiver.

In summary, the particulars of relationship models so far remain unknown. Both the specific cognitive mechanism and the conceptualization are debatable, as are many other issues. It is, for example, uncertain whether there are specific internal working models from each important, formative relationship or a generalized model that is pushed and pulled by various relationship experiences, or whether in fact both types of models exist, perhaps in a hierarchical order.

Although these and other questions remain about internal working models, one may still use the term if sufficiently cautious. For the purposes of this paper and this task, it seems best to look at the internal working model as a useful metaphor. If it serves a purpose in our therapeutic work, such as allowing us to conceptualize change and take the steps to enact change, then we can use the term at the very least as a label for the cognitive processes. In other words, we accept that something is *there*, even if we cannot at this time operationalize whatever is there with the optimal clarity science demands. Evidence for the existence of an actual mental model that agrees in structure with any present or future theories perhaps will come with continued longitudinal and intervention work.

IMPLICATIONS FOR THERAPY

Discussions of the therapeutic implications of attachment theory have been popular but also divergent, loosely structured, and largely speculative. There has been little published discourse on how to measure in a clinical setting the past or present attachment relationships of a client and make use of what is discovered about the attachment relationship. For instance, both the Strange Situation, a popular assessment for young children in a research setting (see Ainsworth et al., 1978) and the AAI are sufficiently accurate when aggregated across a group but are not appropriate for defining individual clients or dyads without other convergent information.

A volume devoted to clinical implications of attachment (Belsky & Nezworski, 1988) produces only a few direct examples of therapeutic "work" around attachment issues. A computer search of peer-reviewed journals reveals an eclectic assortment of attachment-related therapy articles, including group therapy (Schain, 1989), family therapy (Byng-Hall, 1990), and short-term adult work (West, Sheldon, & Reiffer, 1989). Cicchetti, Toth, and Bush (1988) offer recommendations for intervention addressing attachment issues for a number of conditions or disorders of development, including Down syndrome, failure-to-thrive, childhood depression, offspring of depressed parents, and child maltreatment. Most practitioners who make use of attachment theory in their clinical work seem to apply it in idiosyncratic ways. There are no widely accepted guidelines or methods, although the approach pioneered by Selma Fraiberg (Fraiberg et al., 1974), working with parents and infants together and using the infant as the transference object instead of the therapist (see Lieberman, 1991), continues to exert considerable influence.

Although the specific intervention discussed later in this article was a multiservice program, an underlying goal was to focus on the feelings, attitudes, and representations of the parent–child relationship. If we accept the internal working model (whatever it may be) as an important element of the attachment relationship for both parent and child, then the model is a logical place to begin. One assumption for therapeutic work may therefore be stated: To change a maladaptive attachment relationship between parent and child, one must ultimately change the internal working model of the relationship for both parent and child.

In addition, one may hypothesize from the evidence previously discussed that the parent's behavior significantly influences both the child's external attachment behavior patterns and internal conceptualization of the relationship. An assumption that arises from this is that by influencing the parent's internal working model, one may also influence the child's developing model. The parent in this sense is considered the "gatekeeper" to the attachment relationship. Even if the problem is defined in terms of the parent–child relationship and even if the parent and infant are seen together, the parent becomes the primary target for therapeutic intervention.

By calling the cognitions a "working model," Bowlby was highlighting their dynamic, constructive nature and their susceptibility to modification and adaptation. He was, however, at the same time somewhat pessimistic about the extent of change possible once the models stabilize in adulthood (Bowlby, 1980). A single experience is not likely to alter the model in any significant way. In fact, the opposite may be more likely to occur: that the model will "do" something to the event, or the individual's perception of the event, to bring it in line with the individual's conceptualization. In Piagetian terms, the model will assimilate the event to its own structure rather than accommodate its structure to include the event.

We know, however, that accommodation can occur. Egeland et al. (1988), for example, demonstrated that early childhood history is not destiny. Mothers who had a childhood history of maltreatment but were not classified as abusive toward their own children usually had either a positive, additional relationship with an adult as a child or a significant, positive relationship in their adult life. A plausible interpretation of this finding is that a long-term, significant relationship was able to challenge a maladaptive working model brought on by the abuse and change it for the better. One form of long-term relationship shown to be helpful was a therapeutic relationship. With this sample, time spent in therapy separated the parents of abused and nonabused children. Even though it was not in itself an intervention study and never defined the mothers' internal working models, its findings do suggest that successful therapeutic intervention can change a parent's maladaptive working model, with the results seen in improved parent–child relationships.

Some intervention studies have demonstrated success at improving parent–child relationships through psychotherapy. The Clinical Infant Development Program (Greenspan et al., 1987), using the therapeutic model developed by Fraiberg, demonstrated that psychodynamic parent–infant therapy could be used successfully with even "difficult to reach," multiproblem families. Unfortunately, results were presented mostly in case-study format, making an overall evaluation of the program difficult. More recently, Lieberman, Weston, and Pawl (1991), using Fraiberg's parent–infant psychotherapy, demonstrated changes in attachment relationship from insecure to secure, along with increases in maternal sensitivity, in a moderately sized sample of economically disadvantaged mothers and infants through year-long intervention with the parent–child dyad. Another intervention study (Cramer et al., 1990), using short-term psychotherapy (either a psychodynamic or guidance model), also showed successful results with 38 parent–infant dyads referred to a child guidance clinic for a variety of functional and behavioral disorders.

For purposes of simplification, there are two general ways in which we feel psychotherapy might be expected to affect the parent's internal working model (and in turn, hopefully, the parent–child relationship). Borrowing from psychodynamic formulations of therapy, the role of insight is considered vital to intervention. Whether individually with the parent or as part of direct work with the current parent–child relationship, the therapist attempts to make parents aware of how conceptions and assumptions based on early childhood experiences influence how they raise their own child. By making the unconscious conscious, by facilitating the parent's thinking about what was previously automatic or unthought, the therapist hopes to give the parent greater control over actions. Change comes out of this process—understanding and accepting how the internal working model has been operating and influencing behavior will serve a curative function.

One of the contributions of attachment theory to psychotherapy is an emphasis on emotional "understanding" in addition to the cognitive realizations implicit in insight work. Both the intervention work of Fraiberg (Fraiberg et al., 1974) and the research of Main (e.g., Main et al., 1985) demonstrated the role that avoidance and disconnection of feelings from early event memories may play in unhealthy parent–child relationships. Mothers in Main et al. (1985) who dismissed the pain connected to negative childhood memories, remaining affectively neutral or flat when describing these memories, were likely to have insecure relationships with their children. However, as the case studies presented in Fraiberg et al. (1974) demonstrated, the disturbed emotional relationship between mother and child can change when the mother allows herself to experience and remember emotions previously blocked. The feelings released through this exploration can become incorporated into the mother's working model.

The other way in which the intervention may alter the parent's model of relationships is through the therapeutic relationship itself. This last point comes from the acknowledgment that a psychotherapeutic relationship is more than a business relationship or service transaction. In presenting their emotional, cognitive, and behavioral difficulties, clients open themselves up to the therapist. Disclosure such as this requires much trust in the therapist, and for this reason the working alliance has a great deal of intimacy. Moving beyond simple affiliation, it is an important, primary relationship for the client. The client for this reason will react to it based on his or her model or representation of intimate, primary relationships.

The therapist, in short, cannot escape the client's working model. We assume that the parent will unconsciously attempt to assimilate the therapeutic relationship into his or her model of relationships and lay upon it the expectations and assumptions built from earlier attachment experiences. As often pointed out (e.g., West et al., 1989), this bears some similarities to the psychoanalytic concept of transference. Unlike transference, however, the therapist does not present himself or herself as a blank slate upon which the client's relationship with the parent is projected, although the possibility that the therapist may become a parent figure to some clients is not ruled out.

A close relationship, then, allows the therapist an opportunity or opening for change. When the therapeutic relationship is subsumed into the working model, the relationship can be utilized from within. The therapist maintains a healthy, supportive alliance with the parent, proving to the parent that such relationships are possible. The parent also will begin to see himself or herself as someone who deserves support and attention and, by extension, will see his or her child as deserving the same (Lieberman, 1991). In this way, a good, positive therapeutic alliance will necessarily challenge a maladaptive working model. Instead of the attempted assimilation of the relationship to the model occurring, the relationship becomes a powerful enough condition to force accommodation of the model. This is what French and Alexander (1946) label the "corrective emotional experience," and Lieberman a "corrective attachment experience."

The therapeutic alliance, then, serves a dual purpose. The building and maintenance of a positive therapeutic relationship is important to engage in insight work. Borrowing a term Ainsworth used to describe the parent–child relationship, Bowlby (1985) wrote of the client using the therapist as a "secure base" to explore uncomfortable and challenging ideas, feelings, and memories without fear of rejection and criticism. Yet, the actual building of the relationship in itself and the challenge to the parent's model that such building entails is much of the therapeutic work. The client makes use of the alliance to explore his or her models and to have maladaptive models corrected. The relationship, in short, becomes both the means and the end of the therapeutic process.

In the remainder of this article, we discuss some specific ways in which these concepts from attachment theory have been translated into intervention strategies. Keep in mind that while these strategies are logically derived and theory-driven, they are not yet "proven" approaches. We share them as work-in-progress, part of a comprehensive preventive intervention program currently being evaluated in a controlled study at the University of Minnesota. (This 5-year evaluation study was initiated in 1987 with funding from the National Institute of Mental Health.) We have only begun to examine to what extent, and for whom, the STEEP program has been effective. Even when all the data are analyzed, we will not know the relative impact of specific techniques used within this broad program. Our belief is that it would be fruitless to try to attribute effects to one particular aspect of the program, and, in fact, we believe that the different components of the program all may be necessary, working together in a way that creates a whole greater than the sum of its parts.

FROM THEORY TO PRACTICE: THE STEEP PROGRAM

The STEEP program was designed to promote healthy parent–infant relationships and prevent social and emotional problems among children born to first-time mothers who are at risk for parenting problems due to poverty, youth, lack of education, social isolation, and stressful life circumstances. The program begins with home visits initiated during the second trimester of pregnancy, with a focus on helping mothers prepare for the baby's arrival, in terms of both planning for the baby's needs and dealing with the mother's own feelings and expectations about parenthood. Home visits continue every other week until the child's first birthday, and are tailored to the unique needs, strengths, and interests of each family. Also, about the time the babies are born, approximately eight mothers with due dates within a few weeks of each other are brought together for group sessions, which also continue biweekly until the child is 1 year old. In an effort to build trust and ensure continuity of service, the group is led by the same staff person who conducts the home visits. Through demonstration, discussion, and participatory activities, the facilitator provides information about child development and works with the mothers to discover what they know about their child and their relationships. Following an hour of parent–infant activities and a social time for mothers (with a free meal), the mothers have time for mutual support and discussion of their own emotional issues regarding relationships, personal growth, education and work, and general life management.

While the STEEP program certainly can be used with families with more than one child (and, in fact, has been in some community applications of the program), we chose to target first-time mothers in the original implementation and program evaluation, Project STEEP. As described elsewhere (Egeland & Erickson, 1990), we see the time just around the birth of the first child as a special window of opportunity to have an impact on the prospective mother's view of herself, her child, and their relationship. Recruitment of primiparous women during pregnancy allows for a completely proactive approach before the mother can in any way feel that she has "failed" at parenting. Thus, it is a good time to build on the mother's desire to be a good parent and to foster or support her belief that she can be one. Furthermore, the transition to parenthood is a time of dramatic change and usually anxiety, which in our experience creates a certain receptivity to intervention. We generally have found women relatively open to our offer to support and encourage them as they approach the great new adventure of parenthood. Finally, we find that the early weeks of parenting trigger a wide range of emotions that provide good material for therapeutic intervention. While we know of no formal comparative analysis, it seems that memories of childhood may be more accessible to the mother during this time when she is confronted with the needs of her new baby. That notion also has been suggested by Fonagy et al. (1991) in their study examining concordance and discordance between maternal representations of attachment during pregnancy and the mother's subsequent attachment with her infant. Specifically, they identified a small group of mothers whose responses to the AAI were classified as insecure but who later were observed to have a secure attachment with their child. They hypothesized that for those mothers the transition to parenthood may have led to a positive alteration in their mental structure. The impact of parenthood on a mother's access to memories, and her patterns of thought with respect to those memories, is an interesting question for further research.

Toward Insight and Understanding

As discussed earlier, a primary therapeutic goal is to make the unconscious conscious, specifically promoting the client's recognition and understanding of how early experiences influence current thoughts, feelings, and behavior. This involves both a cognitive awareness and a deeper emotional understanding of the links between past and present. In the case of the STEEP intervention, this goal relates primarily to how the parent's early experiences influence his or her interactions with the baby; however, also relevant is the way the parent relates to significant others and deals with other issues in daily life, because those behaviors have at least an indirect impact on the parent–child relationship.

There are several ways in which we have worked to facilitate insight and understanding in the STEEP program, seizing the opportunity presented by the new experience of caring for an infant and finding a new sense of identity as a parent. First of all, we recognize the infant as a trigger for old feelings and we explicitly encourage the mother to link the baby's apparent experience to her own early memories. For example, we might say, "Isn't it amazing how relieved and relaxed your baby seems when you pick her up? Does holding your baby ever make you remember (or wonder) about what it was like for you when you were little and needed someone to hold you?" Or we might draw upon our own experience and comment, "Sometimes when I need to care for my child I find myself just wishing that someone would care for me that way too. Do you have those feelings sometimes, too?"

For many parents, the demands of caring for a new baby may trigger their own feelings of sadness, loss, and anger because they have never really felt cared for. In our experience, some parents will (if given permission and acceptance from the facilitator and/or other group members) acknowledge some resentment that they are expected to respond to their baby in a way that no one ever did for them— really a kind of jealousy or rivalry with the baby. Bringing such emotions into conscious awareness can be the first step toward letting go of those feelings so that they do not interfere with the parent's ability to respond to the baby.

For some parents, the group is a good place to examine memories from their own childhood, facilitated by the discovery that others have had similar experiences and feelings. In one activity, we put out on a table an array of messages that we might have heard from our parents (in words or actions) when we were growing up. Each mother chooses the messages that she remembers hearing or writes her own on blank cards. The facilitator then encourages mothers to remember and talk about how it felt to experience those messages—good, bad, and everything in between. This can be a painful process, but a very useful one for tapping into emotional memories. Next, the mothers are asked to choose messages they wish they had heard in their childhood. Then they are asked to think about which messages they want to pass on to their own child, tearing up the painful ones and keeping the positive ones. At that point in the exercise, mothers and babies move into a free play time, with the mothers urged to practice communicating those positive messages to their babies through words and behavior.

Accessing the feelings of sadness, loss, and anger from their own childhood can be useful tools for helping a parent to see things from the baby's perspective: "If I still feel sad that no one came to me when I cried, I can imagine how my baby feels when he doesn't get the attention he needs." But it seems to us that the intervention process may work in the opposite direction as well. That is, by engaging parents in exercises that promote seeing things from the baby's view, we may help parents retrieve their own suppressed or repressed feelings and recognize the legitimacy of their own emotional needs. We have employed several strategies aimed at promoting the parent's ability to see things from the child's perspective. One technique is "talking for" the baby. For example, when we see a baby pushing the bottle away as the mother insists on feeding her, we may say in a small voice, "Hey, Mom, I've had enough for now." (After several months of speaking for the babies, we began to notice some mothers doing the same with each other's babies—a good sign that they were in a perspective-taking frame of mind.) Another strategy that mothers and other family members reported really made them stop and think (and sometimes cry) was writing letters to the parents from the baby. One letter from an 8-month-old who always wanted Mom in sight said, "You are the most important thing in my life right now. . . . I'd crawl for miles on my hands and knees just to see your face. . . . Sometimes even just hearing your voice is enough to make me feel okay." Finally, we also have made extensive use of videotaping and guided viewing as a way of promoting perspective-taking. During group or home visit, we often videotape parents and babies in a variety of play, feeding, and childcare situations. We then watch the tape with the parent, commenting and questioning in a manner that encourages them to discover what the baby is experiencing and communicating. We might say, "Look at that expression on his face. I wonder what he was feeling then." Or perhaps we would comment, "You knew just what she needed there. How did you know?" This strategy seems useful not only for promoting perspective-taking, but also as a way of helping parents discover and articulate the meaning of their infant's cues and signals.

(As noted before, sensitivity to baby's cues is a major predictor of secure attachment.)

Having at least an indirect bearing on the parent–child relationship is the parent's awareness and understanding of how their early experience influences their response to other life situations. For example, many of the mothers in the STEEP program have learned to play the part of victim in their relationships with others, particularly their male partners. Within the framework of attachment theory, we would say that their internal working models are of others as controlling, rejecting, and hurtful and their reciprocal model of self is as unworthy of care and unable to solicit it. Certainly such relationships can have an impact on the parent's emotional capacity to care for the baby, not to mention the direct impact that witnessing a victim–victimizer relationship between parents can have on the child's development. We have found group sessions to be an especially effective place to address these issues. A mother who has those difficulties in her own life often will seem quite skilled at seeing victimization of others and solving problems about how to change those patterns. It is not long before others in the group point out that she needs to look at her own life, too. In a recent conversation among several women who were just completing the STEEP program, a mother said that one of the most important aspects of the program was discovering that other mothers were struggling with the same issues in their relationships. She went on to say that helping to figure out their problems helped her to figure out her own. It is important to note, though, that recognition of the issues and thinking about how to deal with them are only first steps in the process. Realistically, behavioral change comes much more slowly, and we can only hope that the cognitive and emotional changes will lead to real change in the way these mothers function in their primary relationships. In a few cases we have observed fairly dramatic change, whereas in other cases we hold onto the hope that our program has at least planted a seed for later change.

Therapeutic Relationship as a Pathway to New Models

As discussed earlier, attachment theory would lead us to view the therapeutic relationship between the STEEP facilitator and the mother as a major pathway to new ways of thinking and feeling about self, others, and relationships—new internal working models, in theoretical terms. There are several ways in which the STEEP program tries to help the mothers experience a new way of being in a relationship, in the hope that this will be a step toward generalized change in working models and therefore in the mothers' relationship behavior.

The first and most basic principle is to be consistent and predictable with the mother, carefully following through on what we say we will do with and for the mother. This is easy to say, but sometimes hard to do. It means that, from the very beginning, we must promise no more than we can deliver—even though it is tempting to overpromise in the early stages as a way of trying to entice the mother to engage in the program. It also means that we must always show up when we say we will, even though a mother herself may fail appointments or not be ready when the van picks her up for group. As a policy, we keep going back for a mother, assuming that she will keep her commitment to the program, unless she specifically tells us that she does not want to participate. In other words, we do not drop a mother from the program because of failed appointments. Some mothers have told us that this was their first experience with someone who "hung in there" with them, and some even have admitted later that they "tested" their facilitator early in the program to see what she would do. In one mother's words, "She was the first person who ever thought I could come through."

A second way in which we try to modify working models is by identifying and affirming strengths in both mother and baby. This is not a matter of praising what the mother does; in fact, we have a concern that praise may foster a dependence on external judgments rather than encouraging a mother's self-evaluation and affirmation. Thus, we try to question and comment in a manner that nudges the mother to identify and build on her own—and her baby's—strengths and positive qualities. Guided viewing of her own videotapes, as described earlier, is a useful tool in this process. Likewise, in regard to other aspects of the mother's life, we might say, "You must feel really good about how you dealt with that problem," rather than, "You did a great job."

Empowerment is an underlying theme throughout the STEEP program, and this also can be considered within the framework of internal working models. One of the challenges for STEEP facilitators is to avoid disempowering the mother by doing things for her when she could do them herself. It is easy to feel overwhelmed by the challenges the families face and to want to jump in and solve things for them; however, that can send a clear message to a parent that they are incompetent and powerless—often a message that they have heard in various ways since early childhood. So, for example, rather than making a phone call to connect a mother with a needed resource, we might ask her what she needs in order to make that call. For some mothers, being given a pocket directory of local resources is sufficient. Others may want to role-play how to ask for what they need and how to proceed if they are given the runaround or get bogged down in red tape. (Advocacy in the human service arena to promote more user-friendly services is sometimes the STEEP facilitator's role as well.)

At the heart of good relationships is good communication; thus, communication is an important tool in the therapeutic relationship aimed at modifying working models. Careful listening, reflecting feelings, and giving clear "I" messages can be steps toward helping a mother find new ways of interacting. It can be a major discovery to find that someone can disagree with you or dislike what you say or do, yet still care about you and work through the relationship. It may, for example, be important for a mother to be told honestly that the facilitator feels frustrated and disappointed when the mother is not home at the time of a home visit appointment, and yet not be discarded as a failure or a "bad person." This relates to the important distinction between labeling the behavior and labeling the person, something we hope parents will learn in regard to their child's behavior as well.

Finally, another strategy employed in the STEEP program is to explicitly name the patterns we see a mother using in her relationship with the facilitator and to explore how those patterns evolved in the context of her other relationships. (This requires a high level of trust and would not be done until we already had built a strong alliance with the mother.) For example, many mothers in the STEEP program fall easily into "all or nothing" thinking and may characterize someone as all good or all bad depending on what that person has just done. She may do this with the facilitator, viewing the facilitator as wonderful when things are going smoothly and then rejecting the facilitator if he or she perhaps probes too deeply or confronts a particularly difficult area in the mother's life. The facilitator might say, "Last week you thought I was great, but now that I've done something you don't like, you think I'm terrible."

During group sessions, we also talk specifically about defense mechanisms and how we all use them to protect ourselves from difficult, painful feelings. By sharing some of our own experiences and acknowledging that defense mechanisms serve an important function, we can then move into examining ways that they also can interfere with our own well-being and our relationships with our children and significant others. We also can explore how those defenses developed in the context of our early relationships. For one mother, it was an important discovery to see how she displaced her anger onto her son when her boyfriend treated her badly. As she talked about specific episodes from her own childhood, she could begin to understand why she learned to displace her anger in a home where it was dangerous to express it directly. Hopefully, this will be a step toward changing this pattern in her new family.

Evaluating the Effectiveness of Project STEEP

A rigorous evaluation of the STEEP program, funded by the National Institute of Mental Health, currently is nearing completion. Beginning in 1987, we recruited a sample of 154 primiparous women through obstetric clinics during the second trimester of pregnancy. All of the women were low-income, had no more than a high school education, and were at least 17 years of age. The women were randomly assigned to treatment or control groups, with 74 participating in the STEEP program and the other 80 being in the control group. A variety of assessments were administered during pregnancy, at the completion of the program when the babies were 1 year old, and again at 19 and 24 months. Although data analysis is still under way, preliminary findings suggest that the program was effective in promoting some of the hoped-for changes discussed in this article. For example, STEEP participants demonstrated better understanding of their babies' needs than did the control group, and they were judged to provide a more appropriately stimulating and organized home environment for their child. Mothers in the intervention group also reported fewer depressive symptoms and less anxiety, and they demonstrated better life management skills than mothers in the control group.

We had hoped to find a higher proportion of securely attached children in the intervention group than in the control group, but that has not been the case. We did, however, identify a trend for STEEP participants to move toward a more secure relationship during the second year of life, whereas control group members showed movement in the opposite direction. Ongoing analyses will examine these findings more closely and will also attempt to identify factors that account for differences between participants who show good progress and those who do not. Given the complexity of the parent–child relationship and other aspects of the family's life and circumstances, such research does not lend itself to simple analysis and easy answers.

SUMMARY

Attachment theory, particularly the concepts of internal working models as mediators of behavior, suggests several directions for therapy with mother–infant dyads. A growing body of research has begun to identify important links between attachments past and present, and a meaningful discussion of implications for practice has begun to unfold. Our program, STEEP, is one example of how key concepts from attachment theory and research have guided the development of a therapeutic preventive intervention with new parents, many of whom have a history of attachment problems and various kinds of maltreatment in their own childhood. While the strategies described here are being evaluated as part of a large-scale longitudinal study of the effectiveness of the STEEP program, we will not know with much certainty to what extent change is a result of specific techniques within the broad model. Nevertheless, we believe it is important to inform others of the strategies we have employed based on our current understanding of attachment theory and research. It is our hope that these ideas will help to shape other interventions and research that further explores the role of internal working models in parent–child relationships, how those models appear to change, and how they may influence or mediate parental behavior.

REFERENCES

Ainsworth, M. D. S., Blehar, M. C., Waters, E., & Wall, S. (1978). *Patterns of attachment: A psychological study of the strange situation.* Hillsdale, NJ: Erlbaum.

Belsky, J., & Nezworski, T. (Eds.). (1988). *Clinical implications of attachment.* Hillsdale, NJ: Erlbaum.

Bowlby, J. (1969). *Attachment and loss. Vol. 1: Attachment.* New York: Basic Books.

Bowlby, J. (1973). *Attachment and loss. Vol. 2: Separation.* New York: Basic Books.

Bowlby, J. (1980). *Attachment and loss. Vol. 3: Loss, sadness, & depression.* New York: Basic Books.

Bowlby, J. (1985). The role of childhood experience in cognitive disturbance. In M. J. Mahoney & A. Freeman (Eds.), *Cognitive and psychotherapy* (pp. 181–200). New York: Plenum.

Bretherton, I. (1985). Attachment theory: Retrospect and prospect. In I. Bretherton & E. Waters (Eds.), *Growing points of attachment theory and research. Monographs of the Society for Research in Child Development*, 50(1–2, Serial No. 209), 3–35.

Bretherton, I., & Waters, E. (Eds.). (1985). *Growing points of attachment theory and research. Monographs of the Society for Research in Child Development*, 50(1–2, Serial No. 209), 3–35.

Byng-Hall, J. (1990). Attachment theory and family therapy: A clinical view. *Infant Mental Health Journal*, 11, 228–237.

Cicchetti, D., Toth, S., & Bush, M. (1988). Developmental psychopathology and incompetence in childhood: Suggestions for intervention. In B. Lahey & A. Kazdin (Eds.), *Advances in clinical child psychology* (pp. 1–71). New York: Plenum.

Clarke-Stewart, K. A. (1973). Interactions between mothers and their young children: Characteristics and consequences. *Monographs of the Society for Research in Child Development*, 38(15–6, Serial No. 153).

Cramer, B., Robert-Tissot, C., Stern, D. N., Serpa-Rusconi, S., De Muralt, M., Besson, G., Palacio-Espasa, F., Bachmann, J., Knauer, D., Berney, C., D'Arcus, U. (1990). Outcome evaluation in brief mother–infant psychotherapy: A preliminary report. *Infant Mental Health Journal*, 11, 278–300.

Egeland, B., & Erickson, M. F. (1990, December). Rising above the past: Strategies for helping new mothers break the cycle of abuse and neglect. *Zero to Three*, 11(2), 29–35.

Egeland, B., Jacobvitz, D., & Sroufe, L. A. (1988). Breaking the cycle of abuse. *Child Development*, 59, 1080–1088.

Epstein, S. (1980). The self-concept: A review and the proposal of an integrated theory of personality. In E. Staub (Ed.), *Personality: Basic aspects and current research* (pp. 82–131). Englewood Cliffs, NJ: Prentice-Hall.

Erickson, M. F., Egeland, B., & Sroufe, L. A. (1985). The relationship between quality of attachment and behavior problems in preschool in a high-risk sample. In I. Bretherton & E. Waters (Eds.), *Growing points of attachment theory and research. Monographs of the Society for Research in Child Development*, 50(1–2, Serial No. 209), 147–186.

Fonagy, P., Steele, H., & Steele, M. (1991). Maternal representations of attachment during pregnancy predict the organization of infant–mother attachment at one year of age. *Child Development*, 62, 891–905.

Fraiberg, S., Adelson, E., & Shapiro, V. (1974). Ghosts in the nursery: A psychoanalytic approach to the problems of impaired infant–mother relationships. *Journal of the American Academy of Child Psychiatry*, 13, 387–421.

French, T. M., & Alexander, F. (1946). *Psychoanalytic therapy: Principles and application.* New York: Ronald Press.

Greenberg, M., Cicchetti, D., & Cummings, E. M. (Eds.). (1990). *Attachment in the pre-school years: Theory, research, and intervention.* Chicago: University of Chicago Press.

Greenspan, S., Wieder, S., Lieberman, A. F., Nover, R., Robinson, M., & Lourie, R. (Eds.). (1987). *Infants in multirisk families.* Madison, CT: International Universities Press.

Guidano, V. F., & Liotti, G. (1985). A constructivistic foundation for cognitive therapy. In M. J. Mahoney & A. Freeman (Eds.), *Cognition and psychotherapy* (pp. 101–142). New York: Plenum.

Lieberman, A. F. (1991). Attachment theory and infant–parent psychotherapy: Some conceptual, clinical, and research considerations. In D. Cicchetti & S. L. Toth (Eds.), *Rochester Symposium on Developmental Psychopathology, Vol. 3: Models and integrations* (pp. 261–287). Rochester, NY: University of Rochester Press.

Lieberman, A. F., Weston, D., & Pawl, J. H. (1991). Preventive intervention and outcome with anxiously attached dyads. *Child Development, 62,* 199–209.

Main, M., & Goldwyn, R. (1984). Predicting rejection of her infant from mother's representation of her own experience: Implication for the abused–abusing intergenerational cycle. *Child Abuse and Neglect, 8,* 203–217.

Main, M., & Goldwyn, R. (in press). Interview-based adult attachment classification related to infant–mother and infant–father attachment. *Developmental Psychology.*

Main, M., Kaplan, N., & Cassidy, J. (1985). Security in infancy, childhood, and adulthood: A move to the level of representation. In I. Bretherton & E. Waters (Eds.), *Growing points of attachment theory and research. Monographs of the Society for Research in Child Development, 50*(1–2, Serial No. 209), 66–104.

Ricks, M. H. (1985). The social transmission of parental behavior: Attachment across generations. In I. Bretherton & E. Waters (Eds.), *Growing points of attachment theory and research. Monographs of the Society for Research in Child Development, 50*(1–2, Serial No. 209), 211–227.

Schain, J. (1989). The new infant research: Some implications for group therapy. *Group, 13,* 112–121.

Sroufe, L. A., & Fleeson, J. (1986). Attachment and the construction of relationships. In W. Hartup & Z. Rubin (Eds.), *Relationships and development* (pp. 51–71). Hillsdale, NJ: Erlbaum.

Sroufe, L. A., & Jacobvitz, D. (1989). Diverging pathways, developmental transformations, multiple etiologies and the problem of continuity in development. *Human Development, 32,* 196–203.

Urban, J., Carlson, E., Egeland, B., & Sroufe, L. A. (1991). Patterns of individual adaptation across childhood. *Development and Psychopathology, 4,* 445–460.

West, M., Sheldon, A., & Reiffer, L. (1989). Attachment theory and brief psychotherapy: Applying current research to clinical interventions. *Canadian Journal of Psychiatry, 34,* 369–375.

20

Pharmacokinetically Designed Double-Blind Placebo-Controlled Study of Nortriptyline in 6- to 12-Year-Olds with Major Depressive Disorder

Barbara Geller

Washington University School of Medicine, St. Louis, Missouri

Thomas B. Cooper

Columbia University College of Physicians and Surgeons, New York City

Donna L. Graham, Harriet H. Fetner,

Frederick A. Marsteller, and Janet M. Wells,

University of South Carolina, Columbia

A random assignment, double-blind, placebo-controlled study of nortriptyline in 50 prepubertal 6- to 12-year-olds with Research Diagnostic Criteria and DSM-III major depressive disorder was performed. The protocol included a 2-week placebo wash-out phase and an 8-week double-blind, placebo-controlled phase with weekly plasma level monitoring. Active subjects had their plasma level pharmacokinetically placed at 80 ± 20 ng/ml by using previously developed tables to determine the starting dose from a plasma level 24 hours after a single dose administered at baseline. The mean plasma level was 89.9 ng/ml. The study population was severely depressed; had a chronic, unremitting course of long duration before the study;

Reprinted with permission from *Journal of the American Academy of Child and Adolescent Psychiatry*, 1992, Vol. 31(1), 34–44. Copyright © 1992 by the American Academy of Child and Adolescent Psychiatry.

This study was supported by Grant R01 MH40273 to Dr. Geller from the National Institute of Mental Health. Preliminary results were presented at the National Institute of Mental Health New Clinical Drug Evaluation Unit meeting in Key Biscayne, Florida, May 1988. Early findings were also presented at the Annual Meeting of the American Psychiatric Association, May 1988, Montreal, Canada. Pamelor and placebo capsules were supplied by Sandoz Corporation, Hanover, New Jersey.

had a high percentage of family histories with affective disorder, alco-holism, and suicidality; and had a high rate of comorbidity. None of the subjects had ever received tricyclic antidepressants before this study. There was a poor rate of response in both treatment groups (30.8% active, 16.7% placebo). Active subjects did not evidence the anticholinergic side effects reported in adult samples. The implica-tions of these findings for future pharmacotherapy studies of depressed children are discussed.

The hypothesis of the similarity of major depressive disorder (MDD) across age groups was the basis for investigating tricyclic antidepressants (TCAs) in children (Puig-Antich, 1980). However, in contrast to the numerous controlled studies of TCAs for MDD in older populations (Klein et al., 1980), systematic investigation in children has been limited (Puig-Antich et al., 1987). In spite of multiple, open, uncontrolled trials of TCAs that supported the feasibility of safe administration (Puig-Antich, 1980), there is only one double-blind, placebo-controlled study of a TCA in children that included a statistically adequate number of subjects, that used diagnostic criteria and assessment instruments comparable to those used in studies of MDD in adults, and that monitored plasma levels (Puig-Antich et al., 1987).

In that study, Puig-Antich et al. (1987) investigated a fixed dose of imipramine (IMI) and found that 68% of the placebo group and 56% of the active group responded. The authors also reported that subjects in the active group who had higher IMI plasma levels had a much higher rate of response. Based on their findings, Puig-Antich et al. (1987) recommended that future studies of TCAs in children with MDD include an initial placebo wash-out phase and suggested the usefulness of controlling for plasma level range. Therefore, to optimize response, it seemed imperative for future studies of TCAs in children to include a placebo wash-out phase and to use a "fixed plasma level" design.

This article reports on the first double-blind, placebo-controlled study of nor-triptyline (NT) in pediatric MDD. It is also the first investigation to use a phar-macokinetically derived fixed plasma level design.

The reasons for the selection of NT as the TCA to investigate were the following: feasibility studies supported the hypothesis that the pharmacology and side effects of NT would be similar in children and adults. These studies showed the following: a suggested relationship between NT steady-state plasma levels and response to determine the fixed plasma level range to use in the double-blind, placebo-controlled study (Geller et al., 1986); a plasma level drawn 24 hours after a single dose predicted steady-state plasma levels and, therefore, permitted one-step dosage adjustment in a fixed plasma level design (Geller et al., 1985a); the stability of plasma levels over time (i.e., lack of enzyme induction or other mechanisms that might reduce plasma levels) so that a fixed plasma level could be expected to be maintained for the duration of a double-blind, placebo-controlled study (Geller et al., 1985b); and a sufficiently long half-life so that medication would not need to be administered during school hours (Geller et al., 1987) (i.e., once or twice daily dosing would be sufficient). Because there were reports of significantly less cardiovascular problems with NT than with IMI in geriatric subjects (Thayssen et al., 1981), it was reasoned that NT might also be safer in this respect in the pediatric age group. In adults, NT is less sedative than IMI or amitriptyline (Baldessarini, 1977), an especially important issue in school-aged children. The pilot data suggested that children had low sedative, orthostatic, and anticholinergic effects and had similar EKG changes to those in adults (Geller et al., 1983, 1985c). Finally, the reported higher ratio of desmethylimipramine (DMI) to IMI in children (Puig-Antich et al., 1979) suggested the possibility that the adrenergic metabolite DMI might be responsible for the response to IMI in open, uncontrolled studies. Therefore, investigating another adrenergic drug, i.e., NT, seemed reasonable.

This study was performed from January 1985 to January 1988.

METHOD

Subjects

Subjects were prepubertal boys and girls 6 to 12 years old who met *DSM-III* (American Psychiatric Association, 1980) criteria and Research Diagnostic Criteria (RDC) (Spitzer et al., 1978) for MDD and who were nondelusional. The authors included the RDC in order to provide comparability to the Puig-Antich et al. (1987) study. The *DSM-III* criteria were included to permit comparison with concurrent and future studies. Delusional children were excluded based on data from studies of delusional adults that suggested that adult delusional depressives responded poorly to conventional doses of tricyclic antidepressants (Quitkin et al., 1978). Subjects needed to have a score ≥ 40 (moderate-severe illness) on the unrevised Children's Depression Rating Scale (CDRS) (Poznanski et al., 1979) and to have a duration of illness ≥ 2 months. Although *DSM-III* listed a duration of 2 weeks, a duration of at least 2 months was used because it was thought that it was unreasonable to place children on a 10-week protocol if the duration of illness was only 2 weeks. Exclusion criteria were an IQ < 75; Tanner Stage of pubertal development $\geq$ III (Katchadourian, 1977); autism; childhood onset pervasive developmental disorder; other major medical, psychiatric, or neurological illness; psychotropic drugs in the past month; substance use disorders; or excessive fear of venipuncture.

All subjects were outpatients. Families of suicidal children were instructed in home and school precautions (Geller and Carr, 1988). Parents signed an informed consent form, and children signed an assent form before the study.

Psychiatric Assessments

To provide comparability with data from adult studies, *DSM-III* MDD was established using the pediatric version of the Schizophrenia and Affective Disorders Schedule, i.e., the 1978 version of the Kiddie Schizophrenia and Affective Disorders Schedule–Present State (Kiddie-SADS-P) (Puig-Antich and Chambers, 1978). The Kiddie-SADS-P had good agreement with clinical diagnoses (Apter et al., 1989). Severity was measured with the pediatric version of the Hamilton Depression Rating Scale, the Children's Depression Rating Scale (CDRS) (Poznanski et al., 1979). Poznanski et al. (1979) reported that the CDRS had good agreement with clinician's ratings of the severity of depression. The 1986 version of the Kiddie-SADS-P and the revised CDRS were not available when this study began. The Kiddie-SADS-P was administered at baseline and at Week 10 to the mother and child, separately, in that order. Summary ratings on the Kiddie-SADS-P are based on the rater's best judgement. A rating of $\geqslant 4$ (moderate-severe) was needed on the MDD criteria items. Separation anxiety and antisocial behavior were established if these items, on the Kiddie-SADS, had a score of $\geqslant 4$. The Kiddie-SADS-P was modified to include a duration of illness item of 5 or more years because of the chronicity of MDD in the subjects in the pilot data. The CDRS was administered to the mother and child, together, at baseline and at Weeks 1 to 10, similar to its use during the preliminary study (Geller et al., 1986). The Kiddie Global Assessment Scale (GAS) (Puig-Antich and Chambers, 1978), the pediatric version of the GAS used in adults, was completed at baseline and Week 10. The Kiddie GAS is the last page of the Kiddie-SADS-P. Socioeconomic status was calculated from the Hollingshead and Redlich Two Factor Index (Hollingshead and Redlich, 1958). The Family History–Research Diagnostic Criteria (FH-RDC) (Andreasen et al., 1977) data were obtained for first- and second-degree relatives and from the mother by raters who were not blind to the subjects' diagnoses. Other assessment instruments obtained at baseline and Week 10 were the Child Behavior Checklist–Teacher's Report Form and Parent Version (CBCL-T and CBCL-P) (Achenbach and Edelbrock, 1983); the Psychosocial Schedule for School-Age Children (PSS) (Puig-Antich and Andrews, 1978); and the Children's Depression Inventory (CDI) (Kovacs, 1980–81).

To reduce bias based on rater expectation, different raters gave the baseline and Week 10 instruments than those who gave Weeks 1 to 9. Raters had established interrater reliability before the start of the study, and all raters were blind.

Training of Raters

Raters on the Kiddie-SADS rated taped interviews of mothers and children with MDD, then rated while observing a trained rater administer the interview, and then interviewed while a trained rater observed. Each of the above three types of training was completed when five consecutive interviews with virtual agreement on MDD and comorbidity items had been obtained. Training on the FH-RDC included observing a trained rater and then interviewing while a trained rater observed. Training was complete when there were five consecutive interviews with virtual agreement on diagnostic categories. A consensus conference was held after each study interview with another trained rater to establish final diagnoses. The interclass correlations on the CDRS from 131 ratings by four raters in four pairings was 0.97 (0.96–0.98, 95% confidence interval) for the total score and a range of 0.87 to 1.00 on individual items. The intraclass correlation of 42 paired ratings on the Asberg side effects scale was 0.99 (0.97–0.99, 95% confidence interval), with a range of 0.80 to 1.00 for individual items.

Side Effects and Plasma Level Assessments

Side effects were measured at baseline and weeks 1 to 10 with the Asberg Side Effects Scale (Asberg et al., 1970), which was developed for use in NT studies in adults. The authors had previously modified the scale for use in the pediatric age group (Geller et al., 1986). It was given to the mother and child together. A standard 12 lead EKG was obtained, with Lead II also run at 50 mm/s to enhance interval measurements, at baseline, and at weeks 1 to 10. EKG tracings were interpreted by the study pediatrician in consultation with a pediatric cardiologist. The Food and Drug Administration approved EKG guidelines for this study were P-R interval ≤ 0.21 seconds, QRS interval $\leq$ the baseline QRS value plus 30%, and heart rate < 130 beats per minute. Blood pressure measurement was obtained from the right arm with a Tycos pediatric or adult cuff, depending on the subject's upper arm width (Nelson et al., 1979), recumbent, and after standing for 1 minute at baseline and at weeks 1 to 10. At baseline, good physical health was determined from a physical examination, complete blood count, sequential multichannel autoanalyzer-18, urinalysis, sedimentation rate, medical history, and previous pediatric records. Nortriptyline and total, cis- and trans-10-hydroxy nortriptyline (10-OH-NT) plasma levels were assayed at Nathan Kline Institute by methods previously described (Cooper et al., 1976; Geller et al., 1985a; Suckow and Cooper, 1982). Samples were blindly coded before shipment. Plasma samples were obtained and assayed on all subjects at Weeks 1 to 10.

Study Design and Outcome Criteria

The study included a 2-week, single-blind, placebo, wash-out phase followed by an 8-week, random assignment, double-blind, placebo-controlled phase. Each week subjects were seen for 30 minutes between 4:00 to 6:00 P.M. During this visit, the CDRS, side effects scale, EKG, blood pressure, and plasma level were obtained.

Subjects were categorized as placebo wash-out responders if at the end of Week 1 or Week 2 they had a CDRS score of ≤ 25. At the end of the 8-week, double-blind, placebo-controlled phase (Week 10 of protocol), subjects were categorical responders if they had a CDRS score of ≤ 20 and had items scores of 1 or 2 on all of the *DSM-III* criteria items for MDD on the Kiddie-SADS-P. A higher cut-off point on the CDRS at the end of the placebo wash-out phase was used because it was reasoned that if a subject was already this well at the end of 1 or 2 weeks of placebo they were likely to go on to full response.

Study Medication and Compliance

Plasma levels were used as a compliance check (and as a correct dispensing check) in addition to pill counts. Study medication for each day of the 10-week protocol consisted of eight capsules. Four capsules were taken at 7:00 A.M. and four at 7:00 P.M. to permit plasma levels and EKGs to be taken 9 to 11 hours (between 4:00 and 6:00 P.M.) after the 7:00 A.M. dose. Each dose consisted of two capsules the size of 25-mg Pamelor® (nortriptyline) and two the size of 10-mg Pamelor® to comprise a total daily dose range of zero (i.e., all capsules contained placebo) to a maximum of 70 mg per dose and a maximum total daily dose of 140 mg. Study medication was dispensed from the research pharmacy in the Childhood Affective Disorders Program unit and was packaged in commercially available pillminders (Geller and Fetner, 1989). Each pillminder contained a slot for each day of the week. Two pillminders were dispensed, one for the 7:00 A.M. doses and one for the 7:00 P.M. doses. Each slot contained the four capsules for that dose. The slots were sealed with waterproof tape. At the time the parents gave the medication to the child, they removed the tape and the child received the entire contents of the slot. Parents were instructed to return the pillminders at each visit so that a pill count could be taken, and a new set of pillminders would then be dispensed. Subjects were discontinued for noncompliance if they missed more than two doses in the same week.

Establishing the Fixed Plasma Level

At baseline, subjects received a single dose of NT, and a plasma level was obtained 24 hours later. Subjects 6 to 9 years old were given a 25-mg dose and 10- to 12-year-olds were given a 50-mg dose at 9:00 A.M. (Geller et al., 1985a). Subjects randomized to the active group began receiving a dose needed to obtain steady-state plasma levels of 60 to 100 ng/ml. The starting dose was determined from the previously reported tables of 24-hour plasma levels versus starting dose in children (Geller et al., 1985a). The 60 to 100 ng/ml range was determined from the authors' previous study that suggested that optimal response occurred at steady-state NT plasma levels of 60 to 100 ng/ml (Geller et al., 1986). To achieve these levels, the authors anticipated a total daily dose range of 10 to 140 mg because of the wide variation in the rate of metabolism of NT (Geller et al., 1985b).

Statistical Methods

Interrater reliability for the CDRS and Asberg side effects scale was assessed using intraclass correlations. Categorical data were analyzed using Yates' corrected chi-square statistic, except when expected cell frequencies were < 5, Fisher's Exact test was used. Treatment means for continuous variables were compared using t-tests. Spearman's rank correlations were used to analyze the associations between continuous study variables. Differences between treatment groups in the amount of change of continuous variables were analyzed using repeated measures multivariate analyses of variance. Post-hoc, the associations between study variables and response were analyzed using stepwise multiple linear regression when the outcome measure was final, and CDRS or GAS scores and stepwise linear logistic regression when the outcome measure was categorical response. Significance level for all analyses was $p < 0.05$.

Recruitment of Subjects

Referrals were sought via presentations to school personnel, media feature stories on the Childhood Affective Disorders Program, talks at community mental health centers, and a newspaper ad.

RESULTS

Seventy-two subjects were entered: 12 responded during the placebo washout phase, 50 (26 active, 24 placebo) completed the double-blind, placebo-controlled phase, and 10 were discontinued during the double-blind, placebo-controlled phase (three for noncompliance, three families changed their minds, one family unexpectedly moved out-of-state, one child developed severe pneumonia, one subject needed emergency hospitalization for escalating suicidal behavior, and one for other administrative reasons). Five of the noncompleters were assigned to active drug and five to placebo. There were no statistically significant differences between the demographic characteristics of the placebo wash-out responder, drop-out, or completer groups, nor were there any clinical picture differences observed.

The study was designed for $N = 60$ (30 active, 30 placebo) based on an expected rate of response, after the placebo wash-out period, of 75% to active and 40% to placebo (Fleiss, 1981). Data analysis (see below) at the completion of 50 subjects showed no significant difference in the response rate between the active and placebo groups. Using the multinomial distribution statistic the probability of finding a statistical difference in response rate had the $N = 60$ been completed was only two in 1,000 (Bradley et al., 1968). Therefore, the study was stopped at an $N = 50$.

Subject Recruitment

There were 375 telephone inquiries, and 307 of these were seen at a screening interview. Most of the 152 subjects who were not invited to enter the study after the screening interview were excluded because the child had only dysthymia or had only dysphoric mood. Therefore, the excluded children did not meet the *DSM-III* syndromal criteria and/or did not meet the study severity criteria. The remainder were excluded because of medical reasons. The study was offered to 155 families of whom 108 signed the consent form. Of these 108, 28 were excluded at the baseline evaluation (did not fit *DSM-III* criteria or medical exclusions), eight changed their minds, and 72 entered the study. The 50 subjects who completed the protocol were referred from the following sources: 21 from school personnel, 12 from the newspaper ad, six from media feature stories, five from a relative or friend of another subject's family, five from community mental health professionals, and one from a family practice physician.

Subject Characteristics

Table 1 shows the demographic characteristics of the active and placebo groups. The subjects were largely male; Causasian; middle- and upper-class; suburban; and from small, intact families. The socioeconomic status data in the IMI study, using the four-point Hollingshead and Redlich scale, was presented as mean scores of the active and placebo groups. From these scores, the authors calculated a total sample mean, 32.2 ± 14.8, which corresponds to middle class III. Ten per-

TABLE 1
Demographic Characteristics

	Total (N = 50)	Active (N = 26)	Placebo (N = 24)	Statistic[a]	p
Mean Age ± SD (yrs)	9.7 ± 1.6	9.7 ± 1.6	9.7 ± 1.7	0.05[b]	0.96
Range	(6.0–12.0)	(6.0–12.0)	(6.0–12.0)		
Sex (%)				0.24[c]	0.62
Male	70.0	73.1	66.7		
Female	30.0	26.9	33.3		
Socioeconomic status class (%)[d]				9.73[c]	0.05
I	14.0	3.9	25.0		
II	24.0	38.5	8.3		
III	28.0	30.8	25.0		
IV	30.0	23.1	37.5		
V	4.0	3.9	4.2		
Ethnicity (%)				F.E.[e]	1.00
Caucasian	90.0	88.5	91.7		
Other	10.0	11.5	8.3		
Residence (%)				3.11[c]	0.21
Urban	8.0	3.9	12.5		
Suburban	62.0	73.1	50.0		
Rural	30.0	23.1	37.5		
Family structure (%)				2.31[c]	0.32
Both parents	66.0	57.7	75.0		
Only mother	18.0	19.2	16.7		
Other	16.0	23.1	8.3		
Mean number ± SD in household					
Siblings	1.5 ± 1.2	1.4 ± 0.9	1.7 ± 1.5	−0.91[b]	0.37
Siblings plus parent(s)	3.4 ± 1.4	3.2 ± 0.9	3.7 ± 1.8	−1.16[b]	0.25
Other	0.1 ± 0.5	0.1 ± 0.4	0.2 ± 0.5	−1.03[b]	0.31

[a] Comparison between active and placebo groups.
[b] t-test.
[c] Chi-square.
[d] Hollingshead and Redlich Two Factor Index — Class I is upper class.
[e] Fisher's Exact test.

cent of the NT subjects were non-Caucasian compared with 58% of the IMI study (Puig-Antich et al., 1987).

Tables 2 and 3 show that the two treatment groups did not significantly differ on baseline severity, duration of MDD before the study, or diagnostic categories. They were similar on the percentage of subjects with the family history categories except for a significantly higher percentage of subjects with mania in the first- and second-degree relatives in the placebo group. Both groups were chronically ill (94% had MDD for over 2 years and 50% for over 5 years); were severely depressed; had high endogenicity and melancholia; and had a high percentage of subjects with family histories of mood disorders, alcoholism, and suicidality in first- and second-degree relatives. The baseline mean KGAS corresponded to the description on the KGAS scale of "major impairment" in functioning, including behaviors resulting from depressive symptomatology, such as social withdrawal and poor academic performance. Ninety-four percent of the subjects had moderate-severe academic performance problems, and 80.0% had moderate-severe social withdrawal. The onset of symptoms and signs of separation anxiety occurred after the onset of MDD in 83.3% of the subjects, and all of the onset of the symptoms and signs of antisocial behaviors occurred after the onset of MDD. The 18% of subjects with antisocial behaviors were similar to the 18% in the Puig-Antich et al. (1987) study of IMI (calculated from their Table 3). The 1978 version of the Kiddie-SADS (Puig-Antich and Chambers, 1978) used in this study did not include assessments of other comorbid diagnoses. The Kiddie-SADS-P does not assess two of the symptoms of atypical depression, i.e., rejection sensitivity and leaden paralysis (Stewart et al., 1989). Atypical depressive symptoms (Stewart et al., 1989) that are assessed by the Kiddie-SADS include mood reactivity, hyperphagia, and hypersomnia. No subject had a rating ≥ 4 on all of these items. Only 2% had a reactive mood. Twenty-eight percent had hyperphagia, and 16% had hypersomnia.

Outcome

There was no significant difference in categorical response rate using the criteria described above in the Methods section (30.8% active vs. 16.7% placebo; $\chi^2 = 1.36$, $df = 1$, $p = 0.24$). There was also no significant difference using the Puig-Antich et al. (1987) categorical response criteria that were scores of 1 or 2 on the Kiddie-SADS-P dysphoria and anhedonia items (46.2% active vs. 58.3% placebo; $\chi^2 = 0.74$, $df = 1$, $p = 0.39$). The latter is similar to the 56% active vs. 68% placebo reported for the IMI study.

There were also no significant differences in outcome using the continuous measures (Table 3). The nine-item Kiddie-SADS score was calculated to provide comparability of data to the Puig-Antich et al. (1987) study. The mean Week 10

TABLE 2

Duration of Illness, Diagnostic Characteristics, and Family History Categories

	Total (N = 50)	Active (N = 26)	Placebo (N = 24)	Statistic[a]	p
Duration of MDD before the study (%)					
Less than 1 year	4.0	0.0	8.3	3.93[b]	0.23
1 to 2 years	2.0	0.0	4.2		
2 to 5 years	44.0	42.3	45.8		
More than 5 years	50.0	57.7	41.7		
Diagnostic characteristics (%)					
RDC endogenous	96.0	100.0	91.7	F.E.[c]	0.23
DSM-III melancholia	74.0	73.1	75.0	0.02[b]	0.88
Separation anxiety	84.0	80.8	87.5	F.E.	0.70
Antisocial behavior	18.0	15.4	20.8	F.E.	0.72
Subjects (%) with family history categories[d]					
Affective disorder	87.2	79.2	95.7	F.E.	0.19
Alcoholism	74.5	66.7	82.6	1.57[b]	0.21
Suicide attempts	40.4	33.3	47.8	1.02[b]	0.31
Suicide completion	10.6	8.3	13.0	F.E.	0.67
Mania	34.0	16.7	52.2	6.60[b]	0.01

[a] Comparison between active and placebo groups.
[b] Chi-square.
[c] Fisher's Exact test.
[d] Based on an N = 47 because three subjects were adopted. Family history categories include first- and second-degree relatives.

TABLE 3
Pre-and Postprotocol Continuous Outcome Measures

	Total (N = 50)	Active (N = 26)	Placebo (N = 24)	Statistic[a]	p
CDRS					
Baseline	49.8 ± 4.4	49.9 ± 4.2	49.6 ± 4.6	0.21	0.84
Week 10	32.5 ± 10.6	32.9 ± 11.4	32.0 ± 9.8	0.29	0.77
Change score[b]		0.2 ± 11.6	-0.6 ± 8.6	0.24	0.81
Change (%)		-33.6 ± 23.5	-35.8 ± 16.7	0.37	0.71
KGAS					
Baseline	37.9 ± 3.3	37.7 ± 3.5	38.2 ± 3.0	-0.59	0.56
Week 10	59.0 ± 19.2	57.8 ± 20.7	60.3 ± 17.6	-0.46	0.65
Change Score[b]		81.0 ± 20.5	83.9 ± 17.6	-0.53	0.60
Change (%)		55.7 ± 59.1	59.2 ± 49.9	-0.23	0.82
9-Item KSADS					
Baseline	3.94 ± 0.46	3.98 ± 0.42	3.89 ± 0.50	0.69	0.49
Week 10	2.31 ± 0.80	2.41 ± 0.81	2.20 ± 0.78	0.95	0.34
Change score[b]		0.95 ± 0.88	0.76 ± 0.69	0.81	0.42
Change (%)		-37.90 ± 23.90	-44.00 ± 16.50	1.04	0.30

Note: CDRS = Children's Depression Rating Scale; KGAS = Kiddy Global Assessment Scale; K-SADS = Kiddie Schizophrenia and Affective Disorders Schedule.

[a] *t*-test comparison of treatment groups (active vs. placebo).

[b] Regressed change score = Postscore − [($r \times \frac{SD\ post}{SD\ pre}$) (Prescore)], "where r is the Pearson correlation coefficient between the prescores and postscores in the sample" (Puig-Antich et al., 1979).

KGAS score corresponds to clinically significant psychopathology. The final KGAS score in the Puig-Antich et al. (1987) study, 62.0 ± 16.7, was similar to the final KGAS in the NT study.

Multivariate analyses of variance were performed to test the effects of time (baseline vs. Week 10), treatment group (active vs. placebo), and the interaction between time and treatment on the CBCL-T, CBCL-P, PSS, and CDI. There were no significant effects of active drug on the CBCL-T or CBCL-P total behavior scores, individual behavioral scales, or on the social competency scores on the CBCL-P, nor were there any significant effects of active drug on the PSS relationship scales or the summary CDI scores. Detailed secondary analyses of these scales will be presented elsewhere.

Nortriptyline and 10-Hydroxy Nortriptyline Plasma Levels

Table 4 shows that all subjects receiving active medication achieved steady-state plasma levels in the fixed plasma level range of the study and that there was no significant difference between the responders and nonresponders. The NT plasma levels were the means from Weeks 6 to 9 when subjects were on a stable dose, i.e., after any initial adjustments to obtain plasma levels between 60 to 100 ng/ml. Twenty-two of the 26 subjects receiving active drug had all four samples taken, two subjects had two samplings, and two subjects had three samplings because of poor blood draw. All subjects receiving placebo had zero plasma levels. Table 4 also shows that there were no significant differences between the responder and nonresponder steady-state mean plasma levels from Weeks 6 to 9 of total, cis- or trans-10-hydroxy NT. There were no significant correlations between Week 10 CDRS scores and mean NT or mean total, trans- or cis-10-OH-NT plasma levels (Spearman's $r = 0.05, 0.23, 0.10$, and 0.30, respectively).

Dose of NT

Table 4 shows that there was no significant difference tween the total mean ± SD total daily dose of NT between the responders and nonresponders, even though the design of the protocol was fixed plasma level and not fixed dose. Because many pediatric medications, including IMI, are prescribed on a mg/kg basis (Puig-Antich et al., 1987), the authors also calculated the mean ± SD total daily mg/kg dose of the responders ($1.44 ± 0.65$) and nonresponders ($1.50 ± 0.72$). There was no significant difference ($t = 0.19$, $p = 0.85$). The range of the total daily dose was within the 10 to 140 mg amount that was planned for in the dispensing procedures. The total daily dose did not significantly correlate with Week 10 CDRS scores (Spearman's $r = 0.20$, $p = 0.34$).

TABLE 4

Mean ± SD Nortriptyline and 10-OH-Nortriptyline Plasma Levels (ng/ml) and Total Daily Dose (mg)

	Total (N = 26)	Responders (N = 8)	Nonresponders (N = 18)	r^a	p
NT plasma level	89.9 ± 14.4	87.3 ± 11.8	91.1 ± 15.5	0.61	0.55
Total 10-OH-NT	208.8 ± 145.6	186.9 ± 166.9	218.5 ± 139.1	0.50	0.62
Trans-10-OH-NT	178.9 ± 131.1	162.4 ± 153.7	186.2 ± 123.9	0.42	0.68
Cis-10-OH-NT	29.9 ± 19.3	24.5 ± 15.7	32.3 ± 20.6	0.96	0.35
Total daily dose	54.2 ± 24.0	47.5 ± 22.7	57.2 ± 24.5	0.95	0.35

[a] t-test comparison of responders to nonresponders.

EKG Monitoring

Because of the known wide intrasubject variability in children's heart rates with respect to time of day and to response to environmental stimuli (Nelson et al., 1979), pre- and post-treatment EKG measures were compared in the following manner to have multiple baseline and protocol time points: We used the means of values of Weeks 1 and 2, when all subjects were on placebo, as the baseline measure and the means of Weeks 6 to 9, when all active subjects were at a stable dose, as the treatment measure. These EKG tracings, as noted above, were obtained 9 to 11 hours after the 7:00 A.M. dose (4:00–6:00 P.M.) and at the same time as the plasma level samples were drawn. Table 5 shows that there was a significant increase in heart rate in the active group. This mean increase of 17 beats per minute did not produce clinical symptoms.

Blood Pressure Measures

Blood pressures (BPs) in children have the same intrasubject variability as noted above for heart rate (Nelson et al., 1979). For this reason, the same multiple time points were used for analysis of the BP data as were used for the EKG measures. In children, there is sometimes a dimming of the diastolic BP before disappearance. As is customary, the average of the dimmed diastolic BP and the disappearance of the diastolic BP were used as the value (Nelson et al., 1979). Also, in children, the diastolic BP can sometimes be heard at 20 mm. This occurred seven times in four subjects at Weeks 1 and 2 and twelve times in nine subjects at Weeks 6 to 9. When this occurred, an average of the subject's other diastolic values was used. Table 5 shows that the active group had significantly greater increases of standing systolic and of lying and standing diastolic BPs than the placebo group. However, these increases were 3 to 7 mm Hg and are of no known clinical significance.

Because there was a recent report of a statistically significant correlation between the orthostatic change in baseline BP and positive outcome on NT treatment in a geriatric population (Schneider et al., 1986), the authors tested for a similar relationship in the subjects in the present study. The orthostatic change at baseline in systolic BP did not significantly correlate with Week 10 CDRS scores ($r = 0.218, p = 0.284$) or with Week 10 GAS scores ($r = -0.077, p = 0.708$). The orthostatic change in diastolic BP also did not have a significant correlation with Week 10 CDRS scores ($r = -0.219, p = 0.282$) or with Week 10 GAS scores ($r = 0.235, p = 0.249$).

TABLE 5
Mean ± SD Blood Pressure and Electrocardiogram Measurements

| | Weeks 1–2[a] | | Weeks 6–9[b] | | | |
	Active (N = 26)	Placebo (N = 24)	Active (N = 26)	Placebo (N = 24)	F^c	p
Systolic BP (mm Hg)						
Lying	100.3 ± 6.1	101.2 ± 10.5	103.9 ± 7.1	102.1 ± 9.9	3.60	0.06
Standing	98.2 ± 5.7	100.4 ± 10.9	102.0 ± 5.8	101.2 ± 10.5	4.48	0.04
Diastolic BP (mm Hg)						
Lying	58.8 ± 6.8	60.1 ± 9.2	62.6 ± 7.0	57.5 ± 7.5	6.12	0.02
Standing	62.7 ± 9.2	64.1 ± 8.2	67.8 ± 7.0	63.8 ± 6.9	6.50	0.01
P-R interval (msec[d])	148.0 ± 19.0	145.0 ± 21.0	153.0 ± 16.0	146.0 ± 20.0	2.40	0.13
QRS interval (msec[d])	73.0 ± 9.0	72.0 ± 11.0	75.0 ± 6.0	72.0 ± 10.0	2.46	0.12
Heart rate (beats per minute)	80.8 ± 9.4	82.2 ± 8.2	96.8 ± 7.5	81.4 ± 8.4	92.29	0.00

[a] Mean of weeks 1 and 2 when all subjects were on placebo.
[b] Mean of weeks 6 to 9 when all active subjects were at a stable dose.
[c] Treatment × time multivariate analysis of variance.
[d] Milliseconds.

Side Effects

Table 6 presents a comparison of the modified Asberg Side Effects Scale (Geller et al., 1986) items between the two treatment groups at Weeks 1 and 2 when all subjects were on placebo and Weeks 6 to 9 when all active subjects were at a stable dose. Side effects were counted if they were rated 2, definitely present, or 3, definitely present and functional impairment. Items needed to be present for 2 consecutive weeks to ensure they were not transient effects because of subsyndromal intercurrent illnesses, which are common in pediatrics. The most common side effects reported (i.e., tiredness, sleep problems, and headaches) are all also frequent symptoms of MDD. Notably, none of the subjects had any of the anticholinergic items (i.e., dry mouth, constipation, or micturition problems), which are commonly reported in adults on TCAs.

Weight and Height

Weight and height were log transformed before analyses because of their allometric relationship. The two treatment groups did not significantly differ in mean weight (kg) or height (cm) at baseline ($t = -0.35$, $p = 0.72$ and $t = -0.58$, p

TABLE 6

Comparison of Side Effect Items (%) Between Active and Placebo Groups[a]

	Weeks 1–2[b]		Weeks 6–9[c]	
	Active ($N = 26$)	Placebo ($N = 24$)	Active ($N = 26$)	Placebo ($N = 24$)
Tired	23.1	12.5	23.1	29.2
Sleep	19.2	12.5	23.1	29.2
Headache	7.7	8.3	3.9	12.5
Vertigo	3.9		3.9	
Orthostatic				
Palpitation				
Tremor				
Perspiration				4.2
Dry mouth				
Constipation				
Micturition				

[a] Fisher's Exact tests for differences between active and placebo groups were all nonsignificant.
[b] Rating of 2 or 3 at both weeks 1 and 2, when all subjects were receiving placebo.
[c] Rating of 2 or 3 for any two consecutive weeks between weeks 6 to 9, when all active subjects were receiving a stable dose.

= 0.56, respectively). The mean percentage of change in weight from baseline to Week 10 was significantly less for the actives (2.5 ± 2.9 vs. 4.7 ± 3.1, $t = -2.59$, $p = 0.013$). The mean percentage of change in height was not significantly different ($t = 0.09$, $p = 0.93$). A repeated measures multivariate analysis of covariance of weight at baseline and Week 10, with a baseline height and change in height as covariates, was significant for a change in weight × treatment interaction ($F = 4.1$, $p = 0.049$). Height was included as a covariate; a significant change in height over the 10-week protocol was not expected.

Post-Hoc Analyses

Study variables entered were sex, age, treatment group, melancholia, separation anxiety, antisocial behavior, and the family history categories, including mania. No variable was significant for predicting final CDRS score or categorical response. Duration of illness was significant for predicting a lower GAS score ($\beta = -8.2 ± 3.6$, $R^2 = 0.097$, $p = 0.28$), but only acounted for < 10% of the variance.

COMMENT

The similar results to the Puig-Antich et al. (1987) study, in spite of the addition of a 2-week placebo, wash-out period and of controlled plasma levels, strongly suggest that other issues may be relevant in the poor response to TCAs in prepubertal children.

One of these issues is whether or not the plasma level range selected was appropriate for this population. As noted above, the range chosen was based on pilot data (Geller et al., 1986). The mean plasma level, 89.9 ng/ml, was higher than the mean level of 72 ng/ml in a similar study of NT in adults reported by Murphy et al. (1984). It may be argued that children, because of their more rapid clearance of the drug (Geller et al., 1984), might require higher doses. Before controlled studies at higher plasma levels are undertaken, however, feasibility data to demonstrate the safety and efficacy of higher NT plasma levels in open trials in 6- to 12-year-olds would be necessary. Although the early concerns about increased cardiotoxicity (Hayes et al., 1975; Winsberg et al., 1975) in children have not been supported by the authors' NT data or other placebo-controlled studies (Biederman et al., 1985; Donnelly et al., 1986), none of these reports were from subjects at higher plasma level ranges than those used in adult studies. In this regard, the recent report of three sudden, unexplained deaths in prepubertal children at what had been considered safe plasma levels of DMI suggests the need for continued caution in administering TCAs to children (Sudden Death, 1990).

The fact that NT was effective in the authors' plasma level/response study

(Geller et al., 1986) and not in the double-blind, placebo-controlled study bears comment. This issue is also relevant to the reported effectiveness of TCAs in multiple, uncontrolled studies and case reports in depressed children (Klein et al., 1980; Puig-Antich, 1980). In the NT plasma level/response study, similar to the case reports and open studies, parents and children knew they were receiving a drug that the physicians and/or investigative team considered highly likely to work, based on extrapolation from the adult literature. Parental attitudes very likely are important factors in placebo response in pediatric populations analogous, for example, to children who perform better in school when their parents wish them to (Werner et al., 1971). It is for these reasons that double-blind, placebo-controlled studies are necessary across age groups.

A further question that arises is the difference between the negative outcome in the IMI (Puig-Antich et al., 1987) and NT controlled outpatient studies and the Preskorn et al. (1987) inpatient study of IMI. Even if the Preskorn et al. (1987) inpatient study had included the number of subjects necessary for adequate power and had still shown a positive outcome, the important differences between inpatient and outpatient populations may make comparisons problematic. Recent articles on the psychosocial differences between inpatient and outpatient pediatric populations may bear on this issue (Perrin et al., 1989; Wise and Eisenberg, 1989). It is generally accepted that to be admitted as a child requires not only a diagnosis but some psychosocial situation that prevents parents from providing the adequate care at home. For example, in the NT study, families were able to provide suicidal precautions (Geller and Carr, 1988) in the home setting.

There are several pharmacological issues that may have influenced a negative response in children to TCAs. It was not for this reason that the hydroxy metabolites were measured. Because it was found that the wide interindividual variation in the rate of metabolism of NT to the two hydroxy isomers and that the preponderance of the trans-isomer were similar to that reported for adults (Bertilsson et al., 1982; Young et al., 1984; Ziegler et al., 1976), it appears less likely that this pharmacokinetic issue influenced outcome. Pharmacodynamic factors have not yet been explored, but their importance may be evidenced by the different side effect pattern noted in the prepubertal subjects. The virtual absence of anticholinergic side effects, especially of the prominent dry mouth reported in adults, may indicate age-specific differences in drug–tissue interaction. There are many analogous situations for age-specific effects of drugs used in both the pediatric and the adult age groups. Animal work also supports age-specific differences in the effects of psychoactive drugs (Rinne, 1987; Rinne et al., 1990). In this regard, the absence of a significant relationship between baseline orthostatic blood pressure and outcome, which has been reported for the elderly (Schneider et al., 1986), also suggests age-specific differences in drug action. Additional support for developmental influences on TCA-tissue interaction is the decrement in weight observed in the subjects, quite dissimilar to the weight gain problems noted in older individuals.

Because only the Puig-Antich et al. (1987) and this study have been done, the negative findings may be a cohort effect. In this regard, 33% of TCA studies in adults also did not demonstrate efficacy of the active drug (Klein et al., 1980).

Perhaps, however, the most striking difference between the Puig-Antich et al. (1987) and NT studies and those reported in the adult literatwure were the sample characteristics. The population of children who came to both studies were largely comorbid for separation anxiety and conduct-disordered features and had a severe degree of psychopathology. These two characteristics (i.e., comorbidity and severity) have been reported to predict treatment resistance in some adult samples, although not in others (Hamilton, 1979; Keller, 1990; Kupfer and Spiker, 1981; Liebowitz et al., 1990). Perhaps these characteristics also predict poor response in children. There may be a subgroup of outpatient children with MDD, who have moderate severity and little or no comorbidity, who would be responsive to TCA medications. Future studies could subtype by comorbidity and severity.

Another characteristic of the authors' study population was the unremitting chronicity of the MDD before entering the study, dissimilar to the episodic course often noted in adults (Hamilton, 1979). Unfortunately, the study did not include a lifetime assessment instrument so that "double depression" (dysthymia and MDD) might have been ascertained, an issue that has been related to chronicity in follow-up studies of adults (Keller et al., 1983). Although Kocsis et al. (1989) reported that IMI was effective for chronic double depressives, his subjects were moderately depressed (baseline GAS 56 ± 8) compared with the greater severity in the NT subjects (baseline KGAS 37.9 ± 3). There is literature from adult community samples that suggests comorbidity and severity predict chronicity (Sargeant et al., 1990). If this is also true for the childhood population, it would be consistent with the characteristics of the prepubertal subjects. Future investigations should include lifetime assessment instruments, and future study populations could be subtyped by the chronicity of the index episode.

The family history data need to be addressed from two different perspectives. One is the similarity of the high prevalence in the present study of MDD and alcoholism in the first- and second-degree relatives to that reported by Puig-Antich et al. (1989) for a sample of prepubertal children. Several other investigators have also reported that early age of onset significantly correlates with a high risk for major depression in first- and second-degree relatives (Kupfer et al., 1989; Weissman et al., 1987). Because the family history was used rather than the family study method, it has to be assumed that the prevalence may have been underestimated by as much as 40% (Andreasen et al., 1977). The second perspective addresses the issue that because the subjects were observed during an initial episode of MDD, it is not known whether their future course will be unipolar or bipolar. Theoretically, if all of the subjects had the same familial MDD as their older counterparts, they should have had a similar response to NT, if no other age-specific biological or psychosocial factors were operative. The latter situation would be analogous to the response of bacterial infections to antibiotics across age groups. Another possibility, however, is that the loaded and/or multigenerational family histories, marked psychomotor retardation, and early age of onset in the subjects were predictive of a later course of bipolarity; similar to the predictive value of these factors adolescent populations (Akiskal et al., 1983; Strober and Carlson, 1982). If the latter is the case, subjects were observed who later may go on to a bipolar course. Adults with bipolar depression have been reported to be less responsive to TCAs than unipolar depressives (Himmelhoch et al., 1982). Thus, if the subjects were experiencing bipolar depression, they could be poor responders to TCAs on that basis. To test the hypothesis that pediatric MDD subjects may have bipolar depression, the authors are conducting a controlled study of lithium for 6- to 12-year-olds with MDD and a bipolar or a loaded/multigenerational family history.

The subjects from this study are in an ongoing, controlled follow-up study that potentially can elucidate reasons for the negative NT study and can ascertain whether the NT subjects were sustaining MDD as part of a bipolar course. The follow-up study and other ongoing longitudinal studies of children with MDD (Kovacs et al., 1984a, b, 1988, 1989; Weissman et al., 1984) can provide prospective data on multiple issues including the continuity of MDD across age groups, the relationship between early onset and severity of adult episodes, the course of comorbid diagnoses, and whether children who are resistant to TCAs will respond when they have MDD episodes as adults. These studies can also provide data on childhood predictors of future bipolarity.

Because of the increasingly earlier onset of severe MDD in recent decades (Gershon et al., 1987), the high rate of adolescent suicide (Holinger and Offer, 1982; Morbidity and Mortality Weekly Report, 1985), and the substantial morbidity and poor prognosis of prepubertal MDD (Kovacs et al., 1984a, b, 1988, 1989), it seems crucial to continue studies of therapeutic interventions for MDD in children.

REFERENCES

Achenbach, T. M. & Edelbrock, C. (1983), *Manual for the Child Behavior Checklist and Revised Child Behavior Profile*. Burlington, VT, University of Vermont Department of Psychiatry.

Akiskal, H. S., Walker, P., Puzantian, V. R., King, D., Rosenthal, T. L. & Dranon, M. (1983), Bipolar outcome in the course of depressive illness. *J. Affective Disord.*, 5:115–128.

American Psychiatric Association, Committee on Nomenclature and Statistics (1980), *Diagnostic and Statistical Manual of Mental Disorders*, 3rd ed. Washington, DC: American Psychiatric Association.

Andreasen, N. C., Endicott, J., Spitzer, R. L. & Winokur, G. (1977), The family history method using diagnostic criteria: reliability and validity. *Arch. Gen. Psychiatry*, 34:1229–1235.

Apter, A., Orvaschel, H., Laseg, M., Moses, T. & Tyano, S. (1989), Psychometric properties of the K-SADS-P in an Israeli adolescent inpatient population. *J. Am. Acad. Child Adolesc. Psychiatry*, 28:61–65.

Asberg, M., Cronholm, B., Sjoqvist, F. & Tuck, D. (1970), Correlation of subjective side effects with plasma concentrations of nortriptyline. *Br. Med. J.*, 4:18–21.

Baldessarini, R. J. (1977), *Chemotherapy in Psychiatry*. Cambridge, MA: Harvard University Press.

Bertilsson, L., Mellstrom, B., Nordin, C., Silvers, B. & Sjoqvist, F. (1982), Stereo-specific hydroxylation of nortriptyline. In: *Clinical Pharmacology in Psychiatry*, eds. E. Usdin, S. Dahl & L. Gram. New York: Macmillan.

Biederman, J., Gastfriend, D., Jellinek, M. S. & Goldblatt, A. (1985), Cardiovascular effects of desipramine in children and adolescents with attention deficit disorder. *J. Pediatr.*, 106:1017–1020.

Bradley, R. A., Hunter, J. S., Kendall, D. G. & Watson, G. S. (eds.) (1968), *An Introduction to Probability Theory and Its Applications*. New York: Wiley, pp. 98–111, 114–140.

Cooper, T. B., Allen D. & Simpson, G. M. (1976), A sensitive method for the determination of amitriptyline and nortriptyline in human plasma. *Psychopharmacol. Commun.* 2:105–116.

Donnelly, M., Zametkin, A. J., Rapoport, J. L. et al. (1986), Treatment of childhood hyperactivity with desipramine: plasma drug concentration, cardiovascular effects, plasma and urinary catecholamine levels, and clinical response. *Clin. Pharmacol. Ther.*, 39:72–81.

Fleiss, J. L. (1981), *Statistical Methods for Rates and Proportions*. New York: Wiley, pp. 46, 70.

Geller, B., & Carr, L. G. (1988), Similarities and differences between adult and pediatric depression. In: *Depression and Mania: A comprehensive Textbook*, eds. A. Georgatas & R. M. Cancro. New York: Elsevier Press, pp. 565–580.

——— & Fetnerr, H. H. (1989), Use of pillminders to dispense research medication [letter]. *J. Clin. Psychopharmacol.*, 9:72–73.

——— Perel, J. M., Knitter, E. F., Lycaki, H. & Farooki, Z. Q. (1983), Nortriptyline in major depressive disorder in children: response, steady-state plasma levels, predictive kinetics, and pharmacokinetics. *Psychopharmacol. Bull.*, 19:62–64.

——— Cooper, T. B., Chestnut, E., Abel, A. S. & Anker, J. A. (1984), Nortriptyline pharmacokinetic parameters in depressed children and adolescents: preliminary data. *J. Clin. Psychopharmacol.*, 4:265–269.

——— ——— ——— Anker, J. A., Price, D. T. & Yates, E. (1985a), Child and adolescent nortriptyline single dose kinetics predict steady state plasma levels and suggested dose: preliminary data. *J. Clin. Psychopharmacol.*, 5:154–158.

—————— —————— —————— (1985b), Serial monitoring and achievement of steady state nortriptyline plasma levels in depressed children and adolescents: preliminary data. *J. Clin. Psychopharmacol.*, 5:213–216.

—————— Farooki, Z. Q., Cooper, T. B., Chestnut, E. C. & Abel, A. S. (1985c), Serial ECG measurements at controlled plasma levels of nortriptyline in depressed children. *Am. J. Psychiatry*, 142:1095–1097.

—————— Cooper, T. B., Chestnut, E. C., Anker, J. A. & Schluchter, M. D. (1986), Preliminary data on the relationship between nortriptyline plasma level and response in depressed children. *Am. J. Psychiatry*, 143:1283–1286.

—————— —————— Schluchter, M. D., Warham, J. E. & Carr, L. G. (1987), Child and adolescent nortriptyline single dose pharmacokinetic parameters: final report. *J. Clin. Psychopharmacol.*, 7:321–323.

Gershon, E. S., Hamovit, J. H., Guroff, J. J. & Nurnberger, J. I. (1987), Birth-cohort changes in manic and depressive disorders in relatives of bipolar and schizoaffective patients. *Arch. Gen. Psychiatry*, 44:314–319.

Hamilton, M. (1979), Mania and depression: classification, description, and course. In: *Psychopharmacology of Affective Disorders*, eds. E. S. Paykel & A. Coppen. New York: Oxford University Press, pp. 4–5.

Hayes, T. A., Pavitch, M. L. & Barker, E. (1975), Imipramine dosage in children: a comment on "Imipramine and electrocardiographic abnormalities in hyperactive children." *Am. J. Psychiatry*, 132:546–547.

Himmelhoch, J. M., Fuchs, C. Z. & Symons, B. J. (1982), A double-blind study of tranylcypromine treatment of major anergic depression. *J. Nerv. Ment. Dis.*, 170:628–634.

Holinger, P. C. & Offer, D. (1982), Prediction of adolescent suicide: a population model. *Am. J. Psychiatry*, 139:302–307.

Hollingshead, A. B. & Redlich, F. C. (1958), *Social Class and Mental Illness.* New York: Wiley.

Katchadourian, H. (1977), *The Biology of Adolescence.* San Francisco: W. H. Freeman and Company.

Keller, M. B., Lavori, P. W., Endicott, J., Coryell, W. & Klerman, G. L. (1983), "Double depression": Two-year follow-up. *Am. J. Psychiatry*, 140:689–694.

—————— (1990), Diagnostic and course of illness variables pertinent to refractory depression. In: *APA Annual Review of Psychiatry*, eds. A. Tasman, C. Kaufman & S. Goldfinger. Washington, DC: American Psychiatric Press, pp. 10–32.

Klein, D. F., Gittelman, R., Quitkin, F. & Rifkin, A. (1980), *Diagnosis and Drug Treatment of Psychiatric Disorders: Adults and Children.* Baltimore: Williams & Wilkins, pp. 268–408.

Kocsis, J. H., Mason, B. J., Frances, A. J., Sweeney, J., Mann, J. J. & Marin, D. (1989), Prediction of response of chronic depression to imipramine. *J. Affective Disord.*, 17:255–260.

Kovacs, M. (1980–81), Rating scales to assess depression in school age children. *Acta Paedopsychiatr.*, 46:305–315.

———— Feinberg, T. L., Crouse-Novak, M. A., Paulauskas, S. L. & Finkelstein, R. (1984a), Depressive disorders in childhood, I: a longitudinal prospective study of characteristics and recovery. *Arch. Gen. Psychiatry*, 41:229–237.

———— ———— ———— ———— Pollock, M. & Finkelstein, R. (1984b), Depressive disorders in childhood, II: a longitudinal study of the risk for a subsequent major depression. *Arch. Gen. Psychiatry*, 41:643–649.

———— Paulauskas, S., Gatsonis, C. & Richards, C. (1988), Depressive disorders in childhood, III: a longitudinal study of comorbidity with and risk for conduct disorders. *J. Affective Disord.*, 15:205–217.

———— Gatsonis, C., Paulauskas, S. L., & Richards, C. (1989), Depressive disorders in childhood, IV: a longitudinal study of comorbidity with and risk for anxiety disorders. *Arch. Gen. Psychiatry*, 46:776–782.

Kupfer, D. J., & Spiker, D. G. (1981), Refractory depression: prediction of non-response by clinical indicators. *J. Clin. Psychiatry*, 42:307–312.

———— Frank, E., Carpenter, L. L. & Neiswanger, K. (1989), Family history in recurrent depression. *J. Affective Disord.*, 17:113–119.

Liebowitz, M. R., Hollander, E., Schneier, F. et al. (1990), Anxiety and depression: discrete diagnostic entities? *J. Clin. Psychopharmacol.*, 10:61S–66S.

Morbidity and Mortality Weekly Report (1985), (Vol. 34) Atlanta, GA: U.S. Dept. of Health and Human Services, Centers for Disease Control.

Murphy, G. E., Simons, A. D., Wetzel, R. D. & Lustman, P. J. (1984), Cognitive therapy and pharmacotherapy: singly and together in the treatment of depression. *Arch. Gen. Psychiatry*, 41:33–41.

Nelson, W. E., Vaughan, V. C., McKay, R. J. & Behrman, R. E. (eds.) (1979), *Textbook of Pediatrics*. Philadelphia, PA: W. B. Saunders Company.

Perrin, J. M., Homer, C. J., Berwick, D. M., Woolf, A. D., Freeman, J. L. & Wennberg, J. E. (1989), Variations in rates of hospitalization of children in three urban communities. *N. Engl. J. Med.*, 320:1183–1187.

Poznanski, E. O., Cook, S. C. & Carroll, B. J. (1979), A depression rating scale for children. *Pediatrics*, 64:442–450.

Preskorn, S. H., Weller, E. B., Hughes, C. W., Weller, R. A. & Bolte, K. (1987), Depression in prepubertal children: dexamethasone non-suppression predicts differential response to imipramine vs. placebo. *Psychopharmacol. Bull.*, 23:128–133.

Puig-Antich, J. (1980), Affective disorders in childhood. *Psychiatr. Clin. North Am.*, 3:403–424.

———— & Andrews, E. (1978), *Psychosocial Schedule for School-Age Children 6–16*. New York: New York State Psychiatric Institute.

———— & Chambers, W. (1978), *The Schedule for Affective Disorders and Schizophrenia for School-Age Children (Kiddie-SADS)*. New York: New York State Psychiatric Institute.

———— Perel, M. M., Lupatkin, W., Chambers, W. J., Shea, C., Tabrizi, M. A. & Stiller,

R. L. (1979), Plasma levels of imipramine (IMI) and desmethylimipramine (DMI) and clinical response in prepubertal major depressive disorder: a preliminary report. *J. Am. Acad. Child Psychiatry*, 18:616–627.

–––––– Perel, J. M., Lupatkin, W. et al. (1987), Imipramine in prepubertal major depressive disorder. *Arch. Gen. Psychiatry*, 44:81–89.

–––––– Goetz, D. & Davies, M. (1989), A controlled family history study of prepubertal major depressive disorder. *Arch. Gen. Psychiatry*, 46:406–418.

Quitkin, F., Rifkin, A. & Klein, D. F. (1978), Imipramine response in deluded depressive patients. *Am. J. Psychiatry*, 135:806–811.

Rinne, J. O. (1987), Muscarinic and dopaminergic receptors in the aging human brain. *Brain Res.*, 404:162–168.

–––––– Lonnberg, P. & Marjamaki, P. (1990), Age-dependent decline in human brain dopamine D_1 and D_2 receptors. *Brain Res.*, 508:349–352.

Sargeant, J. K., Bruce, M. L., Florio, L. P. & Weissman, M. M. (1990), Factors associated with 1-year outcome of major depression in the community. *Arch. Gen. Psychiatry*, 47:519–526.

Schneider, L. S., Sloane, R. B., Staples, F. R. & Bender, M. (1986), Pretreatment orthostatic hypotension as a predictor of response to nortriptyline in geriatric depression. *J. Clin. Psychopharmacol.*, 6:172–176.

Spitzer, R. L., Endicott, J. & Robins, E. (1978), Research diagnostic criteria: rationale and reliability. *Arch. Gen. Psychiatry*, 35:773–782.

Stewart, J. W., McGrath, P. J., Quitkin, F. M., Harrison, W., Markowitz, J., Wager, S. & Leibowitz, M. R. (1989), Relevance of DSM-III depressive subtype and chronicity of antidepressant efficacy in atypical depression: differenmtial response to phenelzine, imipramine, and placebo. *Arch. Gen. Psychiatry*, 46:1080–1087.

Strober, M. & Carlson, G. (1982), Bipolar illness in adolescents with major depression-clinical, genetic, and psychopharmacologic predictors in a three- to four-year prospective follow-up investigation. *Arch. Gen. Psychiatry*, 39:549–555.

Suckow, R. F. & Cooper, T. B. (1982), Simultaneous determination of amitriptyline, nortriptyline and their respective isomeric 10-hydroxy metabolites in plasma by liquid chromatography. *J. Chromatogr.*, 230:391–400.

Sudden death in children treated with a tricyclic antidepressant (1990), *Med. Lett. Drugs Ther.*, 32:53.

Thayssen, P., Bjerre, M., Kragh-Sorensen, P., Moller, M., Petersen, O. L., Kristensen, C. B. & Gram, L. F. (1981), Cardiovascular effects of imipramine and nortriptyline in elderly patients. *Psychopharmacology*, 74:360–364.

Weissman, M. M., Leckman, J. F., Merikangas, K. R., Gammon, G. D. & Prusoff, B. A. (1984), Depression and anxiety disorders in parents and children: results from the Yale Family Study. *Arch. Gen. Psychiatry*, 41:845–852.

–––––– Gammon, G. D., John, K., Merikangas, K. R., Warner, V., Prusoff, B. A. & Sholomskas, D. (1987), Children of depressed parents: increased psychopathology and early onset of major depression. *Arch. Gen. Psychiatry*, 44:847–853.

Werner, E. E., Bierman, J. M. & French, F. E. (1971), *The children of Kauai*. Honolulu: University of Hawaii Press.

Winsberg, B., Goldstein, S., Yepes, L. & Perel, J. M. (1975), Imipramine and electrocardiographic abnormalities in hyperactive children. *Am. J. Psychiatry*, 132:542–545.

Wise, P. H. & Eisenberg, L. (1989), What do regional variations in the rates of hospitalization of children really mean? [letter] *N. Engl. J. Med.*, 320:1209–1211.

Young, R. C., Alexopoulos, G. S., Shamoian, C. A., Manley, M. W., Dhar, A. K. & Kutt, H. (1984), Plasma 10-hydroxynortriptyline in elderly depressed patients. *Clin. Pharmacol. Ther.*, 35:540–544.

Ziegler, V. E., Fuller, T. A. & Biggs, J. T. (1976), Nortriptyline and 10-hydroxynortriptyline plasma concentrations. *J. Pharm. Pharmacol.*, 28:849–850.

Part VII
PSYCHOSOCIAL ISSUES

The four papers in this section address the impacts of differing environments on social and educational outcomes. In the first paper, Lewis draws on a diverse literature to describe the origins of aggression. She explores how a variety of psychophysiological and familial factors may interact with maltreatment to lead to violence. The impact of environmental influences on aggression, including the intrauterine environment, stressful living conditions, exposure to aggressive adults, and pain and physical abuse are examined. Then the physiological and behavioral consequences of these stressors, including hormonal and neurotransmitter responses, are summarized. The author proposes that biological vulnerability to impulsivity, hypervigilance, expressive difficulties, dissociation, and stressful environments may lead to aggression. Lewis concludes by suggesting that many of these factors can be addressed in intervention studies. Only one important area of recent interest is missing from this provocative paper—the impact of violent neighborhoods and subcultures.

The second paper in this section addresses a major societal concern: academic achievement among minority youth. Steinberg, Dornbusch, and Brown present the results of a large multisite study of ethnic differences in adolescent achievement patterns. Questionnaire data on 15,000 students of diverse socioeconomic backgrounds from nine different high schools in the west and midwest were collected. Approximately 5,000 students were of minority background: African-American, Asian-American, and Hispanic.

To understand adolescent school success, the authors examined the interplay between the major contexts in which teens develop—family, peer group, and school. One critical family variable was parenting style. For all ethnic groups, authoritative parenting was associated with better adjustment across all areas (except school) than nonauthoritative homes. For school performance, however, White and Hispanic youngsters were more likely to benefit from authoritative parenting than African-American or Asian-American teenagers. There were also important ethnic differences in beliefs about the negative consequences of doing poorly in school. Peer support for academic success, highest among Asian-Americans and lowest among African-Americans, was another critical variable. With so little support for academic success among their peers, some high-achieving minority group members affiliated primarily with students from other ethnic groups. For Hispanic students, the authors hypothesize that the high level

503

of authoritarian parenting (emphasizing obedience and conformity) and low level of peer support for academics may hinder performance.

Overall, this is an impressive body of work, which enhances our thinking regarding factors influencing academic achievement among minority youth. The integrative approach to analysis can lead to ideas for intervening on multiple levels—the individual, the family, the school environment, and peer support.

In these difficult economic times, all social service programs require justification to be maintained and/or expanded. In the next article in this section, Chafel describes the issues involved in funding Head Start, one of the best-known early-childhood social programs. The basic issue presented by Chafel is whether additional money should be allocated to reach more children, or to improve upon the quality of existing services.

After providing a brief background on the program, issues such as which children should be served, at what age, and for how long are reviewed. Chafel argues that local communities need to retain options for deciding which families to serve. She also discusses issues that affect the quality of the program, such as salaries and training. These issues are relevant to many preschool programs. However, the lack of teachers specifically trained in child development and work with "troubled" families creates a burden in trying to provide a good program. Many children come to Head Start with difficulty controlling their behavior, having had less than optimal experiences as infants and toddlers. This article does not address the difficulty in dealing with these children; however, it does reiterate the need for experienced teachers. A variety of issues related to Head Start as a program for families are mentioned, including the need that many families have for full-day care. The original plan to improve the parents' lives has been overlooked in many of the programs. The author concludes with a series of recommendations aimed at prioritizing funding needs.

In the last article, Howes, Phillips, and Whitebook focus on the effects of the daycare environment. The paper elegantly demonstrates how we have moved beyond the debate on whether daycare harms children to studying the components that make for the most beneficial experience for those children and families who need day care. The authors argue that correlational studies showing that better quality is linked to more optimal outcomes is frustrating to policymakers, who need specific thresholds to set criteria for care. Thresholds for two aspects of child care are examined: adult-to-child ratio and group size. The authors examine the pathways from ratio and group size to caregiving and attachment with teachers to social competence with peers. This study supports the notion that regulatable variables do affect unregulatable variables, such as quality of care.

The subjects were 414 children, aged 14 to 54 months, enrolled in a variety of child care centers in California and Georgia. They represented the full range of social classes. A variety of measures were completed after observations of each classroom and each child for a two- to three-hour period. Observers completed the Attachment Q-set for the child's behavior with the primary teacher. Social orientation to peers and adults and play behavior with peers were rated. Classrooms were classified according to adult-child ratio, group size, appropriate caregiving, and developmentally appropriate activities. Preschool children in classrooms with the 1:8 ratio were more likely to receive caregiving rated as very good than preschool children in 1:9 classrooms (Federal standard). Children classified as secure were more likely than children classified as anxious to be enrolled in classrooms rated as good in appropriate caregiving. What appears to be a minor difference in ratios (1:8 vs. 1:9) appears to have a major impact on the quality of care provided to children. Results of this study can be used by government, families, and day care centers to provide a better quality of care to infants and preschoolers.

21

From Abuse to Violence: Psychophysiological Consequences of Maltreatment

Dorothy Otnow Lewis

New York University School of Medicine, New York City

This paper reviews the psychophysiological literature related to violent behaviors. It explores the interactions of environmental influences, pain, stressors, hormones, and neurotransmitters. It presents ways in which maltreatment in the form of abuse or neglect exacerbates preexisting psychobiological vulnerabilities. It proposes that whatever forces increase impulsivity and irritability, engender hypervigilance and paranoia, diminish judgment and verbal competence, and curtail the recognition of pain in the self and others, will enhance violence, and presents evidence that maltreatment has all of these effects.

Unlike other species such as rodents, strains of which have been bred for aggressiveness (Ebert, 1973; Lagerspetz and Lagerspetz, 1971), no particular ethnic, racial, or religious group has shown itself to be innately or enduringly more aggressive than any other (although from time to time throughout history, the people of one country or another have attempted to so distinguish themselves). The social and biological sciences have come to recognize that probably the most important influences on the development of violent behavior are environmental or experiential. Although violence does not invariably beget violence (Widom, 1989), there is abundant evidence that a history of maltreatment is often associated with aggressive behaviors. From conception onwards, the ways in which living creatures are treated affect the ways in which they treat others of their species.

Reprinted with permission from *Journal of the American Academy of Child and Adolescent Psychiatry*, 1992, Vol. 31(3), 383–391. Copyright © 1992 by the American Academy of Child and Adolescent Psychiatry.

Just how abusive treatment engenders aggression is not yet entirely understood. The purpose of this paper is to explore some of the most important psychobiological consequences of maltreatment in animals and humans and how they may contribute to aggression.

Aggression in animals and humans is not identical. Animal behavior tends to fall into two categories: affective and predatory (Flynn et al., 1970). Predatory aggression is accomplished with little autonomic activation; it involves carefully stalking and quickly subduing the prey in the interest of providing fast food. Affective aggression, on the other hand, calls forth intense autonomic activation and includes among other behaviors intramale, fear-induced, and irritable aggression.

The nature of human aggression is not easily classified. The behaviors of Jack the Ripper and John D. Rockefeller have both been considered aggressive. For purposes of this discussion, human aggression or violence will be used simply to denote recurrent behaviors intended to cause pain, damage, or destruction to another person. It will not be used as a synonym for ambitiousness or assertiveness.

ENVIRONMENTAL INFLUENCES ON AGGRESSION

Intrauterine Environment

The very position in utero of animals within a litter has been found to influence behavior. Female mice that develop in utero between two males are more aggressive after birth than those positioned between other females (vom Saal, 1984). Thus, animals from the same litter who have shared the same uterus at the same time have not had identical prenatal environments. Maternal stress during pregnancy has also been shown to affect the behavior of offspring (vom Saal, 1984) long after delivery.

In humans, there is strong evidence that different kinds of noxious prenatal influences ranging from minor viral infections to maternal anxiety and psychological stress have been associated with childhood maladaptation (Pasamanick, 1956, 1961; Rutter, 1970; Stott, 1973; Stott and Latchford, 1976). The adverse effects of maternal alcoholism and other substances on fetal development and on subsequent postnatal social and intellectual functioning are well documented. The exposure of the fetus to abnormal levels of certain gonadal hormones has also been associated with behavioral sequelae (Ehrhardt and Money, 1967; Ehrhardt et al., 1968).

Stressful Living Conditions, Isolation, and Neglect

Overheating, crowding, and uncomfortable living conditions have been demonstrated to promote aggression in animals (Griffitt, 1970; Hutchinson, 1972). In humans, noxious odors (Jones and Bogat, 1978; Rotton et al., 1978), high temperatures, and increased population density (Griffitt and Veitch, 1971) also have been shown to provoke hostility and aggression in experimental situations. These kinds of stressors are of special interest because of their possible implications for understanding some of the factors that contribute to aggression in impoverished, crowded urban environments.

Isolation of otherwise gentle animals during critical phases of development, an experience analogous in some ways to the neglect of human infants, is an especially powerful influence on the genesis of aggressive behaviors (Brain and Nowell, 1971; Goldsmith et al., 1976; Luciano and Lore, 1976). The work of Spitz (1946), Bowlby (1969, 1975), and Provence and Lipton (1962) illustrates the devastating developmental consequences of isolation for human infants. Whereas almost total stimulus deprivation of infants can lead to extreme developmental delays, depression, and even death, lesser degrees of neglect have been associated with extremely poor peer relationships and with the development of aggressive behaviors (Cicchetti, 1989; Mueller and Silverman, 1989). In fact, as Widom (1989) has noted, there is a need to study neglect separately from abuse because of the evidence from certain studies that neglected children may be even more dysfunctional and aggressive than children who are physically abused. Noxious stimuli may actually be less detrimental to development than no stimulation at all.

Exposure to Aggressive Adults

The quality of early parenting also affects aggressiveness. Animals bred to have an especially gentle nature, if cross-fostered by adult females of a violent strain, will become more aggressive than is their usual nature (Southwick, 1968). There is evidence that mice reared in the company of their fathers as well as their mothers grow up to be more aggressive than those raised only by mothers (Mugford and Nowell, 1972). On the other hand, the results of cross-fostering aggressive strains of infant rodents with less aggressive adult animals are more variable. Certain strains of aggressive mice retain their aggressiveness even when reared by less aggressive adults (Southwick, 1968), whereas other strains do respond by becoming less aggressive (McCarty and Southwick, 1979; Smith and Simmel, 1977) when cross-fostered by less aggressive parent surrogates. Thus, in certain rodents, exposure to aggressive adults has a more powerful or predictable influence on subsequent adaptive styles than does exposure to more docile parent surrogates.

What are the psychological and behavioral consequences of aggressive parenting? We know that aggression can be learned. There is sound experimental evidence that modeling plays an important role in the development of aggressive behaviors both in animals (Hamburg, 1971) and in humans (Bandura, 1973). We also know that aggressive behaviors (like more adaptive behaviors) can be acquired through reinforcement. Patterson (1977) observed that when children's aggressive behaviors were punished severely by parents, they tended to continue. On the other hand, when positive behaviors were reinforced by praise and aggressive behaviors given less attention, aggressive behaviors diminished (Patterson, 1979). Farrington (1978) also found severe physical punishment to be an antecedent of aggressive delinquency.

The author's own studies comparing extremely aggressive delinquents to their less aggressive delinquent peers indicated that the exposure to extreme violence within the household, particularly between caretakers, was strongly associated with children's violent behaviors (Lewis et al., 1979). When, however, in a follow-up study of these delinquents (Lewis et al., 1989), an attempt was made to distinguish between those children raised in violent households and those who themselves were physically abused, it was found that the more information that was obtained, the clearer it became that abuse and exposure to other family violence tended to go hand in hand, making it difficult to assess the relative importance of each.

Pain and Physical Abuse

Probably the most powerful generator of aggression in animals and possibly in man is the repeated infliction of pain (Berkowitz, 1984). So strong is this response in animals that a conventional experimental method for inducing murderous behaviors in mice and rats involves administering painful shocks to their feet (an ethically questionable practice). Physical torment also is an effective means of engendering viciousness in fighting dogs (e.g., pit bulls). The consequences of maltreatment in animals include the development of hypervigilance. Defeat in animals tends to engender defensiveness (Flannelly et al., 1984), which in turn is generalized to other situations and other opponents (Leschner, 1981; Seward, 1946).

Like animals, children who have been physically abused tend to behave in more aggressive ways than their nonabused peers (Cicchetti, 1989; Widom, 1989). These abused children have been noted to develop a hypervigilance, to misinterpret their surroundings, and, most importantly, to lash out when they perceive ambiguous stimuli as threatening (Dodge et al., 1984; Rieder and Cicchetti, 1989). The author's studies of older children and adolescents revealed that the symptoms most characteristic of very violent youngsters were paranoid ideation and misperceptions, both of which are analogous to the hypervigilance of abused children and animals (Lewis et al., 1979, 1986). The finding of an association between paranoia and violence in delinquents was also consistent with the findings of Yesavage (1983a, b) who reported that the most important symptom distinguishing aggressive from nonaggressive psychiatric patients was paranoia.

Abusive treatment has been observed to have other deleterious effects that are peculiar to humans and that further contribute to aggression. Maltreatment affects expressive skills. Abused children have great difficulty putting their feelings into words (Cicchetti and Beeghly, 1987). Lacking the ability to convey emotions verbally, they tend, rather, to demonstrate their anger and misery through actions. Ironically, abused toddlers speak less about their negative feelings than do children from normal backgrounds. Cicchetti has hypothesized that such children develop overcontrolled styles of coping. However, there may be an alternative explanation for the clinical observations in this study, which suggests that severely abused children repress and totally deny abusive experiences. The most grotesquely and recurrently maltreated children dissociate themselves from the abusive experiences and often do not even recall the abuse. The abused child's inability to identify, much less verbalize, his own distress probably accounts for his observed difficulty in appreciating the distress of others (Main and George, 1985). This lack of empathy noted in abused toddlers is most likely a reflection of their conditioned ability to insulate themselves from any stimuli that might reevoke their own painful experiences.

In summary, studies of human beings indicate that the same kinds of environmental stressors that increase violence in animals (i.e., intrauterine stressors, isolation or neglect, exposure to violent adults, and the infliction of pain) contribute to aggressive behaviors in humans. The question remains how such seemingly different kinds of experiences result in similar kinds of aggressive behavioral changes. Some possible psychophysiological mechanisms by which these kinds of experiences may engender aggression will be explored.

PHYSIOLOGICAL AND BEHAVIORAL CONSEQUENCES OF EXPERIENTIAL STRESSORS

The fact that environmental or experiential influences affect the development of aggression does not mean that these effects are exclusively or even primarily psychodynamic or social. Children probably do not become recurrently violent simply as a result of modeling or reinforcement, although imitation and conditioned responses are contributory. Studies of animals and humans suggest that the environmental conditions and stressors that engender aggression are mediated at least in part physiologically.

Hormonal Responses to Stressors

Environmental stressors affect hormone production. Levels of gonadal hormones are especially critical during fetal and neonatal growth (Goy and McEwen,1980), influencing the development of sexually dimorphic areas of the brain (Hines, 1982). The presence of androgens prenatally has been shown to be crucial to the normal development of aggressive behaviors in such diverse species as fish, lizards, birds, and chimpanzees (Floody and Pfaff,1972). Androgens, which contribute to hypervigilance, are thought to sensitize the parts of the fetal brain that mediate aggression. Sensitized animals subsequently are able to respond rapidly and aggressively to stimuli that elicit surges of testosterone (Kamel et al., 1975). Studies have shown that when pregnant female rats are stressed by abnormal periodic exposure to bright lights, their serum testosterone levels as well as the testosterone levels of their male fetuses rise (vom Saal, 1984). Of note, episodic elevations of testosterone, especially if they occur at critical developmental stages for the fetus, have been associated with increased postnatal aggressiveness. Thus, an environmental stressor affecting the mother has physiological consequences for the fetus and eventual behavioral consequences postnatally.

Some effects of prenatal exposure of humans to abnormally high levels of androgens have been observed in girls with congenital adrenal hyperplasia and in girls exposed in utero to exogenous masculinizing progestins. Their increased energy and athleticism, and their relative lack of interest in the more traditionally feminine concerns are thought to reflect an early in utero sensitization or masculinization of the brain (Ehrhardt et al., 1968; Ehrhardt and Money, 1967).

The early behavioral effects of gonadal hormones are not immutable; rather, hormones and their behavioral concomitants respond to the vicissitudes of life. In animal societies, such as monkey colonies, levels of circulating androgens respond to experiences of success or defeat and affect dominance and submissiveness. For example, when a previously dominant male is bested by another male, his testosterone may fall as much as 80%, and his place in the hierarchy of animals plummet (Rose et al., 1971). In contrast, successful challengers experience elevations of testosterone and may assume more assertive roles in the colony.

One cannot simply extrapolate from the effects of gonadal hormones on animals to their effects on man. There is some evidence that experiences of success, as in winning a tennis match or graduating from medical school, are associated with elevation of serum testosterone levels in men (Mazur and Lamb, 1980). However, for the most part, results of studies regarding the relationship between testosterone levels and aggression in humans have been equivocal (Ehrenkraz et al., 1974; Kreuz and Rose, 1972; Meyer-Bahlburg, 1974; Monti et al., 1977; Rada et al., 1976). The use of anabolic steroids in body builders has been associated with extremes of aggressive behavior (Pope and Katz, 1988) and with the development of paranoid symptoms (Pope and Katz, 1987; Tennant et al., 1988). Of note, although diminishing levels of circulating androgens in men by means of chemical or surgical castration has been found to reduce sexual aggression (i.e., rape) (Tupin, 1987), it has *not* been demonstrated to be an effective biological treatment for the suppression of other kinds of nonsexual violent behaviors. Its effectiveness as a deterrent, no doubt, would be considerable.

Gonadal hormones are not the only hormones affected by environmental stressors. Defeat, which tends to lower testosterone levels, causes circulating corticosteroids to rise (Christian, 1955, 1959). When an animal has been repeatedly exposed to defeat, even exposure to a potential aggressor will cause a surge of corticosteroids (Bronson and Elftheriou, 1965a, b). Similarly, the administration of high doses of corticosteroids to a dominant male will induce submissive behavior (Flannelly et al., 1984).

The relationship of endocrine status to behavior is complex and far from fully understood. The effects of androgens, estrogens, progestins, and corticosteroids, as well as myriad other hormones, vary tremendously. The discussion of testosterone and corticosteroids is but an illustration of some of the ways in which experiences can affect physiological state, and physiological state, in turn, affect behavior. These interactions demonstrate the important fact that the biological state of the organism, animal or man, is not fixed but is, rather, continually changing and responding to the environment. Thus what may appear to be an inherent aggressive temperament can, in fact, be the reflection of a physiological state induced and reinforced by environmental stressors.

Neurotransmitter Responses to Stressors

Just as environmental stressors affect hormone levels, so there is an ever-growing literature documenting the effects of stress on brain levels of neurotransmitters. What is more, studies of animals and humans suggest that certain neurotransmitters such as norepinephrine, dopamine, and serotonin play important roles in both the genesis and suppression of aggressive behaviors.

For example, aggressive behaviors in animals have been induced by administering precursors of norepinephrine and by administering noradrenergic mimetic drugs (Lal et al., 1968, 1970; Randrup and Munkvad, 1966; Reis, 1972). Although the ways in which norepinephrine enhances aggression are not known, it is thought that its presence in specific parts of the brain inhibits certain brain stem neurons known to suppress aggression (Reis, 1972). Thus, it is thought to inhibit inhibitors. (It is important to recall that there are different kinds of aggression in animals. Norepinephrine has been found to facilitate affective or intermale aggression while inhibiting the predatory behaviors associated with food acquisition. Similarly, substances that increase intermale aggression suppress infantici-dal behaviors [vom Saal, 1979]. Thus, when considering behavioral effects on animals of particular neurotransmitters, it is essential that the type of aggression be specified.)

Dopamine is also thought to play a role in the affective or intermale aggression of animals. For example, when mice are given methylparatyrosine, an inhibitor of dopamine synthesis, their aggressiveness diminishes (Lycke et al., 1969). The behavioral effects on humans of fluctuations in norepinephrine and dopamine are uncertain. Whereas the calming, focusing effects of stimulant medication suggest that increases in central nervous system dopamine and norepinephrine diminish hyperactivity and consequently lessen aggressive behaviors, the tranquilizing effects of the antipsychotic medications that block dopamine receptors suggest an opposite behavioral effect of dopamine. In short, at this time, it is impossible to generalize about the role of these kinds of neurotransmitters on human aggression.

One of the most studied neurotransmitters in terms of its influence on aggres-sive behaviors in animals and man is serotonin. For example, Sahakian (1981) reported low concentrations of serotonin in the cerebrospinal fluid of hyperaggressive rats. Others have demonstrated increased aggression in mice and rats whose brains for one reason or another have been depleted of serotonin (Alpert et al., 1981; Lycke et al., 1969). When mice are isolated at critical devel-opmental stages, their concentration of brain serotonin diminishes, and these serotonin-depleted mice become aggressive (Garattini et al., 1969; Valzelli, 1974). Conversely, substances that potentiate serotonin have been demonstrated to diminish aggression (Alpert et al., 1981).

In humans there is a growing body of literature suggesting a relationship between diminished levels of brain serotonin and self-injurious (Asberg et al., 1976, 1987) as well as outwardly aggressive behaviors (Brown et al., 1979). Based on studies of violent offenders and impulsive fire setters, Linnoila and col-leagues (1983) suggested that low cerebral serotonin concentration (as reflected in low CSF-5-HIAA) may be associated with impulsive behaviors in general rather than aggressiveness or violence in particular. In a follow-up study of these subjects, Virkkunen and his colleagues (1989) reported diminished concentrations of both 5-HIAA and HVA (metabolites of serotonin and dopamine) in recidivists as compared to nonrecidivists. Recently, Coccaro and colleagues (1989) demon-strated diminished prolactin responses to fenfluramine (a serotonin-releasing agent) in impulsive-aggressive patients diagnosed as having personality disorders and in depressed suicidal patients. Consistent with these data is the fact that many of the antidepressant medications increase serotonin and relieve agitation and sui-cidal behavior. Coccaro and colleagues (1989) hypothesize the existence of a psy-chobiological susceptibility to impulsive-aggressive behavior, secondary to insufficient serotonin in the brain. This theory, however, does not explain why some individuals with diminished amounts of serotonin simply become unhappy and irritable whereas others become aggressive. What else is necessary to cause a person in a serotonin-depleted, irritable state to aggress against another person rather than bite his own nails or tear at his own flesh?

BRAIN FUNCTION AND THE INTERACTIONS OF HORMONES AND NEUROTRANSMITTERS

Neuroanatomy, hormones, and neurotransmitters cannot really be studied separately. A few examples of their interactions are offered:

1. In vitro studies of the effects of hormones on the embryonic rat brain show that both estrogen and progesterone enhance the growth of mesencephalic dopamine neurons (Reisert et al., 1987). Thus, hormones actually affect brain structure.
2. Studies of rats and hamsters reveal that hormones associated with aggression, such as estradiol and testosterone, concentrate in specific limbic system neucleii (Floody and Pfaff, 1972).
3. The introduction of testosterone into particular hypothalamic nuclei of castrated rats causes them to resume those aggressive behaviors that were previously suppressed by castration (Herbert, 1989). In this study, testosterone seems to act as a neurotransmitter.
4. In vitro studies of the effect of neurotransmitters on testicular tissue in hamsters reveal the role of catecholamine in the production of testosterone (Mayerhofer et al., 1989).
5. Serotonin agonists, releasers, precursors, and uptake inhibitors have been found to elevate corticosterone levels in rats (Fuller, 1981).

Clearly the actions of hormones cannot be studied without considering their interactions with neurotransmitters and vice versa.

Where in the brain do the neurophysiological interactions related to aggression occur? Clinical data and data from experimentation with animals have shown that three areas of the brain are especially important in terms of the modulation of violent behaviors. MacLean (1985) and Weiger and Bear (1988) have conceptualized a hierarchy of neural controls that involves particularly the hypothalamus, amygdala, and orbital prefrontal cortex. The hypothalamus, which receives input from osmo and chemoreceptors and from the amygdala, affects endocrine responses through its influence on the pituitary. For example, damage to the anterior hypothalamus and male rats reduces sexual and aggressive behaviors (Floody and Pfaff, 1972).

In addition, hypothalamic projections to the brain stem control stereotyped behaviors, a phenomenon illustrated by the sham rage of decorticate cats (Bard, 1928). Aggressive behaviors can be elicited or suppressed, depending on which parts of the hypothalamus are stimulated or ablated. Acetylcholine has been shown to be an important neurotransmitter in this area of the brain (Bandler, 1970; Bear et al., 1986; Smith et al., 1970). In humans, lesions in the hypothalamus have been associated with unplanned animal-like attacking behaviors.

In contrast with the hypothalamus, the amygdala receives input from all sensory modalities. It has projections to the hypothalamus and plays a role in the association of particular sensory stimuli with aggressive responses (Downer, 1961; Weiger and Bear, 1988). Lesions in the amygdala have been shown to impair an animal's ability to distinguish between appropriate and inappropriate objects for satisfying hunger and sexual drives (Keating, 1971; Kluver and Bucy, 1939).

Experiments on animals suggest that stimulation of the amygdala, located deep within the temporal lobe, is involved in the kind of aggression that occurs in response to fear (Egger and Flynn, 1963; Siegel and Flynn, 1968). On the other hand, damage to the amygdala has been reported to result in a diminution of aggressive behaviors in response to novel stimuli. In humans, lesions in the amygdaloid area have been associated with apathy and hyposexuality, whereas abnormal electrical activity in this area has been associated with aggression. Whether or not directed aggression ever occurs during an actual seizure originating in the amygdala or in other limbic structures of the brain remains a topic of debate. However, interictally, many patients with epileptic disorders experience irritability, intensification of feelings, fearfulness, and outright paranoia (Bear and Fulop, 1987; Lewis, 1976; Lewis et al., 1982).

This finding—that a particular part of the brain involved in aggression is especially responsive to stimuli that elicit fear—is important because, as previously discussed, paranoid misperceptions, i.e., fearfulness, hypervigilance, and an unwarranted sense of threat, play such an important role in the etiology of violent behavior in human beings. It is during these kinds of emotionally intense interictal periods that planned, purposeful interpersonal violence can occur. It is important to recognize that intentionally violent behaviors can and do occur as a result of brain dysfunction and that premeditation is not necessarily an indication of sanity.

The frontal cortex, that part of the brain so essential for abstract thought, planning, and judgment, interacts with the rest of the neocortex as well as the amygdala and hypothalamus. Lesions of the frontal cortex have been associated with apathy, impulsivity, and irritability, depending on their location. Damage to the dorsolateral convexity has been linked with apathetic, irresponsible behaviors, whereas damage to the orbital area is more commonly linked with impulsive, inappropriate behaviors (Blumer and Benson, 1975; Luria, 1980).

Although attempts have been made to explain specific kinds of criminally aggressive behaviors in terms of the localization of lesions, as yet there are no hard and fast rules that apply invariably to specific human behaviors. The above examples of brain function and dysfunction are, in fact, gross oversimplifications. No part of the brain works in isolation, and, as noted, the structures involved in aggression have widespread connections to other parts of the brain. The essential principle to keep in mind is that in real life the expression of violence is not simply the outcome of localized stimulation. Different parts of the brain are continuously interacting with each other, and violent behaviors reflect the result of the equilibrium achieved between the stimulation and suppression of particular areas at specific points in time.

ARE ALL PEOPLE CREATED EQUAL IN TERMS OF AGGRESSIVE RESPONSES TO MALTREATMENT?

Are we all created equal or are some of us innately more aggressive than others? Studies of infants indicate that we do not enter the world as temperamentally identical blank slates. Some infants are more tense and irritable than others and are more given to temper tantrums when stressed by the ordinary vicissitudes of life (Chess and Thomas, 1984). The same squeaky chalk will feel more abrasive to some slates than others. However, early temper tantrums are not predictive of a life of violent crime (Kagan and Moss, 1962), and, although aggressive behaviors subsequent to age 3 years are often associated with ongoing interpersonal problems, the majority of aggressive young children do not become violent adults.

Are there any genetic abnormalities that impart a specific tendency toward violence? With the exception of Lesch Nyhan Syndrome (Palmour, 1983), no genetic abnormality has yet been identified that predisposes an individual specifically to violent behavior.

The findings reported during the 1960s and 1970s suggesting that certain chromosomal abnormalities (e.g., XYY and XXY anomalies) were associated with a predisposition to violence (Casey et al., 1966; Forssman and Hambert, 1967; Hook, 1973; Nielson, 1968; Telfer, 1968; Witkin et al., 1976) have been reevaluated, and their conclusions questioned (Baker et al., 1970; Gerald, 1976; Jacobs et al., 1971; Schiavi et al., 1984). Most probably, these abnormal constellations of chromosomes, like other abnormal conditions, predispose an individual to a variety of different kinds of adaptational problems which, depending on upbringing and stressors, may or may not be manifested by aggression.

The only chromosomal constellation or syndrome that has repeatedly been demonstrated to be associated with aggressive behavior is the "XY Syndrome." A major feature of the XY Syndrome is a diminished violence threshold, and this characteristic is true of most animals as well as man. What is it about the male condition that creates this tendency to respond aggressively? Given the fact that this quality of temperament is not peculiar to humans, but rather is equally characteristic of animals, it makes no sense to conclude that physiological rather than simply societal influences are at play. It would seem that boys, with their testosterone-sensitive masculinized brains and their physiological capacity to secrete large amounts of androgen in response to particular stimuli, are, from the outset, more susceptible than girls to the aggression-promoting effects of maltreatment.

What other physiological conditions or states lower the threshold for violent responses to stressful stimuli? After al, not all abused children, not even all abused boys, become violent. What makes one boy more susceptible than the next to the "slings and arrows of outrageous fortune?"

The author's studies of violent individuals suggest that some children are indeed more susceptible than others to the violence engendering effects of abuse and neglect. For example, the studies found that among abused boys, those with psychiatric, neurological, and cognitive impairments are far more likely to act aggressively than those whose central nervous system functions are intact (Lewis et al., 1989). Severely neuropsychiatrically impaired girls, on the other hand, even when abused, are far less violent than boys (Lewis et al., 1991). It seems reasonable, therefore, to conclude that impaired boys, who for any number of reasons already have neurophysiological vulnerabilities, who either start with abnormal neurotransmitter concentrations or abnormal physiological responses to stress, are more likely than their impaired female counterparts or their more neuropsychiatrically intact male counterparts to be affected adversely by the psychobiological consequences of abuse or neglect. The boy who is already intrinsically vulnerable to paranoid misperceptions by virtue of an inherent neurophysiological predisposition to major psychiatric illness, or the boy who suffers from some sort of central nervous system dysfunction that increases irritability and impulsivity, might be expected to respond especially aggressively to the additional psychological and neurophysiological insults imposed by neglectful or abusive treatment.

We do know that once a physiological response has been established it is easily reevoked by exposure to similar stimuli. It is, therefore, reasonable to hypothesize that ongoing abuse and neglect, especially in early childhood, have conditioning effects, setting up the kinds of neurophysiological circuits and responses that contribute to violence. The more vulnerable the child is to begin with, the more likely that maltreatment will set up these kinds of circuits and result in recurrent aggressive behavior.

What are the most common characteristics of violent individuals? The literature has tended to focus separately on different concomitants of aggression. Some have concentrated primarily on impulsivity and the biochemical abnormalities associated with it; others have stressed the importance of paranoia in repeatedly antisocial individuals; still others have focused on cognitive or intellectual deficits. In spite of these findings, it is important to remember that most brain-damaged, impulsive children are not violent; most psychotic, paranoid children are not violent; and most cognitively impaired, learning disabled, or retarded children are not violent. These separate vulnerabilities do not, in and of themselves, seem to create violence. Furthermore, most abused children do not turn into violent criminals (Widom, 1989).

On the other hand, work by the author over the years has suggested that when neuropsychiatric and cognitive deficits exist together, maltreatment is an especially potent precipitant of aggression. That is, when impulsivity, hypervigilance, and cognitive expressive deficits coexist, the psychophysiological stage is set for violence to occur. What is it about these kinds of vulnerabilities that create a matrix for violence? First, brain dysfunction of almost any kind is often associated with irritability, impatience, and mood lability. Second, paranoid ideation and misperceptions, symptoms associated with so many different kinds of psychiatric disorders, increase fearfulness and a tendency to retaliate for both genuine and imagined threats. Finally, cognitive deficits not only impair judgment but also diminish the ability to conceptualize feelings and put them into words rather than actions.

How might one understand the ways in which maltreatment in the form of abuse or neglect exacerbates these vulnerabilities and encourages violence? Certainly, maltreatment has psychodynamic consequences, engendering rage and providing a model of violent behavior. In addition, extrapolating from the research on animals, maltreatment modified the physiology of the organism itself. It is reasonable to hypothesize that abusive, neglectful treatment diminishes concentrations in the brain of substances such as serotonin that ordinarily help to modulate feelings; maltreatment seems to increase the outpouring of substances such as dopamine and testosterone that enhance competitive and retaliatory aggression. These same substances also contribute to hypervigilance, and thus increase the fearfulness and paranoia that give rise to violent acts.

There is also another way in which these kinds of physiological reactions to maltreatment may possibly contribute to aggression. We know that testosterone and other hormones affect the very structure of the brain. The delayed verbal skills of boys compared to girls is thought to be a reflection in part of the action of testosterone on the developing brain (Hines, 1982). The special difficulties that abused toddlers have expressing feelings in words may not be simply a reflection of psychological intimidation but rather a manifestation of neuroanatomical and neurophysiological changes secondary to abusive or neglectful treatment.

Furthermore, the apparent lack of empathy of abused aggressive children noted previously may be a manifestation of a centrally mediated expressive deficit coupled with a conditioned imperviousness to certain painful stimuli and not simply a reflection of nastiness or character pathology. Studies of abused young children indicate that they do not suffer from a lack of moral development. Abused children, as well as normal children, consider it wrong to cause physical harm (Smetana and Kelly, 1989). It would seem, rather, that abused children are unable to act on their intellectual understanding of moral principles when they are stressed. When such traumatized children also happen to be paranoid (which is frequently the case), they tend to adopt defensive, contemptuous attitudes toward the rest of the world, thus seeming to complete the picture of sociopathy.

In short, whatever increases impulsivity and irritability, engenders hypervigilance and paranoia, diminishes judgment and verbal competence, and curtails the ability to recognize one's own pain and the pain of others, also enhances the tendency toward violence. Abusive, neglectful caretaking does all of these things. In a resilient child, maltreatment (i.e., abuse or neglect) may not engender aggression. In an already vulnerable child with tendencies toward impulsivity, hypervigilance, expressive difficulties, and dissociation from painful feelings, maltreatment is often sufficient to create a very violent individual. To the extent that testosterone contributes to this constellation of vulnerabilities, persons with the XY Syndrome are at special risk.

What are the implications of the above psychobiological phenomena for the treatment and prevention of violence? Clearly, interventions that help control impulsivity, diminish irritability, enhance a child's sense of security, alleviate paranoid feelings, improve cognition and verbal expressiveness, and encourage recognition of one's own pain and the pain of others, will diminish the likelihood of violence. To date, programs addressing each of these issues individually and specifically do not exist.

On the other hand, ironically, our correctional system reproduces all of the ingredients known to promote violence: isolation, discomfort, exposure to other aggressive individuals, insecurity, and lack of intellectual stimulation. If in our prisons we have demonstrated our ability to make a laboratory which predictably produces and reinforces aggressive behavior, surely the possibility exists that with a little ingenuity we might, just as reliably, be able to create an environment to produce and encourage the opposite.

REFERENCES

Alpert, J. E., Cohen, D. J., Shaywitz, B. A. & Piccirillo, M. (1981), Neurochemical and behavioral organization: disorders of attention, activity, and aggression. In: *Vulnerabilities to Delinquency*, ed. D. O. Lewis. New York: Spectrum, pp. 109–171.

Asberg, A., Traskman, L. & Thoren, P. (1976), 5-HIAA in cerebrospinal fluid: a biochemical suicide predictor? *Arch. Gen. Psychiatry* 33:1193–1196.

Asberg, M., Schalling, D., Traksman-Bendz, L. & Wagner, A. (1987), A psychobiology of suicide, impulsivity, and related phenomena. In: *Psychopharmacology: Third Generation of Progress*, ed. H. Y. Meltzer. New York: Raven Press, pp. 655–688.

Baker, D., Telfer, M. A., Richardson, C. E. & Clark, G. R. (1970), Chromosome errors in men with antisocial behavior: comparison of selected men with "Klinefelter's syndrome" and XYY chromosome pattern. *JAMA*, 214:869–878.

Bandler, R. J. (1970), Cholinergic synapses in the lateral hypothalamus for the control of predatory aggression in the rat. *Brain Res.* 20:409–424.

Bandura, A. (1973), *Aggression: A Social Learning Analysis*. Englewood Cliffs, NJ: Prentice-Hall.

Bard, P. (1928), A diencephalic mechanism for the expression of rage with special reference to the sympathetic nervous system. *Am. J. Physiol.* 84:490–515.

Bear, D. M. & Fulop, M. (1987), The neurology of emotion. In: *Behavioral Biology in Medicine*, ed. A. Hobson. South Norwalk, CT: Meduration, Inc.

————Rosenbaum, J. F. & Norman, R. (1986), Aggression in cat and man precipitated by a cholinesterase inhibitor. *Psychosomatics* 26:535–536.

Berkowitz, L. (1984), Physical pain and the inclination to aggression. In: *Biological Perspectives on Aggression*, eds. K. J. Flannelly, R. J. Blanchard & D. C. Blanchard. New York: Liss, pp. 27–47.

Blumer, D. & Benson, D. F. (1975), Personality changes with frontal and temporal lobe lesions. In: *Psychiatric Aspects of Neurologic Disease*, eds. D. F. Benson & D. Blumer. New York: Grune and Stratton, pp. 151–170.

Bowlby, J. (1969), *Attachment and Loss*, vol. 1. New York: Basic Books.

————(1975), *Attachment and Loss*, vol. 2. Harmondsworth: Penguin.

Brain, P. F. & Nowell, N. W. (1971), Isolation versus grouping effects on adrenal and gonadal function in albino mice. 1. The male. *Gen. Comp. Endocrinol.*, 16:149.

Bronson, F. H. & Eleftheriou, B. E. (1965a), Adrenal response to fighting in mice: separation of physical and psychological causes. *Science* 147:627.

————————(1965b), Relative effects of fighting on bound and unbound corticosterone. *Proc. Soc. Exp. Biol. Med.* 118:146.

Brown, G. L., Ballenger, J. C., Minichiello, M.D. & Goodwin, F. K. (1979), Human aggression and its relationship to cerebrospinal fluid 5-hydroxy-indoleacetic acid, 3-methoxy-4-hydroxy-phenyl-glycol, and homovanillic acid. In: *Psychopharmacology of Aggression*, ed. M. Sandler. New York: Raven Press, pp. 131–148.

Casey, L. J., Segall, D. R., Street, K. & Blank, C. E. (1966), Sex chromosomes abnormalities in two state hospitals for patients requiring special security. *Nature*, 209:641–642.

Chess, S. E. & Thomas, A. (1984), *Origins and Evolution of Behavior Disorders*. New York: Brunner/Mazel.

Christian, J. J. (1955), Effect of population size on the adrenal glands and reproductive organs of male mice in populations of fixed size. *J. Physiol.* (Lond.) 182:292.

————(1959), Lack of correlation between adrenal weight and injury from fighting in grouped male albino mice. *Proc. Soc. Exp. Biol. Med.* 101:166.

Cicchetti, D. (1989), How research on child maltreatment has informed the study of child development: perspectives from developmental psychopathology. In: *Child Maltreatment: Theory and Research on the Causes and Consequences of Child Abuse and Neglect*, eds. D. Cicchetti & V. Carlson. New York: Cambridge University Press, pp. 377–431.

————& Beeghly, M. (1987), Symbolic development in maltreatment youngsters: an organizational perspective. In: *Atypical Symbolic Development*, eds. D. Cicchetti & M. Beeghly. San Francisco: Jossey-Bass.

Coccaro, E. F., Siever, L. J., Klar, H. M., Maurer, G. et al. (1989), Serotonergic studies in patients with affective and personality disorders. *Arch. Gen. Psychiatry*, 46:587–598.

Dodge, K., Murphy, R. & Buchsbaum, K. C. (1984), The assessment of intention-cue detection skills in children: implications for developmental psychopathology. *Child Dev.* 55:163–173.

Downer, J. L. (1961), Changes in visual gnostic functions and emotional behaviour following unilateral temporal pole damage in the "split-brain" monkey. *Nature*, 191:50–51.

Ebert, P. D. (1983), Selection for aggression in a natural population. In: *Aggressive Behavior: Genetic and Neural Approaches*, eds. E. C. Himmel, M. E. Hahn & J. K. Walters, Hillsdale, NJ: Laurence Erlbaum, pp. 103–127.

Egger, M. D. & Flynn, J. P. (1963), Effects of electrical stimulation of the amygdala on hypothalamically elicited attack behavior in cats. *J. Neurophysiol.*, 26:705–720.

Ehrenkranz, J., Bliss, E. & Sheard, M. H. (1974), Plasma testosterone: correlation with aggressive behavior and social dominance in man. *Psychosom. Med.* 36:469–475.

Ehrhardt, A. A. & Money, J. (1967), Progestin-induced hermaphroditism: IQ and psychosexual identity in a sample of ten girls. *Journal of Sex Research*, 3:83–100.

————Epstein, R. & Money, J. (1968), Fetal androgens and female gender identity in the early treated adrenogenital syndrome. *Johns Hopkins Medical Journal*, 122:160–167.

Farrington, D. P. (1978), The family backgrounds of aggressive youths. In: *Aggression and Antisocial Behavior in Childhood and Adolescence*, eds. L. A. Hersov, M. Berger & D. Shaffer. Oxford: Pergamon, pp. 73–93.

Flannelly, K. J., Flannelly, L. & Blanchard, R. J. (1984), Adult experience and the expression of aggression: a comparative analysis. In: *Biological Perspectives on Aggression*, eds. K. J. Flannelly, R. J. Blanchard & D. C. Blanchard. New York: Liss, pp. 207–259.

Floody, O. R. & Pfaff, D. W. (1972), Steroid hormones and aggressive behavior: approaches to the study of hormone-sensitive brain mechanisms for behavior, S. H. Frazier. *Aggression*, 52:149–184.

Flynn, J. P., Vanegas, H., Foote, W. & Edward, S. (1970), Neural mechanisms involved in a cat's attack on a rat. In: *Neural Control of Behavior*, eds. R. E. Whalen et al., New York: Academic Press. p. 135.

Forssman, H. & Hambert, G. (1967), Chromosomes and antisocial behavior. *Exerpta Criminologica*, 7:113–117.

Fuller, R. W. (1981), Serotonergic stimulation of pituitary-adrenocortical functions in rats. *Neuroendocrinology*, 32:118–127.

Garattini, S., Giacolone, E. & Valzelli, L. (1969), Biochemical changes during isolation-induced aggressiveness in mice. In: *Aggressive Behavior*, eds. S. Garattini & E. Sigg. New York: Wiley.

Gerald, P. S. (1976), Current concepts in genetics: sex chromosome disorders. *New England Journal of Medicine*, 294:706.

Goldsmith, J. F., Brain, P. F. & Benton, D. (1976), Effects of age at differential housing and the duration of individual housing/grouping on intermale fighting behavior and adrenocortical activity in T. O. strain mice. *Aggressive Behavior*, 2:307–323.

Goy, R. W. & McEwen, B. S. (1980), *Sexual Differentiation of the Brain*. Cambridge, MA: MIT Press.

Griffitt, W. (1970), Environmental effects on interpersonal affective behavior: ambient effective temperature and attraction. *J. Pers. Soc. Psychol.*, 15:240.

———& Veitch, R. (1971), Hot and crowded, influence of population density and temperature on interpersonal affective behavior: ambient effective temperature and attraction. *J. Pers. Soc. Psychol.* 17:92–98.

Hamburg, D. A. (1971), Psychobiological studies of aggressive behaviour. *Nature*. 230:19–23.

Herbert, J. (1989), The physiology of aggression. In: *Aggression and War: Their Biological and Social Bases*, eds. J. Groebel & R. A. Hinde. New York: Cambridge University Press, pp. 58–71.

Hines, M. (1982), Prenatal gonadal hormones and sex differences in human behavior. *Psychol. Bull.* 92(1):56–80.

Hook, E. B. (1973), Behavioral implications of the human XYY genotype. *Science*, 179:139–150.

Hutchinson, R. R. (1972), The environmental causes of aggression. In: *Nebraska Symposium on Motivation*, eds. J. K. Cole & D. D. Jensen. Lincoln: University of Nebraska Press.

Jacobs, P. A., Price, W. H., Richmond, S. & Ratcliff, R. A. W. (1971), Chromosomes surveys in penal institutions and approved schools. *J. Med. Genet.* 8:49–58.

Jones, J. W. & Bogat, G. A. (1978), Air pollution and human aggression. *Psychol. Rep.* 43:721.

Kagan, J. & Moss, H. (1962), *From Birth to Maturity*. New York: Wiley.

Kamel, F., Mock, E. J., Wright, W. W. & Frankel, A. I. (1975), Alterations of plasma concentrations of testosterone, LH, and prolactin associated with mating in the male rat. *Horm. Behav.* 6:277.

Keating, E. G. (1971), Somatosensory deficit produced by parietotemporal disconnection. *Anat. Rec.* 169:353–354.

Kluver, H. & Bucy, P. C. (1939), Preliminary analysis of functions of the temporal lobes in monkeys. *Archives of Neurology and Psychiatry* 42:979–1000.

Kreuz, L. E. & Rose, R. M. (1972), Assessment of aggressive behavior and plasma testosterone in a young criminal population. *Psychosom. Med.* 34:321–332.

Lagerspetz, K. M. J. & Lagerspetz, K. Y. H. (1971), Changes in the aggressiveness of
mice resulting from selective breeding, learning and social isolation. *Scand. J.
Psychol.* 12:241–248.

Lal, H., De Feo, J. J. & Thut, P. (1968), Effect of amphetamine on pain-induced aggression. *Communications in Behavioral Biology*, 1:333.

————Nesson, B. & Smith, N. (1970), Amphetamine-induced aggression in mice pre-
treated with dihydroxyphenylalanine (DOPA) and/or reserpine. *Biol. Psychiatry*,
2:299.

Leshner, A. I. (1981), The role of hormones in the control of submissiveness. In: *A
Multidisciplinary Approach to Aggression Research*, eds. P. F. Brain & D. Benton.
Amsterdam: Elsevier/North Holland Press, pp. 309–322.

Lewis, D. O. (1976), Delinquency, psychohmotor epileptic symptoms, and paranoid ideation: a triad. *Am. J. Psychiatry*, 133:1395–1398.

————Shanok, S., Pincus, J. & Glaser, G. (1979), Violent juvenile delinquents: psychiatric, neurological, psychological and abuse factors. *J. Am. Acad. Child Adolesc.
Psychiatry*, 18:307–319.

————Pincus, J., Shanok, S. & Glaser, G. (1982), Psychomotor epilepsy and violence in
a group of incarcerated adolescent boys. *Am. J. Psychiatry*, 139:882–887.

————Lovely, R., Yeager, C. & Della Femina, D. (1989), Toward a theory of the genesis
of violence: a follow-up study of delinquents. *J. Am. Acad. Child Adolesc. Psychiatry*
28:431–436.

————Pincus, J. H., Feldman, M., Jackson, L. & Bard, B. (1986), Psychiatric, neurological, and psychoeducational characteristics of 15 death row inmates in the United
States. *Am. J. Psychiatry*, 143:838–845.

————Yeager, C., Cobham-Portorreal, C. S., Klein, N., Showalter, C. & Anthony, A.
(1991), A follow-up female delinquents: maternal contributions to the perpetuation of
deviance. *J. Am. Acad. Child Adolesc. Psychiatry*, 30:197–201.

Linnoila, M., Virkkunen, M., Scheinin, M., Nuutila, A., Rimon, R. & Goodwin, F. K.
(1983), Low cerebrospinal fluid 5-hydroxyindoleacetic acid concentration differentiates impulsive from nonimpulsive violent behavior. *Life Sci.* 33:2609–2614.

Luciano, D. & Lore, R. (1975), Aggression and social experience in domesticated rats. *J.
Comp. Physiol. Psychol.*, 88:917.

Luria, A. R. (1980), *Higher Cortical Functions in Man*. New York: Basic Books.

Lycke, E., Modigh, K. & Roos, B. E. (1969), Aggression in mice associated with changes
in the monoamine-metabolism of the brain. *Experientia* 25:951–953.

MacLean, P. (1985), Brain evolution relating to family, play and the separation call. *Arch.
Gen. Psychiatry*, 42:405–417.

Main, M. & George, C. (1985), Response of abused and disadvantaged toddlers to distress
in agitates: a study in the day care setting. *Developmental Psychology*, 21:407–
412.

Mayerhofer, A., Bartke, A. & Steger, R. W. (1989), Catecholamine effects on testicular testosterone production in the gonadally active and the gonadally regressed adult golden hamster. *Biol. Reprod.* 40:752–761.

Mazur, A. & Lamb, T. A. (1980), Testosterone, status and mood in human males. *Horm. Behav.* 14:236–246.

McCarthy, R. & Southwick, C. H. (1979), Parental environment: effects on survival, growth and aggressive behaviors of two rodent species. *Dev. Psychobiol.* 12:269–279.

Meyer-Bahlburg, H. F. L. (1974), Aggression, and androgens and the XYY syndrome. In: *Sex Differences in Behavior*, eds. R. C. Friedman, R. M. Richart & R. L. Vande Wiele. New York: Wiley, pp. 433–453.

Monti, P. M., Brown, W. A. & Corriveau, M. A. (1977), Testosterone and components of aggressive and sexual behavior in man. *Am. J. Psychiatry,* 134:692–694.

Mueller, E. & Silverman, N. (1989), Peer relations in maltreated children. In: *Child Maltreatment: Theory and Research on the Causes and Consequences of Child Abuse and Neglect*, eds. D. Cicchetti, & V. Carlson. New York: Cambridge University Press, pp. 529–578.

Mugford, R. A. & Nowell, N. W. (1972), Paternal stimulation during infancy: effects upon aggression and open-field performance of mice. *Journal of Comparative and Physiological Psychology,* 79:30–36.

Nielson, J. (1968), The XXY syndrome in a mental hospital. *British Journal of Criminology*, 8:186–203.

Owen, D. R. (1972), The 47XYY male: a review. *Psychol. Bull.* 79:209–233.

Palmour, R. M. (1983), Genetic models for the study of aggressive behavior. *Prog. Neuropsychopharmacol. Biol. Psychiatry* 7:513–517.

Pasamanick, B. (1956), Pregnancy experience and the development of behavior disorders in children. *Am. J. Psychiatry* 112:613–617.

———(1961), Epidemiological investigations of some prenatal factors in the production of neuropsychiatric disorder. In: *Comparative Epidemiology for Mental Disorders*, eds. P. H. Hoch & J. Zubin. New York: Grune & Stratton, pp. 260–275.

Patterson, G. R. (1977), Accelerating stimuli for two classes of coercive behaviors. *J. Abnorm. Child Psychol.*, 5:335–350.

———(1979), A performance theory for coercive family interaction. In: *The Analysis of Social Interactions: Methods, Issues, and Illustrations*, ed. R. B. Caines. Hillsdale, NJ: Laurence Erlbaum.

Pope, H. G. & Katz, D. L. (1987), Bodybuilder's psychosis. *Lancet*, I:863.

———(1988), Affective and psychotic symptoms associated with anabolic steroid use. *Am. J. Psychiatry,* 145:487–490.

Provence, S. & Lipton, R. (1962), *Infants in Institutions*. New York: International Universities Press.

Rada, R. T., Laws, D. R. & Kellner, R. (1976), Plasma testosterone levels in the rapist. *Psychosom. Med.* 38:257–268.

Randrup, A. & Munkvad, I. (1966), DOPA and other naturally occurring substances as causes of stereotype and rage in rats. *Acta. Psychiatr. Scand.* 42[Suppl. 19]:193.

Reis, D. J. (1972), Central Neurotransmitters in Aggression, S. F. Frazier. *Aggression*, 52:119–147.

Reisert, I., Han, V., Lieth, E., Toran, A. D., Pilgrim, C. & Lauder, J. (1987), Sex steroids promote neurite growth in mesencephalic tyrosine hydroxylase immunoreactive neuron in vitro. *International Journal of Developmental Neuroscience*, 5:91–98.

Rieder, C. & Cicchetti, D. (1989), An organizational perspective on cognitive control functioning and cognitive-affective balance in maltreated children. *Developmental Psychology*, 25:382–393.

Rose, R., Holaday, J. & Bernstein, I. (1971), Plasma testosterone, dominance rank and aggressive behaviour in male rhesus monkeys. *Nature,* 231:366.

Rotton, J., Barry, T., Frey, J. & Soler, E. (1978), Air pollution and interpersonal attraction. *J. Appl. Soc. Psychol*, 8:57.

Rutter, M. (1970), Sex differences in response to family stress. In: *The Child and His Family*, eds. E. J. Anthony & C. Kompernik. New York: Wiley.

Sahakian, B. J. (1981), The neurochemical basis of hyperactivity and aggression induced by social deprivation. In: *Vulnerabilities to Delinquency*, ed. D. O. Lewis. New York: Spectrum, pp. 173–186.

Schiavi, R., Theilgaard, A., Owen, D. et al. (1984), Sex chromosome anomalies, hormones and aggressivity. *Arch. Gen. Psychiatry*, 41:93–99.

Seward, J. P. (1946), Aggressive behavior in the rat: IV. Submission determined by conditioning, extinction and disuse. *J. Comp. Psychol.*, 39:51.

Siegel, A. & Flynn, J. P. (1968), Differential effects of electrical stimulation and lesions of the hippocampus and adjacent regions upon attack behavior in cats. *Brain Res.* 7:252–267.

Smetana, J. G. & Kelly, M. (1989), Social cognition in maltreated children. In: *Child Maltreatment*, eds. D. Cicchetti & V. Carlson. Cambridge: Cambridge University Press, pp. 620–646.

Smith, D. E., King, M. D. & Hoebel, B. G. (1970), Lateral hypothalamic control of killing: evidence for a cholinoceptive mechanism. *Science* 167:900–901.

Smith, M. L. & Simmel, E. C. (1977), Paternal effects on the development of social behavior in *Mus Musculus*. In: *Child Maltreatment: Theory and Research on the Causes and Consequences of Child Abuse and Neglect,* eds. D. Cicchetti & V. Carlson. New York: Cambridge University Press, pp. 620–646.

Southwick, C. H. (1968), Effect of maternal environment on aggressive behavior of inbred mice. *Communications in Behavioral Biology*, 1:129–132.

Spitz, R. A. (1946), Anaclitic depression. *Psychoanal. Study Child*, 2:313–342.

Stott, D. H. (1973), Follow-up study from birth of the effects of prenatal stresses. *Dev. Med. Child Neurol.* 15:770–787.

———& Latchford, S. A. (1976), Prenatal antecedents of child health, development and behavior. *J. Am. Acad. Child Adolesc. Psychiatry* 15:161–191.

Telfer, M. A. (1968), Are some criminals born that way? *Think*, 34:24–28.

Tennant, F., Black, D. L. & Voy, R. O. (1988), Anabolic steroid dependence with opioid-type features. *N. Engl. J. Med.* 319–578.

Tupin, J. P. (1987), Psychopharmacology and aggression. In: *Clinical Treatment of the Violent Person*, ed. L. H. Roth, pp. 79–94.

Valzelli, L. (1974), 5-Hydroxytryptamine in aggressiveness. In: *Advances in Biochemical Psychopharmacology*, eds. E. Costa, G. Gessa & M. Sandler. New York: Raven.

Virkkunen, M., DeJong, J., Bartko, J., Goodwin, F. K. & Linnoila, M. (1989), Relationship of psychobiological variables to recidivism in violent offenders and impulsive fire setters. *Arch. Gen. Psychiatry* 46:600–603.

vom Saal, F. S. (1979), Prenatal exposure to androgen influences morphology and aggressive behavior of male and female mice. *Horm. Behav.* 12:1.

———(1984), The intrauterine position phenomenon: effects on physiology, aggressive behavior and population dynamics in house mice. In: *Biological Perspectives on Aggression*. eds. K. J. Flannelly, R. J. Blanchard & D. C. Blanchard. New York: Liss. pp. 135–179.

Weiger, W. A. & Bear, D. M. (1988), An approach to the neurology of aggression. *J. Psychiat. Res.* 22:85–98.

Widom, C. S. (1989), The cycle of violence. *Science*, 244:160–166.

Witkin, H. A., Mednick, S. A., Schuylsinger, F., et al. (1976), Criminality in XYY and XXY men. *Science* 193:547–555.

Yesavage, J. A. (1983a), Bipolar illness: correlates of dangerous inpatient behavior. *Br. J. Psychiatry* 143:554–557.

———(1983b), Correlates of dangerous behavior of schizophrenics in hospital. *J. Psychosom. Res.* 18:225–231.

22

Ethnic Differences in Adolescent Achievement: An Ecological Perspective

Laurence Steinberg

Temple University, Philadelphia, Pennsylvania

Sanford M. Dornbusch

Stanford University, Stanford, California

B. Bradford Brown

University of Wisconsin, Madison

Using data collected from a large sample of high school students, the authors challenge three widely held explanations for the superior school performance of African- and Hispanic-American adolescents: group differences in (a) parenting practices, (b) familial values about education, and (c) youngsters' beliefs about the occupational rewards of academic success. They found that White youngsters benefit from the combination of authoritative parenting and peer support for achievement, whereas Hispanic youngsters suffer from a combination of parental authoritarianism and low peer support. Among Asian-American students, peer support for academic excellence offsets the negative consequences of authoritarian parenting. Among African-American youngsters, the absence of peer support for achievement undermines the positive influence of authoritative parenting.

One of the most consistent and disturbing findings in studies of adolescent achievement concerns ethnic differences in school performance. Many studies

Reprinted with permission from *American Psychologist*, 1992, Vol. 47(6), 723–729. Copyright © 1992 by the American Psychological Association.

Lewis P. Lipsitt serviced as action editor for this article.

This article is based on an invited address by Laurence Steinberg to Division 7 (Developmental Psychology) of the American Psychological Association, Boston, August 12, 1990. Work on this article was supported by a grant to the author from the Lilly Endowment. The research described herein was supported by a grant to Laurence Steinberg and B. Bradford Brown from the U.S. Department indicate that African-American students "generally earn lower grades, drop out more often, and attain less education than do whites" (Mickelson, 1990, p. 44). Although less research has focused on direct comparisons between other ethnic groups, recent reports on adolescent achievement in America suggest that the performance of Hispanic adolescents also lags behind that of their White counterparts, but that the performance of Asian-American students exceeds that of White, African-American, and Hispanic students (see Sue & Okazaki, 1990). Despite the widely held assumption that ethnic differences in achievement are accounted for by group differences on other variables, such as socioeconomic status and family structure, research indicates quite clearly that these patterns of ethnic differences in achievement persist even after important third variables are taken into account.

Although there is considerable agreement that these ethnic differences in school performance are genuine, there is little consensus about the causes of these differences, and a variety of explanations for the pattern have been offered. Among the most familiar are that (a) there are inherited differences between ethnic groups in intellectual abilities, which are reflected in differences in school performance (e.g., Lynn, 1977; Rushton, 1985); (b) that ethnic differences in achievement-related socialization practices in the family lead youngsters from some ethnic groups to develop more positive achievement-related attitudes and behaviors (e.g., Mordkowitz & Ginsburg, 1987); (c) that there are ethnic differences in cultural values, and especially in the value placed on educational success (see Sue & Okazaki, 1990, for a discussion); and (d) that there are ethnic differences in perceived and actual discrimination within educational and occupational institutions (e.g., Mickelson, 1990; Ogbu, 1978).

This article focuses on ethnic differences in school achievement, a phenomenon that, as a recent article in this journal put it, is "in search of an explanation" (Sue & Okazaki, 1990, p. 913). Because the genetic hypothesis has received so little support in studies of school achievement (see Sue & Okazaki, 1990; Thompson, Detterman, & Plomin, 1991), we focus instead on the various environmental accounts of the phenomenon. To do so, we present and integrate several sets of findings from the first wave of data collected as part of a program of research on a large, multiethnic sample of high school students. The research is aimed at understanding how different contexts in youngsters' lives affect their behavior, schooling, and development.

of Education, through the National Center on Effective Secondary Schools at the University of Wisconsin—Madison, and by a grant from the Spencer Foundation to Sanford M. Dornbusch and P. Herbert Leiderman at the Stanford University Center for the Study of Families, Children, and Youth. The contributions of Nancy Darling, Sue Lamborn, Mindy Landsman, Nina Mounts, Phil Ritter, and Lance Weinmann are gratefully acknowledged.

OVERVIEW OF THE RESEARCH PROGRAM

During the 1987–1988 school year, we administered a 30-page, two-part questionnaire with a series of standardized psychological inventories, attitudinal indices, and demographic questions to approximately 15,000 students at nine different high schools. The schools were selected to provide a window on the contrasting social ecologies of contemporary American adolescents. They included an inner-city school in Milwaukee, Wisconsin, serving a substantially Black population; a San Jose, California, school serving a large number of Hispanic students; a small rural Wisconsin school in a farming community; a semirural California school with youngsters from farm families, migrant workers, and recently arrived Asian refugees; and several suburban schools serving mixtures of working-class and middle-class adolescents from a variety of ethnic backgrounds. All told, our sample was approximately one third non-White, with nearly equal proportions of African-American, Hispanic, and Asian-American youngsters—much like the adolescent population in the United States today (Wetzel, 1987). The sample was quite diverse with respect to socioeconomic status and household composition.

The questionnaires, which were administered schoolwide, contained numerous measures of psychosocial development and functioning, as well as several measures of social relations in and outside of school. The outcome variables fell into four general categories: *psychosocial adjustment* (including measures of self-reliance, work orientation, self-esteem, and personal and social competence); *schooling* (including measures of school performance, school engagement, time spent on school activities, educational expectations and aspirations, and school-related attitudes and beliefs); *behavior problems* (including measures of drug and alcohol use, delinquency, susceptibility to antisocial peer pressure, and school misconduct); and *psychological distress* (including measures of anxiety, depression, and psychosomatic complaints).

This outcome battery is more or less standard fare in the field of adolescent social and personality development. What makes our database different, however, is that it is equally rich in measures of the contexts in which our adolescents live. We have tried to move beyond the simple "social address" models that are pervasive in survey research, in which measures of the environment do not go beyond checklists designed to register the number of persons present in the setting and their relationship to the respondent (see Bronfenbrenner, 1986, for a critique of such models). Accordingly, our measures of family relationships include a number of scales tapping such dimensions as parental warmth, control, communication style, decision making, monitoring, and autonomy granting. Our peer measures include affiliation patterns, peer crowd membership, perceptions of peer group norms, and time spent in various peer activities. Our measures of extracurricular and work settings provide information on the activities the adolescents engage in outside of school. Our measures of the school environment concern the classes the adolescents are taking and the classroom environments they encounter. For each student, we also have information on the family's ethnicity, composition, socio-economic status, marital history, immigration history, and patterns of language use. For some of these variables, the questionnaire data was supplemented with interviews with both students and parents from a cross section of the schools.

Our large and heterogeneous sample permits us to examine a number of questions about the importance of contextual variations in shaping and structuring youngsters' lives and behavior during the high school years. Because the youngsters in our sample are growing up under markedly different circumstances, we can ask whether and how patterns of development and adjustment differ across these social addresses. Because we have detailed information on processes of influence within these social addresses, we can look more specifically at mechanisms of influence, both across and within contexts. And because we have information on more than one context in youngsters' lives, we can look at the interactions between contexts and how variations in the way in which contexts are themselves linked affect youngsters' development. Indeed, as we shall argue, ethnic differences in school performance can be explained more persuasively by examining the interplay between the major contexts in which youngsters develop—the family, the peer group, and the school—than by examining any one of these contexts alone.

SOCIALIZATION OF ACHIEVEMENT IN THE FAMILY

According to familial socialization explanations of ethnic group differences of achievement discussed above, we should be able to account for achievement differences among ethnic groups by taking into account the extent to which they use different sorts of parenting practices. Although psychologists have only recently begun examining ethnic differences in adolescent development (Spencer & Dornbusch, 1990), interest among developmentalists in the relation between parenting practices and youngsters' school performance has quite a lengthy history (see Maccoby & Martin, 1983). This literature indicates that adolescent competence, virtually however indexed, is higher among youngsters raised in *authoritative* homes—homes in which parents are responsive and demanding (see Baumrind, 1989)—than in other familial environments (Steinberg, 1990). Presumably, better performance in school is just one of many possible manifestations of psychosocial competence. Researchers writing in this tradition have hypothesized that parental authoritativeness contributes to the child's psychosocial development, which in turn facilitates his or her school success (e.g., Steinberg, Elmen, & Mounts, 1989).

Recently, it has been suggested that three specific components of authoritativeness contribute to healthy psychological development and school success during adolescence: parental acceptance or warmth, behavioral supervision and strictness, and psychological autonomy granting or democracy (Steinberg, 1990; Steinberg et al., 1989; Steinberg, Mounts, Lamborn, & Dornbusch, 1991). This trinity—warmth, control, and democracy—parallel the three central dimensions of parenting identified by Schaefer (1965) in his pioneering work on the assessment of parenting practices through children's reports. These components are also conceptually similar to dimensions of parental control proposed by Baumrind (1991a, 1991b) in her recent reports: supportive control (similar to warmth), assertive control (similar to behavioral supervision and strictness), and directive/conventional control (similar to the antithesis of psychological autonomy granting).

The parenting inventory embedded in our questionnaire contained scales designed to assess parental warmth, behavioral control, and psychological autonomy granting. In our model, authoritative parents were defined as those who scored high in acceptance, behavioral control, and psychological autonomy granting. Not surprisingly, these parenting dimensions are moderately intercorrelated with each other and with other aspects of the parent–child relationship. For example, authoritative parents not only are warmer, firmer, and more democratic than other parents, but they are also more involved in their children's schooling, are more likely to engage in joint decision making, and are more likely to maintain an organized household with predictable routines. In view of this, we have used a categorical approach to the study of parenting, in which we used scores on each of our three dimensions to assign families to one of several categories. Using this general model of authoritative parenting, we have documented in several different studies that adolescents who are raised in authoritative homes do indeed perform better in school than do their peers (Dornbusch, Ritter, Leiderman, Roberts, & Fraleigh, 1987; Lamborn, Mounts, Steinberg, & Dornbusch, 1991; Steinberg et al., 1989; Steinberg et al., 1991).

Can ethnic differences in school performance be explained by ethnic differences in the use of authoritative parenting? According to Dornbusch's earlier work (Dornbusch et al., 1987; Ritter & Dornbusch, 1989), the answer is no. For example, although Asian-American students have the highest school performance, their parents are among the least authoritative. Although African-American and Hispanic parents are considerably more authoritative than Asian-American parents, their children perform far worse in school on average. Given the strong support for the power or authoritative parenting in the socialization literature, these findings present somewhat of a paradox.

One explanation for this paradox is that the effects of authoritative parenting may differ as a function of the ecology in which the adolescent lives. Some writers have speculated that parental authoritarianism may be more beneficial than authoritativeness for poor minority youth (e.g., Baldwin & Baldwin, 1989; Baumrind, 1972). To examine this possibility, we used three demographic variables to partition our sample into 16 ecological niches, defined by ethnicity (four categories: African-American, Asian-American, Hispanic, and White), socioeconomic status (two categories: working class and below versus middle class and above), and family structure (two categories: biological two-parent and nonintact; for details, see Steinberg et al., 1991).

After ensuring that the reliability of each of our three parenting scales was adequate in every ecological niche, we categorized families as authoritative and nonauthoritative. Families who scored above the entire sample median on warmth, behavioral control, and psychological autonomy granting were categorized as authoritative. Families who had scored below the entire sample median on any of the three dimensions were categorized as nonauthoritative. Consistent with previous research (e.g., Dornbusch et al., 1987), we found that authoritativeness is more prevalent among White households than minority households. Also consistent with previous work, we found that Asian-American youngsters are least likely to come from authoritative homes. Again, in light of the superior performance of Asian-American students, this finding runs counter to the family socialization hypothesis.

We contrasted the adolescents from authoritative and nonauthoritative homes within each niche on several outcome variables, including our indices of school performance. Across the outcome variables that are not related to school (psychosocial development, psychological distress, and behavior problems), we found that youngsters from authoritative homes fared better than their counterparts from nonauthoritative homes, in all ethnic groups. When we looked at youngsters' school performance, however, we found that White and Hispanic youngsters were more likely to benefit from authoritative parenting than were African-American or Asian-American youngsters. Within the African-American and Asian-American groups, youngsters whose parents were authoritative did not perform better than youngsters whose parents were nonauthoritative. Virtually regardless of their parents' practices, the Asian-American students in our sample were receiving higher grades in school than other students, and the African-American students were receiving relatively lower grades than other students. Indeed, we found that African-American students' school performance was even unrelated to their parents' level of education (Dornbusch, Ritter, & Steinberg, in press)—a finding that is quite surprising, given the strong association between parental social class and scholastic success reported in the sociological literature on status attainment (e.g., Featherman, 1980).

GLASS CEILING EFFECT

Why would authoritativeness benefit Asian-American and African-American youngsters when it comes to psychological development and mental health, but not academic performance? One possibility we explored derives from the work of urban anthropologist John Ogbu and his colleagues (e.g., Fordham & Ogbu, 1986; Ogbu, 1978). Ogbu has argued that African-American and Hispanic youngsters perceive the opportunity structure differently than White and Asian-American youngsters do. Because adolescents from what he has called "caste-like" minorities believe that they will face a job ceiling that prohibits them from "receiving occupational rewards commensurate with their educational credentials" (Mickelson, 1990, p. 45), they put less effort into their schoolwork. According to this view, the lower school performance of African-American and Hispanic youngsters is a rational response to their belief that, for them, educational effort does not pay off.

Although Ogbu's (1978) thesis has received a great deal of popular attention, it has been subjected to very little empirical scrutiny. The main tests of his hypothesis have come from ethnographic studies focusing on single peer groups of Black adolescents. Although important in their own right, these studies have not permitted the crucial cross-ethnic comparisons that are at the heart of Ogbu's thesis, because it is impossible to determine from these studies whether the beliefs expressed by the students in these samples are unique to minority adolescents. As several commentators (e.g., Steinberg, 1987) have pointed out, the notion that it is admirable to work hard in school is not widespread among contemporary American adolescents, whatever their color.

On one of our questionnaires, students responded to two questions designed to tap their beliefs about the likelihood of school success: (a) "Suppose you *do* get a good education in high school. How likely is it that you will end up with the kind of job you hope to get?"; and (b), "Suppose you *don't* get a good education in high school. How likely is it that you will still end up with the kind of job you hope to get?" Interestingly, responses to these two questions were only modestly correlated.

When we examined the correlations between our two measures of beliefs about the value of school success and our indices of school performance and school engagement, we found results that are generally consistent with one of the central assumptions of Ogbu's (1978) theory—namely, that the more students believe that doing well in school pays off, the more effort they exert in school and the better they perform there. Of particular interest, however, is the finding that the extent to which students believe that there are *negative* consequences of school failure is a better predictor of their school performance and engagement than the extent to which they believe that there are positive consequences of school success. That is, across ethnic groups, the more youngsters believe that not getting a good education hurts their chances, the better they do in school.

We then looked at ethnic differences in the extent to which youngsters endorse these beliefs. The results were quite surprising. We found no ethnic differences in the extent to which youngsters believe that getting a good education pays off. From the point of view of educators, the news is good: Virtually all students in our sample, regardless of their ethnicity, endorsed the view that getting a good education would enhance their labor market success. However, on the second of these questions—concerning students' beliefs about the consequences of not getting a good education—we found significant variability and significant ethnic differences. Much more than other groups, Asian-American adolescents believe that it is unlikely that a good job can follow a bad education. Hispanic and African-American students are the most optimistic. In other words, what distinguishes Asian-American students from others is not so much their stronger belief that educational success pays off, but their stronger fear that educational failure will have negative consequences. Conversely, unwarranted optimism, rather than excessive pessimism, may be limiting African-American and Hispanic students' school performance.

We noted earlier that academic success and school engagement are more strongly correlated with the belief that doing poorly in school will have negative repercussions than with the belief that doing well will have positive ones. The pattern of ethnic differences on our measures of school performance and engagement is generally consistent with this general principle. In general, Asian-American students, who in our sample were the most successful in school and were most likely to believe that doing poorly in school has negative repercussions, devote relatively more time to their studies, are more likely to attribute their success to hard work, and are more likely to report that their parents have high standards for school performance. Asian-American students spend twice as much time each week on homework as do other students and report that their parents would be angry if they came home with less than an A-. In contrast, African-American and Hispanic students, who do less well in school, are more cavalier about the consequences of poor school performance, devote less time to their studies, are less likely than others to attribute their success to hard work, and report that their parents have relatively lower standards.

In sum, we found that students' beliefs about the relation between education and life success influence their performance and engagement in school. However, it may be students' beliefs about the negative consequences of doing poorly in school, rather than their beliefs about the positive consequences of doing well, that matter. Youngsters who believe that they can succeed without doing well in school devote less energy to academic pursuits, whereas those who believe that academic failure will have negative repercussions are more engaged in their schooling. Although African-American and Hispanic youth earn lower grades in school than their Asian-American and White counterparts, they are just as likely as their peers to believe that doing well in school will benefit them occupationally.

In essence, our findings point to an important discrepancy between African-American and Hispanic students' values and their behavior. In contrast to the differential cultural values hypothesis outlined earlier—which suggests that ethnic differences in achievement can be explained in terms of ethnic differences in the value placed on education—we found that African-American and Hispanic students are just as likely as other students to value education. Their parents are just as likely as other parents to value education as well. Yet, on average, African-American and Hispanic youth devote less time to homework, perceive their parents as having lower performance standards, and are less likely to believe that academic success comes from working hard.

These ethnic differences in student behaviors have important implications for how students are perceived by their teachers and may help illuminate the relation between ethnicity and student performance. A recent paper by George Farkas and his colleagues (Farkas, Grobe, & Shuan, 1990) helps to make this link more understandable. In a large-scale study of Dallas students, they found that teachers assigned grades to students in part on the basis of such noncognitive factors as their work habits. The lower relative performance of African-American and Hispanic students and the higher relative performance of Asian-American students may be in large measure due to differences in these groups' work habits, which affect performance both directly, through their influence on mastery, and indirectly, through their effects on teachers' judgments.

We noted earlier that our analysis of the influence of authoritative parenting on psychosocial development, including youngsters' work orientation, indicated similar effects across all ethnic groups. Because earlier work had indicated that work orientation is a very strong predictor of school performance, and authoritative parenting a strong predictor of work orientation (Patterson, 1986; Steinberg et al., 1991), we were left with somewhat of a mystery. Why should youngsters who say they value school success, who believe in the occupational payoff of school success, and whose parents rear them in ways known to facilitate a positive work orientation, perform less well in school than we would expect? For African-American students in particular, where was the slippage in the processing linking authoritative parenting, work orientation, and school success? To understand this puzzle, we turned to yet another context—the peer group—and examined how it interacts with that of the family.

PEERS AND PARENTS AS INFLUENCES ON ACHIEVEMENT

Many of the items on our questionnaire asked students directly about the extent to which their friends and parents encouraged them to perform well in school. We used a number of these items to calculate the degree to which a student felt he or she received support for academic accomplishment from parents and, independently, from peers. We then used these indices of support to predict various aspects of students' attitudes and behaviors toward school.

We found, as have others (e.g., Brittain, 1963), that although parents are the most salient influence on youngsters' long-term educational plans, peers are the most potent influence on their day-to-day behaviors in school (e.g., how much time they spend on homework, whether they enjoy coming to school each day, and how they behave in the classroom). There are interesting ethnic differences in the relative influence of parents and peers on student achievement, however. These differences help to shed light on some of the inconsistencies and paradoxes in the school performance of minority youngsters.

For reasons that we do not yet understand, at least in the domain of schooling, parents are relatively more potent sources of influence on White and Hispanic youngsters than they are on Asian-American or African-American youngsters (Brown, Steinberg, Mounts, & Philipp, 1990). This is not to say that the mean levels of parental encouragement are necessarily lower in minority homes than in majority homes. Rather, the relative magnitude of the correlations between parental encouragement and academic success and between peer encouragement and academic success is different for minority than for majority youth. In comparison with White youngsters, minority youngsters are more influenced by their peers, and less by their parents, in matters of academic achievement.

Understanding the nature of peer group norms and peer influence processes among minority youth holds the key to unlocking the puzzle about the lack of relation between authoritative parenting and academic achievement among Asian-American and African-American youth. To fully understand the nature of peer crowds and peer influence for minority youth, it is essential to recognize the tremendous level of ethnic segregation that characterizes the social structure of most ethnically mixed high schools. We discovered this quite serendipitously. To map the social structure of each school, we interviewed students from each ethnic group in each grade level about the crowds characteristic of their school and their classmates' positions in the crowd structure (Schwendinger & Schwendinger, 1985).

For the most part, students from one ethnic group did not know their classmates from other ethnic groups. When presented with the name of a White classmate, for instance, a White student could usually assign that classmate to one of several differentiated peer crowds—"jocks," "populars," "brains," "nerds," and so forth.

When presented with the name of an African-American classmate, however, a White student would typically not know the group that this student associated with, or might simply say that the student was a part of the "Black" crowd. The same was true for Hispanic and Asian-American students. In other words, within ethnic groups, youngsters have a very differentiated view of their classmates; across ethic groups, however, they see their classmates as members of an ethnic group first, and members of a more differentiated crowd second, if at all.

The location of an adolescent within the school's social structure is very important, because peer crowd membership exerts an effect on school achievement above and beyond that of the family (Steinberg & Brown, 1989). Across all ethnic groups, youngsters whose friends and parents both support achievement perform better than those who receive support only from one source but not the other, who in turn perform better than those who receive no support from either. Thus, an important predictor of academic success for an adolescent is having support for academics from both parents and peers. This congruence of parent and peer support is greater for white and Asian-American youngsters than for African-American and Hispanic adolescents.

For White students, especially those in the middle class, the forces of parents and peers tend to converge around an ethic that supports success in school. Working with our data set, Durbin, Steinberg, Darling, and Brown (1991) found that, among White youth, youngsters from authoritative homes are more likely to belong to peer crowds that encourage academic achievement and school engagement—the "jocks" and the "populars." For these youngsters, authoritative parenting is related to academic achievement not only because of the direct effect it has on the individual adolescent's work habits, but because of the effect it has on the adolescent's crowd affiliation. Among White youngsters, authoritatively raised adolescents are more likely to associate with other youngsters who value school and behave in ways that earn them good grades.

The situation is more complicated for youngsters from minority backgrounds, because the ethnic segregation characteristic of most high schools limit their choices for peer crowd membership. We recently replicated Drubin et al.'s (1991) analyses on the relation between parenting practices and peer crowd affiliation separately within each ethnic group. Surprisingly, among African-American and Asian-American students, we found no relation between parenting practices and peer crowd membership. In other words, authoritatively raised minority youngsters do not necessarily belong to peer groups that encourage academic success. Those whose peers and parents do push them in the same direction perform quite well in school, but among authoritatively reared minority youth who are not part of a peer crowd that emphasizes achievement, the influence of peers offsets the influence of their parents.

In ethnically mixed high schools, Asian-American, African-American, and, to a lesser extent, Hispanic students find their choices of peer groups more restricted than do White students. But the nature, and consequently, the outcome of the restriction vary across ethnic groups. More often than not, Asian-American students belong to a peer group that encourages and rewards academic excellence. We have found, through student interviews, that social supports for help with academics—studying together, explaining difficult assignments, and so on—are quite pervasive among Asian-American students. Consistent with this, on our surveys, Asian-American youngsters reported the highest level of peer support for academic achievement. Interestingly, and in contrast to popular belief, our survey data indicate that Asian-American parents are less involved in their children's schooling than any other group of parents.

African-American students face quite a different situation. Although their parents are supportive of academic success, these youngsters, we learned from our interviews, find it much more difficult to join a peer group that encourages the same goal. Our interviews with high-achieving African-American students indicated that peer support for academic success is so limited that many successful African-American students eschew contact with other African-American students and affiliate primarily with students from other ethnic groups (Liederman, Landsman, & Clark, 1990). As Fordham and Ogbu (1986) reported in their ethnographic studies of African-American teenagers, African-American students are more likely than others to be caught in a bind between performing well in school and being popular among their peers.

Understanding African-American and Asian-American students' experiences in their peer groups helps to account for the finding that authoritative parenting practices, although predictive of psychological adjustment, appear almost unrelated to school performance among these youngsters. For Asian-American students, the costs to schooling of nonauthoritative parenting practices are offset by the homogeneity of influence in favor of academic success that these youngsters encounter in their peer groups. For African-American youngsters, the benefits to schooling of authoritative parenting are offset by the lack of support for academic excellence that they enjoy among their peers. Faced with this conflict between academic achievement and peer popularity, and the cognitive dissonance it must surely produce, African-American youngsters diminish the implications of doing poorly in school and maintain the belief that their occupational futures will not be harmed by school failure. This, we believe, is one explanation for the apparent paradox between African-American students' espoused values and their actual school behavior.

The situation of Hispanic students is different still. Among these youngsters, as among White youngsters, the family exerts a very strong influence on school performance and the relative influence of the peer group is weaker. Yet Hispanic students report grades and school behaviors comparable with those of African-

American students. This illustrates why the influence of the family must be evaluated in terms of the other contexts in which youngsters are expected to perform. Although Hispanic youngsters may be influenced strongly by what goes on at home (at least as much as White youngsters), what goes on in many Hispanic households may not be conducive to success in school, at least as schools are presently structured. As is the case in Asian-American homes, in Hispanic homes, the prevalence of authoritative parenting is relatively lower, and the prevalence of authoritarian parenting relatively higher. In a school system that emphasizes autonomy and self-direction, authoritarian parenting, with its emphasis on obedience and conformity and its adverse effects on self-reliance and self-confidence, may place youngsters at a disadvantage. Without the same degree of support for academics enjoyed by Asian-American students in their peer group, the level of parental authoritarianism experienced by Hispanic students may diminish their performance in school.

CONCLUSION

These findings illustrate the complex mechanisms through which the contexts in which adolescents live influence their lives and their achievement. We began by looking at one process occurring in one context: the relation between authoritative parenting and adolescent adjustment. We found, in general, that adolescents whose parents are warm, firm, and democratic achieve more in school than their peers. At the same time, however, our findings suggest that the effects of authoritative parenting must be examined within the broader context in which the family lives and in which youngsters develop. Our findings suggest that the effect of parenting practices on youngsters' academic performance and behavior is moderated to a large extent by the social milieu they encounter among their peers at school.

The nature of this moderating effect depends on the nature of the peers' values and norms: Strong peer support for academics offsets what might otherwise be the ill effects of growing up in a nonauthoritative home, whereas the absence of peer support for academics may offset some of the benefits of authoritativeness. Whether such offsetting and compensatory effects operate in other outcome domains is a question we hope to investigate in further analyses of these data.

We do not believe that we have explained the phenomenon of ethnic differences in achievement in any final sense. We do believe that the ecological approach, with its focus on the multiple contexts in which youngsters live, offers promise as a foundation for future research on this important social issue. Any explanation of the phenomenon of ethnic differences in adolescent achievement must take into account multiple, interactive processes of influence that operate across multiple interrelated contexts.

REFERENCES

Baldwin, C., & Baldwin, A. (1989, April). *The role of family interaction in the prediction of adolescent competence.* Symposium presented at the meeting of the Society for Research in Child Development, Kansas City, MO.

Baumrind, D. (1972). An exploratory study of socialization effects on Black children: Some Black–White comparisons. *Child Development, 43,* 261–267.

Baumrind, D. (1989). Rearing competent children. In W. Damon (Ed.), *Child development today and tomorrow* (pp. 349–378). San Francisco: Jossey-Bass.

Baumrind, D. (1991a). Parenting styles and adolescent development. In J. Brooks-Gunn, R. Lerner, & A. C. Petersen (Eds.), *The encyclopedia of adolescence* (pp. 746–758). New York: Garland.

Baumrind, D. (1991b). Effective parenting during the early adolescent transition. In P. A. Cowan & E. M. Hetherington (Eds.), *Advances in family research* (Vol. 2, pp. 111–163). Hillsdale, NJ: Erlbaum.

Brittain, C. V. (1963). Adolescent choices and parent–peer cross-pressures. *American Sociological Review, 28,* 385–391.

Bronfenbrenner, U. (1986). Ecology of the family as a context for human development: Research perspectives. *Developmental Psychology, 22,* 723–742.

Brown, B., Steinberg, L., Mounts, N., & Philipp, M. (1990, March). The comparative influence of peers and parents on high school achievement: Ethnic differences. In S. Lamborn (Chair), *Ethnic variations in adolescent experience.* Symposium conducted at the biennial meetings of the Society for Research on Adolescence, Atlanta.

Dornbusch, S. M., Ritter, P. L., Liederman, P., Roberts, D., & Fraleigh, M. (1987). The relation of parenting style to adolescent school performance. *Child Development, 58,* 1244–1257.

Dornbusch, S., Ritter, P., & Steinberg, L. (in press). Differences between African Americans and non-Hispanic Whites in the relation of family statuses to adolescent school performance. *American Journal of Education.*

Durbin, D., Steinberg, L., Darling, N., & Brown, B. (1991). *Parenting style and peer group membership in adolescence.* Manuscript submitted for publication.

Farkas, G., Grobe, R., & Shuan, Y. (1990). Cultural differences and school success: Gender, ethnicity, and poverty groups within an urban school district. *American Sociological Review, 55,* 127–142.

Featherman, D. L. (1980). Schooling and occupational careers: Constancy and change in worldly success. In O. Brim, Jr., & J. Kagan (Eds.), *Constancy and change in human development* (pp. 675–738). Cambridge, MA: Harvard University Press.

Fordham, S., & Ogbu, J. U. (1986). Black students' school success: Coping with the burden of "acting White." *Urban Review, 18,* 176–206.

Lamborn, S. D., Mounts, N. S., Steinberg, L., & Dornbusch, S. M. (1991). Patterns of competence and adjustment among adolescents from authoritative, authoritarian, indulgent, and neglectful families. *Child Development, 62,* 1049–1065.

Liederman, P. H., Landsman, M., & Clark, C. (1990, March). *Making it or blowing it:*

Coping strategies and academic performance in a multiethnic high school population. Paper presented at the biennial meetings of the Society for Research on Adolescence, Atlanta.

Lynn, R. (1977). The intelligence of the Japanese. *Bulletin of the British Psychological Society, 40*, 464–468.

Maccoby, E., & Martin, J. (1983). Socialization in the context of the family: Parent–child interaction. In E. M. Hetherington (Ed.), *Handbook of child psychology: Vol. 4. Socialization, personality, and social development.* (pp. 1–101). New York: Wiley.

Mickelson, R. (1990). The attitude–achievement paradox among Black adolescents. *Sociology of Education, 63*, 44–61.

Mordkowitz, E., & Ginsberg, H. (1987). Early academic socialization of successful Asian-American college students. *Quarterly Newsletter of the Laboratory of Comparative Human Cognition, 9*, 85–91.

Ogbu, J. (1978). *Minority education and caste.* San Diego, CA: Academic Press.

Patterson, G. (1986). Performance models for antisocial boys. *American Psychologist, 41*, 432–444.

Ritter, P., & Dornbusch, S. (1989, March). *Ethnic variation in family influences on academic achievement.* Paper presented at the American Education Research Association Meeting, San Francisco.

Rushton, J. (1985). Differential K theory: The sociobiology of individual and group differences. *Personality and Individual Differences, 6*, 441–452.

Schaefer, E. (1965). Children's reports of parental behavior: An inventory. *Child Development, 36*, 413–424.

Schwendinger, H., & Schwendinger, J. (1985). *Adolescent subcultures and delinquency.* New York: Praeger.

Spencer, M., & Dornbusch, S. (1990). Challenges in studying minority youth. In S. Feldman & G. Elliot (Eds.), *At the threshold: The developing adolescent* (pp. 123–146). Cambridge, MA: Harvard University Press.

Steinberg, I. (1987, April 25). Why Japan's students outdo ours. *The New York Times*, p. 15.

Steinberg, L. (1990). Autonomy, conflict, and harmony in the family relationship. In S. Feldman & G. Elliot (Eds.), *At the threshold: The developing adolescent.* (pp. 255–276). Cambridge, MA: Harvard University Press.

Steinberg, L., & Brown, B. (1989, March). *Beyond the classroom: Family and peer influences on high school achievement.* Paper presented to the Families as Educators special interest group at the annual meetings of the American Educational Research Association, San Francisco.

Steinberg, L., Elmen, J., & Mounts, N. (1989). Authoritative parenting, psychosocial maturity, and academic success among adolescents. *Child Development, 60*, 1424–1436.

Steinberg, L., Mounts, N., Lamborn, S., & Dornbusch, S. (1991). Authoritative parenting and adolescent adjustment across various ecological niches. *Journal of Research on Adolescence, 1*, 19–36.

Sue, S., & Okazaki, S. (1990). Asian-American educational achievements: A phenomenon in search of an explanation. *American Psychologist, 45*, 913–920.

Thompson, L., Detterman, D., & Plomin, R. (1991). Association between cognitive abilities and scholastic achievement: Genetic overlap but environmental differences. *Psychological Science, 2*, 158–165.

Wetzel, J. (1987). *American youth: A statistical snapshot*. New York: William T. Grant Foundation Commission on Work, Family, and Citizenship.

23

Funding Head Start: What Are the Issues?

Judith A. Chafel

Indiana University, Bloomington

Despite its current popularity in Congress, budgetary constraints dictate that future appropriations for Head Start will inevitably fall short of the amount needed to provide increased access to the program and sufficient improvement of its services. Issues are examined, competing policy options are analyzed, and a hierarchy of needs for future funding is proposed.

As Head Start celebrates its 25th anniversary, liberals and conservatives alike are extolling its virtues *(Rovner, 1990)*. Ex-president Bush sees it as a "paradigm of kindness and gentleness" (*"Bring Back," 1989*), the nation's business leaders view it as a key to resolving the shortage of skilled labor *(Rovner, 1990)*, and the governors agree that the states and the federal government should share responsibility for its funding (*"Governor's Panel," 1990*). As a *Newsweek* article aptly put it, "Everybody likes Head Start" *(1989, p. 49)*. Behind the bipartisan declarations of support, however, political controversy is brewing. Clearly, Head Start is earmarked for increased funding. Among the policy options that are vying for attention, many hard choices need to be made. Given limited financial resources, should additional money be allocated to reach more children or to improve upon the quality of existing services *(Rovner, 1990)*?

Budgetary constraints dictate that future appropriations will inevitably fall short of the amount needed to meet fully the demands of doing both. This article examines the issues, analyzes competing policy options, and offers recommenda-

Reprinted with permission from *American Journal of Orthopsychiatry*, 1992, Vol. 62(1), 9–21, Copyright © 1992 by American Orthopsychiatric Association, Inc.

A revised version of a paper submitted to the Journal in September 1990. Work on the paper was completed while the author served as Congressional Science Fellow under the sponsorship of the Society for Research in Child Development in the U.S. House of Representatives.

tions. By drawing on relevant research, it provides a conceptual framework for assessing the policy options, generating a hierarchy of needs for future funding. A rationale is developed about where the money should go first, since funds are limited.

Numerous recommendations for future funding have been presented in the literature (*"Head Start in the 1980s," 1980; "Head Start: The Nation's Pride," 1990*), but have not been ranked in any order of priority. Policymakers need this type of guidance from advocates as legislators grapple with the difficult task of balancing unrestricted wants with limited resources. As the review of relevant research in this article demonstrates, Head Start's future is in jeopardy, despite the fact that it is enjoying a veritable "lovefest" in Congress.

BACKGROUND

Launched in 1965 under the general authority of the Economic Opportunity Act (1964), Head Start is a comprehensive child development program whose primary goal is to enhance the social competence of 3–5-year-old children from low-income families. Social competence pertains to "the child's everyday effectiveness in dealing with both present environment and later responsibilities in school and life" *(Head Start Bureau, 1984, p. 1)*. Zigler and Trickett *(1978)* identified four classes of variables that constitute social competence: achievement, formal cognitive ability, motivational and emotional factors, and physical health and well-being. The performance standards of the Head Start program *(Head Start Bureau, 1984)* play an important role in advancing social competence, as well as in sustaining the overall quality of the program. They specify that Head Start must deliver a wide range of services to ensure comprehensive care: health, education, parental involvement, and social services (*"Head Start: The Nation's Pride," 1990*).

Originally administered by the Office of Economic Opportunity, the Head Start program is now run by the Administration for Children, Youth, and Families (ACYF), Department of Health and Human Services (DHHS) *(National Health Policy Forum, 1990)*. Federal regulations (*"Eligibility Requirements," 1989*) require that 90% of the children enrolled must fall below the poverty level defined by the guidelines of the Office of Management and Budget, with the neediest families receiving preference. Up to 10% of those enlisted in local programs may be from families who do not meet the criterion of low income, although the Head Start regulations state that "If applications for admission . . . are received for more children from low-income families than the Head Start program can accommodate, the children from the lowest income families shall be given preference" (*"Eligibility Requirements," 1989, p. 231*). Ten percent of the places available for each state must be accessible to handicapped children. Once accepted, a child remains eligible for that year and the following one, regardless of any changes in family income.

In 1989, 3% of Head Start enrollees were under age 3, 8% were 5-year-olds, 25% were 3-year-olds, and 64% were 4-year-olds. Approximately 13% were handicapped. In 1990, Head Start was calculated to enroll approximately 20% of the total population of 3–5-year-olds whose family income fell below the poverty line, with a projected appropriation of $1.386 billion serving an estimated 488,470 children *(Stewart & Robinson, 1990)*.

A substantial body of research attests to the effectiveness of the Head Start program. Using a statistical technique known as meta-analysis, McKey, Condelli, Ganson, Barrett, McConkey, and Plantz *(1985)* analyzed 210 reports of research on the effects of Head Start on children, families, and communities. Representing one of the most definitive and comprehensive statements of Head Start's impact ever published, the study concluded that children who were enrolled in the program experienced immediate gains in cognitive and socioemotional test scores, as well as in health status. Over time, gains in cognitive and socioemotional development did not remain superior by comparison with disadvantaged children who did not attend Head Start. A small subset of studies verified that former Head Start children were more likely to be promoted to the next grade and less likely to be assigned to special education classes. Other findings indicated that Head Start assisted families by furnishing education, health, and social services and by linking them with available resources in the community. Furthermore, economic, educational, health care, social service, and other institutions were influenced by Head Start staff and parents in a way that yielded benefits to Head Start and non-Head Start families in their respective communities.

REACHING MORE CHILDREN

During his 1988 campaign, President Bush vowed to provide "full funding" for Head Start *(Rovner, 1990)*. As submitted to Congress on January 29, 1990, his budget sought to increase financing of the program by $500 million in fiscal year 1991 to an overall allocation of $1.9 billion. The 36% increase over the 1990 level, the largest in the program's history, would enable Head Start to enroll an estimated additional 180,000 4-year-olds *("Budget of the United States Government," 1990)*. As the administration has maintained, the added funds "could allow us to serve up to 70 percent of eligible children for at least 1 year and bring within reach our goal of a universal Head Start program" (Rovner, 1990, p. 1194). According to Wade Horn of DHHS, full funding for Head Start would eventually mean one year of the program for 90% of those eligible, with an emphasis on 4-year-olds. The administration did not stipulate when it would reach that goal or at what cost *(Rovner, 1990)*.

On May 16, 1990, the House passed a four-year Head Start reauthorization bill. That legislation (HR 4151) authorized $2.4 billion in fiscal 1991 ($1 billion more than currently funded and $500 million more than the president's request). Full funding would be reached in fiscal 1994 at a cost of $7.7 billion *(Perez, 1990)*. HR 4151 would permit the Head Start program to serve all eligible 3- and 4-year-olds and the 30% of 5-year-olds who are not enrolled in kindergarten *(Rovner, 1990)*.

IMPROVING SERVICES

Many advocates of Head Start maintain that the quality of existing programs should be improved before expansion occurs. Administration officials, on the other hand, insist that expanding enrollment should come before considerations of quality. Yale psychologist Edward F. Zigler, an architect of the original program, pointed out, "I see a tremendous decline in the quality of Head Start from 25 years ago. . . . I'd rather serve fewer children well than more children badly" *(quoted in Rovner, 1990, p. 1191)*. According to Wade Horn of DHHS, "Quality is at its highest level in the history of the program" *(quoted in Rovner, 1990, p. 1194)*.

With legislative jurisdiction over Head Start, the House Education and Labor Subcommittee on Human Resources is determined to improve its quality, as well as to expand enrollment. As provided by HR 4151, the four-year reauthorization of Head Start, passed on May 16, 1990, 10% of the total funding in the first fiscal year and 25% in each subsequent year are designated for improving quality, provided that appropriations grow sufficiently to cover inflation and to furnish a cushion (yet to be specified). Half the set-aside would go for improving salaries and benefits, with the remainder earmarked for hiring support staff; improving facilities; and paying for insurance, staff training, and transportation *(HR 4151, 1990)*.

RESOLVING ISSUES

In resolving the competing policy options as they pertain to the quantity versus quality dilemma, several essential questions must be addressed: 1) Who should be served? 2) For how long? and 3) Are there threats to the quality of the program?

Who Should Be Served?

Current Head Start policy is focused on providing a single year of service for 4-year-olds. The rationale for the policy is threefold. First, it targets limited resources. Second, it reaches a higher percentage of the eligible population, with eligibility limited to 4-year-olds *("Head Start: The Nation's Pride," 1990)*. Third, it provides services for children in the year before they begin school *(National Health Policy Forum, 1990).*

Since its inception, Head Start has emphasized flexibility in operation of the program by local communities *(Stewart & Robinson, 1990).* Any future expansion of Head Start enrollment should respect this orientation. The recruitment process should continue to seek out children from the "most disadvantaged homes," as currently specified by Head Start's program performance standards *(Head Start Bureau, 1984, p. 53).* Targeting specific age groups should be left to the discretion of local grantees. This approach to expansion recognizes that the question of who should be served is best decided at the local level, based upon an assessment of a community's needs.

For How Long?

Current Head Start policy, as stated previously, is focused on providing a single year of service. As James Renier, a trustee of the Committee for Economic Development (CED), cogently testified, "All by itself, one year of preschool is not going to instill children, buffeted and battered by the culture of poverty, with the . . . values and drive needed to help them compete successfully in school" *(quoted in Rovner, 1990, p. 1195).* In fact, Head Start staff report that they frequently need two years to provide the benefits reported by high-quality early childhood programs. For multiple-problem families, it may take the entire first year of enrollment to get to know the children and parents well enough to provide adequate services. Moreover, a second year is often critical for children whose primary language is not English *("Head Start: The Nation's Pride," 1990; National Health Policy Forum, 1990).* Both these groups represent a growing proportion of the Head Start population *("Head Start: The Nation's Pride," 1990; Kusserow, 1989).*

In addition, Head Start provides nutritious meals, medical and dental care, and other services to children who might not otherwise receive them. A second year in the program would magnify these benefits. The potential for reaching children and families more effectively and for promoting healthy development both point to the need for extending Head Start beyond a single year of service. Unless exceptions are warranted on the basis of an assessment of a local community's needs, it is preferable to reach fewer children more effectively with multiple years of service than a higher percentage of the eligible population for a single year, as the current policy prescribes.

The Bush administration has justified its policy of providing a single year of service for 4-year-olds on the basis of a study which showed that a second year of preschool for children in poverty is less cost-effective than is the first *("Head Start Endures," 1990).* Although the study was not named, at least two investigations furnished partial support for the administration's position. While a study of the Perry Preschool program in Ypsilanti, Michigan, found that two years of preschool were no more beneficial than was one *(Barnett, 1985; Weber, 1975; Weber, Foster, & Weikart, 1978)*, the sample was too small to place much confidence in the data *(Barnett & Escobar, 1987)*. In addition, the generalizability of that study was limited by the characteristics of the program as well as of the sample, and by the context of the experiment *(Barnett & Escobar, 1987)*. Working with a comfortably larger sample, a study of Home Start found no meaningful effects pertaining to the length of intervention, whether children entered at age 3 or 4. Two years of the program were indisputably twice as expensive as one *(Love, Nauta, Coelen, Hewlett, & Ruopp, 1976)*. However, Home Start is sufficiently different from Head Start for the generality of these findings to be questionable. Furthermore, as Barnett and Escobar *(1987)* pointed out, confidence in the data is lessened by a 57% attrition rate over two years.

For children of disadvantaged backgrounds, "the more intervention the better" hypothesis is a reasonable assertion, even if it is not supported by existing data *(Washington & Oyemade, 1987; Zigler & Valentine, 1979)*. Although scientific evidence would lend greater weight to the hypothesis, the lack of it should not preclude the recommendation advanced here. The point at issue is not that intervention efforts should be implemented, but that they should be implemented *effectively*. Intuition and the insights of practitioners in the field, as argued earlier, suggest that a two-year, rather than a single-year, model is preferable, the lack of research notwithstanding.

Are There Threats to the Program's Quality?

Several points merit consideration in addressing this question. First, to be effective, the Head Start program should provide good early childhood services, as reflected by several important indicators of program quality commonly agreed upon in the field of early childhood education *(Bredekamp, 1990; "Head Start: The Nation's Pride," 1990; Weikart, 1989)*. Second, it should provide for continuity with and transition into the public schools *("Head Start: The Nation's Pride," 1990; McKey et al., 1985)*. Third, it should respond flexibly to the changing needs of Head Start parents for full-day, year-round care, as well as to the growing number of dysfunctional families whose children are enrolled in the program. *("Head Start: The Nation's Pride," 1990)*.

Regarding the first point—that the program must provide good early childhood services: on a cost-per-child basis, Head Start has a long history of inadequate funding *(Bolce, 1990)*. According to data provided by the High Scope Educational Research Foundation, per-child funding of Head Start in constant dollars declined by 13% in the eighties, from $3,084 in 1981 to $2,672 in 1989 *(Rovner, 1990)*.

By comparison, the Perry Preschool program, often cited as a successful intervention model for disadvantaged children, is funded at a level more than double that of Head Start: about $4,963 per child per year in 1981, which translates to $6,287 in 1989 dollars *(Danziger & Stern, 1990)*.

The low cost per child in the Head Start program is reflected in a number of important indicators of program quality: 1) salaries and benefits, 2) staff training, 3) class size, 4) staffing, and 5) transportation and facilities *(Bolce, 1990)*.

Salaries and benefits. The inability to pay competitive salaries is making it increasingly difficult both to recruit and to retain qualified staff *(Collins, 1990)*. Stephan *(1986)* reported a 19% turnover rate in urban areas. The current expansion of non-Head Start early childhood programs in the public schools is a major factor that has fueled the high turnover rate. Non-Head Start programs, in general, offer higher salaries and better benefit packages than do Head Start programs *(Slaughter, Washington, Oyemade, & Lindsey, 1988)*. A study by the Administration for Children, Youth, and Families in 1988 reported that 47% of Head Start teachers earned less than $10,000 per year *("Head Start: The Nation's Pride," 1990)*. In 1988, the average annual beginning salary of a Head Start teacher with a bachelor of arts degree was $12,074, a figure well below a public school teacher's salary. Inadequate salaries are not limited to teachers, but affect coordinators and aides, as well *("Head Start: The Nation's Pride," 1990)*.

Whitebook, Howes, and Phillips *(1989)* examined how teachers and their work environment affect the quality of programs. They found that teachers provided more sensitive and appropriate caregiving if they received higher wages and better benefits and *worked in centers in which a higher percentage of the operating budget was allocated to teaching personnel.* With respect to the adult work environment, the most important predictor of the quality of care that children received was the wages of staff. Teaching staff who earned the lowest wages were twice as likely to leave their jobs as were those who earned the highest wages. *Turnover is harmful to children.* Children in centers with higher rates of turnover spent less time engaged in social activities with peers, spent more time in aimless wandering, and scored lower on a test of language development than did children in centers with more stable teaching staff.

Staff training. Research indicates that a well-trained staff is a critical component of a high-quality early childhood program *(Whitebook et al., 1989)*. Although Head Start's overall program budget has increased by over 80% in the past decade, the set-aside for training has increased only slightly during that time *(National Health Policy Forum, 1990)*. An analysis of Head Start Fact Sheets done by the National Head Start Association, has shown that funding for training and career development as a percentage of the Head Start budget declined from approximately 5.25% in 1974 to 2.10% in 1989 *("Head Start: The Nation's Pride," 1990)*. With the Head Start program experiencing a high turnover rate and depending heavily on parent volunteers, a reduction in training and technical assistance has had serious consequences *(Slaughter et al., 1988).* At a time when Head Start staff are struggling to find ways of assisting families who are faced with serious problems (e.g., substance abuse, homelessness), adequate training is more important than ever *(National Health Policy Forum, 1990).*

Class size. Research strongly suggests that smaller groups and higher teacher–child ratios have positive benefits for children *(Bredekamp, 1990).* Currently, the average size of a Head Start classroom is 18, with a range of 12 to 22 children *(Federal Register, 1988).* Although the figures appear to be acceptable, Bolce *(1990)* reported that to reduce costs, many Head Start programs have been forced to increase the size of their classes. The National Day Care Study *(Ruopp, Travers, Glantz, & Coelen, 1979)* reported on the advantages for children of preschool classrooms having small group sizes. In classrooms with a small number of children, teachers engaged in more social interaction with children and less passive observation of activities, with children showing greater gains on assessments of cognitive skill, cooperation with peers, verbal initiative in offering opinions, supplying information, expressing preferences, and reflective or innovative behavior in play or in assigned tasks. Moreover, children exhibited less negative behavior—hostility or conflict—with others and were less likely to wander aimlessly around the classroom or to be disengaged from activities.

The teacher–child ratio is an important determinant of the quality of a program because it facilitates individualized care *(Bredekamp, 1990).* Exemplary early childhood programs tend to have high teacher–child ratios *(Grubb, 1989).* Grubb reported a ratio of 1:7.5 for Head Start classrooms, an acceptable proportion. Some consensus has emerged among professionals about the outer limit of what is considered adequate. The National Day Care Study found that above the ratio of 1:10, quality deteriorates, with children displaying less persistence as well as less interest in activities *(Ruopp et al., 1979).* In future, care must be taken to ensure that class sizes and teacher–child ratios in Head Start programs are held consistent with what is suggested by the findings of research, the recommendations of professionals in the field, and information on what is considered to be "good" practice.

Staffing. Limited funding has forced many programs to cut back on staff that are required for the delivery of Head Start's comprehensive services. A recent analysis revealed that 71% of Head Start programs nationwide had social service caseloads of more than 60 to 1; 17% of Head Start grantees lacked a full-time social service coordinator, 12% lacked a full-time health coordinator, and 18% lacked a full-time parent involvement coordinator *(Bolce, 1990).* In addition, insufficient staff and travel funds have impaired the ability of regional Head Start offices to monitor local programs and to offer technical assistance *("Head Start: The Nation's Pride," 1990; National Health Policy Forum, 1990).*

ACYF estimated that in 1988 about 20% of Head Start programs were monitored *(Stewart & Robinson, 1990)*.

Transportation and facilities. Limited funding has caused many programs to decrease or eliminate transportation services for children and families. Without such services, those who are most in need of Head Start may be unable to participate *(Bolce, 1990)*. In their responses to the Silver Ribbon Panel survey, many parents reported that lack of transportation was a barrier to their involvement, as well as to medical services and job opportunities *("Head Start: The Nation's Pride," 1990)*. Another serious problem is the shortage of affordable and appropriate facilities *("Head Start: The Nation's Pride," 1990)*. An expanding preschool population has forced many public schools to take back space that they had either given or rented to Head Start programs in the past *(Goodman & Brady, 1988)*. The trend is disturbing, given that the General Accounting Office estimated that 29% of Head Start's facilities are situated in public school buildings *("Head Start: The Nation's Pride," 1990)*. Today, many Head Start programs operate in facilities that were not designed originally for use by children. Bolce *(1990, p. 2)* testified that such accommodations may be "inappropriate, inadequate, or in some instances even unsafe.'

The second point to be considered is that the Head Start program must provide for continuity with and transition into the public schools. Research has verified that Head Start has immediate positive effects on the cognitive and socioemotional development of young children, but questions remain about long-term gains *(Gamble & Zigler, 1989; McKey et al., 1985; Schweinhart & Weikart, 1986)*. As noted in the final report of the Head Start Evaluation, Synthesis and Utilization Project, one of the most definitive and comprehensive statements of Head Start's impact ever published: "It may be that cognitive and socioemotional differences diminish over time because the educational environment in elementary schools does not support and stimulate the children as effectively as Head Start did" *(McKey et al., 1985, p. 21)*. McKey et al. compared long-range cognitive effects on Head Start children found by studies before and after 1970. Gains by Head Start children for the first two years after they left the program were greater when measured by studies carried out after 1970 than before. According to the researchers, these findings suggest that changes that were made in Head Start after 1970 (e.g., converting summer Head Start to full-year programs, initiating training and technical assistance, and implementing Head Start performance standards) were having positive effects. Several small-scale studies of Follow Through programs (whose aim is to pick up where Head Start leaves off) have substantiated that the continuation of compensatory education in the first three grades of school can maintain cognitive gains through these grades *(Abelson, Zigler, & DeBlasi, 1974)*.

Innovative efforts to sustain the early developmental benefits of Head Start are warranted to ensure that the effects of early intervention do not fade *(Copple, Cline, & Smith, 1987; McKey et al., 1985)*. One such attempt was Project Developmental Continuity, a demonstration model begun in 1974 by the Office of Child Development, to ensure the continuity of goals *after* Head Start. The program offered continuous services to children throughout the first three years of primary school *(Zigler & Valentine, 1979)*. Since the philosophy and curriculum of the public schools are often at variance with the Head Start program, intervention efforts like Project Developmental Continuity are critical to Head Start's success and should be revived.

The third point is that the program must respond flexibly to the changing needs of Head Start families for full-day, year-round care, which is necessary to accommodate the schedules of a growing number of Head Start parents in the work force, as well as the growing number of dysfunctional families whose children are enrolled in the program. About 90% of Head Start families are headed by a single parent *(Slaughter et al., 1988)*, who has no choice but to work outside the home to achieve economic self-sufficiency. The National Head Start Association reported that in 1988, 32% of Head Start parents worked full time and another 19% worked part time, performed seasonal work, or were enrolled in school or training programs *("Head Start: The Nation's Pride" 1990)*. Yet, the number of full-day Head Start programs is too small to meet the needs of these families *(National Health Policy Forum, 1990)*. Today, Head Start is primarily a half-day program. For many low-income families, especially those headed by a single-parent or teenage mother, the availability of affordable, high-quality child care can make the difference between choosing and not choosing to pursue educational and employment opportunities *(Slaughter et al., 1988)*.

The Family Support Act of 1988 makes the case for full-day care even more compelling *(Committee on Ways and Means, 1990; National Health Policy Forum, 1990)*. The law mandates that mothers with children over age 3 must enter job training programs or risk losing their payments from Aid to Families with Dependent Children (AFDC). The JOBS program, established under the Family Support Act of 1988, guarantees child care assistance to any welfare parent who engages in education, training, or work. The major purpose of the child care component is to free parents to enroll in JOBS. Forty-seven percent of Head Start families receive AFDC *(Stewart & Robinson, 1990)*. Many families who are enrolled in JOBS and who are eligible for Head Start may choose not to enroll in the latter program if their needs for full-day, full-year care are not met *(Stewart & Robinson, 1990)*. The coordination of child care with local welfare agencies is essential if Head Start is to retain its client base *(Head Start Bureau, 1990; National Health Policy Forum, 1990)*. Without such coordination, a growing number of children may be placed in low-quality child care programs that lack Head Start's comprehensive services *(National Health Policy Forum, 1990)* and, consequently, may be placed at further risk of developmental harm.

Head Start must respond to the growing number of dysfunctional families whose children are enrolled in the program. DHHS has reported an increase in the number of serious problems afflicting Head Start families—problems so severe that they alter the ability of many families to participate in Head Start services *(Kusserow, 1989)*. As defined by the DHHS report, "dysfunctional families" are those with problems so virulent that the family is not able to fulfill the physical, psychological, and social needs of children and other family members. The study's survey of Head Start programs found that the problems that multiproblem families most frequently face are substance abuse, the lack of parenting skills by teenage single mothers, child abuse, domestic violence, and inadequate housing. Some programs reported having no such families, but others estimated that they constituted as much as 85% of their programs and that community services for these families were either "inaccessible" or "inadequate" *(Kusserow, 1989, p. 15)*. Concern was expressed about the additional demands that such families place on Head Start programs and their staff.

SERVICE WITHIN THE FAMILY CONTEXT

During the seventies, Head Start experimented with a model of service delivery known as the Child and Family Resource Program (CFRP) *(Comptroller General, 1979)*. The CFRPs provide a way of addressing many of the threats to program quality discussed earlier. A family-focused approach, the CFRPs served children from birth through age 8 within the context of their families. A broad range of services were provided, such as home visiting for infants, early intervention for developmentally delayed children, and referrals to much-needed social services *(National Health Policy Forum, 1990)*.

Family services were furnished by the CFRPs on the assumption that a child cannot develop optimally in the presence of serious unresolved family problems *(Zigler & Seitz, 1980)*. A distinctive feature of the CFRP was its attempt to tailor services to individual families' needs *(Comptroller General, 1979)*. The program engaged in both formal and informal assessment and goal setting, with different families receiving services, as indicated. By dealing with the full scope of each family's needs, the CFRPs endeavored to bring coherence to the fragmented system of public and private social services with which low-income families typically must cope. They were designed to supplement, rather than duplicate, existing community resources.

Services were offered within the context of three components: 1) the Infant-Toddler Component, 2) the Head Start Component, and 3) the Preschool-School Linkage Component, each designed to serve families with children in a specific age group *(Comptroller General, 1979)*. Taken together, the three components were intended to provide developmental and educational continuity from before birth to the primary grades of school.

The first component served families with children from birth to age 3. Two types of activities were offered to families: home visits and sessions at CFRP centers. Home visits provided needs assessments and goal setting, parental education and counseling, and child development activities. Sessions at centers delivered parental education activities (e.g., lectures and discussions of common problems) and infant-toddler activities (e.g., group experiences that, in some cases, were educational or even therapeutic). In addition, families received special services (e.g., crisis intervention, counseling) on an "as-needed" basis.

The second component served families with children from age 3 until the children entered elementary school. At this stage, children received developmental services through the Head Start program itself. Parents continued to receive home visits, attend sessions at centers, and participate in other support services.

The third component established linkages with the public schools. There were five goals: 1) parental involvement with the teacher, 2) an enhanced sense of belonging in the school system, 3) expanded parental involvement in the child's academic development, 4) better attendance at school, and 5) augmented academic skills. Linkages were generally limited to establishing contact, finding out about registration procedures, and informing schools that children would enter. Other activities included orientation of Head Start children, their parents, and school personnel; troubleshooting in response to requests from parents and school personnel; tutoring children; sharing children's records with the schools and assisting in the placement of children with special needs; and, in some programs, home visits. The CFRPs' efforts to ease the transition of at-risk children into the public schools and to boost parents' interest and involvement in their education have a strong basis in research, given Rist's *(1970)* documentation of how a child's first few months in school can establish a negative pattern that endures for years.

Travers, Nauta, and Irwin *(1982)* reported that the evaluators of CFRPs found significant effects on mothers' self-reported control of events and general coping, participation in job training and employment, and use of community resources. These significant effects did not translate into immediately measurable benefits for children, a finding that can be explained by the fact that much of the program's effort was devoted to family support rather than to child development *(Nauta & Travers, 1982)*. No effects were observed on child development and only modest gains were found in certain parental teaching skills.

A study by the General Accounting Office (GAO) *(Comptroller General, 1979)* found the CFRPs to be cost-effective. Documented benefits of the program included better preventive health care and nutrition for young children, speedy assistance to families in times of crisis, the correction of problems (such as inadequate housing) through referrals to existing agencies, and improvement in the overall quality of life. The GAO report emphasized that "The CFRPs, as designed, contain the components necessary for a successful early childhood and family development program" *(p. 53)*. In spite of GAO's recommendation that the CFRPs be expanded, they were terminated in 1983 under the Reagan administration. The concept was revived with modest demonstration funding by Congress in 1988, with passage of legislation enacting the Comprehensive Child Development Centers *(National Health Policy Forum, 1990)*. Given the nature of the CFRP and its documented positive effects, it warrants funding in any future appropriations devoted to Head Start.

RECOMMENDATIONS

Research has confirmed that early childhood programs can help children from impoverished families achieve both cognitively and socially and overcome school failure *(Berrueta-Clement, Schweinhart, Barnett, Epstein, & Weikart, 1984; McKey et al., 1985; Lazar, Darlington, Murray, Royce, & Snipper, 1982)*. These positive effects occur, *provided that programs are of high quality (Ruopp et al., 1979)*. Today, Head Start is struggling to maintain the quality of its program. As Congress contemplates the possibility of broadening access to Head Start, the issue of quality must be addressed. Deriving from research and "best" professional practice, a number of recommendations for future funding are presented. All are critical to the well-being of the Head Start program. Given budgetary constraints, it is highly unlikely that Congress can address them all. Therefore, the recommendations should be targeted for funding according to a hierarchy of needs, as follows:

1. If Head Start enrollments are increased at a time when staff is declining because of turnover, it will be unprepared to accommodate more children. Excessive staff turnover is not only harmful to children *(Whitebook et al., 1989)*, but increases the costs of staff training, as newly prepared staff leave for better paying jobs elsewhere *("Head Start: The Nation's Pride," 1990)*. To reverse the trend in staff turnover, salaries and benefits must be increased.

2. Research has long suggested that "the quality of child care can be no better than the quality of the care giver" *("Head Start in the 1980s," 1980, p. 14)*. Therefore, funding for the training of caregivers and the appropriate incentives to obtain that training must be allocated to ensure that Head Start children receive effective services.

3. Money should be targeted to guarantee that programs continue to be in compliance with acceptable staff–child ratios and class sizes, as suggested by the findings of research, the recommendations of professionals in the field, and information on what is considered to be "good" practice.

4. Resources should be provided for the gradual establishment of minimums (as specified by the Social Services Task Force *[Head Start Bureau, 1989])* for family–staff ratios in the areas of health, services for the handicapped, the involvement of parents, and social services. They should also permit training of the corresponding personnel, as well as provision of technical assistance and over-sight to maintain and improve the program's quality.

5. Funding should be provided to phase the CFRP into Head Start. The CFRP model would do the following:

a. Tailor services to the needs of individual families and link families with a broad array of social services, building on already-existing community resources.

b. Enable Head Start programs to attend to prenatal and toddler services, par-ticularly for children of teenage parents. Outreach services to teenagers during pregnancy and immediately after the birth of a child would be enhanced. Head Start's successful nutrition component could be extended to the prenatal and immediate postnatal period, a time when good nutrition is critical for child devel-opment *("Head Start in the 1980s, 1980).*

c. Reach out to severely "troubled" families, providing speedy assistance in times of crisis (for example, when families are afflicted by substance abuse, domestic violence, inadequate housing, or child abuse), and help them to cope better with the daily tasks of survival.

d. Ease the transition of at-risk children into the public schools and elevate par-ent's interest and involvement in their education.

6. Options should be explored and developed for providing full-day, year-round care for the children of working families, who compose a large proportion of the population that is in poverty *("Head Start in the 1980s," 1980).* Ways should be examined to collaborate with welfare agencies in providing full-day services to Head Start families, falling under the JOBS program. Among these ways are "wraparound" (coordinated) arrangements with existing funding sources and ser-vices in the community *(Head Start Bureau, 1990; Wrap-around Funding," 1989–90).* Wraparound arrangements can extend Head Start services without additional financial outlays by combining Head Start funding with other federal, state, or local sources (e.g., Title XX, state departments of education, the United Way). Steps should be taken to ensure that continuity of care is provided for chil-dren with any wraparound arrangement and that Head Start's high standards are maintained.

7. Head Start is experiencing a lack of space, a situation that will be worsened by the need to serve more children. Therefore, funds should be designated for facilities, and possible incentives for public and private investment in Head Start should be explored *("Head Start: The Nation's Pride," 1990).*

8. Because of limited funding, Head Start has reduced transportation services, another problem that will be exacerbated by expanding enrollments. To make it

possible to serve wider geographic boundaries and families situated in distant locales (e.g., in rural areas), funds should be earmarked for transportation costs.

9. Access for more children should be increased:

a. The recruitment process should continue to seek out children from "the most disadvantaged homes," as currently specified by the Head Start Program Performance Standards *(Head Start Bureau, 1984, p. 53)*.

b. Targeting of specific age groups should be left to the discretion of local grantees.

c. Unless exceptions are warranted on the basis of an assessment of local community needs, it is preferable to reach fewer children more effectively with multiple years of service than a higher percentage of the eligible population for a single year, as current policy prescribes.

d. Future legislation ought to contain specific language to ensure that any decisions regarding the ages of children served, as well as the length of service, should remain the prerogative of local Head Start programs, since these programs best understand the needs of the children and families who are residing in their communities *(Human Services Reauthorization Act, 1990)*.

10. Research and evaluation efforts should be funded to assess which features of Head Start are most effective for which types of families. These efforts are needed to guide program planning and to assist Head Start in offering the most cost-effective match of services *("Head Start in the 1980s," 1980)*, as well as to ascertain what is necessary for sustaining Head Start's positive effects on children *("Head Start: The Nation's Pride," 1990)*.

11. Funding should be provided to develop and test innovative strategies for serving dysfunctional families and to collect and disseminate information on what is successful *(Kusserow, 1989)*.

12. Innovative arrangements with state and local governments and with businesses to share responsibility for financing Head Start should be explored. The nation's governors have agreed that the states and the federal government should participate in its support *("Governor's Panel," 1990)*. The CED (1987), an independent organization of over 200 business executives and educators, has called for "full funding of the program," asserting that if present trends persist, the nation will face a severe employment crisis in the years ahead. The CED concluded that Head Start's effects on children can lead to success in formal schooling and the workplace. Enlisting the support of the business community is a logical extension of this idea.

Many of the recommendations made by Washington and Oyemade *(1987)* are consistent with those just advanced. Specifically, they pertain to the following: 1) staff training, salary, and benefits; 2) class size and child–staff ratios; 3) technical assistance; 4) parenting by teenagers; 5) services for children under age 3; 6) transition into the public schools; 7) full-day care; 8) transportation; and 9) access.

While Washington and Oyemade *(1987)* did not rank these options for future funding, they averred that the first priority should be "to maintain and improve the quality of Head Start programs" *(p. 146).*

As Head Start undertakes its second quarter of a century, it faces serious challenges. In an era of budgetary constraint, advocates of the program must shift from pleading for the satisfaction of all its needs, even if they are essential, to accepting that hard choices can and will be made. Fortunately, research provides some guidance for deciding among the options. Advocates of the program must see to it that policymakers are so informed.

REFERENCES

Abelson, W., Zigler, E., & DeBlasi, C. (1974). Effects of a four-year follow through program on economically disadvantaged children. *Journal of Educational Psychology, 66,* 756–771.

Barnett, W. (1985). Benefit-cost analysis of the Perry Preschool Program and its long-term effects. *Educational Evaluation and Policy Analysis, 7,* 333–342.

Barnett, W., & Escobar, C. (1987). The economics of early educational intervention: A review. *Review of Educational Research, 57,* 387–414.

Berrueta-Clement, J., Schweinhart, L., Barnett, W., Epstein, A., & Weikart, D. (1984). Changed lives: The effects of the Perry Preschool Program on youths through age 19. *Monographs of the High/Scope Educational Research Foundation, 8.* Ypsilanti, MI: High/Scope Press.

Bolce, D. (1990, February 1). Informal briefing by the Director of Information Services, National Head Start Association, to the staff of the Subcommittee on Children, Family, Drugs and Alcoholism of the Committee on Labor and Human resources, 101st Cong., 2nd sess., U.S. Senate, Washington, DC.

Bredekamp, S. (Ed.). (1990). *Accreditation criteria and procedures of the National Academy of Early Childhood programs.* Washington, DC: National Association for the Education of Young Children.

Bring back big spending. (1989, March 27). *New Republic, 200,* pp. 7–8.

Budget of the United States Government, Fiscal year 1991 (041 001 00349 5). (1990). Washington, DC: U.S. Government Printing Office.

Collins, R. (1990). *National Head Start Association 1989–90 staff salary survey: Preliminary findings for 7 states.* Unpublished manuscript, National Head Start Association, Alexandria, VA.

Committee for Economic Development. (1987). *Children in need: Investment strategies for the educationally disadvantaged.* New York: Author.

Committee on Ways and Means. (1990). *Overview of entitlement programs. 1990 Green Book: Background material and data on programs within the jurisdiction of the Committee on Ways and Means.* Washington, DC: U.S. Government Printing Office.

Comptroller General of the United States. (1979, February 6) (No. HRD 79-40). *Report to the Congress: Early childhood and family development programs improve the quality of life for low-income families.* Washington, DC: U.S. Government Accounting Office.

Copple, C., Cline, M., & Smith, A. (1987). *Path to the future: Long-term effects of Head Start in the Philadelphia School District.* Washington, DC: Head Start Bureau, U.S. Department of Health and Human Services.

Danziger, S., & Stern, J. (1990, September). *The causes and consequences of child poverty in the United States.* Paper prepared for UNICEF, International Child Development Center, Project on Child Poverty and Deprivation in Industrialized Countries.

Eligibility requirements and limitations for enrollment in Head Start (45 CFR, part 1305). (1989, October 1). Washington, DC: Office of Human Development Services.

Everybody likes Head Start. (1989, February 20). *Newsweek*, pp. 49–50.

Federal Register. (1988, December 8). Washington, DC: U.S. Government Printing Office.

Gamble, T., & Zigler, E. (1989). The Head Start Synthesis Project: A critique. *Journal of Applied Developmental Psychology, 10,* 267–274.

Goodman, I., & Brady, J. (1988). *The challenge of coordination.* Unpublished manuscript, Education Development Center, Newton, MA.

Governor's panel urges full funding of Head Start. (1990, February 25). *Washington Post*, p. A3.

Grubb, W. (1989). Young children face the State: Issues and options for early childhood programs. *American Journal of Education, 97,* 358–397.

HR 4151. (1990, March 1). Washington, DC: U.S. House of Representatives, 101st Cong., 2nd sess.

Head Start Bureau. (1984, November). *Head Start program performance standards* (45-CFR 1304). Washington, DC: U.S. Department of Health & Human Services.

Head Start Bureau. (1989, March 29). *Information Memorandum: Final Report, Commissioner's Task Force on Social Services* (ACYF-IM-89-07). Washington, DC: U.S. Department of Health & Human Services.

Head Start Bureau. (1990). *Information memorandum: Head Start coordination with child care programs* (ACYF-IM-90-02). Washington, DC: U.S. Department of Health and Human Services.

Head Start endures, Making a difference. (1990, April 22). *Washington Post*, p. A1.

Head Start in the 1980s: Review and recommendations (DHHS Publication No. [OHDS] 81-31164). (1980, September). Washington, DC: U.S. Department of Health and Human Services.

Head Start: The nation's pride, A nation's challenge: Recommendations for Head Start in the 1990s. (1990). Alexandria, VA: National Head Start Association.

Human Services Reauthorization Act of 1990. Report together with supplemental and additional views (Report 101-480). (1990, May 9). Washington, DC: U.S. House of Representatives, 101st Cong., 2nd sess.

Kusserow, R. (1989, November). *Dysfunctional families in the Head Start Program: Meeting the challenge* (OAI-09-89-01000). Washington, DC: U.S. Department of Health & Human Services.

Lazar, I., Darlington, R., Murray, H., Royce, J., & Snipper, A. (1982). Lasting effects of early education. *Monographs of the Society for Research in Child Development, 47* (2-3, Serial No. 195).

Love, J., Nauta, M., Coelen, C., Hewlett, K., & Ruopp, R. (1976). *National Home Start evaluation final report: Findings and implications.* Cambridge, MA: Abt Associates.

McKey, R., Condelli, L., Ganson, H., Barrett, B., McConkey, C., & Plantz, M. (1985). *The impact of Head Start on children, families and communities. Executive summary* (DHHS Publication No. [OHDS] 85-31193). Washington, DC: U.S. Government Printing Office.

National Health Policy Forum. (1990). *The future of Head Start* (Issue Brief No. 544). Washington, DC: Author.

Nauta, M., & Travers, J. (1982). *The effects of a social program: Executive summary of CFRP's infant-toddler component.* Cambridge, MA: Abt Associates.

Perez, R. (1990, April 7). House subcommittee approves big Head Start expansion. *Congressional Quarterly, 48*(14), 1081.

Rist, R. (1970). Student social class and teacher expectations: The self-fulfilling prophecy in ghetto education. *Harvard Educational Review, 40*, 411–451.

Rovner, J. (1990, April 21). Head Start is one program everyone wants to help. *Congressional Quarterly, 48*(16), 1191–1195.

Ruopp, R., Travers, J., Glantz, F., & Coelen, C. (1979). *Children at the center: Summary findings and their implications. Final report of the National Day Care Study* (Vol. 1). Cambridge, MA: Abt Associates.

Schweinhart, L., & Weikart, D. (1986). What do we know so far? A review of the Head Start Synthesis Project. *Young Children, 41*, 49–55.

Slaughter, D., Washington, V., Oyemade, U., & Lindsey, R. (1988, Summer). *Head Start: A backward and forward look* (Social Policy Report, 3 [2]). Washington, DC: Society for Research in Child Development.

Stephan, S. (1986, January). *Head Start issues in FY 1986: Funding, administration, and recent evaluations.* Washington, DC: Library of Congress, Congressional Research Service.

Stewart, A., & Robinson, D. (1990). *The Head Start Program: Background information and issues.* Washington, DC: Library of Congress, Congressional Research Service.

Travers, J., Nauta, M., & Irwin, N. (1982). *The effects of a social program; Final report of the Child and Family Resource Program's infant-toddler component.* Cambridge, MA: Abt Associates.

Washington, V., & Oyemade, U. (1987). *Project Head Start: Past, present, and future trends in the context of family needs.* New York: Garland.

Weber, C. (1975). *An economic analysis of the Ypsilanti Perry Preschool Project.* Unpublished doctoral dissertation, University of Maryland, College Park.

Weber, C., Foster, P., & Weikart, D. (1978). *An economic analysis of the Ypsilanti Perry Preschool Project.* Ypsilanti, MI: High/Scope Press.

Weikart, D. (1989). *Quality preschool programs: A long-term social investment.* New York: Ford Foundation.

Whitebook, M., Howes, C., & Phillips, D. (1989). *Who cares? Child care teachers and the quality of care in America*. Oakland, CA: Child Care Employees Project.

Wrap-around funding/services in Head Start. Some advantages/some disadvantages (Fall 1989–Winter 1990). Alexandria, VA: National Head Start Association.

Zigler, E., & Freedman, J. (1987). Early experience, malleability, and Head Start. In J. Gallagher & C. Ramey (Eds.), *The malleability of children*. Baltimore: Paul H. Brooks.

Zigler, E., & Seitz, V. (1980). Early childhood intervention programs: A reanalysis. *School Psychology Review, 9*, 354–368.

Zigler, E., & Trickett, P. (1978, September). I.Q., social competence and evaluation of early childhood intervention programs. *American Psychologist, 32*, 789–798.

Zigler, E., & Valentine, J. (1979). *Project Head Start: A legacy of the war on Poverty*. New York: Free Press.

24

Thresholds of Quality: Implications for the Social Development of Children in Center-Based Child Care

Carollee Howes
University of California, Los Angeles
Deborah A. Phillips
University of Virginia, Charlottesville
Marcy Whitebook
Child Care Employee Project, Oakland, California

We assessed the quality of center child care relationships with adults and peers for 414 children (ages 14 to 54 months). Classrooms were classified by ratio and group size provisions of the Federal Interagency Day Care Requirements (FIDCR) and by the Early Childhood and Infant and Toddler Environmental Rating Scales. Children cared for in classrooms meeting FIDCR ratios were more likely to be in classrooms rated as good or very good in caregiving and activities. Children in classrooms rated as good or very good in caregiving were more likely to be securely attached to teachers. Securely attached children were more competent with peers. Children cared for in classrooms meeting FIDCR group size were more likely

Reprinted with permission from *Child Development*, 1992, Vol. 63, 449–460. Copyright © 1992 by the Society for Research in Child Development, Inc.

Thanks to the Atlanta NCCSS research staff, Mary Zurn, Myritice Dye, Vernessa Clark, Joyce Cross, Christine Drea, Ellery Hill, Elizabeth St. Andre, Sandra Cay Westfall, and Ann Zavitkovsky, for their work in recruiting the centers and collecting the data. Thanks also to the California research team: Kristin Droege, Darlene Galluzzo, Annette Groen, Claire Hamilton, Lisabeth Meyers, Catherine Matheson, and Ellen Wolpow. The children in the second California sample were originally part of a dissertation completed by Carol Rodning. We appreciate her foresight in establishing this longitudinal study. We are especially grateful to the child care center directors and teachers who permitted us to observe in their centers. The NCCSS was funded by a group of foundations including Ford, Foundation for Child Development, Smith-Richardson, Spunk, and Mailman Family Fund. The California studies were funded by the Spencer Foundation.

to be in classrooms rated higher in activities. Children in classrooms rated high in activities were likely to orient to both adults and peers. Children with social orientations to adults and peers were more competent with peers.

Relations between child care quality and children's social and cognitive development are well established. Children who experience high-quality child care score higher than children who experience low-quality child care on a variety of child development measures (see Phillips & Howes, 1987, for a review of this literature). However, research studies that simply suggest that better quality is linked to more optimal outcomes have frustrated policymakers. If child care is to be optimally regulated based on current knowledge of child development and child care, research must provide thresholds for quality variables as well as demonstrate linear relations between quality and outcome. The purpose of the current analysis is to examine thresholds for two aspects of child care: adult:child ratio and group size. We examine associations among different levels of these variables, quality of care, and children's social development.

We define threshold as the point between child care that harms children or hinders their development and child care that does not create detectable harm. We selected the Federal Interagency Day Care Requirements (FIDCR) as our quality threshold. The FIDCR were developed by child development experts and policymakers a decade ago but never fully implemented. We expected classrooms that met the FIDCR standards to provide higher quality care than classrooms that failed to meet these standards.

Child care quality can be defined with either structural or process variables. Structural variables included in the FIDCR were adult:child ratios, group size, and the training of the teachers. These structural variables can be regulated. A state can decide, for example, to limit the adult:child ratio in classrooms for children under 2 years of age to one adult for every three children. Process variables include the behavior of the teacher and the provision of activities for the children. Process variables require interpretation and judgment by experts and thus are more difficult, if not impossible, to regulate. For example, requiring that infant teachers be warm and attentive would require both a clear behavioral definition of the constructs warm and attentive and enforcement personnel trained to judge these behaviors.

Structural variables are assumed to influence process variables. Specifically in the current study we expected adult:child ratio to be linked to caregiving and to the provision of developmentally appropriate activities (Bruner, 1980; Clarke-Stewart & Gruber, 1984; Cummings & Beagles-Ross, 1983; Howes, 1983; Howes & Rubenstein, 1985; Roupp, Travers, Glantz, & Coelen, 1979). If a teacher is responsible for a small number of children, she is more likely to individualize care and to be able to attend to their social bids than if she is responsible for more children. Developmentally appropriate activities for young children are hands-on and experiential with an element of child initiation rather than teacher imposed (Bredekamp, 1987). Developmentally appropriate activities require both that children move around the room at will and that an orderliness prevails so that children are not interrupted as they pursue their interests. Therefore, smaller teacher-to-child ratios and smaller groups are more conducive to developmentally appropriate activities than are larger groups and many children per teacher.

Reviews of child care children's development suggest that detrimental effects of child care enrollment are most likely to be in the area of social outcomes (Belsky, 1988). We focused our analysis of child outcomes on children's relationships with teachers and peers.

We assessed two aspects of children's relationships with adults: their attachment behaviors and their social orientation. Attachment behaviors reflect children's sense that they can trust the adult to care for them in a responsive and sensitive manner (Ainsworth, Blehar, Waters, & Wall, 1978). Recent research on children enrolled in child care implies that teachers as well as parents function as attachment figures (Goossens & van Ijzendoorn, 1990; Howes & Hamilton, 1990; Howes, Rodning, Galluzzo, & Meyers, 1988). We expected that children in classrooms rated higher in appropriate caregiving would be more likely to direct secure attachment behaviors to their primary teacher.

With regard to social orientation to adults and peers, children in low-quality child care centers wander aimlessly rather than becoming involved in interaction with toys, teachers, or peers (Vandell & Powers, 1983). This aimless behavior predicts later adjustment problems when the children are school age (Vandell, Henderson, & Wilson, 1988). Harper and Huie (1987) suggest that orientation to peers as well as aimless wandering may be problematic for later school success. We expected social orientation to vary as a function of developmentally appropriate activities. If the teacher provides interesting activities, the child is less likely to wander and more likely to engage in them with others. If the activities are developmentally appropriate, children will often work cooperatively with peers and adults rather than alone.

One of the tasks that child care children face is to develop reasonably pleasant ways of relating to peers. Engaging with peers can be complex from a social-cognitive perspective as well as an emotional perspective. There are two major explanations for the antecedents of competent relationships with peers: experiences with peers and adult attachment relationships (Belsky, 1988; Harper & Huie, 1987; Howes, 1988). Children who have daily contact with stable peer groups from fairly young ages appear most socially competent with peers (Howes, 1988). Furthermore, within child care samples the children observed to be the most competent with peers are peer-oriented rather than solitary or adult-oriented

(Galluzzo, Matheson, Moore, & Howes, 1988). Children who feel emotionally secure with adults are positively oriented to peers (Jacobson, Tianen, Wille, & Aytch, 1987; Sroufe, 1983). Therefore, we expected that both children's social orientation and their attachment behaviors to teachers' security would influence their social peer behaviors.

In summary, we expected children enrolled in classrooms meeting the FIDCR ratio and group size standards to receive acceptable ratings for appropriate caregiving and developmentally appropriate activities. We then expected children with acceptable caregiving to be securely attached to teachers and children with acceptable developmental activity ratings to be socially oriented to both teachers and peers. Finally, we expected children with secure attachment behaviors and social orientations that include peers to be socially competent with peers.

METHOD

Sample

Three independent samples of children were included in this research. Two samples were drawn from southern California and one from Atlanta, Georgia. All of the children were enrolled at least 20 hours a week in child care centers. All of the children were enrolled for at least 2 months in the center before we observed them. One California sample entered child care prior to their first birthdays and participated in a longitudinal study of relationships with adults and peers from infancy through preschool. The sample was initially recruited from five child care centers; however, the children frequently changed their child care centers throughout the course of the study. For the purposes of the current analysis, we selected a single data-collection point for each child in the longitudinal study, making sure, as far as possible, that each of these children was enrolled in a different classroom. The 72 children, age range 14 to 47 months, who contributed data to the current study were enrolled in 30 different child care classrooms. Approximately one-third of the children were enrolled in subsidized centers, which were required to meet the most stringent of the California licensing requirements. These centers integrate tuition paying and subsidized children.

The second southern California study consisted of 87 children enrolled in preschool child care centers. This sample was recruited through birth records and was also an infancy-to-preschool longitudinal study. We selected the 4-year child care observation for these children because many of these children either did not enter child care until late preschool or were only enrolled part time at earlier ages. In 15 cases, the 4-year-old observation was not available and we used the 3-year-old child care observation. The children in this sample were enrolled in 68 different child care classrooms. There was no overlap in subjects or child care classrooms between the first and second southern California samples.

The third sample were the children of the National Child Care Staffing Study (NCCSS) (Whitebook, Howes, & Phillips, 1990). This sample was recruited using a random sampling strategy to select 45 child care centers in the Atlanta metropolitan area. The sample of centers matched the proportion of full-time, licensed, center-based child care based on low-, middle-, or high-income U.S. Census tracts and urban and suburban neighborhoods. Within each center we randomly selected three classrooms, one each from among all infant, toddler, and preschool classrooms. Two children, preferably a girl and a boy, were randomly selected from each target classroom (n = 255, age range = 14 to 62 months).

The sample of the current study consisted of 414 (190 girls) children. The children ranged in age from 14 to 54 months. Sixty-eight children (17%) were infants (14 to 24 months), 175 (42%) were toddlers (25 to 36 months), and the remaining 171 (41%) children were preschoolers (37 to 54 months). Twenty-one percent (87) of the children were African-American, 73% (302) of the children were European-American, and the remainder were from other ethnic and racial groups. The children represented the full range of social classes, including children enrolled in subsidized child care centers because of family poverty or disorganization and children from two-parent, relatively wealthy homes.

California and Georgia have very different licensing standards for child care centers. On the average the California samples had better quality scores. However, there also was considerable overlap between the samples on these measures.

Procedures

Each child was observed in his or her classroom for at least 2 hours and as much as 3 hours. In 83% of the cases, the child was visited on more than one day; in all cases, the time a child was observed covered both morning and afternoon activities.

In the Atlanta sample, one observer observed the classroom while a second collected child behavior observations. In the two California samples, two observers each independently collected both measures.

In the Atlanta and second California sample, each child was observed for six 5-min blocks evenly distributed over a 2-hour period. In the first California sample, 12 5-min blocks were collected for each child over a total of 4 hours of observation. To make the data comparable, the Atlanta and second California sample frequencies were doubled.

Measures

Indices of quality. Adult:child ratios and group size were recorded every 15 min during the observation. These were averaged across the 15-min blocks to create a single ratio and a single group size score for each child.

Process quality was assessed with the Early Childhood Environmental Rating Scale (ECERS) (Harms & Clifford, 1980) for each observed preschool classroom and the Infant-Toddler Environmental Rating Scale (ITERS) (Harms & Clifford, 1986) for each of the observed infant and toddler classrooms. These scales comprehensively assess the day-to-day quality of care provided to children. Individual items are rated from a low of 1 to a high of 7. The ECERS is widely used in child development research and has predicted optimal child outcomes in a number of studies (Phillips & Howes, 1987). The ITERS was derived from the ECERS and has been extensively field tested in infant and toddler classrooms. These scales were completed by the classroom observers at the conclusion of the observation.

Interrater reliabilities for structural and process quality were established in the NCCSS to a criterion of 80% agreement prior to data collection. At midpoint of data collection interrater reliability within Atlanta was 94% agreement. Interrater reliability in the California samples was established to a criterion of 85% agreement prior to data collection. Interrater reliability was checked bimonthly during data collection (median interrater reliability was kappa $= .91$).

We used a maximum likelihood factor analysis, with oblique rotation, of the ECERS and ITERS scale items for the entire NCCSS sample of 313 preschool and 330 infant and toddler classrooms (Whitebook et al., 1990). This resulted in two subscales of quality. The first subscale, appropriate caregiving, captured the items pertaining to child-adult interactions, supervision, and discipline. It accounted for 52% of the variance in the ECERS and 56% of the variance in the ITERS. The second subscale, developmentally appropriate activity, captures the items pertaining to the materials, schedule, and activities of the classroom. It accounted for 48% of the variance in the ECERS and 44% of the variance in the ITERS. The two scales were intercorrelated; infants $r = .82$, toddlers $r = .81$, and preschoolers $r = .78$. Appropriate caregiving and developmentally appropriate activity scores were generated for the California and Atlanta samples by summing the items with a factor loading of .50 or higher on each of the subscales.

Children's relationships with teachers and behaviors with peers

Attachment behavior. Following the observation the observer completed the Deane Attachment Q-Set (1985) for the child's primary teacher. This Q-Set assesses the child's attachment behaviors with caregivers. It is an observational alternative to the Ainsworth Strange Situation (Ainsworth et al., 1978). The Q-Set yields a security score, which is the correlation between the child's item scores and an ideal child item score. There is reasonable correspondence between

Strange Situation classifications and Q-Set security scores (Vaughn & Waters, 1990; Waters & Deane, 1985). Interrater reliability on the Q-Set was kappa = .85 in Atlanta, and kappa = .93 and kappa = .89 in the California samples.

We classified the children as secure, avoidant, or ambivalent in their emotional security with their primary teacher, using clusters derived from a Wards cluster analysis of the Waters and Deane Attachment Q-Set (Howes & Hamilton, 1990). Item distributions, security scores, and measures of adult involvement differentiate the clusters in theoretically meaningful ways (Howes & Hamilton, 1990).

Social orientation. Based on work by Galluzzo and colleagues (Galluzzo et al., 1988), we identified four social orientations: to adults, to peers, to adults and peers, and solitary. Frequency of proximity to a peer (within 3 feet) and proximity to an adult (within 3 feet) varied by the age, sex, and race of the child. Therefore, we created standardized residual scores for adult and peer proximity by regressing out the variance attributable to age, age squared, sex, and race. Children with standard scores greater than 0 in adult proximity and less than 0 in peer proximity were classified as adult oriented. Children with standard scores of greater than 0 in peer proximity and less than 0 in adult proximity were classified as peer oriented . Children classified as adult and peer oriented had standard scores of greater than 0 for both peer and adult proximity. Children classified as solitary had standard scores of less than 0 for both peer and adult proximity.

Interaction with peers. In the entire sample, interactions with peers were rated every 20 sec using a revised version of the Peer Play Scale (Howes, 1980). The Peer Play Scale has acceptable stability over time (Howes, 1988). The revised scale measures complexity of social pretend play as well as social play and is appropriate for the infant to preschool age range. Kappa Interobserver reliabilities for the scale were .88 in the Atlanta sample and .92 and .94 in the two California samples. Interactions with teachers were rated on the same schedule as peer interaction using an adult involvement scale (Howes & Stewart, 1987). For the purposes of the current analysis, only the measure of adult proximity (the child is within 3 feet of the teacher) was used. Interrater reliability was .92 in Atlanta, and .89 and .93 in the California samples.

Five measures of peer interaction were derived from the Peer Play Scale: percent uninvolved, percent of peer contact the child is an onlooker, percent of peer contact the child engages in interaction, percent of peer contact the child engages in competent social play, and percent of peer contact the child engages in competent social pretend play. Uninvolved was the frequency of solitary play separated from peers. Onlooking is merely watching another child without making or responding to a social bid or participating in parallel activity. Peer contact is activity with other children that at least includes parallel activity with some mutual awareness. Competent social play was defined as at least complementary and reciprocal action based role reversals (Howes, Unger, & Seidner, 1989).

Competent social pretend play was defined as at least cooperative social pretend play in which children act out nonliteral roles (Howes et al., 1989). Previous work on the development of peer interaction suggests that social play and social pretend play are related to other measures of competence with peers, including sociometric and teacher ratings (Howes, 1988).

All five of these peer interaction variables varied significantly as a function of the child's age, sex, and race. Therefore, we created standardized residual scores for each variable by regressing out the variance attributable to age, age squared, sex, and race. These standardized scores were used in further analysis.

Classification of Classrooms

Regulatable quality of care

Adult:child ratio. Adult:child ratio categories corresponded to the Federal Interagency Day Care Requirements (FIDCR). There were three infant categories: three children per adult (46% of sample), more than three but no more than four children per adult (17% of sample), and more than four children per adult (37% of sample). The toddler categories were: no more than four children per adult (39% of sample), more than four but no more than six children per adult (31% of sample), and more than six children (30% of sample). The preschool categories were: no more than eight children per adult (85% of sample), more than eight but no more than nine children per adult (6% of sample), and more than nine children per adult (9% of sample). The 1:8 ratio is the California ratio for subsidized centers. Infants were defined as children under 24 months of age, toddlers as children age 25 to 36 months, and preschoolers as children between 37 and 54 months of age.

Group size. We used the FIDCR to create categories of group size. Infant categories were: six children or less (FIDCR, 28% of sample), seven to 12 children (48% of sample), and more than 12 children (24% of sample). Toddler categories were: 12 children or less (FIDCR, 65% of sample), 13 to 18 children (28%), and more than 18 children (7% of sample). Preschool categories were 18 children or less (FIDCR, 85% of sample) or more than 18 children (15% of sample).

Process quality. We created the following appropriate caregiving and developmentally appropriate activity categories: inadequate (1 to 2.9; 18% of sample caregiving, 33% activities; 31% of sample caregiving, 41% activities); barely adequate (3 to 3.9); good (4 to 4.9; 27% of sample caregiving, 21% activities); and very good (5 and above; 24% of sample caregiving, 5% activities). There was a significant association between appropriate caregiving and age, $x^2(6) = 22.23$, $p = .001$. Infants and toddlers received less adequate care than preschoolers. Seventy percent of infants and 52% of the toddlers were in classrooms rated as barely adequate or inadequate. There was no association between developmentally appropriate activities and age, $x^2(6) = 5.12$, N.S. Larger percentages of children received good or very good caregiving scores than good or very good activity scores, $x^2(1) = 6.14$, $p < .05$.

RESULTS

Relations between Regulatable and Process Quality Variables

We expected children in classrooms with better adult:child ratios and group sizes to receive higher appropriate caregiving and developmentally appropriate activities scores. To examine this hypothesis, we first plotted ratio and group size against the percent of children in classrooms rated as inadequate in caregiving and activities. To be considered inadequate on the ECERS or ITERS, the rating must be less than 3. To test our predictions, we conducted a chi-square analysis between regulatable and process quality classifications using the FIDCR and California cut-off points.

Adult:child ratio. We plotted ratio against inadequate caregiving and activities. When five or more children were cared for by one adult in infant classrooms and nine children in toddler and preschool classrooms, at least 50% of the children were in classrooms rated as inadequate in caregiving. When five or more children were cared for by one adult in infant groups, eight or more children in toddler groups, and preschool groups, at least 50% of the children were in classrooms rated as inadequate in activities. Children in infant classrooms with 1:3 or less ratios, and preschool classrooms with 1:9 or less were more likely than children in classrooms with worse (higher) ratios to experience both caregiving and activities rated as good or very good. Preschool children meeting the more stringent ratios (1:8 or less) prescribed by California standards were more likely to receive caregiving rated as very good than preschool children meeting the less stringent (1:9) FIDCR standards (Fisher Exact Test = .05). Table 1 presents the distribution of process quality ratings by each category of ratio.

Group size. We then plotted group size against inadequate caregiving and activities. When 11 or more children were in infant groups, 18 or more in toddler groups, and 20 or more in preschool groups, at least 50% of the children were in classrooms rated as inadequate in caregiving. When 11 or more children were in infant groups, 15 or more children in toddler groups, and 19 or more children in preschool groups, at least 50% of the children were in classrooms rated as inadequate in activities. Group size appears to have a curvilinear relationship with developmentally appropriate activities in preschool classrooms. Fifty percent or more of children in classrooms with group sizes of seven or smaller were also in classrooms rated as inadequate in activities. Children in infant classrooms with six or less children, toddler classrooms with 12 or less children, and preschool

TABLE 1
Relations between Adult:Child Ratio and Process Quality

	PROCESS QUALITY				
RATIO	Inadequate	Barely Adequate	Good	Very Good	χ^2
Appropriate caregiving:					
Infant:					
3 or less	10	10	69	11	
3 to 4	45	37	18	0	
More than 4	57	23	12	8	14.21*
Toddler:					
4 or less	4	30	48	18	
4 to 6	26	30	26	19	
More than 6	39	29	23	8	21.66**
Preschool:					
8 or less	9	20	35	36	
8 to 9	52	35	13	0	
More than 9	54	14	32	0	18.58*
Developmentally appropriate activities:					
Infant:					
3 or less	7	7	80	6	
3 to 4	50	50	0	0	
More than 4	46	42	13	0	39.23**
Toddler:					
4 or less	2	21	54	24	
4 to 6	41	32	24	4	
More than 6	42	36	17	4	13.31*
Preschool:					
8 or less	7	23	44	26	
8 to 9	50	25	25	0	
More than 9	50	38	12	0	13.40*

NOTE.—Numbers in table are percent of children in each ratio category. Chi-square completed on raw numbers. Underlined categories are FIDCR standards.
* $p < .05$.
** $p < .01$.

classrooms with 18 or less children were more likely than children in classrooms exceeding these standards to experience developmentally appropriate activities. There was no association between group size and appropriate caregiving. Distributions are in Table 2.

Relations between Process Quality and Teacher Security and Social Orientation

We expected children enrolled in classrooms classified as higher in appropriate caregiving would be more likely to create secure relationships with their teachers. We also expected children enrolled in classrooms classified as higher in developmentally appropriate activities to be oriented to both adults and peers rather than being solitary or peer oriented. To test these predictions, we conducted chi-square

TABLE 2
Relations Between Group Size and Process Quality

	PROCESS QUALITY				
GROUP SIZE	Inadequate	Barely Adequate	Good	Very Good	χ^2
Appropriate caregiving:					
Infant:					
6 or less	11	61	22	6	
6 to 12	32	45	10	13	
More than 12	13	53	7	27	8.17
Toddler:					
12 or less	18	37	25	20	
12 to 18	22	29	22	26	
More than 18	58	25	17	0	9.43
Preschool:					
18 or less	9	18	38	35	
More than 18	18	36	36	10	6.01
Developmentally appropriate activities:					
Infant:					
6 or less	11	17	65	7	
6 to 12	32	55	13	0	
More than 12	54	21	25	0	13.24*
Toddler:					
12 or less	4	16	45	35	
12 to 18	37	31	24	8	
More than 18	50	25	25	0	14.72*
Preschool:					
18 or less	6	20	50	24	
More than 18	50	33	8	8	8.28*

NOTE.—Numbers in table are percent of children in each ratio category. Chi-square completed on raw numbers. Underlined categories are FIDCR standards.
* $p < .05$.
** $p < .01$.

analyses between process quality and relationship classifications and between process quality and social orientation classifications.

Attachment security. Fifty-one percent of the children in our sample were categorized as secure, 36% avoidant, and 13% ambivalent in security. There was no significant association between age group and relationship classification, $x^2(4) = 7.89$, N.S. Children classified secure were more likely than children classified as avoidant or ambivalent to be enrolled in classrooms rated as good or very good in appropriate caregiving. Table 3 presents this distribution. There was no significant association between security and developmentally appropriate activities.

Social orientation. Forty-four percent of the children were classified as adult oriented, 27% as peer oriented, 21% as adult and peer oriented, and the remaining 8% as solitary. There was no significant association between age group and social orientation, $x^2(6) = 2.75$, N.S. Children classified as both adult and peer oriented were more likely to be enrolled in classrooms rated higher in developmen-

TABLE 3
Relations Between Teacher Relationships and Process Quality

| | PROCESS QUALITY | | | | |
RELATIONSHIP CATEGORIES	Inadequate	Barely Adequate	Good	Very Good	χ^2
Appropriate caregiving:					
Secure (B)	11	32	26	31	
Avoidant (A)	28	32	21	19	
Ambivalent (C)	22	49	17	12	15.55*
Developmentally appropriate activities:					
Secure (B)	25	46	23	6	
Avoidant (A)	36	42	20	2	
Ambivalent (C)	22	56	20	2	7.95

NOTE.—Numbers in table are percent of each attachment category. Chi-square completed on raw numbers.
* $p < .05$.
** $p < .01$.

tally appropriate activities than children classified as solitary. See Table 4 for this distribution. There was no significant association between social orientation and appropriate caregiving.

Differences in Peer Behaviors of Children with Different Attachment Security Classifications and Social Orientations

Our final prediction concerned the antecedents of social competence with peers. We expected children who were secure with their teachers and children whose social orientation was toward peers to be more socially competent than children who either were insecure with their teachers and/or were solitary or adult oriented.

To test this prediction, we conducted a multivariate two-way analysis of variance comparing the peer behavior of children with different relationship and social orientation classifications. There were significant multivariate main effects for both security, $F(10,664) = 3.04$, $p < .05$, and social orientation, $F(15,949) = 6.95$, $p < .01$, but not for the interaction of security and social orientation, $F(30,950) = 1.09$, N.S.

Children secure with teachers were more likely than children insecure with teachers to spend more of their peer contact engaged with peers, $F(2,409) = 3.08$, $p < .05$, Scheffé: B > A,C. Secure children spent a larger proportion of their peer contacts in competent social play than children with avoidant relationships, $F(2,409) = 3.70$, $p < .01$, Scheffé: B > A, and a larger proportion of their peer contacts in competent social pretend play than children with ambivalent relationships, $F(2,409) = 3.43$, $p < .05$, Scheffé: B > C. Children with ambivalent relationships spent a greater proportion of their peer contacts being onlook-

TABLE 4
Relations between Social Orientation and Process Quality

	PROCESS QUALITY				
SOCIAL ORIENTATION	Inadequate	Barely Adequate	Good	Very Good	χ^2
Appropriate caregiving:					
Adult	20	31	27	22	
Peer	6	40	30	24	
Adult and peer	25	28	25	23	
Solitary	13	29	29	29	12.61
Developmentally appropriate activities:					
Adult	35	36	23	6	
Peer	14	69.	13	4	
Adult and peer	1	25	39	34	
Solitary	40	28	32	0	35.20**

NOTE.—Numbers in table are percent of each social orientation category. Chi-squares completed on raw numbers.
* $p < .05$.
** $p < .01$.

ers than children with secure relationships, $F(2,409) = 3.50$, $p < .05$, Scheffé: C > B, and were uninvolved with peers more often than children with secure and avoidant teacher relationships, $F(2,409) = 6.89$, $p < .01$, Scheffé: C > A, B.

Children classified as solitary in orientation were the least involved with peers, $F(3,409) = 10.23$, $p < .61$, Scheffé: AP, P > A, S. Children classified as adult oriented were less involved with peers than children classified as peer or adult and peer oriented. Children classified as peer or as adult and peer oriented spent a greater proportion of their peer contacts engaged and in competent social play than children classified as adult or solitary in orientation, $F(3,409) = 6.29$, $p < .01$, Scheffé: P > AP > A, S. Children classified as adult and peer oriented spent a larger proportion of their peer contacts in competent social pretend play than any other classification, $F(3,409) = 6.42$, $p < .01$, Scheffé: AP > P > S, A. Children classified as peer oriented spent a larger proportion of their peer contacts in competent social pretend play than children classified as solitary or adult oriented.

From Regulatable Quality Variables to Peer Competence

As a final step in our analysis, we tested the strength of the paths in our model using path analysis. This analysis allows us to examine direct as well as mediating influences of regulatable and process measures of quality of child care. The paths that were tested are represented in Figure 1. As the unit of analysis for this procedure, we created several classroom average composite measures for child outcomes. Teacher relationships was the average security score for children in the

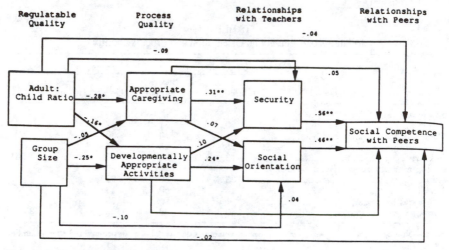

Figure 1. From regulatable quality to peer competence

classroom. Social orientation was represented by the average standardized residual score for proximity to peers. Social competence with peers was represented by a composite measure created after a principal component analysis of the five standardized measures of behavior with peers. The formula for this score was percent of peer contact engaged + percent of peer contact competent social play + percent of peer contact pretend play – percent uninvolved – percent of peer contact as onlooker. These scores were averaged within classrooms. Beta weights for each path are included in Figure 1. This analysis suggests that the influence of regulatable quality on social competence with peers is mediated through process quality and through children's relationships with adults and peers rather than directly influencing peer competence. Likewise, process quality is mediated through children's relationships with adults and peers rather than directly influencing peer competence.

DISCUSSION

Relationships between Regulatable and Process Quality: Are There Thresholds?

Our findings suggest that licensing standards for ratios do make a difference in the quality of care provided for children. The California 1:8 standard for preschoolers was associated with higher levels of appropriate caregiving than the FIDCR 1:9 standard. It appears that even with stringent regulations it is possible to further define quality. Policymakers sometimes believe that simply adding one more child can't make that much of a difference. Our results suggest otherwise.

Ratio and group size may serve as marker variables for other unmeasured influences, including teacher training and the commitment of the child care center's sponsoring organization to provide quality care. It is frequent in studies of American child care to find that "good things go together" (Phillips & Howes, 1987). Thus, centers that maintain adequate adult:child ratios and group sizes also tend to hire well educated teachers and pay relatively higher salaries (Whitebook et al., 1990).

Most research studies of structural variables in child care include teacher training as well as ratio and group size (Phillips & Howes, 1987). Unfortunately, we did not have measures of teacher training in the California portion of our sample. Other research from the NCCSS does find teacher training to influence child care process, especially in infant and toddler classrooms. The NCCSS nationally representative sample (Whitebook et al., 1990) found that teacher training had deteriorated since the last survey of training in the mid-1970s. While most teachers report some training in early childhood education, the majority of teachers received such training in high school or vocational school. In the NCCSS, only college level training was associated with effective teaching. We suspect that even with favorable ratios and group sizes, an untrained teacher would find it difficult to provide developmentally appropriate activities.

In our current sample, a child was more likely to receive appropriate caregiving than developmentally appropriate activities. This finding also may be related to teacher training. Although teachers with high levels of early childhood education training are more likely than those with less training to engage in appropriate caregiving (Whitebook et al., 1990), it may be more difficult for a teacher with no training to provide appropriate activities than to be warm and sensitive in her caregiving.

From Quality Indicators to Child Outcomes

Our findings support our predicted pathways from regulatable to process quality to relationships with teachers to relationships with peers. Children whose caregiving was rated as good or very good were more likely to be emotionally secure with teachers, while children whose caregiving was inadequate or barely adequate were more likely to be avoidant or ambivalent with teachers. Children who were more secure with caregivers were more competent with peers than children with insecure caregivers.

The large percentage of teacher-avoidant children in this study is disturbing, particularly as attachment behaviors are linked to behavior with peers. Children who are less competent with peers are at risk for peer rejection. Peer rejection appears as a powerful predictor of later negative outcomes, including early withdrawal from school and delinquency (Parker & Asher, 1987).

The pathway from group size to developmentally appropriate activities to social orientation and then to social competence with peers is less well established in the literature than the pathway from adult:child ratio through appropriate caregiving and attachment to social competence with peers. Our findings do support such a path, and we hope that they will stimulate future research in this area. These links suggest that children do not become competent with peers simply from extended contact and experience, but that by the provision of materials and the organization of the classroom the teacher can provide a context for the acquisition of peer social skills.

There is an important limitation of this study. We know little about the processes families used to enroll their children in these child care centers. If there were choices between child care arrangements for families, we would expect to find links between family characteristics and the quality of care provided for their children. Some parental choice is constrained by income. However, we know that children from all social classes are found in all kinds of programs (Whitebook et al., 1990).

CONCLUSION

The child care teacher and the context of teaching emerge as important in this study. When teachers teach in child care centers meeting reasonably high standards of quality, they are likely to engage in appropriate caregiving and provide developmentally appropriate activities. When teachers teach in centers that fail to meet these standards, they are less likely to be as effective.

Child care regulation also emerges as important in this study. The variations in quality of care attributable to structural variables in this study highlight the importance of examining variability in policy-level variables in future research. For example, examining compliance with state standards and comparing child care across states with different regulatory standards would be a fruitful direction (Phillips, Howes, & Whitebook, in press).

REFERENCES

Ainsworth, M. S., Blehar, M., Waters, E., & Wall, S. (1978). *Patterns of attachment.* Hillsdale, NJ: Erlbaum.

Belsky, J. (1988). The effects of infant day care reconsidered. *Early Childhood Research Quarterly, 3*, 237–272.

Bredekamp, S. (1987). *Developmentally appropriate practice in early childhood programs serving children from birth through age 8.* Washington, DC: National Association for the Education of Young Children.

Bruner, J. (1980). *Under fire in Britain.* Ypsilanti, MI: High Scope.

Clarke-Stewart, K. A., & Gruber, C. (1984). Day-care forms and features. In R. C. Ainslie (Ed.), *Quality variations in day care* (pp. 35–62). New York: Praeger.

Cummings, M. E., & Beagles-Ross, J. (1983). Towards a model of infant day care: Studies of factors influencing responding to separation in day care. In R. C. Ainslie (Ed.), *Quality variations in day care* (pp. 159–182). New York: Praeger.

Galluzzo, D., Matheson, C., Moore, J., & Howes, C. (1988). Social orientation to adults and peers in infant child care. *Early Childhood Research Quarterly, 3*, 417–426.

Goossens, F. A., & van Ijzendoorn, M. H. (1990). Quality of infant's attachment to professional caregivers: Relation to infant-parent attachment and day-care characteristics. *Child Development, 61*, 832–837.

Harms, T., & Clifford, R. (1980). *Early childhood environmental rating scale.* New York: Teachers College Press.

Harms, T., & Clifford, R. (1986). *Infant-toddler environmental rating scale.* Unpublished document, University of North Carolina, Chapel Hill.

Harper, C., & Huie, F. (1987). Relations among preschool children's adult and peer contacts and later academic achievements. *Child Development, 58*, 1051–1065.

Howes, C. (1980). The peer play scale as an index of complexity of peer interaction. *Developmental Psychology, 16*, 371–372.

Howes, C. (1983). Caregiver behavior in center and family day care. *Journal of Applied Developmental Psychology, 4*, 99–107.

Howes, C. (1988). Peer interaction of young children. *Monographs of the Society for Research in Child Development, 53*(1, Serial No. 217).

Howes, C., & Hamilton, C. E. (1990). *Children's relationships with child care teachers.* Los Angeles: University of California Press.

Howes, C., Rodning, C., Galluzzo, D., & Meyers, L. (1988). Attachment and child care: Relationships with mother and caregiver. *Early Childhood Research Quarterly, 3*, 417–426.

Howes, C., & Rubenstein, J. (1985). Determinants of toddlers' experiences in daycare: Age of entry and quality of setting. *Child Care Quarterly, 14*, 140–150.

Howes, C., & Stewart, P. (1987). Child's play with adults, toys, and peers: An explanation of family and child care influences. *Developmental Psychology, 23*, 423–430.

Howes, C., Unger, O., & Seidner, L. (1989). Social pretend play in toddlers: Parallels with social play and social pretend. *Child Development, 60*, 77–84.

Jacobson, J. L., Tianen, R. L., Wille, D. E., & Aytch, D. M. (1987). Infant-mother attachment and early peer relations: The assessment of behavior in an interactive context. In E. Mueller & C. Cooper (Eds.), *Process and outcome in peer relations* (pp. 55–78). New York: Academic.

Parker, J. G., & Asher, S. R. (1987). Peer relations and later personal adjustment: Are low accepted children at risk? *Psychology Bulletin, 102*, 357–389.

Phillips, D. A., & Howes, C. (1987). Indicators of quality in child care: Review of research.

In D. A. Phillips (Ed.), Quality in child care: What does research tell us? *Research Monograph of the National Association for the Education of Young Children: Vol. 1.* Washington, DC: NAEYC.

Phillips, D. A., Howes, C., & Whitebook, M. (in press). Policy determinants of quality: The role of regulation. *American Journal of Community Psychology.*

Roupp, R., Travers, J., Glantz, F., & Coelen, C. (1979). *Children at the center: Final report of the National Day Care Study.* Cambridge, MA: Abt Associates.

Sroufe, L. A. (1983). Infant-caregiver attachment and patterns of adaptation in preschool: Roots of maladaption and competence. In M. Perlmutter (Ed.), *Minnesota symposium on child psychology* (Vol. 16, pp. 41–81). Hillsdale, NJ: Erlbaum.

Vandell, D., Henderson, V. K., & Wilson, K. S. (1988). A longitudinal study of children with varying quality day care experiences. *Child Development, 59,* 1286–1292.

Vandell, D., & Powers, C. (1983). Day care quality and children's free play activities. *American Journal of Orthopsychiatry, 53,* 293–500.

Vaughn, B., & Waters, E. (1990). Attachment behavior at home and in the laboratory: Q-sort observations and Strange Situation classifications of one-year-olds. *Child Development, 61,* 1965–1973.

Waters, E., & Deane, K. E. (1985). Defining and assessing individual differences in attachment relationships: Q-methodology and the organization of behavior in infancy and early childhood. In I. Bretherton & E. Waters (Eds.), Growing points in attachment theory and research (pp. 41–65). *Monographs of the Society for Research in Child Development, 50*(1–2, Serial No. 209).

Whitebook, M., Howes, C., & Phillips, D. A. (1990). *Who cares? Child care teachers and the quality of care in America.* The National Child Care Staffing Study. Oakland: Child Care Employee Project.